PREVENTIVE STRATEGIES FOR LIVING IN A CHEMICAL WORLD

A SYMPOSIUM IN HONOR OF IRVING G. SELIKOFF

The purpose of the Collegium is to be that of a bridge between the world of scientific discovery and those social and political centers which must act on these discoveries to conserve life and prevent disease.

Bylaws of the Collegium Ramazzini

Article I, Section 2

ANNALS OF THE NEW YORK ACADEMY OF SCIENCES
Volume 837

PREVENTIVE STRATEGIES FOR LIVING IN A CHEMICAL WORLD

A SYMPOSIUM IN HONOR OF IRVING J. SELIKOFF

Edited by Eula Bingham and David P. Rall

The New York Academy of Sciences
New York, New York
1997

Library of Congress Cataloging-in-Publication Data

Preventive strategies for living in a chemical world: a symposium in honor of Irving J. Selikoff / edited by Eula Bingham and David P. Rall.
p. cm. — (Annals of the New York Academy of Sciences ; v. 837)
Includes bibliographical references and index.
ISBN 1-57331-074-3 (cloth : alk. paper). — ISBN 1-57331-075-1 (pbk : alk. paper)
1. Environmental toxicology—Congresses. 2. Chemical carcinogenesis—Congresses. 3. Health risk assessment—Congresses. 4. Industrial toxicology—Congresses. I. Bingham, Eula. - II. Rall, David P. III. Series.
Q11.N5 vol. 837
[RA1226]
500 s—dc21
[615.9′02] 97-39041
CIP

PCP
Printed in the United States of America
ISBN 1-57331-074-3 (cloth)
ISBN 1-57331-075-1 (paper)
ISSN 0077-8923

ANNALS OF THE NEW YORK ACADEMY OF SCIENCES

Volume 837
December 26, 1997

PREVENTIVE STRATEGIES FOR LIVING IN A CHEMICAL WORLD

A SYMPOSIUM IN HONOR OF IRVING J. SELIKOFF[a]

Editors and Conference Organizers
EULA BINGHAM AND DAVID P. RALL

CONTENTS

Dedication. *By* CESARE MALTONI xi

Welcome. *By* EULA BINGHAM xiii

Foreword. *By* BILL BOLAND xv

Ramazzini Lecture

Biomedical Research as a Science for Development: The Case of Gasoline. *By* CESARE MALTONI 1

Identification and Control of Environmental Risks

Motor Fuels

Results of Long-term Experimental Carcinogenicity Studies of the Effects of Gasoline, Correlated Fuels, and Major Gasoline Aromatics on Rats. *By* CESARE MALTONI, ADRIANO CILIBERTI, CARMINE PINTO, MORANDO SOFFRITTI, FIORELLA BELPOGGI, and LORETTA MENARINI 15

Carcinogenicity of Gasoline: A Review of Epidemiological Evidence. *By* JOHN M. DEMENT, LISA HENSLEY, and AMY GITELMAN 53

Results of Long-term Experimental Studies on the Carcinogenicity of Methyl *tert*-Butyl Ether. *By* FIORELLA BELPOGGI, MORANDO SOFFRITTI, FEDERICA FILIPPINI, and CESARE MALTONI 77

Methyl Tertiarty-Butyl Ether Antibodies among Gasoline Service Station Attendants. *By* ARISTO VOJDANI, GALAL NAMATALLA, and NACHMAN BRAUTBAR 96

[a]This volume is a result of an international symposium entitled **Preventive Strategies for Living in a Chemical World,** which was dedicated to the memory of Irving J. Selikoff, M.D. Sponsored by the Collegium Ramazzini, the symposium was held in Washington, D.C. on November 2-5, 1995.

Industrial and Environmental Chemicals

Scientific Update on Benzene. *By* URVASHI RANGAN and ROBERT SNYDER. 105

Validation of Benzene Exposure Assessment. *By* M. DOSEMECI, N. ROTHMAN, S.-N. YIN, G.-L. LI, M. LINET, S. WACHOLDER, W.-H. CHOW, and R. B. HAYES. 114

Immune Function in n-Hexane-Exposed Workers. *By* A. KARAKAYA, B. YÜCESOY, S. BURGAZ, and A. E. KARAKAYA. . . 122

Industrial Contamination with Glycol Ethers Resulting in Teratogenic Damage. *By* DOLORES SAAVEDRA, MANUEL ARTEAGA, and MARTHA TENA. 126

Mortality of Power Workers Exposed to Phenoxy Herbicides and Polychlorinated Biphenyls in Waste Transformer Oil. *By* ALASTAIR HAY and JOHN TARREL. 138

Lymphohematopoietic Cancers and Butadiene and Styrene Exposure in Synthetic Rubber Manufacture. *By* G. MATANOSKI, E. ELLIOTT, X. TAO, M. FRANCIS, A. CORREA-VILLASENOR, and C. SANTOS-BURGOA. 157

Underestimating Risk for Three Important Human Carcinogens: Vinyl Chloride, Benzene, and Butadiene. *By* MARVIN S. LEGATOR. 170

Living in a Chemical World: Health Impact of 1,3-Butadiene Carcinogenesis. *By* CARLOS SANTOS-BURGOA, ROCÍO ALATORRE EDEN-WYNTER, HARACIO RIOJAS-RODRÍGUEZ, and GENEVIEVE M. MATANOSKI. 176

Results of Long-term Carcinogenicity Studies of Chlorine in Rats. *By* MORANDO SOFFRITTI, FIORELLA BELPOGGI, AND ANGELA LENZI, and CESARE MALTONI. 189

Results of a Long-term Experimental Study on the Carcinogenicity of Vinyl Acetate Monomer in Mice. *By* CESARE MALTONI, ADRIANO CILIBERTI, GIUSEPPE LEFEMINE, and MORANDO SOFFRITTI. 209

Mercurial Uncertainties in Environmental Health. *By* PHILIPPE GRANDJEAN. 239

Insecticides

Long-term Health Effects of the Occupational Exposure to DDT: A Preliminary Report. *By* PIERLUIGI COCCO, AARON BLAIR, PATRIZIA CONGIA, GIOVANNA SABA, ANNA R. ECCA, and COSTANTINO PALMAS. 246

Surveillance of Occupational, Accidental, and Incidental Exposure to Organophosphate Pesticides Using Urine Alkyl Phosphate and Phenolic Metabolite Measurements. *By* JOHN E. DAVIES and JAMES C. PETERSON 257

Agricultural Sustainability, Pesticide Exposures, and Health Risks: Israel, the Palestinian National Authority, and Jordan. *By* ELIHU D. RICHTER, STEPHEN GASTEYER, SAMIR EL HAJ, M. JAQHABIR, and J. SAFI 269

Occupational Exposure to Pentachlorophenol: The Portuguese Situation. *By* ANTÓNIO JORGE FERREIRA, DUARTE N. VIEIRA, ESTELA P. MARQUES, and ISABEL S. PEDRO 291

Dibromochloropropane: Epidemiological Findings and Current Questions. *By* JOHN R. GOLDSMITH 300

Occupational Health

Liver and Kidney Function Tests as a Tool for Periodic Health Evaluation of Laboratory Workers. *By* A. PINES, D. ALKASLASSY, M. KLEBANOV, C. LEMESCH, J. RIBAK, and Y. LERMAN 307

Two NIOSH Resources for Implementing Workplace Safety and Health Surveillance. *By* LEELA I. MURTHY 319

Molecular Epidemiology and Occupational Health. *By* FREDERICA P. PERERA and CHRISTOPHER DICKEY 353

Risk Assessment and Prevention

The Historical Basis for Ecological Risk Assessment. *By* JOANNA BURGER 360

Paradigms for Ecological Risk Assessment. *By* JOANNA BURGER and MICHAEL GOCHFELD 372

Probabalistic Risk Assessment: Lessons from Four Case Studies. *By* LAURA C. GREEN and EDMUND A. C. CROUCH 387

Disconnect Brain and Repeat after Me: Risk Assessment is Too Conservative. *By* ADAM M. FINKEL 397

A Memoir on Risk Assessment and Environmental Policy. *By* SHELDON WILFRED SAMUELS 418

Economic Aspects of Environmental Protection

The Use of Economics in Environmental Decision Making. *By* HOLLY STALLWORTH 433

A National Estimate of the Cost of Occupationally Related Disease in 1992. *By* MARIANNE C. FAHS, STEVEN B. MARKOWITZ, J. PAUL LEIGH, CHONG-GAK SHIN, and PHILIP J. LANDRIGAN. 440

Can Protecting Human Health and the Environment Be Justified on Cost-Benefit Grounds? *By* RUTH RUTTENBERG. 456

Carcinogenesis

Mechanistic Modeling of Multiple Tumorigenesis: An Application to Data on Lung Tumors in Mice Exposed to Urethane. *By* A. Y. YAKOVLEV and L. V. PAVLOVA. 462

Results of Three Life-Span Experimental Carcinogenicity and Anticarcinogenicity Studies on Tamoxifen on Rats. *By* CESARE MALTONI, FRANCO MINARDI, CARMINE PINTO, FIORELLA BELPOGGI, and LUCIANO BUA. 469

Breast Cancer

Recent Developments on the Avoidable Causes of Breast Cancer. *By* DEVRA LEE DAVIS, MONTIRA J. PONGSIRI, and MARY WOLFF 513

Dietary Fiber, Hispanics, and Breast Cancer Risk? *By* LOVELL A. JONES, ROSIE GONZALEZ, PATRICIA C. PILLOW, SARAH A. GOMEZ-GARZA, CATHERINE J. FOREMAN, JANICE A. CHILTON, ADRIANA LINARES, JOHN YICK, MAYHAR BADREI, and RICHARD A. HAJEK. 524

Reproductive Determinants of Breast Cancer in Mexican Women. *By* LIZBETH LÓPEZ-CARRILLO, JAIME BRAVO-ALVARADO, OFELIA POBLANO-VERASTEGUI, and DORIS ORTEGA ALTAMIRANO. 537

Ethical Issues

Building Community Networks for Environmental Health. *By* JANET A. PHOENIX.. 551

Ethical Issues in Genetic Screening and Genetic Monitoring of Employees. *By* KAREL VAN DAMME, PAOLO VINEIS, and MARJA SORSA. 554

Genetic Testing: A Technology Assessment Perspective. *By* PAOLO VINEIS. 566

Irving J. Selikoff Memorial Lecture

The Long-lasting Legacy of Industrial Carcinogens: The Lesson of Asbestos. *By* CESARE MALTONI. 570

***

Index of Contributors 587

Financial assistance was received from:

- THE CENTERS FOR DISEASE CONTROL AND PREVENTION
    - THE NATIONAL INSTITUTE FOR OCCUPATIONAL SAFETY AND HEALTH
    - THE NATIONAL CENTER FOR ENVIRONMENTAL HEALTH
    - THE AGENCY FOR TOXIC SUBSTANCES AND DISEASE REGISTRIES
- THE INTERNATIONAL BROTHERHOOD OF HEATING, FROST AND ASBESTOS WORKERS UNION
- THE OCCUPATIONAL SAFETY AND HEALTH ADMINISTRATION OF THE DEPARTMENT OF LABOR
- THE NATIONAL INSTITUTE FOR ENVIRONMENTAL HEALTH SCIENCES OF THE NATIONAL INSTITUTES OF HEALTH
- THE COCA COLA COMPANY

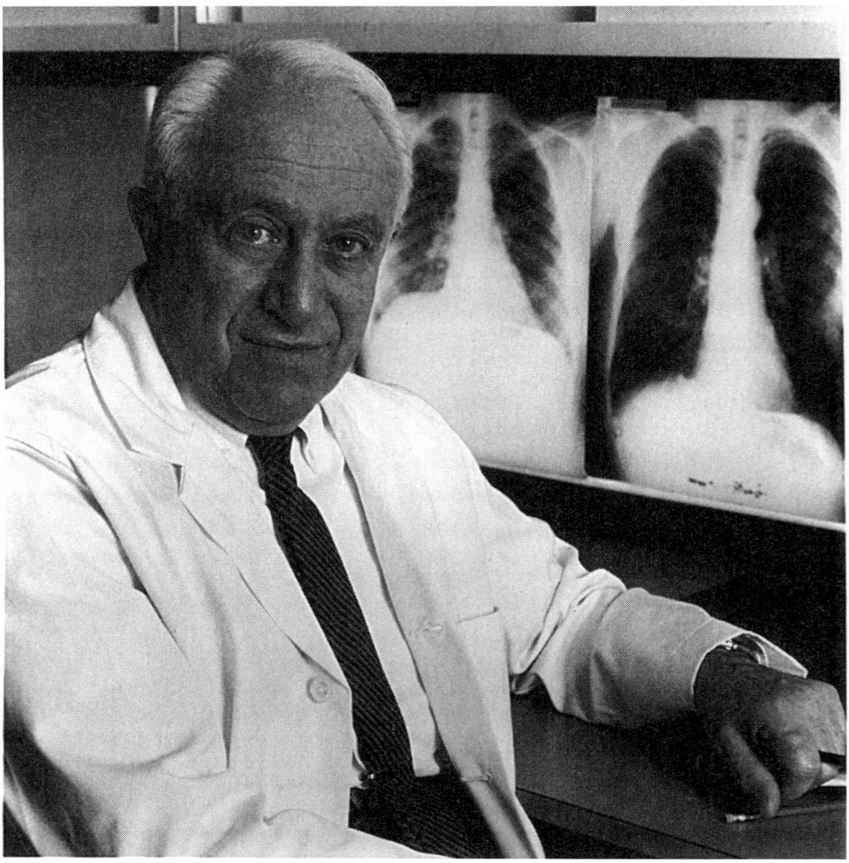

IRVING J. SELIKOFF
1915–1992

Dedication

This volume is dedicated to the memory of Irving J. Selikoff, Founder and first President of the Collegium Ramazzini.

It has been said that, like the living, the dead have their destiny. To see themselves diminished in stature, sinking into oblivion; or else burgeoning, towering across the vistas of the future. This seal alone history sets on the true worth of men.

The figure of Selikoff continues to grow with time. His scientific rigor stands as a great lesson to today's researchers; his moral rigor as an example to today's intellectuals. Many of the things he foresaw have come to pass in scientific reality.

It is a profound satisfaction to his friends to know that this figure will now outlive the witness of their words, immune against oblivion.

CESARE MALTONI
SECRETARY GENERAL
COLLEGIUM RAMAZZINI

Welcome

TO OUR COLLEAGUES FROM AROUND THE WORLD:

The Collegium Ramazzini is an international group of scientists, physicians, and a few lawyers and social scientists, dedicated to scientific inquiry into the causes of environmental and occupational disease and committed to bringing about the changes that will reduce the toll of illness and death from environmental agents.

The preventive strategies around which this volume is organized include identifying agents causing disease, determining exposures, setting priorities for change based on risk assessments, educating citizens and workers, and regulatory approaches.

Identifying Causative Agents. This means catching up with the backlog of chemicals that are untested and speaking out when a chemical is introduced without adequate tests. The first step in prevention is to know the *disease* and the *agent.*

Exposure Assessment. In an earlier New York Academy of Sciences meeting (1976), I quoted Wilhelm Hueper, who said, ''without an environmental carcinogen there is no environmental cancer.'' This statement still holds true; if we can reduce the exposure to, or in some cases eliminate the use of, environmental agents causing disease, the risk of environmental disease will be minimal.

Risk Assessment. We need to determine what action to take first, and how much action should be taken. The most objective way to accomplish this is through formally assessing risks.

Education. One of the most powerful preventive strategies is education of citizens and workers, and involving them in a prevention plan. Recognition of the right-to-know has been an important public health policy decision.

Regulations, Guidelines, and Enforcement. These strategies are not popular among certain leaders in the United States Congress. Yet, standards that would protect people from cancer or other illnesses languish at federal agencies. A worker or citizen may not have a choice as to where to work or live. These concepts are important as the government moves toward environmental justice and equity. These topics are reflected in our volume.

Finally, one last preventive strategy—courage and dedication to duty. During this period many seem to be afraid to be true to the principles that Dr. Selikoff stood for. We as scientists are timid in speaking out on public health issues, because it is not ''in fashion.'' The voices of many in the government are muted and defensive. There are a few in government speaking out—concerned about communities living on dumps, concerned about citizens without environmental equity or justice in their lives. But the silence among many so called environmental leaders is deafening. We are chilled by the lack of fire and the opportunities being missed day after day.

Dr. Selikoff used to tell us this story. When workers would develop asbestos disease, toward the end of their lives their physical condition would deteriorate. When this happened, the workers would be pale, weak, emaciated, would gasp for breath. His union brothers who came faithfully to visit every day would turn all the mirrors in the house around to face the wall so their dying brother could not see his life fading away. I implore you to stop the need for this ritual of kindness. Prevent the diseases so there is no need to hide the mirrors.

EULA BINGHAM
PRESIDENT
COLLEGIUM RAMAZZINI

Foreword

Irving J. Selikoff had a long and productive association with the New York Academy of Sciences. An Academy member for 43 1/2 years, he served as its President in 1969 and was an Honorary Life Governor from 1970 until his death. He was awarded the Academy's Sarah L. Poiley Award and Medal for Biological Research in 1974.

Dr. Selikoff generated and was involved in several Academy and non-Academy conferences, serving as organizer, consultant, and participant. The resulting *Annals* volumes in which he had a hand ranged from the classic *Biological Effects of Asbestos* (Volume 132, Article 1, 1965) and *Toxicity of Vinyl Chloride-Polyvinyl Chloride* (Volume 246, 1975) to *The Third Wave of Asbestos Disease: Exposure to Asbestos in Place: Public Health Control* (Volume 643, 1991) and included the pioneering *Acquired Immune Deficiency Syndrome* (Volume 437, 1984). He was coeditor with Professor Cesare Maltoni of *Living in a Chemical World: Occupational and Environmental Significance of Industrial Carcinogens* (Volume 534, 1988), the precursor of the present volume.

We are honored to be publishing the proceedings of this memorial symposium sponsored by the Collegium Ramazzini, to which Dr. Selikoff contributed so much.

Dr. Selikoff was always interested in the health of workers, even when this cause was politically unpopular; indeed, he had great respect for the ordinary working person. He imbued others with a sense of *vocation*, inspiring them to work to their maximal ability in aid of the common good.

Among my vivid memories of Dr. Selikoff is finding him at 7:30 one morning sitting at my desk correcting proofs. He looked up and said, "Oh, starting late today?"

BILL M. BOLAND
EXECUTIVE EDITOR, THE *ANNALS*
NEW YORK ACADEMY OF SCIENCES

Biomedical Research as a Science for Development: The Case of Gasoline

Ramazzini Lecture, 1995

CESARE MALTONI

Cancer Research Center
European Ramazzini Foundation
of Oncology and Environmental Sciences
Bentivoglio Castle
40010 Bentivoglio (BO), Italy

In the tradition of Bernardino Ramazzini
to honor the memory of Irving J. Selikoff

PREAMBLE

Before presenting my Ramazzini Lecture I wish to thank the President and the Executive Council of the Collegium Ramazzini and the Town of Carpi for the great honor of being chosen as Ramazzini Lecturer, 1995.

I also wish to say how proud I am to be included in the list of scientists who have preceded me as Ramazzini Lecturers. Finally, I wish to dedicate my presentation to the founder of our Collegium and unforgettable friend, Dr. Irving J. Selikoff.

THE BACKGROUND

The industrial era began in the second half of the nineteenth century. In little more than a century it has caused greater changes to the planet Earth and the life of mankind than had taken place in the entire course of previous human history.

The pattern of industrial development has brought man undoubted progress and benefit, but has exacted a heavy price, which humankind at this end of the second millennium is forced to reckon with. Items in that price are: the plundering of the earth's resources, life-threatening changes in the environment, dire alterations to biological equilibria, and last, damage to the health of man (as prophesied by the lone voice of Bernardino Ramazzini some three centuries ago).

In the early years of industrial development, the cost of this technological trend was ignored in the name of progress. Only later, above all after the Second World War, did this cost begin to stare us in the face. But though it could no longer be misconstrued, the name of progress again caused it to be played down.

In more recent times the idea has arisen of a cost/benefit analysis of progress, though the benefit is still being emphasized and the cost still underestimated. If properly applied, the cost/benefit approach may yield fruit and curtail the damage;

however, with time, the depleting of the resources, the degrading of the environment and the perils to human health have created a borderline situation calling for more radical solutions than are contained within the narrow confines of cost/benefit philosophy.

Time is running out, if we are to preserve such resources as the planet still holds, if we are to safeguard life on earth and an already jeopardized biosphere, and if we are to protect the health of mankind from the endless hazards created by the industrial model of development.

Against this background, biomedical research and, above all, preventive research are coming to represent one of the main tools for the protection of man and, indirectly, the environment and its resources. For such research has the task of pinpointing the risks and weighing the costs of the modern development paradigm in terms of the damage to public health. In other words, biomedical research steps into the role of advocate for mankind's right to soundness of mind and limb, and indeed for life itself.

HOW BIOMEDICAL RESEARCH NOW STANDS IN RELATION TO POWER

Biomedical research into the prevention of industrial, environmental, and occupational disease has gained momentum in our century; yet its weight, past and present, has fallen dramatically short of the weight of interested parties, whose political, economic, and technological maneuvres go under the name of power.

The reality is that the wielders of power have curbed the development of biomedical research in the preventive field by every means available, for in it they clearly see their dialectical antagonist.

The ruses adopted by power are numerous indeed, but may I cite a few:

- the repeated, quite spurious, claim that our current paradigm of development, which buttresses the interests of power, is "in line with the development of evolution and the profound unrolling of history"—to quote Julien Benda in 1928 in his prophetic book *The Treason of the Intellectuals;*
- underestimating the cost (risks);
- curtailing resources to preventive biomedical research, which, in today's world, has access to funds the extent of which is derisory when measured against the weight of problems confronting such research;
- the ensuing difficulty in recruiting and training researchers or creating adequate centers, facilities, and research schemes;
- the setting up of alternative biomedical research designed entirely to show that power is based on science. The main task of this pseudoresearch is to play down or deny the cost of today's development model, in return for which it enjoys lavish funding and privileges;
- the creation of unholy temples of bureaucracy in which are pitted, in unequal line-up, the direct representatives of power, the representatives of servile science, bureaucrats (aseptic if only in their detached Byzantine mode of speech),

and, as an afterthought but not always, some timid representative of proper research.

And yet, however mortified, biomedical preventive research may be seen to have a great future. This forecast rests on several facts: (1) the unshelvable urgency of the problems hanging over us; (2) the self-awareness of the true scientific community and its pride in its own role; (3) the selection of a collegium of researchers, albeit small, who are immunized against the blandishments or snares of power; and (4) the grasping by these last of certain inalienable basic principles by which the role of biomedical preventive research is to be safeguarded.

INALIENABLE RIGHTS OF BIOMEDICAL PREVENTIVE RESEARCH

In fulfilling its purpose, biomedical research must lay claim to these inalienable rights:

(1) to choose its own priorities among research sectors;
(2) to plan research for itself;
(3) to draw up the protocols of research;
(4) to interpret the results of research and weigh the repercussions of such results on public health and development model planning; and
(5) to broadcast its findings among the scientific community and, if necessary, to enlist public opinion.

THE TIME LAG OF BIOMEDICAL PREVENTIVE RESEARCH

In this context, for all the efforts of its "saints and martyrs," biomedical preventive research is off to a late start. The delay lies not in its potential, for such research possesses the scientific and technological tools to perform its task. The real cause of delay has been the failure to accord it a proper primary role, the withholding of any realistic resources with which to meet the risk situations already on us or on the horizon, the attempts to muzzle its freedom, and a concerted strategy of intimidation and defamation.

A mere fraction of the tens of thousands of technological processes, agents, consumer goods, and pollutants spawned by industry, with lifestyles to match, have been properly investigated to assess the degree of health hazard or otherwise. Yet what we do know points to an urgent need to fill the gaps in our knowledge of the whole arsenal of industrial development.

One insight may serve as an example: it regards the risks of cancer attaching to industrial/exogenous agents. To our knowledge the two main projects to ascertain the cancer risks of exogenous/industrial agents are: the U.S. National Toxicology Program (NTP) and the Program of the Cancer Research Center at the Castle of

TABLE 1. Results of the Completed Long-term Carcinogenicity Bioassays Performed in the Framework of NTP and BT Projects.

	Agents Studied at NTP		Agents Studied at BT	
Results	No.	%	No.	%
Clear evidence of carcinogenicity at least in 1 test system	138	46.7	50[a]	45.9
Limited evidence of carcinogenicity at least in 1 test system	50	17.0	17[b]	15.6
No evidence of carcinogenicity in the tested system(s)	107	36.3	42	38.5
Total test compounds	295	100.0	109	100.0

[a] Strong and intermediate carcinogen.
[b] Weak and borderline carcinogen.

Bentivoglio (BT) by our Foundation. These two projects have taken a largely random sample of such agents for carcinogenicity testing and have found a high percentage to be carcinogenic. The finding takes on particular significance if one notes the close correspondence of results from one scheme to the other, although different compounds were tested and some differences occurred in the experimental conditions (TABLE 1).

What hazards lurk, one wonders, in the tens of thousands of technological agents, consumer goods, pollutants, and lifestyles met with in daily life, that have never, or only cursorily, been vetted by biomedical research? No one can say, though presumably many have a shrewd idea. This gray area in our knowledge urgently needs exploring, for in the meantime, by light of day or cover of dark, the risk factors will go on sowing disease among humankind.

A case in point is the increase of cancer among industrialized countries. This can only partly be attributed to the aging population. Side by side with the overall increase, we are witnessing a gearing forward of the subject age group and the emergence of new types of neoplasia.

THE EXAMPLE OF GASOLINE

General Details

Motor vehicles and petroleum fuels (of all kinds) together form a sector of the industrial world whose technological and economic impact is enormous, whose repercussions in terms of the depletion of resources, pollution of the environment, and danger to public health are colossal.

More specifically, cars and gasolines (a term covering a range of such fuels, varying in composition) represent two of the main consumer goods by which our modern era is marked.

At the end of the eighties the world car population stood at 403,493,465, with 144,375,000 in the United States alone, 127,979,276 in the EEC, 32,621,046 in Japan, 30,152,400 in Germany, and 26,378,000 in Italy.

The annual consumption of gasoline has been estimated at over 600,000,000 tonnes throughout the world—some 290 million in the United States, over 130 million in the EEC, and around 15 million in Italy.

With its vapors and combustion products, gasoline nowadays contributes in a decisive way to polluting the biosphere, as is apparent when one takes into account the size of the biosphere itself, the amount of gasoline consumed across the globe, and the number of cars in circulation.

The problem of pollution from gasoline and its combustion products takes on an even greater magnitude when summed with the other atmospheric contaminants with which the planet abounds—namely, those connected with: (1) the use of other liquid fuels for automobile and other motor transport, heating, and energy production; (2) the use of gas and solid fuels for motor vehicles and/or heating and/or energy production; (3) the mining industries; (4) waste disposal by burning (including agricultural waste); (5) the production of active volatile chemical substances of various kinds (including pesticides, propellants, and solvents); and (6) the volatile or powdery materials used in the building and metalworking trades.

The gasoline-car combination has thus turned progressively into an ecological and health problem affecting the physical, chemical, and, by extension, biological equilibria of the earth's biosphere, with a parallel effect, to the best of our current knowledge, on the health of man.

In recent years the problem has gained in complexity through the introduction of new kinds of gasoline. The pressure to reduce and halt the use of lead octane optimizers; the need to optimize gasoline in relation to the various types of motor-engine, and, indeed, containment system; the progress made in refining techniques; the availability and employment of artificial additives in the optimization process; the trend towards using recycled products, or those from replenishable (agricultural) sources, as components of gasoline itself; and likewise the prospect of producing gasoline from alternative sources to petroleum—all these mean that nowadays the gasolines produced range widely in their composition, performance, and type of combustion products.

As things stand, gasolines may be classified, in order of toxicology, as:

A) Conventional gasolines
   (a) Lead-added gasoline
   (b) Unleaded gasoline, high in aromatic hydrocarbon content (especially benzene and alkylbenzenes—i.e., toluene, a mixture of ortho-meta- and par-axylene, ethyl benzene, propyl benzene, 1,2,4 trimethylbenzene, etc.), obtained in the process of petroleum refining and/or subsequent mixing (used above all in Europe).
   (c) Unleaded gasoline, lower in aromatic hydrocarbons than the European form, high in isoparaffin and especially trimethylpentane, obtained by

a special type of petroleum refining (alkylation) that employs special catalysts (used above all in the United States).

B) Gasolines containing oxygenated additives

By oxygenated additive gasolines one means those in which a significant amount of oxygenated (non-petroleum-derived) compounds have been introduced, with a view to optimizing octanes, and also as fuel proper. When the amount of oxygenated additive exceeds a certain level, one has a considerable rearrangement of the other components of the final product; in this case one talks of reformulated gasolines.

The oxygenates hitherto used or recommended are methyl alcohol, ethyl alcohol, methyl-ter-butyl-ether (MTBE), ethyl-ter-butyl-ether (ETBE), di-isopropyl-ether (DIPE) and tert-amyl-methyl-ether (TAME).

In the face of the planetary problem of the potential health effects of gasolines, our biomedical information on the effects of gasoline on health is woefully inadequate. No systematic, integrated study plan has been promoted by organs or institutions of hygiene and public health, or by the producers themselves of gasoline and its additives. There is thus no basis for quantitative analysis of the risks of the various gasolines, their components and their combustion products, such as to guide the decision-making process.

What information there is is piecemeal and often anecdotal. The research behind such information has been performed in separate laboratories, with differing criteria. Often it provides no data for any precise evaluation of the risks, let alone serving for the comparison of toxicity/carcinogenicity among the various gasolines.

To sift the research in the field is to conclude that biomedical investigations have here been left to chance, or else have been undertaken to suit the ends of economic competition.

One clear fact emerges from this situation: the information is scanty, insufficient, exploitable; yet, paradoxically, in this warped context in which no data equates with negative data, what are favored are precisely those gasolines on which no data at all are available.

Recent history is instructive here. After the toxic effects of lead had sunk home, all the unleaded gasolines began to be publicized as "new and ecological," creating in the popular mind the fallacy that by simply removing lead one rendered gasoline risk free and safe (including, for instance, those richest in aromatic hydrocarbons). Subsequently, with the growth of the market for oxygenated additives (as substitutes for lead) and the trend towards the use of alcohols, especially ethyl alcohol, we reached the absurdity of the "green gasoline" slogan to denote fuels containing ethyl alcohol additive, this alcohol being vegetable in origin. All this without there being, then or now, adequate data available on the toxicity/carcinogenicity of oxygenates per se, oxygenate-added gasolines, and the combustion products of them.

On the subject of the unsystematic and utterly amateur nature of gasoline research, the case of MTBE stands as a classic. This long-known component has been in use industrially since 1985 and is used today to the tune of millions of tonnes. Levels of this additive are kept high in cold areas, above all in the winter months. A few years ago, some users (especially in Alaska) reported symptoms including a series of ailments typical of hypersensitization syndrome to chemical agents. The public alarm generated by these reports and by the size of the interests involved brought MTBE suddenly to the forefront of toxicological research in the months that followed. Yet at the same time it stands on record that, despite the massive production of this compound, despite its widespread diffusion and the accordingly dense ranks of those exposed to it, and despite the weight of economic interests involved, there exist to date only two long-term carcinogenicity research studies: one conducted in the United States by the Task Force of MTBE producers, the results of which are not yet published in the scientific literature; and one, unsolicited by any interested party, private or public, conducted by our own institute, supported partly by public funds and for the most part by the generosity of the private citizen. The results of this last study have recently been published in a scientific journal.[1]

Last, and even more puzzlingly, one finds that the occasional spontaneously promoted studies, which may have their shortcomings (understandable in view of the official lack of liaison); but which objectively bring to light unsuspected dangers to public health, encounter an attitude of arrogant opposition or contestation directed at the studies and at the scientists responsible, by industry and the public authorities themselves; yet these groups have never promoted valid research of their own, but instead counter the facts with opinion and criticism, or cite the findings of slanted studies ill-equipped to reach any assessment of specific end-point pathologies, as well as being ill-controlled and not uncommonly devoid of the minimum scientific requirements—all this in an attempt to suppress the "unwelcome news," by suppressing its scientific messengers.

Among the major potential risks of gasoline, its components and its combustion products, carcinogenicity is certainly the gravest pathological effect.

The Carcinogenicity of Gasoline: A Story

There was no substantial information on the carcinogenicity of gasoline until the mid seventies, apart from the observation of an increase in leukemias among workers not belonging to the petrol industry, exposed to benzene used as a solvent—a minor instance, since benzene is mainly a major component of gasoline and a key compound of the petrochemical industry. It should be added that this conclusion stemmed from anecdotal case reports, not systematic epidemiological surveys[2] and came in for considerable criticism. Note that in those days the risks of benzene were not referred to gasoline or to the petrochemical industry, or even to tobacco smoke, which has benzene as one of its main components. The aim was to avoid any gasoline-leukemia association or even that of gasoline-tobacco when the latter was a known carcinogenic factor. At the time, besides, it was thought from the inadequate evidence of the results available that benzene was not carcinogenic to experimental animals.[2]

This was the context in 1975, when our Foundation's Cancer Research Center embarked on its wide-ranging experimental project to assess the carcinogenic effect of various kinds of petroleum fuel, especially gasoline and its components, beginning with research on benzene (BT project).

The results of the project came out in the second half of the seventies, the eighties, and the early nineties. They documented the carcinogenicity of benzene,[3–7] the carcinogenic risks of some alkylbenzenes,[6] and of MTBE.[1]

TABLE 2. BT Project of Experimental Bioassays on Gasoline Carcinogenicity: Plan of the Experiments.

Material		Type of Exposure (route)	Animal System		
Category	Specific Material		Species	Strain	Sex
Petrol Fuels	Unleaded gasoline	Gavage	Rat	Sprague-Dawley	M, F
	Leaded gasoline	Gavage	Rat	Sprague-Dawley	M, F
	Diesel	Gavage	Rat	Sprague-Dawley	M, F
	Kerosene	Gavage	Rat	Sprague-Dawley	M, F
Aromatic hydrocarbons	Benzene	Gavage	Rat	Sprague-Dawley	M, F
				Wistar	M, F
			Mouse	Swiss	M, F
				RF/J	M, F
		Inhalation	Rat	Sprague-Dawley	M, F
	Toluene	Gavage	Rat	Sprague-Dawley	M, F
	Xylenes	Gavage	Rat	Sprague-Dawley	M, F
	Ethylbenzene	Gavage	Rat	Sprague-Dawley	M, F
	1,2,4-Trimethylbenzene	Gavage	Rat	Sprague-Dawley	M, F
Isoparaffins	Trimethylpentane	Gavage	Rat	Sprague-Dawley	M, F
Oxygenated additives	Methyl alcohol	Drinking water	Rat	Sprague-Dawley	M, F
		Gavage	Rat	Sprague-Dawley	M, F
	Ethyl alcohol	Drinking water	Rat	Sprague-Dawley	M, F
		Gavage	Rat	Sprague-Dawley	M, F
	Methyl-ter-butyl-ether (MTBE)	Gavage	Rat	Sprague-Dawley	M, F
	Ethyl-ter-butyl-ether (ETBE)	Gavage	Rat	Sprague-Dawley	M, F
	Di-isopropyl-ether (DIPE)	Gavage	Rat	Sprague-Dawley	M, F
	Tert-amyl-methyl-ether (TAME)	Gavage	Rat	Sprague-Dawley	M, F

TABLE 2. BT Project of Experimental Bioassays on Gasoline Carcinogenicity: Plan of the Experiments (*Continued*)

Material		Type of Exposure (route)	Animal System		
Category	Specific Material		Species	Strain	Sex
Mixtures	Gasoline + Methyl alcohol	Gavage	Rat	Sprague-Dawley	M, F
	Gasoline + Ethyl alcohol	Gavage	Rat	Sprague-Dawley	M, F
	Gasoline + MTBE	Gavage	Rat	Sprague-Dawley	M, F
	Gasoline + ETBE	Gavage	Rat	Sprague-Dawley	M, F
Combustion products	Formaldehyde	Drinking water	Rat	Sprague-Dawley	M, F
	Acetaldehyde	Drinking water	Rat	Sprague-Dawley	M, F
	Particulated	Subcutaneous injection	Rat	Sprague-Dawley	M, F
			Mouse	Swiss	M, F
Catalyzers	Z-Zeolytes	Intrapleural, intraperitoneal, and subcutaneous injection	Rat	Sprague-Dawley	M, F

TABLE 3. BT Project of Experimental Bioassays on Gasoline Carcinogenicity: Available Results

Material			Results	
Category	Specific Material	Animal System	Carcinogenicity	Tumors with Increased Incidence
Petrol fuels	Unleaded gasoline[a]	Sprague-Dawley rats	+	Total malignant tumors
				Mammary cancers
				Head cancers
				Uterus and vagina malignant tumors[b]
	Leaded gasoline	Sprague-Dawley rats	+	Total malignant tumors
				Mammary cancers
				Head cancers
				Uterus and vagina malignant tumors[b]
	Diesel	Sprague-Dawley rats	+	Total malignant tumors
				Head cancers
				Uterus and vagina malignant tumors[b]
	Kerosene	Sprague-Dawley rats	+	Total malignant tumors
				Mammary cancers
				Head cancers
				Uterus and vagina malignant tumors[b]
Aromatic hydrocarbons	Benzene	Sprague-Dawley rats	+	Total malignant tumors
				Mammary cancers
				Oral cavity carcinomas
				Zymbal gland carcinomas
				Nasal cavities carcinomas
				Skin carcinomas
				Forestomach carcinomas
				Hepatomas
				Liver angiosarcomas
				Hemolymphoreticular neoplasias

TABLE 3. BT Project of Experimental Bioassays on Gasoline Carcinogenicity: Available Results (*Continued*)

Material			Results	
Category	Specific Material	Animal System	Carcinogenicity	Tumors with Increased Incidence
	Benzene	Wistar rats	+	Total malignant tumors Oral cavity carcinomas Zymbal gland carcinomas Nasal cavities carcinomas
		Swiss mice	+	Total malignant tumors Mammary cancers Zymbal gland carcinomas Lung tumors
		RF/J mice	+	Total malignant tumors Mammary cancers Lung tumors Hemolymphoreticular neoplasias
	Toluene	Sprague-Dawley rats	+	Total malignant tumors Mammary cancers Head cancers Hemolymphoreticular neoplasias
	Xylenes	Sprague-Dawley rats	+	Total malignant tumors Mammary cancers Head cancers Hemolymphoreticular neoplasias
	Ethylbenzene	Sprague-Dawley rats	+	Total malignant tumors Head cancers
	1,2,4-Trimethylbenzene	Sprague-Dawley rats	+	Total malignant tumors Head cancers

TABLE 3. BT Project of Experimental Bioassays on Gasoline Carcinogenicity: Available Results (*Continued*)

Material			Results	
Category	Specific Material	Animal System	Carcinogenicity	Tumors with Increased Incidence
Oxygenated additives	MTBE	Sprague-Dawley rats	+	Hemolymphoreticular neoplasias
				Leydig cell testicular tumors
	ETBE	Sprague-Dawley rats	(+)	(Total malignant tumors)
Combustion products	Formaldehyde	Sprague-Dawley rats	+	Total malignant tumors
				Mammary cancers
				Stomach cancers
				Intestine cancers
				Hemolymphoreticular neoplasias
				Leydig cell testicular tumors
	Acetaldehyde	Sprague-Dawley rats	+	Total malignant tumors
				Mammary cancers
				Head cancers
				Lung tumors
				Stomach cancers
				Intestine cancers
				Uterus cancers
				Hemolymphoreticular neoplasias

[a] With high level of aromatics.
[b] Also neurinosarcomas.

Meanwhile a study produced by the American Petroleum Institute (API) showed the carcinogenic effect of a cross section of gasolines representative of American gasolines in the eighties.[8] There was also a study by the NTP confirming our results on the carcinogenicity of benzene,[9] and epidemiological studies confirming the leukemic effect of benzene on man, even in low doses.[10,11]

The biophase of most of the BT experiments is now over, and the data from the whole project are being prepared for publication.

It goes without saying that none of the BT project experiments have received government or industry financing.

I would like to use this opportunity to present the BT study plan and some of the main results available.

The BT Project of Experimental Studies on the Carcinogenicity of Gasoline

This project comprises long-term carcinogenicity bioassays on petrol-fuels, including gasoline, leaded gasoline, gasoline with high aromatic content, gasoline aromatics (benzene, toluene, xylenes, ethylbenzene, 1,2,4-trimethylbenzene), the isoparaffin trimethylpentane (TMP), oxygenated additives (MTBE, ETBE, DIPE, TAME) alone or blended with gasoline, products of combustion (formaldehyde, acetaldehyde, particulate exhausts), and also solid catalysts of petrol refining (zeolites). The plan of the project is shown in TABLE 2. For this project more than 15,500 animals were kept under observation until spontaneous death.

The already-published or not-yet-published results available from the project are summarized in TABLE 3.

Our data indicate the carcinogenic risk of gasoline, of some of its components, including additives, and of some of its exhaust. Since several of the agents studied turned out to be carcinogens, from the public health angle one must consider possible syncarcinogenic effects.

Besides the information they afford, our data show the need for further studies to define and quantify the carcinogenic risk of gasoline. They also stress the requirement that all new modifications to gasoline composition be submitted to appropriate biomedical research to screen them from potential risks, or at least reduce the risks, before they go into the production cycle and onto the market.

CONCLUSIONS

In the preventive sector, biomedical research must grow. It is an irreplaceable link in the strategy that society must adopt to defend natural resources, the environment, health, and, in a word, life on earth.

To promote the growth of biomedical research into development research, and its indisputable role in the decision making that shapes the trends of development itself, is, in fact, the prime reason why the Collegium Ramazzini came into being.

REFERENCES

1. Belpoggi, F., M. Soffritti & C. Maltoni. 1995. Methyl-tertiary-butyl ether (MTBE)—a gasoline additive—causes testicular and lymphohaematopoietic cancers in rats. Toxicol. Ind. Health **11**(2): 119-149.
2. IARC. 1974. Some anti-thyroid and related substances, nitrofurans and industrial chemicals. IARC Monograph on the Carcinogenic Risk of Chemicals to Man, Vol. 7. International Agency for Research on Cancer. Lyon.
3. Maltoni, C. & C. Scarnato. 1977. Le prime prove sperimentali dell'azione cancerogena del benzene. Gli Ospedali della Vita **4:** 111-113.
4. Maltoni, C. & C. Scarnato. 1979. First experimental demonstration of the carcinogenic effects of benzene. Long-term bioassays on Sprague-Dawley rats by oral administration. Med. Lav. **70:** 352-357.
5. Maltoni, C., B. Conti & G. Cotti. 1983. Benzene: A multipotential carcinogen. Results of long-term bioassays performed at the Bologna Institute of Oncology. Am. J. Ind. Med. **4:** 589-630.
6. Maltoni, C., B. Conti, G. Cotti *et al.* 1985. Experimental studies on benzene carcinogenicity at the Bologna Institute of Oncology: Current results and ongoing research. Am. J. Ind. Med. **7:** 415-446.
7. Maltoni, C., C. Ciliberti, G. Cotti *et al.* 1989. Benzene, an experimental multipotential carcinogen: Results of the long-term bioassays performed at the Bologna Institute of Oncology. Environ. Health Perspect. **82:** 109-124.
8. Kitchen, D. N. 1984. Neoplastic renal effects of unleaded gasoline in Fischer 344 rats. *In* Advances in Modern Environmental Toxicology, Renal Effects of Petroleum Hydrocarbons, Vol. VII. M. A. Mehlman, G. P. Hemstreet III, J. J. Thrope & N. K. Weaver, Eds.: 65-72. Princeton Scientific Publishers. Princeton, NJ.
9. Huff, J. E. 1986. Toxicology and carcinogenesis studies of benzene (CAS No. 71-43-2) in F344/N rats and B6C3F_1 mice (gavage studies). Technical report No. 289, National Toxicology Program. US Department of Health and Human Services. Washington, DC.
10. Infante, P. & M. White. 1985. Projections of leukemia risk associated with occupational exposure to benzene. Am. J. Ind. Med. **7:** 403-413.
11. Rinsky, R., A. Smith, R. Hornung *et al.* 1986. Benzene and leukemia: An epidemiologic risk assessment, Vol. 24. National Institute for Occupational Safety and Health. Cincinnati, OH.

Results of Long-term Experimental Carcinogenicity Studies of the Effects of Gasoline, Correlated Fuels, and Major Gasoline Aromatics on Rats

CESARE MALTONI, ADRIANO CILIBERTI, CARMINE PINTO, MORANDO SOFFRITTI, FIORELLA BELPOGGI, AND LORETTA MENARINI

Cancer Research Center
European Ramazzini Foundation
of Oncology and Environmental Sciences
Bentivoglio Castle
40010 Bentivoglio (BO), Italy

INTRODUCTION

Up to the midseventies the experimental information on the possible carcinogenic potential of gasolines and their components, with particular regard to aromatic hydrocarbons, was unsubstantial. In the laboratories of the Cancer Research Center (CRC), at the Bentivoglio (BT) Castle of the European Ramazzini Foundation of Oncology and Environmental Sciences, a series of experimental studies was started, aimed at evaluating the carcinogenic burden of gasolines, correlated fuels, and gasoline aromatics.

As early as 1977, it was shown for the first time that benzene was a multipotential carcinogen.[1] Those results were then confirmed in successive studies.[2–6] A study conducted by the American Petroleum Institute in the early eighties showed that a cross section of significant samples of American gasolines was causing kidney tumors in rats exposed by inhalation.[7]

There are no data in the literature on the carcinogenicity of the European type of gasoline, of diesel oil, and of kerosene. The studies on aromatics other than benzene are inadequate or missing.

The experimental carcinogenicity studies on toluene, reported up to 1989, have been considered inadequate.[8] This compound was then tested by inhalation on Fischer 344/N rats and B6C3F1 mice within the framework of the National Toxicology Program (NTP) in two year-long bioassays, with negative results.[9]

The only two experimental carcinogenicity studies on xylenes, performed within the framework of the NTP, in which the compound was given in corn oil by stomach tube to Fischer 344/N rats and B6C3F1 mice, gave negative results.[10,11] Again these bioassays were truncated after two years.

No experimental carcinogenicity studies have been performed to our knowledge on ethylbenzene and on 1,2,4-trimethylbenzene.

TABLE 1. Weight Percent Composition Analysis of Tested Unleaded Gasolines, as Evaluated in Two Different Laboratories

Constituents	I analysis (%)	II analysis (%)
Total saturates	48.0	49.0
N-paraffins	11.0	24.0
Isoparaffins	28.0	25.0
2,2,4-TMP	?	0.2
Olefins	3.3	3.0
Total aromatics	48.0	48.0
Benzene	5.0	5.6

This lack of proper information on these mixtures and compounds is surprising. The production, consumption and distribution of these fuels is enormous. Toluene, xylenes, ethylbenzene, and 1,2,4-trimethylbenzene are present at a high concentration in gasoline. Toluene and xylenes are widely used in the petrochemical industry, and for the production of numerous consumer goods.

This report refers the results of our early studies on European unleaded gasoline with high content of aromatics; leaded gasoline; gasoil (diesel) and kerosene; and toluene, xylenes, ethylbenzene, and 1,2,4-trimethylbenzene.

Preliminary results on toluene, xylenes and ethylbenzene were already published in 1985.[4]

MATERIALS AND METHODS

Gasolines, the other fuels, and the aromatic hydrocarbons were supplied by an Italian petrol industry and by an Italian petrochemical industry, respectively.

The weight percent composition analysis of the tested unleaded gasolines, evaluated in two different laboratories, was as shown in TABLE 1.

The analytical characterization of the tested aromatic hydrocarbons resulted in percent, w/w:

toluene: toluene: 98.34; paraffin: 0.83; benzene: 0.28; ethylbenzene: 0.52; m-xylene and p-xylene: 0.029
xylenes: xylenes: 99.45 (o-xylene: 26.90; m-xylene: 50.31; p-xylene: 22.24); toluene: 0.29; paraffin: 0.05
ethylbenzene: ethylbenzene: 99.57; benzene: 0.07; toluene: 0.20; cumene: 0.06; paraffin: 0.06; unidentified: 0.04
1,2,4-trimethylbenzene: 1,2,4-trimethylbenzene: >99.

Male (M) and female (F) Sprague-Dawley rats of the colony of the CRC/BT were used. This colony of rats has been employed for various experiments in the

BT laboratory for nearly 25 years. Historical data are available on more than 10,000 historical controls, kept under observation for life span and submitted to systematic necropsies and standardized histopathological examinations. Therefore, data on the expected incidence of the different types of tumors in the control animals and on its fluctuations are available.

After weaning, at 4–5 weeks of age, the experimental animals were identified by ear punch, randomized in order to have no more than one male and one female of each litter in the same group, and housed 5 per cage. The animals were 7 weeks old at the start of the experiments.

The plan of the experiments are shown in TABLE 2. Unleaded and leaded gasoline, gasoil (diesel), and kerosene were tested at two dose levels within the same experiment. Toluene, xylenes, and ethylbenzene were tested at two dose levels, with two experiments, each one with its own control group. 1,2,4-trimethylbenzene was tested only at one dose.

Every single dose was administered by stomach tube as 1 ml of extra virgin olive oil solution, 4 days weekly (Monday and Tuesday; Thursday and Friday), for 104 weeks. A 5–6-dose weekly administration of the compound at a higher dose would not have been tolerated by the rats. The solutions were prepared weekly and maintained at 4°C. Control animals were given 1 ml of extra virgin olive oil alone.

The animals were kept under observation until death, under highly standardized housing and diet conditions identical to those used in the CRC/BT; the animals were usually allowed to live until natural death. By doing so, it was possible to develop all the neoplastic potentialities. Mean daily feed and drinking water consumption were determined once weekly for the first 13 weeks from the start of the experiments, then every 2 weeks, until 111 weeks of age. Individual animal weight was measured once weekly from 7 weeks of age for the first 13 weeks, every 2 weeks until 111 weeks of age, and then every 8 weeks until the end of the experiments. In order to detect and register all gross lesions, the animals were examined every week for the first 13 weeks, and then every 2 weeks until the end of the experiments.

The biophase of the experiments either was truncated after 123 weeks (in the experiment studying fuels and the higher doses of aromatics), or else lasted for the life span, up to 145 weeks (in the experiments studying the aromatics at the lower doses).

Upon death, the animals were submitted to systematic necropsy. Histopathology was routinely performed on brain, pituitary gland, Zymbal glands, salivary glands, Harderian glands, head, tongue, thymus and mediastinal lymph nodes, lung, heart, diaphragm, liver, spleen, pancreas, kidneys and adrenal glands, esophagus, stomach, intestine (4 levels), bladder, prostate, uterus, vagina, gonads, interscapular fat pad, subcutaneous and mesenteric lymph nodes, sternum, femur, spinal cord, and any other organs and tissues with pathological lesions.

All organs and tissues were immediately preserved in 70% ethyl alcohol, except bones, which were fixed in 10% formalin and then decalcified with 10% formaldehyde and 20% formic acid in water solution. The normal specimens were trimmed, following the standard procedures of the BT Laboratory: i.e., parenchymal organs were dissected through the hilus to expose the widest surface, and hollow organs were sectioned across the greatest diameter(s). The pathological tissue was trimmed through the largest surface, including normal adjacent tissues. The trimmed specimens were

TABLE 2. Long-term Carcinogenicity Bioassays on Unleaded Gasoline with High Content of Aromatics, Leaded Gasoline, Gasoil (Diesel), Kerosene, Toluene, Xylenes, Ethylbenzene, and 1,2,4-Trimethylbenzene: Plan of the Experiments

Test Compound	Experiment	Daily Dose (mg/kg b.w.)	Animals	
			Sex	No.
Unleaded gasoline with high content of aromatics	BT951	800	M	50
			F	50
			M + F	100
		500	M	50
			F	50
			M + F	100
		0[a,b]	M	50
			F	50
			M + F	100
Leaded gasoline	BT952	800	M	50
			F	50
			M + F	100
		500	M	50
			F	50
			M + F	100
		0[a,b]	M	50
			F	50
			M + F	100
Gasoil (diesel)	BT954	800	M	50
			F	50
			M + F	100
		500	M	50
			F	50
			M + F	100
		0[a,b]	M	50
			F	50
			M + F	100
Kerosene	BT953	800	M	50
			F	50
			M + F	100
		500	M	50
			F	50
			M + F	100
		0[a,b]	M	50
			F	50
			M + F	100
Toluene	BT910	800	M	50
			F	50
			M + F	100
		0[a,c]	M	50
			F	50
			M + F	100

TABLE 2. Long-term Carcinogenicity Bioassays on Unleaded Gasoline with High Content of Aromatics, Leaded Gasoline, Gasoil (Diesel), Kerosene, Toluene, Xylenes, Ethylbenzene, and 1,2,4-Trimethylbenzene: Plan of the Experiments (*Continued*)

Test Compound	Experiment	Daily Dose (mg/kg b.w.)	Animals	
			Sex	No.
	BT903	500	M	40
			F	40
			M + F	80
		0[a,d]	M	50
			F	50
			M + F	100
Xylenes	BT911	800	M	50
			F	50
			M + F	100
		0[a,c]	M	50
			F	50
			M + F	100
	BT904	500	M	40
			F	40
			M + F	80
		0[a,d]	M	50
			F	50
			M + F	100
Ethylbenzene	BT912	800	M	50
			F	50
			M + F	100
		0[a,c]	M	50
			F	50
			M + F	100
	BT905	500	M	40
			F	40
			M + F	80
		0[a,d]	M	50
			F	50
			M + F	100
1,2,4-Trimethylbenzene	BT913	800	M	50
			F	50
			M + F	100
		0[a,c]	M	50
			F	50
			M + F	100

[a] Olive oil alone.
[b] The same control group.
[c] The same control group.
[d] The same control group.

TABLE 3. Effects of Treatments on Survival of Male and Female Rats

Test Compound	Daily Dose (mg/kg b.w.)	Survival[a]	
		M	F
Unleaded gasoline with high content of aromatics	800	+	++
	500	+	+
Leaded gasoline	800	++	+
	500	–	+
Gasoil (diesel)	800	+	++
	500	–	+
Kerosene	800	+	++
	500	+	+
Toluene	800	+	+
	500	–	–
Xylenes	800	++	++
	500	+	–
Ethylbenzene	800	+(+)	+(+)
	500	+	–
1,2,4-Trimethylbenzene	800	+(+)	+

[a] –: unaffected; +: slight reduction; ++: sharp reduction; +(+): intermediate reduction.

processed as paraffin blocks, and 3-5-micron sections of every specimen were obtained. Sections were routinely stained with hematoxylin-eosin. Specific stainings were performed when needed. All slides were examined microscopically by the same group of pathologists; a senior pathologist reviewed all the tumors and any other lesion of oncological interest. All pathologists followed the same criteria of histopathological evaluation and classification.

RESULTS

Survival

Survival was affected by treatment as shown in TABLE 3. The reduction of survival for several compounds appears clearly correlated to the dose, and seems to be influenced to some extent by the sex. The different survival rates may have affected the incidence of tumors.

Tumors

Multiple tumors of the same site (monolateral and bilateral organs) and type were plotted only once.

TABLE 4. Results of Long-term Carcinogenicity Bioassays of Unleaded Gasoline with a High Content of Aromatics, Administered by Gavage to Sprague-Dawley Rats: Total Tumors

Group No.	Dose (mg/kg b.w.)	Animals		% of Animals Bearing Tumors		No. of Malignant Tumors per 100 Animals
		Sex	No.	TBMT[a]	MT[b]	
I	800	M	50	52.0	30.0	34.0
		F	50	62.0	32.0	40.0
		M + F	100	57.0	31.0	37.0
II	500	M	50	54.0	14.0	16.0
		F	50	64.0	36.0	46.0
		M + F	100	59.0	25.0	31.0
	0		50	54.0	24.0	
III	(control)	M/F	50	70.0	22.0	23.0/26.0
		M + F	100	62.0	23.0	24.0

[a] TBMT: total benign and malignant tumors.
[b] MT: malignant tumors.

TABLE 5. Results of Long-term Carcinogenicity Bioassays of Unleaded Gasoline with a High Content of Aromatics, Administered by Gavage to Sprague-Dawley Rats: Mammary Cancers

Group No.	Dose (mg/kg b.w.)	Animals		% of Animals Bearing Cancers
		Sex	No.	
I	800	F	50	16.0
II	500	F	50	10.0
III	0 (control)	F	50	6.0

Unleaded Gasoline

An increase of total malignant tumors was found in males treated with the higher dose, and in females treated with both doses (but not dose related) (TABLE 4). A dose-related increase of mammary cancers was found among treated females (TABLE 5). A slight increase of head cancers was observed in male rats treated with the higher dose (TABLE 6). A higher onset of malignant tumors of the uterus-vagina was found in females treated with both doses, although it was not dose related (TABLE 7). Of particular significance is the observation of uterine-vaginal neurinosarcomas

TABLE 6. Results of Long-term Carcinogenicity Bioassays of Unleaded Gasoline with a High Content of Aromatics Administered by Gavage to Sprague-Dawley Rats: Head Cancers

		Animals		% of Animals Bearing Cancers					
Group No.	Dose (mg/kg b.w.)	Sex	No.	Zymbal Gland CA[a]	Ear Duct CA	Nasal Cavities CA	Oral Cavity CA	Head SA[b]	Total
I	800	M	50	—	—	6.0	—	2.0[c]	8.0
		F	50	—	2.0	2.0	2.0	—	6.0
		M + F	100	—	1.0	4.0	1.0	1.0	7.0
II	500	M	50	2.0	—	—	—	—	2.0
		F	50	—	2.0	—	2.0	—	4.0
		M + F	100	1.0	1.0	—	1.0	—	3.0
III	0 (control)	M	50	2.0	—	—	—	—	2.0
		F	50	2.0	2.0	—	2.0	—	6.0
		M + F	100	2.0	1.0	—	1.0	—	4.0

[a] CA: cancer.
[b] SA: sarcoma.
[c] Fibrosarcoma of oral cavity.

TABLE 7. Results of Long-term Carcinogenicity Bioassays of Unleaded Gasoline with a High Content of Aromatics, Administered by Gavage to Sprague-Dawley Rats: Malignant Tumors of Uterus and Vagina

		Animals		% of Animals Bearing Malignant Tumors				
Group No.	Dose (mg/kg b.w.)	Sex	No.	Uterus CA[a]	Vagina CA	Uterus-Vagina Neurino SA[b]	Uterus: Other SA	Total
I	800	F	50	2.0	—	6.0	—	8.0
II	500	F	50	—	4.0	4.0	2.0	10.0
III	0 (control)	F	50	—	—	—	2.0	2.0

[a] CA: cancer.
[b] SA: sarcoma.

(all grossly detected), which are rarely observed in the historical controls. These tumors seem to arise from the nerves related to the *ganglia cervicalia.*

Leaded Gasoline

An increase of total malignant tumors was found among females treated at both doses, particularly with the lower one; in males an increase was observed only among the animals treated with the lower dose (TABLE 8). An increase of mammary cancers was found in the females treated with both doses, but was not dose related (TABLE 9). A slight dose-related increase of head cancers was detected among treated males (TABLE 10). A sharp increase of malignant uterine-vaginal tumors (including neurinosarcomas) was found in the females treated with the lower dose (TABLE 11).

Gasoil (Diesel)

A non-dose-related increase of total malignant tumors was found among treated males and females (TABLE 12). The treatment did not affect the incidence of female mammary cancers (TABLE 13). An increase in the incidence of head cancer in males was observed in the group treated with the lower dose (TABLE 14). A sharp, dose-related increase of malignant uterine-vaginal tumors (including neurinosarcomas) was found in treated females (TABLE 15).

Kerosene

A dose-related increase of total malignant tumors was observed in treated females and, to a lesser extent, in males exposed to the higher dose (TABLE 16). Mammary cancers and head cancers appeared to be increased among females exposed to the higher dose (TABLES 17 and 18). An increased incidence, not dose-related, of malignant uterine-vaginal tumors (including neurinosarcomas) was found among treated females (TABLE 19).

Toluene

There was a non-dose-related increase of the total malignant tumors among males and females treated with both doses (TABLE 20); of mammary cancers in females-treated with the lower dose (TABLE 21); of head cancers among males treated with the higher dose and, to a lesser extent, in females treated with the lower dose (TABLE 22); and of lymphomas and leukemias among males treated with the higher dose and among females treated with both doses (not dose related) (TABLE 23).

Xylenes

A non-dose-related increase of total malignant tumors was found in males and females treated with both doses (TABLE 24). An increase of mammary cancers was

TABLE 8. Results of Long-term Carcinogenicity Bioassays of Leaded Gasoline with a High Content of Aromatics, Administered by Gavage to Sprague-Dawley Rats: Total Tumors

Group No.	Dose (mg/kg b.w.)	Animals		% of Animals Bearing Tumors		No. of Malignant Tumors per 100 Animals
		Sex	No.	TBMT[a]	MT[b]	
I	800	M	50	38.0	18.0	24.0
		F	50	62.0	34.0	42.0
		M + F	100	50.0	26.0	33.0
II	500	M	50	70.0	34.0	42.0
		F	50	68.0	44.0	60.0
		M + F	100	69.0	39.0	51.0
III	0 (control)	M	50	54.0	24.0	26.0
		F	50	70.0	22.0	22.0
		M + F	100	62.0	23.0	24.0

[a] TBMT: total benign and malignant tumors.
[b] MT: malignant tumors.

TABLE 9. Results of Long-term Carcinogenicity Bioassays of Leaded Gasoline with a High Content of Aromatics, Administered by Gavage to Sprague-Dawley Rats: Mammary Cancers

Group No.	Dose (mg/kg b.w.)	Animals Sex	Animals No.	% of Animals Bearing Cancers
I	800	F	50	12.0
II	500	F	50	16.0
III	0 (control)	F	50	6.0

observed among females treated with the lower dose (TABLE 25). There was a non-dose-related increase of head cancers and of lymphomas and leukemias among males and females treated with both doses (TABLES 26 and 27).

Ethylbenzene

A non-dose-related increase of total malignant tumors was found in males and females treated with both doses (TABLE 28). An increase of head cancers was observed among males and females treated at the higher dose (TABLE 29).

1,2,4-Trimethylbenzene

A slight increase of total malignant tumors was found among treated males and females (TABLE 30). An increase of the incidence of head cancers was observed among the treated males (TABLE 31).

CONCLUSIONS

The results indicate that, although to a varying extent, all the tested materials appear to be carcinogenic (TABLE 32). An increase of total malignant tumors and of head cancers was found among animals treated with all fuels and aromatics, in males and/or in females. An increase of mammary cancers was observed in females treated with tested gasoline, kerosene, toluene, and xylenes. Malignant tumors of the uterus and vagina showed an increase in the animals treated with all types of the tested fuels. Lymphomas and leukemias were increased among males and females treated with toluene and xylenes.

In several instances no dose-response relationship has been observed. These results may be due, among other experimental factors (low number of animals per group; the fact that, in the case of the aromatics, the two doses were tested with two different experiments; in some cases the different length of the biophase of the

TABLE 10. Results of Long-term Carcinogenicity Bioassays of Leaded Gasoline with a High Content of Aromatics, Administered by Gavage to Sprague-Dawley Rats: Head Cancers

		Animals		% of Animals Bearing Cancers					
Group No.	Dose (mg/kg b.w.)	Sex	No.	Zymbal Gland CA[a]	Ear Duct CA	Nasal Cavities CA	Oral Cavity CA	Head SA[b]	Total
I	800	M	50	2.0	2.0	—	—	2.0[c]	6.0
		F	50	2.0	—	—	—	4.0[c]	6.0
		M + F	100	2.0	1.0	—	—	3.0	6.0
II	500	M	50	—	—	2.0	2.0	—	4.0
		F	50	2.0	—	—	—	2.0[c]	4.0
		M + F	100	1.0	—	1.0	1.0	1.0	4.0
III	0 (control)	M	50	2.0	—	—	—	—	2.0
		F	50	2.0	2.0	—	2.0	—	6.0
		M + F	100	2.0	1.0	—	1.0	—	4.0

[a] CA: cancer.
[b] SA: sarcoma.
[c] Osteosarcoma.

TABLE 11. Results of Long-term Carcinogenicity Bioassays of Leaded Gasoline with a High Content of Aromatics, Administered by Gavage to Sprague-Dawley Rats: Malignant Tumors of Uterus and Vagina

Group No.	Dose (mg/kg b.w.)	Animals		% of Animals Bearing Malignant Tumors				
		Sex	No.	Uterus CA[a]	Vagina CA	Uterus-Vagina Neurino SA[b]	Uterus: Other SA	Total
I	800	F	50	4.0	—	—	—	4.0
II	500	F	50	12.0	4.0	4.0	—	20.0
III	0 (control)	F	50	—	—	—	2.0	2.0

[a] CA: cancer.
[b] SA: sarcoma.

TABLE 12. Results of Long-term Carcinogenicity Bioassays of Gasoil (Diesel) Administered by Gavage to Sprague-Dawley Rats: Total Tumors

Group No.	Dose (mg/kg b.w.)	Animals		% of Animals Bearing Tumors		No. of Malignant Tumors per 100 Animals
		Sex	No.	TBMT[a]	MT[b]	
I	800	M	50	56.0	32.0	38.0
		F	50	58.0	42.0	56.0
		M + F	100	57.0	37.0	47.0
II	500	M	50	72.0	48.0	56.0
		F	50	70.0	38.0	50.0
		M + F	100	71.0	43.0	53.0
III	0 (control)	M	50	54.0	24.0	26.0
		F	50	70.0	22.0	22.0
		M + F	100	62.0	23.0	24.0

[a] TBMT: total benign and malignant tumors.
[b] MT: malignant tumors.

TABLE 13. Results of Long-term Carcinogenicity Bioassays of Gasoil (Diesel) Administered by Gavage to Sprague-Dawley Rats: Mammary Cancers

Group No.	Dose (mg/kg b.w.)	Animals: Sex	Animals: No.	% of Animals Bearing Cancers
I	800	F	50	4.0
II	500	F	50	6.0
III	0 (control)	F	50	6.0

experiments testing two doses of the same compound), mainly to the higher toxicity of the higher tested doses.

The carcinogenicity of the fuels is also supported by the observation of neurinosarcomas of the uterus-vagina in treated animals; and the carcinogenicity of ethylbenzene and 1,2,4-trimethylbenzene is supported by the observation in treated males and females of neuroesthesioepitheliomas. These two tumors are, in fact, quite rare in the colony of Sprague-Dawley rats used for these experiments.

The fact that the experimental study performed by NTP on toluene and xylenes gave negative results[8–11] may be due to the different experimental conditions in which these compounds were tested, and particularly to the fact that in those bioassays the experiments were truncated after 104 weeks.

Since the experiments were performed in a standardized way, our data allow us to rank the relative carcinogenic potency of toluene, xylenes, and ethylbenzene using the results obtained with a lower dose, which does not noticeably affect the survival rate; and also to compare the carcinogenic potential of these aromatics with that of benzene, which was also tested in the same experimental conditions in our laboratories (TABLE 33). It must be stressed that benzene causes the onset of a wider range of different cancers (TABLE 34).

Our results call for further research to better assess the level of carcinogenicity potential of the tested compounds and also for preventive measures.

SUMMARY

Unleaded gasoline, with high aromatic content, leaded gasoline, gasoil (diesel), kerosene, toluene, xylenes, ethylbenzene, and 1,2,4-trimethyl-benzene were submitted to long-term experimental carcinogenicity bioassays. The mixtures and the compounds were administered by stomach tube, in olive oil, once daily, 4 days weekly, for 104 weeks, to male and female Sprague-Dawley rats. The animals were kept under control until the end of the experiments. With varying degrees of evidence, all the tested materials were found to increase the total number of malignant tumors and of some site-specific tumors. They must therefore be considered carcinogenic. On the basis of our results the rank of carcinogenic potency of the tested aromatic hydrocarbons increases in the following order: 1,2,4-trimethylbenzene, ethylbenzene, xylenes, toluene (benzene).

TABLE 14. Results of Long-term Carcinogenicity Bioassays of Gasoil (Diesel) Administered by Gavage to Sprague-Dawley Rats: Head Cancers

		Animals		% of Animals Bearing Cancers					
Group No.	Dose (mg/kg b.w.)	Sex	No.	Zymbal Gland CA[a]	Ear Duct CA	Nasal Cavities CA	Oral Cavity CA	Head SA[b]	Total
I	800	M	50	2.0	2.0	—	—	—	4.0
		F	50	—	2.0	—	2.0	—	4.0
		M + F	100	1.0	2.0	—	1.0	—	4.0
II	500	M	50	—	4.0	—	4.0	—	8.0
		F	50	—	—	—	2.0	—	2.0
		M + F	100	—	2.0	—	3.0	—	5.0
III	0	M	50	2.0	—	—	—	—	2.0
	(control)	F	50	2.0	2.0	—	2.0	—	6.0
		M + F	100	2.0	1.0	—	1.0	—	4.0

[a] CA: cancer.
[b] SA: sarcoma.

TABLE 15. Results of Long-term Carcinogenicity Bioassays of Gasoil (Diesel) Administered by Gavage to Sprague-Dawley Rats: Malignant Tumors of Uterus and Vagina

		Animals		% of Animals Bearing Malignant Tumors[a]				
Group No.	Dose (mg/kg b.w.)	Sex	No.	Uterus CA[a]	Vagina CA	Uterus-Vagina Neurino SA[b]	Uterus: Other SA	Total
I	800	F	50	18.0	—	8.0	—	26.0
II	500	F	50	6.0	—	6.0	—	12.0
III	0 (control)	F	50	—	—	—	2.0	2.0

[a] CA: cancer.
[b] SA: sarcoma.

TABLE 16. Results of Long-term Carcinogenicity Bioassays of Kerosene Administered by Gavage to Sprague-Dawley Rats: Total Tumors

Group No.	Dose (mg/kg b.w.)	Animals		% of Animals Bearing Tumors		No. of Malignant Tumors per 100 Animals
		Sex	No.	TBMT[a]	MT[b]	
I	800	M	50	60.0	32.0	36.0
		F	50	72.0	40.0	50.0
		M + F	100	66.0	36.0	43.0
II	500	M	50	56.0	24.0	28.0
		F	50	68.0	26.0	40.0
		M + F	100	62.0	25.0	34.0
III	0 (control)	M	50	54.0	24.0	26.0
		F	50	70.0	22.0	22.0
		M + F	100	62.0	23.0	24.0

[a] TBMT: total benign and malignant tumors.
[b] MT: malignant tumors.

TABLE 17. Results of Long-term Carcinogenicity Bioassays of Kerosene Administered by Gavage to Sprague-Dawley Rats: Mammary Cancers

Group No.	Dose (mg/kg b.w.)	Animals		% of Animals Bearing Cancers
		Sex	No.	
I	800	F	50	10.0
II	500	F	50	6.0
III	0 (control)	F	50	6.0

TABLE 18. Results of Long-term Carcinogenicity Bioassays of Kerosene Administered by Gavage to Sprague-Dawley Rats: Head Cancers

		Animals		% of Animals Bearing Cancers					
Group No.	Dose (mg/kg b.w.)	Sex	No.	Zymbal Gland CA[a]	Ear Duct CA	Nasal Cavities CA	Oral Cavity CA	Head SA[b]	Total
I	800	M	50	—	2.0	—	—	—	2.0
		F	50	—	2.0	2.0	4.0	2.0[c]	10.0
		M + F	100	—	2.0	1.0	2.0	1.0	6.0
II	500	M	50	—	2.0	—	2.0	2.0[c]	6.0
		F	50	—	2.0	—	2.0	—	4.0
		M + F	100	—	2.0	—	2.0	1.0	5.0
III	0 (control)	M	50	2.0	—	—	—	—	2.0
		F	50	2.0	2.0	—	2.0	—	6.0
		M + F	100	2.0	1.0	—	1.0	—	4.0

[a] CA: cancer.
[b] SA: sarcoma.
[c] Osteosarcoma.

TABLE 19. Results of Long-term Carcinogenicity Bioassays of Kerosene Administered by Gavage to Sprague-Dawley Rats: Malignant Tumors of Uterus and Vagina

Group No.	Dose (mg/kg b.w.)	Animals		% of Animals Bearing Malignant Tumors				
		Sex	No.	Uterus CA[a]	Vagina CA	Uterus-Vagina Neurino SA[b]	Uterus: Other SA	Total
I	800	F	50	2.0	—	8.0	—	10.0
II	500	F	50	4.0	6.0	2.0	2.0	14.0
III	0 (control)	F	50	—	—	—	2.0	2.0

[a] CA: cancer.
[b] SA: sarcoma.

TABLE 20. Results of Long-term Carcinogenicity Bioassays of Toluene Administered by Gavage to Sprague-Dawley Rats: Total Tumors

Group No.	Dose (mg/kg b.w.)	Animals: Sex	Animals: No.	% of Animals Bearing Tumors: TBMT[a]	% of Animals Bearing Tumors: MT[b]	No. of Malignant Tumors per 100 Animals
I	800	M	50	60.0	40.0	42.0
		F	50	58.0	30.0	46.0
		M + F	100	59.0	35.0	44.0
II	0 (control)	M	50	54.0	24.0	26.0
		F	50	70.0	22.0	22.0
		M + F	100	62.0	23.0	24.0
I	500	M	40	77.5	45.0	57.5
		F	40	90.0	52.5	80.0
		M + F	80	83.8	48.8	68.8
II	0 (control)	M	50	58.0	24.0	24.0
		F	50	60.0	20.0	22.0
		M + F	100	59.0	22.0	23.0

[a] TBMT: total benign and malignant tumors.
[b] MT: malignant tumors.

TABLE 21. Results of Long-term Carcinogenicity Bioassays of Toluene Administered by Gavage to Sprague-Dawley Rats: Mammary Cancers

Group No.	Dose (mg/kg b.w.)	Animals: Sex	Animals: No.	% of Animals Bearing Cancers
I	800	F	50	6.0
II	0 (control)	F	50	6.0
I	500	F	40	25.0
II	0 (control)	F	50	14.0

TABLE 22. Results of Long-term Carcinogenicity Bioassays of Toluene Administered by Gavage to Sprague-Dawley Rats: Head Cancers

Group No.	Dose (mg/kg b.w.)	Animals: Sex	Animals: No.	% of Animals Bearing Cancers: Zymbal Gland CA[a]	Ear Duct CA	Nasal Cavities CA	Oral Cavity CA	Total
I	800	M	50	—	2.0	2.0	14.0	18.0
		F	50	—	—	—	6.0	6.0
		M + F	100	—	1.0	1.0	10.0	12.0
II	0 (control)	M	50	2.0	—	—	—	2.0
		F	50	2.0	2.0	—	2.0	6.0
		M + F	100	2.0	1.0	—	1.0	4.0
I	500	M	40	2.5	—	—	—	2.5
		F	40	—	—	2.5	2.5	5.0
		M + F	80	1.3	—	1.3	1.3	3.8
II	0 (control)	M	50	2.0	—	—	—	2.0
		F	50	—	—	—	—	—
		M + F	100	1.0	—	—	—	1.0

[a] CA: cancer.

TABLE 23. Results of Long-term Carcinogenicity Bioassays of Toluene Administered by Gavage to Sprague-Dawley Rats: Lymphomas and Leukemias

Group No.	Dose (mg/kg b.w.)	Animals: Sex	Animals: No.	% of Animals Bearing Lymphomas and Leukemias
I	800	M	50	16.0
		F	50	10.0
		M + F	100	13.0
II	0 (control)	M	50	10.0
		F	50	6.0
		M + F	100	8.0
I	500	M	40	7.5
		F	40	17.5
		M + F	80	12.5
II	0 (control)	M	50	6.0
		F	50	2.0
		M + F	100	4.0

TABLE 24. Results of Long-term Carcinogenicity Bioassays of Xylenes Administered by Gavage to Sprague-Dawley Rats: Total Tumors

Group No.	Dose (mg/kg b.w.)	Animals		% of Animals Bearing Tumors		No. of Malignant Tumors per 100 Animals
		Sex	No.	TBMT[a]	MT[b]	
I	800	M	50	58.0	38.0	44.0
		F	50	62.0	36.0	48.0
		M + F	100	60.0	37.0	46.0
II	0 (control)	M	50	54.0	24.0	26.0
		F	50	70.0	22.0	22.0
		M + F	100	62.0	23.0	24.0
I	500	M	40	57.5	35.0	45.0
		F	40	85.0	57.5	65.0
		M + F	80	71.3	46.3	55.0
II	0 (control)	M	50	58.0	24.0	24.0
		F	50	60.0	20.0	22.0
		M + F	100	59.0	22.0	23.0

[a] TBMT: total benign and malignant tumors.
[b] MT: malignant tumors.

TABLE 25. Results of Long-term Carcinogenicity Bioassays of Xylenes Administered by Gavage to Sprague-Dawley Rats: Mammary Cancers

Group No.	Dose (mg/kg b.w.)	Animals		% of Animals Bearing Cancers
		Sex	No.	
I	800	F	50	2.0
II	0 (control)	F	50	6.0
I	500	F	40	27.5
II	0 (control)	F	50	14.0

TABLE 26. Results of Long-term Carcinogenicity Bioassays of Xylenes Administered by Gavage to Sprague-Dawley Rats: Head Cancers

Group No.	Dose (mg/kg b.w.)	Animals		% of Animals Bearing Cancers				
		Sex	No.	Zymbal Gland CA[a]	Ear Duct CA	Nasal Cavities CA	Oral Cavity CA	Total
I	800	M	50	2.0	2.0	—	8.0	12.0
		F	50	—	4.0	—	8.0	12.0
		M + F	100	1.0	3.0	—	8.0	12.0
II	0 (control)	M	50	2.0	—	—	—	2.0
		F	50	2.0	2.0	—	2.0	6.0
		M + F	100	2.0	1.0	—	1.0	4.0
I	500	M	40	2.5	—	—	5.0	7.5
		F	40	—	—	—	10.0	10.0
		M + F	80	1.3	—	—	7.5	8.8
II	0 (control)	M	50	2.0	—	—	—	2.0
		F	50	—	—	—	—	—
		M + F	100	1.0	—	—	—	1.0

[a] CA: cancer.

TABLE 27. Results of Long-term Carcinogenicity Bioassays of Xylenes Administered by Gavage to Sprague-Dawley Rats: Lymphomas and Leukemias

Group No.	Dose (mg/kg b.w.)	Animals: Sex	Animals: No.	% of Animals Bearing Lymphomas and Leukemias
I	800	M	50	14.0
		F	50	14.0
		M + F	100	14.0
II	0 (control)	M	50	10.0
		F	50	6.0
		M + F	100	8.0
I	500	M	40	12.5
		F	40	7.5
		M + F	80	10.0
II	0 (control)	M	50	6.0
		F	50	2.0
		M + F	100	4.0

TABLE 28. Results of Long-term Carcinogenicity Bioassays of Ethylbenzene Administered by Gavage to Sprague-Dawley Rats: Total Tumors

Group No.	Dose (mg/kg b.w.)	Animals		% of Animals Bearing Tumors		No. of Malignant Tumors per 100 Animals
		Sex	No.	TBMT[a]	MT[b]	
I	800	M	50	44.0	24.0	36.0
		F	50	60.0	38.0	48.0
		M + F	100	52.0	31.0	42.0
II	0 (control)	M	50	54.0	24.0	26.0
		F	50	70.0	22.0	22.0
		M + F	100	62.0	23.0	24.0
I	500	M	40	67.5	35.0	35.0
		F	40	75.0	35.0	42.5
		M + F	80	71.3	35.0	38.8
II	0 (control)	M	50	58.0	24.0	24.0
		F	50	60.0	20.0	22.0
		M + F	100	59.0	22.0	23.0

[a] TBMT: total benign and malignant tumors.
[b] MT: malignant tumors.

TABLE 29. Results of Long-term Carcinogenicity Bioassays of Ethylbenzene Administered by Gavage to Sprague-Dawley Rats: Head Cancers

Group No.	Dose (mg/kg b.w.)	Animals		% of Animals Bearing Cancers					
		Sex	No.	Zymbal Gland CA[a]	Ear Duct CA	Nasal Cavities CA	Nasal Cavities NEP[b]	Oral Cavity CA	Total
I	800	M	50	—	2.0	—	6.0	2.0	10.0
		F	50	2.0	2.0	2.0	2.0	6.0	14.0
		M + F	100	1.0	2.0	1.0	4.0	4.0	12.0
II	0 (control)	M	50	2.0	—	—	—	—	2.0
		F	50	2.0	2.0	—	—	2.0	6.0
		M + F	100	2.0	1.0	—	—	1.0	4.0
I	500	M	40	—	—	—	—	—	—
		F	40	2.5	—	—	—	—	2.5
		M + F	80	1.3	—	—	—	—	1.3
II	0 (control)	M	50	2.0	—	—	—	—	2.0
		F	50	—	—	—	—	—	—
		M + F	100	1.0	—	—	—	—	1.0

[a] CA: cancer.
[b] NEP: neuroesthesioepitheliomas.

TABLE 30. Results of Long-term Carcinogenicity Bioassays of 1,2,4-Trimethylbenzene Administered by Gavage to Sprague-Dawley Rats: Total Tumors

Group No.	Dose (mg/kg b.w.)	Animals		% of Animals Bearing Tumors		No. of Malignant Tumors per 100 Animals
		Sex	No.	TBMT[a]	MT[b]	
I	800	M	50	62.0	26.0	34.0
		F	50	66.0	24.0	32.0
		M + F	100	64.0	25.0	33.0
II	0 (control)	M	50	54.0	24.0	26.0
		F	50	70.0	22.0	22.0
		M + F	100	62.0	23.0	24.0

[a] TBMT: total benign and malignant tumors.
[b] MT: malignant tumors.

TABLE 31. Results of Long-term Carcinogenicity Bioassays of 1,2,4-Trimethylbenzene Administered by Gavage to Sprague-Dawley Rats: Head Cancers

		Animals		% of Animals Bearing Cancers					
						Nasal Cavities			
Group No.	Dose (mg/kg b.w.)	Sex	No.	Zymbal Gland CA[a]	Ear Duct CA	CA	NEP[b]	Oral Cavity CA	Total
I	800	M	50	4.0	2.0	—	2.0	2.0	10.0
		F	50	2.0	—	—	4.0	—	6.0
		M + F	100	3.0	1.0	—	3.0	1.0	8.0
II	0 (control)	M	50	2.0	—	—	—	—	2.0
		F	50	2.0	2.0	—	—	2.0	6.0
		M + F	100	2.0	1.0	—	—	1.0	4.0

[a] CA: cancer.
[b] NEP: neuroesthesioepitheliomas.

TABLE 32. Tumors in Which an Increase Was Observed Following Treatment with the Tested Fuels and Aromatics

		Increased Tumors							
		Total Malignant Tumors		Mammary Cancers	Head Cancers		Uterus-Vagina Malignant Tumors	Lymphomas and Leukemias	
Test Compound	Daily Dose (mg/kg b.w.)	M	F	F	M	F	F	M	F
Unleaded gasoline with high content of aromatics	800	+	+	+DR[a]	+		+		
	500		+	+			+		
Leaded gasoline	800		+	+	+DR				
	500	+	+	+	+		+		
Gasoil (diesel)	800	+	+				+DR		
	500	+	+		+		+		
Kerosene	800	+	+DR	+		+	+		
	500		+				+		
Toluene	800	+	+		+			+	+
	500	+	+	+		+			+
Xylenes	800	+	+		+	+		+	+
	500	+	+	+	+	+		+	+
Ethylbenzene	800	+	+		+	+			
	500	+	+						
1,2,4-Trimethylbenzene	800	+	+		+				

[a] DR: dose related.

TABLE 33. Long-term Carcinogenicity Bioassays of Benzene, Toluene, Xylenes, and Ethylbenzene Administered at 500 mg/kg b.w.: Comparative Results

Test Compound	Total Malignant Tumors/ 100 Animals (M + F)	Carcinogenicity Index[a]
Benzene[b]	160.8	6.56
Toluene	68.8	2.81
Xylenes	56.4	2.30
Ethylbenzene	40.3	1.64
Olive oil alone (control)	24.5	1.00

[a] Ratio between observed and expected total malignant tumors.
[b] See Reference 4.

TABLE 34. Tumors Associated with Benzene Exposure on the Basis of the Experimental Project of the Cancer Research Center of the European Ramazzini Foundation of Oncology and Environmental Sciences[a]

	Animals/Route of Administration				
	Sprague-Dawley Rat		Wistar Rat	Swiss Mouse	RF/J Mouse
Tumors	Ingestion	Inhalation	Ingestion	Ingestion	Ingestion
Total malignant tumors	+	+	+	+	+
Carcinomas of Zymbal gland	+	+	+	+	
Carcinomas of oral cavity	+	+	+		
Carcinomas of nasal cavities	+	(+)	+		
Carcinomas of the skin	+				
Carcinomas of the forestomach	+				
Carcinomas of the mammary gland	(+)	(+)		+	+
Hepatomas	(+)	(+)			
Angiosarcomas of the liver	+				
Hemolymphoreticular neoplasias	(+)				+
Tumors of the lung				+	+

[a] See Reference 4.

REFERENCES

1. Maltoni, C. & C. Scarnato. 1977. Le prime prove sperimentali dell'azione cancerogena del benzene. Osp. Vita **4:** 111–113.
2. Maltoni, C. & C. Scarnato. 1979. First experimental demonstration of the carcinogenic effects of benzene. Long-term bioassays on Sprague-Dawley rats by oral administration. Med. Lav. **70:** 352–357.
3. Maltoni, C., B. Conti & G. Cotti. 1983. Benzene: A multipotential carcinogen. Results of long-term bioassays performed at the Bologna Institute of Oncology. Am. J. Ind. Med. **4:** 589–630.
4. Maltoni, C., B. Conti, G. Cotti *et al.* 1985. Experimental studies on benzene carcinogenicity at the Bologna Institute of Oncology: Current results and ongoing research. Am. J. Ind. Med. **7:** 415–446.
5. Huff, J. E. 1986. Toxicology and carcinogenesis studies of benzene (CAS No. 71-43-2) in F344/N rats and B6C3F1 mice (gavage studies). Technical Report No. 289. National Toxicology Program. US Department of Health and Human Services. Washington, DC.
6. Maltoni, C., A. Ciliberti, G. Cotti *et al.* 1989. Benzene, an experimental multipotential carcinogen: Results of the long-term bioassays performed at the Bologna Institute of Oncology. Environ. Health Perspect. **82:** 109–124.
7. Kitchen, D. N. 1984. Neoplastic renal effects of unleaded gasoline in Fischer 344 rats. *In* Advances in Modern Environmental Toxicology, Renal Effects of Petroleum Hydrocarbons, Vol. VII. M. A. Mehlman, G. P. Hemstreet III, J. J. Thrope & N. K. Weaver, Eds.: 65–72. Princeton Scientific Publishers. Princeton, NJ.
8. International Agency for Research on Cancer. 1989. Monographs on the evaluation of carcinogenic risks to humans, Vol. 47. Some organic solvents, resin monomers and related compounds, pigments and occupational exposure in paint manufacture. IARC. Lyon.
9. National Toxicology Program. 1990. Toxicology and carcinogenesis studies of toluene (CAS No. 108-88-3) in F344/N rats and B6C3F1 mice (inhalation studies). NTP TR 371, NIH Publ. No. 90-2826. US Department of Health and Human Services. Research Triangle Park, NC.
10. National Toxicology Program. 1986. Toxicology and carcinogenesis studies of xylenes (mixed) (60% m-xylene, 14% p-xylene, 9% o-xylene, and 17% ethylbenzene) (CAS No. 1330-20-7) in F344/N rats and B6C3F1 mice (gavage studies). NTP TR 327, NIH Publ. No. 87-2583. US Department of Health and Human Services. Research Triangle Park, NC.
11. Huff, J. E., W. Eastin, J. Roycroft *et al.* 1988. Carcinogenesis studies of benzene, methylbenzene, and dimethylbenzenes. Ann. N.Y. Acad. Sci. **534:** 427–440.

Carcinogenicity of Gasoline: A Review of Epidemiological Evidence

JOHN M. DEMENT,[a] LISA HENSLEY, AND AMY GITELMAN

Duke University Medical Center
Department of Community and Family Medicine
Division of Occupational and Environmental Medicine
Box 3834
Durham, North Carolina 27710

INTRODUCTION

In 1989, the United States used approximately 140 billion gallons of gasoline.[1] The United States consumes approximately 310 million gallons of gasoline daily.[2] This large volume of production and use results in widespread occupational and nonoccupational exposure to gasoline and its components.

Gasoline (CAS # 8006-61-9) is a complex mixture of volatile hydrocarbons containing as many as 1,000 chemical substances, with substantial variation depending on the source of crude oil, refinery process, geographic region, season, performance requirements (octane rating), and blending of stock.[1] The hydrocarbon content of gasoline is approximately 63% alkanes, 9% alkenes, and 28% aromatics on a volume basis.[3] The alkanes contain hydrocarbon chains ranging from C4 to C12,[4] and the aromatic hydrocarbon groups include several carcinogenic chemicals including benzene.[5] TABLE 1 provides a list of the major hydrocarbon classes in gasoline on a percent weight and volume basis.

Gasoline is produced by a series of refining processes beginning with the distillation of crude petroleum into fractions of different boiling ranges. Typical refinery fractions are light naphtha, heavy naphtha, kerosene, light gas oil, heavy gas oil, and reduced crude, with unleaded gasoline being largely blended from the naphtha fractions.[2] Gasoline, a middle distillate of petroleum, contains more than 150 hydrocarbons with a boiling range of approximately 40 to 180 degrees centigrade.[5] Catalytic cracking, coking, alkylation, and catalytic reforming are used to modify gasoline to required specifications.[1,2]

Some important toxic constituents of gasoline include benzene, 1,3 butadiene, 1,2 dibromoethane (a lead scavenger additive), toluene, ethyl benzene, and the antiknock agents, tetraethyllead and tetramethyllead. Benzene constitutes up to 4% of gasoline by weight.[6] Leaded gasoline has been phased out in the United States and many other parts of the world. The gasoline additive, MTBE (methyl-tertiary-butyl ether), an oxygenator added to gasoline during the winter months to reduce carbon monoxide

[a] Phone: 919/286-3232; fax: 919/286-1021. e-mail: demen001@mc.duke.edu

TABLE 1. Automotive Gasoline Composition by Hydrocarbon Class[a]

Hydrocarbon	Range
Alkanes	4-8 wt %
Alkenes	2-5 wt %
Isoalkanes	25-40 wt %
Cycloalkanes	3-7 wt %
Cycloalkenes	1-4 wt %
Total aromatics	20-50 wt %
Benzene	0.5-2.5 wt %
Paraffins (naphthenes)	30-90 vol %
Olefins	0-30 vol %
Aromatics	10-50 vol %

[a] Source: IARC, 1989.[6]

pollution from motor vehicles, is a possible carcinogen.[7,8] MTBE typically constitutes up to 4% of gasoline by weight; however, some metropolitan areas (e.g., Phoenix, Arizona; Denver, Colorado) have seasonal requirements to use 12-15% MTBE.[6,7]

The Occupational Health and Safety Administration (OSHA), the American Conference of Governmental Industrial Hygienists (ACGIH), and the National Institute for Occupational Safety and Health (NIOSH) have established occupational exposure limits for gasoline and several of its constituents. TABLE 2 contains a listing of time-weighted average exposure limits (TWA), short-term exposure limits (STEL), and ceiling limits established by OSHA, ACGIH, and NIOSH for gasoline and components.[9] Neither the OSHA permissible exposure limit (PEL) for gasoline nor the ACGIH threshold limit value (TLV) are based on consideration of gasoline's carcinogenicity. The National Toxicology Program (NTP) classifies benzene as a known human carcinogen and 1,3 butadiene and 1,2 dibromoethane as substances reasonably anticipated to be carcinogens.[10] Gasoline is classified by the International Agency for Research on Cancer (IARC) as possibly carcinogenic in humans (Group 2B).[6] The Environmental Protection Agency (EPA) has also classified gasoline as a probable human carcinogen based on sufficient animal evidence and inadequate epidemiological evidence.[1]

OCCUPATIONAL EXPOSURE TO GASOLINE

Once gasoline is produced at a refinery, it is distributed through a series of transport and storage pathways. Gasoline is transported by barge, pipeline, tanker, and tank truck and is stored first at the refinery, and then at bulk terminals, bulk plants, and service stations. A bulk terminal serves as a primary distribution center for petroleum products.[11]

Each time gasoline is loaded or unloaded, gasoline vapors are released into the atmosphere. Three types of "loading" are used: top loading, bottom loading and off loading. During top loading, petroleum products are loaded into a tank truck through

TABLE 2. OSHA, ACGIH, and NIOSH Exposure Limits for Gasoline and Some of Its Constituents

	TWA			STEL/Ceiling		
Substance	OSHA[a] mg/m^3	ACGIH[b] mg/m^3	NIOSH[c] mg/m^3	OSHA mg/m^3	ACGIH mg/m^3	NIOSH mg/m^3
Gasoline	none (900)	890	Ca: lowest feasible concentration	none (1500)	1480	–
Partial List of Gasoline Components						
Benzene	3.25	32, A2; 0.96, A1 proposed	0.32	16	–	3.2
1,3 Butadiene	2200	4.4, A2	Ca: lowest feasible concentration			–
1,2 Dibromoethane	none	A2	–			–
Methyl-tert butyl ether	none	144, A3	–	–	–	–
Toluene	753 (375)	188	375	1130 (560)	–	560
Xylene	435	434	435	(655)	651	435
Ethyl benzene	435	434	435	(545)	543	545
n-Hexane	1800 (180)	176	180	–	–	–
Naphthalene	50	52	50	(75)	79	75

[a] OSHA values presented in parentheses ( ) are vacated 1989 OSHA PELs.
[b] ACGIH carcinogen classifications:
A1 = Human carcinogen
A2 = Suspected human carcinogen
A3 = Animal carcinogen.
[c] Ca = NIOSH potential occupational carcinogen.

a hatch at the top of the truck using a pipe or loading arm resulting in hydrocarbon vapor release from the hatch opening. Bottom loading involves pumping petroleum products into a tank using a loading arm that is connected to the bottom of the tank truck and typically results in less hydrocarbon release than top loading. During off loading, petroleum products are unloaded from a tank truck into a storage tank using a hose.[11]

The EPA has instituted the use of vapor controls to reduce gasoline vapor emissions and to protect human health and the environment.[1] The EPA estimated that at least 40% of gasoline vapor emissions occurred at retail service stations in 1982.[1] Stage 1 controls collect and recover gasoline vapors released when gasoline is transferred from a barge, pipeline, or tanker to a bulk terminal or when gasoline is transferred from a bulk terminal to a tank truck. Stage 2 controls collect and recover gasoline

TABLE 3. Service Station Attendants' Occupational Exposure to Gasoline[a]

Occupation	Exposure and Sampling Duration	Concentration (mg/m³)[b] Total Hydrocarbons, Range; Mean	Benzene, Range; Mean	Reference
Service station attendants (Western Europe)	8 h	7.9-101; 29.3	ND-1.3; 0.35	IARC, 1989[6]
Service station attendants (UK)	3.5-14 h		0.96-7.7	Parkinson, 1971[49]
Service station attendants (USA)	7-8 h	12.2-106; 94.5	0.65	Rappaport, 1987[12]
		—	0.4	Hartle, 1980[7]
	400 min	1.9-14.3; 4.6	—	Kearney, 1986[50]
		1.2-336.6; 28.4[c]	<0.03-6.6; 0.3[c]	McDermott, 1979[51]
	8 h	1.1-130.3; 4.0[d]	0.0-4.2; 0.7[d]	Halder, 1986[52]
Self-service customer	0.5-2 min	—	0.5	Ellis, 1984[53]
	avg	11.8-9452.8 w	0.2-55.2 w	Tironi, 1986[54]
		14.7-3592.6 s	0.3-44.9 s	
		68.91	0.73	Bond, 1986[55]
	10 min	3.9-63.5; 12.7		Kearney, 1986[51]
	2 min	48-320; 155.2	1.3-5.8; 3.1	Clayton, 1983[56]
Retail filling station	3-14 h	—	0.6—10.2; 4.4[a]	Parkinson, 1971[49]

[a] Highest overall 8-h TWA concentrations were observed for drum filling (858 mg/m³ total hydrocarbons, 27.2 mg/m3 benzene) and marine loading operations (246-263 mg/m3 total hydrocarbons, 2.3-4.7 mg/m3 benzene), while service station attendants have the lowest exposure levels.[6]

[b] ND = not detected; w = winter, s = summer.

[c] Mean was calculated as follows: (Σ (# of TWA samples per location * mean of TWA samples)) / total # of samples.

[d] Average of geometric means.

vapors released when gasoline is transferred from a tank truck to a service station and when gasoline is pumped from a service station storage tank into a motor vehicle.

Several studies have measured occupational exposures to gasoline vapors (as total hydrocarbons) and its constituents (e.g., benzene, 1,3 butadiene, MTBE) during various phases of gasoline distribution. The highest occupational gasoline exposures typically occur among bulk terminal operators, truck drivers, marine loading operators, and service station attendants according to the petroleum industry.[11] Due to gasoline's chemical complexity, many studies have reported total hydrocarbon concentrations as a substitute for airborne exposure to all compounds in gasoline.[12] This approach provides a general characterization of airborne contaminants, but lacks specificity and ignores differing toxicities among compounds.

TABLES 3, 4, and 5 contain occupational exposure data for service station attendants. Since those exposure data have widely varying sample durations, it is difficult to compare these studies to each other. Process-related variables (type of fuel dispensed,

TABLE 4. Personal Exposures to 1,3 Butadiene Associated with Gasoline[a]

Operation	Exposure and Sampling Duration	Range; Mean mg/m³
Service station attendant (dispensing fuel)	8-h TWA	ND-1.1; 0.3
Self-service station (filling tank)	2-min TWA	ND-10.6; 1.6

[a] Source: IARC, 1989.[6]

TABLE 5. Personal Exposures to MTBE and Benzene Associated with Gasoline

	Concentration (mg/m³)		
Occupation	MTBE Mean; Range	Benzene Mean; Range	Reference
Service station attendants (Phoenix)	1.08; 0.14-13.99	0.16; 0.03-1.66	Hartle, 1993[8]
Service station attendants (Los Angeles; vapor recovery)	0.50; 0.07-2.63	0.19; 0.03-0.61	Hartle, 1993[8]
Automotive mechanics or gasoline pumpers	ND-5.4 using vapor badge	ND-0.176 ug/m³	Mannino, 1995[14]

volume, type of vapor recovery) and environmental variables (temperature, season of the year, ventilation rate, wind speed) affect exposures and limit comparison between studies. Available data show service station attendants' time-weighted average exposures to total hydrocarbons to range from 1.9 mg/m³ to 101 mg/m³ in studies reviewed by IARC;[6] and TWA exposure to benzene ranged from not detected to 7.7 mg/m³. Although most studies reported TWA benzene exposures below OSHA's permissible exposure limit of 3.25 mg/m³ (1 ppm), higher peak exposures have been documented.[13] Compared to other occupations involving gasoline exposure (e.g., drum filling, marine loading operations), service station attendants have lower gasoline exposures.[6]

IARC data on exposure of service station attendants to 1,3 butadiene are given in TABLE 4. Although peak exposures exceed ACGIH exposure limits for 1,3 butadiene, eight-hour time-weighted average exposures were considerably lower. TABLE 5 presents additional data concerning service station attendants' exposure to MTBE

TABLE 6. Personal Exposures to Total Hydrocarbons and Benzene Associated with Gasoline Bulk Loading

Operation and Controls	Exposure and Sampling Duration	Concentration (mg/m^3) Total Hydrocarbons, Range; Mean	Concentration (mg/m^3) Benzene, Range; Mean	Reference
Top loading of road tankers, no vapor recovery				IARC, 1989[6]
Western Europe	<1 h	6.6–3030	ND–60.5	
USA	8 h	9.9–109	0.1–2.3	
Bottom loading of road tankers, no vapor recovery				IARC, 1989[6]
Western Europe	<1 h	8.2–234	ND–5.5	
USA	8 h	21.9–184	0.2–5.9	
Workers on oil product tankers	variable	Total PAH[a] <0.005–288 ug/m^3	<0.01–1.18	Moen, 1995[57]
Rail tanker loading, bottom loading	5–15 min			Nordlinder & Ramnas, 1987[58]
Operator on top of tank			0.2–1.6; 0.7	
Operator on the ground			1.4–10; 4.4	
Road tanker loading	5–15 min			Nordlinder & Ramnas, 1987[58]
Top Loading				
Open terminal building			1.0–13; 4.3	
Closed terminal building			7.0–54; 22.0	
Bottom loading				
Open terminal building			0.5–4.0; 3.0	
Closed terminal building			0.2–24; 6.9	

TABLE 6. Personal Exposures to Total Hydrocarbons and Benzene Associated with Gasoline Bulk Loading (*Continued*)

Operation and Controls	Exposure and Sampling Duration	Concentration (mg/m^3) Total Hydrocarbons, Range; Mean	Benzene, Range; Mean	Reference
Ship loading	5–15 min			Nordlinder & Ramnas, 1987[58]
Manual sounding			19–365; 107	
Crew on deck			2.7–20; 9.6	
Top loading, no vapor recovery	20 min		7.30	Irving, 1979[59]
Bottom loading, no vapor recovery	18 min		3.3	
Bottom loading with vapor recovery	15 min		1.82	
Bottom loading with vapor recovery	8 h	9.4–195.1; 22.4	0.2–8.9; 0.8	Halder, 1986[52]
	8 h	1.3–237.6; 11.3	0.1–2.1; 0.5	
	8 h	17.6–127.0; 37.5	0.2–2.6; 0.7	
Bottom loading, no vapor recovery	8 h	21.9–183.5; 72.6	0.2–5.9; 0.8	
Top loading without vapor recovery	8 h	9.9–109.2; 37.3	0.1–2.3; 0.7	

[a] PAH = polynuclear aromatic hydrocarbons.

TABLE 7. Personal Exposures to 1,3 Butadiene Associated with Gasoline Bulk Loading[a]

Operation	Mean mg/m^3	Range mg/m^3	Exposure Duration
Bulk loading road tankers			
Top loading <1 h	1.4	ND-32.3	<1-h
Top loading >1 h	0.4	ND-4.7	8-h TWA
Bottom loading <1 h	0.2	ND-3.0	<1-h
Bottom loading >1 h	0.4	ND-14.1	8-h TWA
Loading ships			
Closed system	6.4	ND-21.0	8-h TWA
Open system	1.1	ND-4.2	8-h TWA

[a] Source: IARC, 1989.[6]

and benzene.[8,14] In these studies, MTBE and benzene exposures were clearly measurable but generally below established exposure limits.

Exposures to total hydrocarbons and benzene during bulk loading are presented in TABLE 6. Although short-term concentrations were high during bulk loading, lower concentrations were observed over the full working day. Short-term concentrations tended to be higher during top loading than bottom loading. Bulk loading exposures to 1,3 butadiene are presented in TABLE 7. Short-term top loading concentrations were higher than short-term bottom loading concentrations, and 1,3 butadiene exposures for workers during bulk loading are higher than those for service station attendants.

EPIDEMIOLOGY OF GASOLINE-EXPOSED POPULATIONS

Although not shown in every study, refinery worker mortality studies have generally shown increased risks for a number of cancer sites including leukemia, brain, skin, kidney, and the pancreas as well as several other sites. Several reviews of refinery worker epidemiological data have been published.[6,15,16] As the focus of this review is kidney cancer and cancers of the hematopoietic system in relation to exposures to gasoline, general mortality studies of refinery workers are not included for several reasons. First, many of these studies did not analyze mortality by refinery unit, job, and/or exposure and thus did not specifically address health effects of gasoline exposures. Second, there are multiple possible confounding exposures present in the refinery work environment. As a result of these limitations, most studies of refinery populations provide limited information to directly assess the carcinogenicity of gasoline. Also not included in this review are studies that focus on combustion products of gasoline and not the fuel itself.

Kidney and Urothelial Cancers

Several cohort studies have examined the association between exposure to petroleum products and/or gasoline and the risk of kidney cancer. TABLE 8 provides a summary of these studies, and a brief review of each study follows.

A retrospective cohort study examining deaths among 6,672 male petroleum marketing and distribution workers employed for at least one year between 1946 and 1983 (or who were annuitants as of 1946) was conducted by Schnatter *et al.*[17] Based on nine deaths, these investigators found marketing and distribution workers to have a moderately elevated risk of kidney cancer (standardized mortality ratio, SMR = 135; 95% CI = 62-257). When analyses were restricted to only those workers with known hydrocarbon exposure, an increased SMR of 158 (95% CI = 63-325; $n = 7$) was observed. Analyses by exposure frequency (i.e., nonexposed, less than daily exposure, daily exposed) found kidney cancer SMRs of 91, 99, and 208 (95% CI = 67-485; $n = 5$), respectively. For tank-truck drivers with the highest reported exposures in the cohort, a non-statistically significant elevated SMR of 210 was observed. Cancer by latency and by length of employment was also examined by Schnatter *et al.*,[17] with latency defined as the time from the first exposure and length of employment defined as the time from the first date employed in the marketing distribution area. Deaths from kidney cancer appeared to be concentrated in the 20-29 years worked category, with an SMR of 260 occurring in this category.

Schnatter used a Poisson regression model for internal comparisons in an attempt to control for the healthy worker effect and other variables. A model was constructed comparing those exposed daily to those exposed less than daily while controlling for any, some, or all of the following: age, socioeconomic status, the year of hire (pre-/post-1974). An increased relative risk (RR = 3.86) was observed for those exposed to gasoline daily after adjustment for other parameters in the models; however, these relative risks were based on small numbers. The increasing risk of kidney cancer in this study with increasing exposure provides useful information on possible exposure response.

In the study by Schnatter *et al.*, as in many of the occupational studies, the healthy worker effect must be considered in interpretation of the results. An overall significantly reduced SMR of 88 (95% CI = 84-94; $n = 1154$) was observed for all causes of death for the entire study population, and an SMR of 90 (95% CI = 83-96; $n = 767$) for those study members classified as hydrocarbon exposed. While the study has a sizable number of overall deaths, the analyses of kidney cancer mortality is based on only seven deaths with hydrocarbon exposure; this limits the power of the study. In addition, the follow-up period was relatively short, and the cohort under study was relatively young, as is reflected in the small number of overall observed deaths. Also, the authors reported that they were unable to obtain a complete work history for approximately 50% of the cohort, and in some instances only the last job classification was available. Further, the authors reported some inconsistencies in information on the first date of exposure. These inconsistencies and the lack of detailed job histories would result in exposure misclassification, which would likely bias toward the null effect. Finally, it has been reported that workers in the petroleum industry may smoke less than average, resulting in an overestimation of expected kidney cancer deaths and a reduction in the SMR.

TABLE 8A. SMR and PMR Studies of Gasoline-Exposed Worker Populations: Description of Studies

Author	Location	Minimum Employment	Examination Latency	Assessment by Length of Employment	Exposure Assessment
Rushton (1993)[18]	United Kingdom	≥ 1 year	No	No	Exposure assessment based on dates of employment and last or present job.
Schnatter (1993)[17]	Canada	≥ 1 year	No	Yes	Work history information obtained from company computerized database (location, job title, and code for job function).[a]
Wong (1993)[20]	United States	≥ 1 year	Yes	Yes	Exposure assessment through employment records.
Schwartz (1987)[21]	New Hampshire, United States	—	No	No	Occupation and industry information abstracted from death certificates.
Lagorio (1994)[22]	Latium region, Italy	≥ 1 year	No	Yes	Based on length of employment, number of attendants, amount of fuel sold, and the number of fuel deliveries.

[a] Authors report the quality of this information varied from location to location as well as according to the date this database was implemented at these various locations.

TABLE 8B. SMR and PMR Studies of Gasoline-Exposed Worker Populations: Summary of Results

Author	Population Studied	Cohort Size	Number of Deaths	Reference Group(s)	Results
Rushton (1993)[18]	Males employed >1 y at 750 distribution centers 1950–1975, follow up to 1989	22,306	8743	U.K. population	Increased SMR for kidney cancer, leukemia, acute myeloid and acute lymphatic cancer. None statistically significant.
Schnatter (1993)[17]	Males employed > 1 y in marketing/distribution, 1964–1983	6,672	1154	Canadian population	Increased SMR for kidney cancer, leukemia, and multiple myeloma. None statistically significant.
Wong (1993)[20]	Land-based terminal and marine vessel workers employed > 1 y, 1964–1985	18,135	4761	U.S. general population	Overall no excess deaths were observed for kidney cancer, leukemia, or lymphomas. Increased SMR for kidney cancer for both land and marine employees and increased SMR for leukemia and lymphatic cancer in land-based employees employed 10–19 years.[a]
Schwartz (1987)[21]	Male deaths in New Hampshire, 1975–1985	PMR study	587	U.S. general population	PMRs for kidney cancer, leukemia, and lymphatic cancers increased for service station attendants. Leukemia and lymphatic cancers increased for mechanics.
Lagorio (1994)[22]	Service station managers in 1980 and followed in 1992	2,665	270	Regional population in Italy	Study is too small and the follow up too short to provide meaningful data on the carcinogenicity of gasoline.

[a] No trends by latency or employment date.

One of the largest cohort studies focusing on persons involved in either the refinery or petrol industry with potential gasoline exposures was published by Rushton *et al.* (1993) and included more than 8,000 deaths.[18] This study included men employed for one continuous year or more between 1950 and 1975 in eight refineries and approximately 750 distribution centers in the United Kingdom. Only the distribution data was summarized for assessment of workers exposed to gasoline. An increased SMR of 141 (95% CI = 91–208; n = 25) was observed for malignant neoplasms of the kidney among distribution center workers, with an increasing trend in risk with time since first exposure. The mortality among drivers due to neoplasms of the kidney tended to decrease as the year of entry increased and was shown to increase with time since first exposure until 30–39 years since first exposure.

While the Rushton study is of reasonable size and has excellent follow-up, several weaknesses exist. The mortality from all causes of death was significantly lower compared to the national population (SMR 87, 95% CI = 84–90), indicating the presence of a notable healthy worker effect. The SMR was also significantly reduced for all neoplasms (SMR 89, 95% CI = 84–95), reflecting a significant deficit in malignant neoplasms of the lung (SMR 88, 95% CI = 83–94). In addition, only the most recent job title was used for exposure classification. Similar to Schnatter *et al.*, no information was collected or available on lifestyle. Cigarette smoking has been linked to kidney cancer in several studies;[19] therefore, as with the Schnatter study, if the study population smoked less than the comparison population, the expected number of deaths from kidney cancer may be overestimated, thereby lowering the calculated SMR. The significantly reduced risk for lung cancer among this cohort strongly supports a lowered prevalence of smoking. Finally, Rushton reported that there may have been underreporting of kidney cancers based on the ratio of reported malignant neoplasms and neoplasms of the kidney and bladder in England and Wales.

Wong *et al.* (1993) conducted a cohort study of 18,135 distribution employees with potential exposure to gasoline for at least one year at land-based terminals or on marine vessels between 1946 and 1985.[20] The authors found no statistically significant increased mortality from kidney cancer among marketing employees (SMR = 65.4; 95% CI = 33.7–114.1; n = 12) or marine distribution employees (SMR = 83.7; 95% CI = 45.8–140.5; n = 12) compared to the general population. The authors reported no association between mortality from kidney cancer and duration of employment, duration of exposure, age at first exposure, year of first exposure, job category, cumulative exposure, frequency of peak exposure, or average intensity of exposure. Excess kidney cancer was observed for those employed 10–19 years (SMR = 119.6); however, the SMR was not statistically significant. Among the marine workers an increase was reported for those employees who were classified as working on the deck.

Although the size of the population examined by Wong *et al.* and the quantitative assessment of gasoline exposure are reasonable, several factors limit the utility of this study. The overall SMR for the land-based workers was 51 (95% CI = 49.1–53.6; n = 2066); that for marine workers was 76.9 (95% CI = 73.9–79.9; n = 2695). In addition, the SMR for all malignant neoplasms for land-based employees was 66.4 (95% CI = 60.7–72.5; n = 520) based on United States population death rates. There is a clear healthy worker effect in this study, particularly among the land-based employees, as is evident by the overall SMR of 51. By comparison, limited analyses of mortality among those employed less than six months and not included in the cohort demonstrated an overall SMR of 312, suggesting a strong cohort selection bias based on health status at the time of hire as well as improved health maintenance required by the employer. The authors reported less drinking and smoking for the drivers in 1984 and an above-average socioeconomic status for blue collar employees. In addition, race information was unknown for approximately half of the marine employees and just over a quarter of the land-based workers. The authors also reported that they were unable to obtain death certificates for 14.8% of their marine workers.

Schwartz *et al.* (1987) examined all white male deaths in the state of New Hampshire that occurred between 1975 and 1985.[21] Information concerning usual industry and job for decedents was obtained from death certificates and served as the sole exposure classification. Schwartz *et al.* reported a non-statistically increased proportionate mortality ratio (PMR)(PMR = 152, 22-1057; n = 1) for kidney cancer among service station workers and a decreased PMR (PMR = 45, 7-299; n = 1) for automobile mechanics. Neither of these findings was statistically significant, and the small number of deaths precludes additional analyses.

Lagorio *et al.* (1994) conducted a cohort study of self-employed service station attendants in Italy.[22,23] However, the study size was too small and the follow-up too short to provide meaningful data concerning the carcinogenicity of gasoline.

Several case-control studies have examined the relationship between gasoline exposure and the risk of kidney cancer, and these are summarized in TABLE 9. McLaughlin *et al.* (1985) conducted a population-based case-control study of kidney cancer.[19] Cases diagnosed between January 1, 1974 and June 30, 1979 were ascertained from records of all hospitals in the Minneapolis-St. Paul standard metropolitan area. Controls under the age of 65 were chosen through a telephone sample of all telephone subscribers in the metropolitan area. Controls over the age of 65 were chosen from lists provided by the Health Care Financing Administration of the Social Security Administration. Overall, an odds ratio (OR) of 1.0 (95% CI = 0.7-1.4) was reported for persons with petroleum-related employment. McLaughlin found a slight increase in risk for those classified as ever working as a service station attendant (OR = 1.2, 95% CI = 0.6-2.3; n = 20). Although there was a slight upward trend with duration of employment, this trend was not found to be significant. While this study reported no overall association between the risk of renal cell cancer and employment in jobs with potential exposure to gasoline products, it should be noted that due to the small numbers the investigators would be able to detect only a four-fold increase (power = 80%) in kidney cancer risk associated with the longest duration classification (>10 years).

Kadamani *et al.* (1989) conducted a population-based case-control study to evaluate the association with hydrocarbon exposure and renal cell carcinoma.[24] Men and women over the age of 20 with diagnosed cases of renal cell carcinoma were identified through admissions to 23 Oklahoma hospitals between July 1981 and August 1983. Controls were selected by random-digit dialing from the population of Oklahoma. In addition to exposure information, information on body mass index (BMI) was collected and used as a measure for "degree of fatness." A positive association was found for hydrocarbon exposure in males (OR = 1.6, 95% CI = 0.8-3.2; n = 39), and the highest risk of renal cell carcinoma was found in men less than 60 years of age with moderate hydrocarbon exposure (OR = 3.0, $p \leq 0.05$). For the females in this same age group, an OR of 1.1 was reported, which was not statistically significant.

TABLE 9A. Case-Control Studies of Kidney Cancers: Descriptions of Studies

Author	Location	Minimum Employment	Examination Latency	Assessment by Length of Employment/ Exposure	Exposure
McLaughlin (1985)[19]	Minneapolis-St. Paul, United States	–	No	Yes	Based on occupational coding of employment history.
Domiano (1985)[26]	Buffalo, New York, United States	–	No	No	Patients' occupational history, title, and industry.
Steineck (1990)[28]	Stockholm, Sweden	–	No	Yes	Participant reported work history (industry), education, and military service.
Kadamani (1989)[24]	Oklahoma, United States	≤ 1 year	No	Yes	Scored from 0–5; none–high, based on job history.
Partanen (1991)[25]	Finland	–	Yes	Yes	Based on lifelong job histories.
Poole (1991)[27]	Study population taken from combined cohorts in 36 refinery locations	6 months to 5 years	Yes	Yes	Persons grouped into two categories; hydrocarbon; emphasis on those in gasoline and chemical and physical agents.
Gamble (1996)[29]	Cohort from oil refinery & chemical plants	>1 month 1/1/70–12/31/92	Yes	Yes	Exposure from histories and grouped by type of hydrocarbon exposure.

TABLE 9B. Case-Control Study of Kidney Cancers: Summary of Results

Author	Population Studied	No. of Cases	Ratio Cases to Controls	Comparison Group	Results
McLaughlin (1985)[19]	Renal cancer cases in population-based study	500	1 : 1.4	Population of Minneapolis-St. Paul	Increased OR for gasoline attendants.
Domiano (1985)[26]	Hospital-based patients 1957–1965 (Roswell Park Memorial Inst.)	92	1 : 17.25	Hospital patients age 30–89 admitted during study period	OR = 0.52 for gasoline exposure. Smoking and gasoline possibly interactive.
Steineck (1990)[28]	Urothelial cancer in Stockholm 1985–1987	254	1 : 1.12	Population of Stockholm	OR = 1.4 for gasoline exposure. OR = 2.5 for highest annual dose. Benzene associated with increased risk.
Kadamani (1989)[24]	Population-based study in 23 Oklahoma hospitals	210	1 : 1	General population State of Oklahoma	OR = 1.6 for hydrocarbon exposure. Weak positive trend with exposure.
Partanen (1991)[25]	Newly diagnosed cases in Finland 1977–1978	338	1 : 2	General population Finland	OR = 1.72 for gasoline. Gasoline alone OR = 2.05. OR = 7.39 for highest gasoline exposure.
Poole (1991)[27]	Data from petroleum industry cohorts in 36 refineries	100	1 : 4	Internal	OR = 2.4 for receipts, storage, and movement work. Increased OR for > 35 age at hire and exposed to nonaromatic compounds.
Gamble (1996)[29]	Cohort study population	37	1 : 4	Internal	OR = 4.08 (95% CI = 0.24–68.72) for those employed > 38 years. OR = 4.17 for "gasoline" exposure.

When examined by duration of exposure, although no effect was observed with females, a borderline statistically significant increase was reported for males with more than 15 years of exposure (OR = 2.8 for highest exposure and >30 years latency). Hydrocarbon exposure and percent standard BMI demonstrated statistically significant increases in kidney cancer risk for both males and females, with the highest risks reported for those workers with the greatest percentage of standard BMI and with the greatest hydrocarbon exposure; OR = 11.4 ($p < 0.01$) for males and OR = 7.1 ($p \leq 0.05$) for females. After adjusting for weight and education, an increased OR was found in males reporting a smoking history and who were exposed to hydrocarbons. Little joint effect for hydrocarbon exposure and smoking was noted for the females. Wine consumption was reported to lower risks for both sexes in all hydrocarbon exposure categories. Persons in the moderate exposure category who did not consume wine were at the highest risk.

Although the study by Kadamani *et al.* was well conducted, the study is limited in that exposure assessment was based only on occupational classifications. Hydrocarbon exposures have varied quantitatively over time for many of the occupations listed, and exposure misclassification would likely minimize the estimates of risk.

Partanen *et al.* (1991) conducted a case-referent study of kidney cancer among Finnish residents who had ever been employed, including entrepreneurs.[25] All cases (n = 338) were Finnish residents over the age of 20 who were newly diagnosed between 1977 and 1978; they were identified through the Finnish Cancer Registry. Controls (n = 484) were identified from the Population Register Centre. Lifelong job histories were collected. In addition, information on smoking history, coffee consumption, and obesity were obtained. The authors reported an elevated risk for exposure to gasoline for both men and women combined (OR = 1.72, 95% CI = 1.03–2.87; n = 39 cases) and for men separately (OR = 1.63, 95% CI = 0.97–2.75; n = 39 cases). Men exposed to gasoline, and not to diesel or other distilled fuels, had a kidney cancer OR of 2.1 (95% CI = 1.1–4.0; n = 23 cases). When the author simultaneously adjusted for occupational exposures that they found to be associated with exposure to gasoline (diesel and other distilled fuels (positive correlation), oil mist (positive correlation), animal exposure (negative correlation), smoking, coffee consumption, and obesity, an OR of 1.2 (95% CI = 0.6–2.5) was observed. Although no clear trend was identified for duration of exposure, the authors did find an exposure-response relationship. The risk of renal cell carcinoma was highest in those persons with the highest level of exposure, as approximated by benzene-equivalent concentrations (OR = 7.39, 95% CI = 1.58–34.6; n = 10 cases). Increasing cumulative exposure, estimated by the level and duration of exposure, displayed an upward trend in renal cancer risk, with the greatest risk (OR = 4.34, 95% CI = 1.15–16.4; n = 9 cases) seen in the highest exposure category of 14–102 ppm-year. In addition, the observed excess risk was reported to be greatest among those with a latency period of approximately 30 years.

The Partanen *et al.* study is well designed and analyzed and provides strong evidence for an association between gasoline exposure and kidney cancer while controlling for multiple confounders by logistic regression. Exposure-response analyses based on exposure level and cumulative exposure are more limited, due to the small number of cases in each exposure stratum.

Domiano *et al.* (1985) conducted a hospital-based case-control study of kidney cancer.[26] Cases (n = 92) and controls (n = 1,588) were white males selected from patients admitted to the Roswell Park Memorial Institute in Buffalo, New York from 1957 to 1965. Domiano *et al.* examined the separate and combined effects of smoking and gasoline exposure and found an increased risk for renal cell carcinomas for those definitely exposed to gasoline and who had 21 or more pack-years of smoking (OR = 1.6). Analyses by gasoline exposure found that four of their 92 cases and 122 of their 1,588 controls were exposed, producing a non-statistically significant age-adjusted OR of 0.53, suggesting to the authors that there is no independent effect of gasoline exposure on the risk of renal cell carcinoma. A possible interactive effect of smoking and gasoline exposure was suggested by the authors.

Poole *et al.* (1993) conducted a nested case-control study of kidney cancers among refinery workers.[27] Cases (n = 102) and controls (n = 408) were taken from a cohort of 100,000 male refinery workers employed by five petroleum companies, with cases identified by review of death certificates. Job histories were obtained for 98% of the cases and 94% of the controls. The overall relative risk for gasoline exposure was found to be 1.0 (95% CI = 0.51–1.94; n = 100 cases). Non-statistically significant increased OR's were reported for those workers employed in the receipt, storage, and movement departments (OR = 2.49, 95% CI = 0.95–6.56; n = 9 cases), for laborers (OR = 1.94, 95% CI = 0.96–3.92; n = 24 cases), and for unit cleaners (OR = 2.28, 95% CI = 0.53–9.93; n = 3 cases). In addition, non-statistically significant increased OR's were reported for those ≥35 years of age at hire (OR = 2.50, 95% CI = 0.72–8.72; n = 37 cases) and for those workers exposed to nonaromatic gasoline components.

Misclassification of exposure must be considered in the study by Poole *et al.*, given that exposure assessment was based on jobs and exposure ratings by hygienists. In addition, potential confounders such as obesity, smoking history, and other lifestyle variables were not addressed. The small number of workers in the various job categories for the longest-held job make detection of increased risk difficult, although several trends in increased risk were apparent.

Steineck *et al.* (1990) reported an increased risk of urothelial cancer in Stockholm, Sweden following exposure to benzene and exhausts based on a population-based case-referent study of urothelial cancer.[28] Cases (n = 254) were identified from a study of men born between 1911 and 1945 in the county of Stockholm. Incident cases occurring between September 15, 1985 and November 30, 1987 were included in the study. Controls were obtained by stratified random sampling from a computer registry of the Stockholm population. An overall OR of 1.4 (95% CI = 0.7–2.9; n = 18 cases) was reported for exposure to petrol. For those with the highest annual exposure, an OR of 2.5 (95% CI = 0.8–7.5) was observed. For exposure to petrol exhaust and for benzene, OR's of 1.0 (95% CI = 0.5–1.9; n = 24) and 2.0 (95% CI = 1.0–3.8; n = 26), respectively, were observed. When cases were examined by annual exposure, an OR of 3.0 (95% CI = 1.0–8.7) was observed for benzene exposure, and an OR of 3.9 (95% CI = 0.4–35.5) was observed for exposure to petrol exhausts in the highest exposure categories.

Gamble *et al.* (1996) reported results of a nested case-control study of kidney cancer among refinery and petrochemical workers.[29] Kidney cancer cases (n = 37) were identified among a previous cohort mortality study of three refineries and chemical plants. Four controls were selected from the cohort and were frequency matched on sex, race, date of birth, and at-risk status. Regression analyses controlling for body mass index, blood pressure, and smoking demonstrated an increasing risk of renal cancer with increasing tenure, with an OR of 4.08 (95% CI = 0.24-68.72) for those employed 38 years or more. An adjusted OR of 4.17 ($p < 0.17$) was observed for exposure to the petroleum hydrocarbon fraction judged to most resemble unleaded gasoline

Leukemia and Cancers of the Hematopoietic System

In the Rushton *et al.* study,[18] a slightly elevated SMR for leukemia was reported for distribution workers (SMR = 108, 95% CI = 83-140; *n* = 61). When leukemias were analyzed by cell type, elevated SMRs were reported for acute lymphatic (SMR = 133, 95% CI = 43-309; *n* = 5), chronic lymphatic (SMR = 115, 95% CI = 66-187; *n* = 16), all lymphatic (SMR = 115, 95% CI = 71-176; *n* = 21), acute myeloid (SMR = 121, 95% CI = 78-179; *n* = 25), other myeloid (SMR = 113, 95% CI = 3-629; *n* = 1), and all myeloid (SMR = 109, 95% CI = 75-152; *n* = 34). There were no observed deaths from other lymphatic leukemias. The authors further reported elevations with various jobs and with specific locations, based on small numbers of observed cases.

In the mortality study by Schnatter *et al.,* the SMR for leukemia was found not to be elevated for the hydrocarbon-exposed workers (SMR = 101, 95% CI = 40-208; *n* = 7); however, a slight increase was observed for all workers (SMR = 135, 95% CI = 83-226; *n* = 14). Non-statistically significant decreased SMRs for myeloid leukemia (SMR = 84, 95% CI = 40-208; *n* = 7) and lymphoid leukemias (SMR = 98, 95% CI = 39-202; *n* = 1) were observed. Nonsignificantly elevated SMRs for leukemia were reported for those persons employed 10-19 years (SMR = 144) and for those employed for 20-29 years (SMR = 132). For myeloid/lymphoid leukemia, an elevated SMR of 156 was reported for persons in the 20-29 years employed classification. For persons with the highest reported exposures (tank truck drivers) statistically significant raised SMRs were reported for all leukemias (SMR = 335, 95% CI = 108-781; *n* = 5) and for myeloid/lymphoid leukemias (SMR = 387, 95% CI = 106-992; *n* = 4). When age, socioeconomic status (SES), year hired, hire before or after 1974 were placed in the authors' model and examined, no elevated SMRs were observed comparing those exposed daily and less than daily. The small number of leukemia cases in this study precludes meaningful exposure-response analyses.

Several occupational exposures, including benzene, have been found to increase the risk of multiple myeloma. When Schnatter *et al.* examined multiple myeloma in their mortality study, elevated SMRs were reported both for all workers (SMR = 183, 95% CI = 73-377; *n* = 7) and for hydrocarbon-exposed workers (SMR = 199, 95% CI = 64-463; *n* = 5).[17] Analyses by exposure frequency demonstrated a slight upward trend. For those not exposed, an SMR of 154 was reported; for those exposed less than daily, an SMR of 167; and for those exposed daily, an SMR of 228. Multiple myeloma deaths were more frequent among the longer-tenured employees. For those employed 20-29 years and greater than 30 years, there was a greater than two-fold increased risk, but this increase was not statistically significant.

The Wong *et al.* mortality study of distribution workers reported decreased SMRs for leukemia and aleukemia in both the land-based (SMR = 89.1, 95% CI = 59.4-

128.8, $n = 27$) and marine cohort (SMR = 70, 95% CI = 42.2-109.4; $n = 16$).[20] When the cases were assessed by length of exposure, a non-statistically significant elevated SMR for land-based employees was reported in the 10-19 years category (SMR = 107.6; $n = 7$). Analyses by time since first exposure demonstrated a slightly elevated, although not statistically significant, SMR for leukemia for both the marine and land-based employees in the 10-19 years since first exposure category. Analyses by job category demonstrated an elevated SMR for operators in the land-based cohort. A slightly elevated SMR (103.5; $n = 3$) was reported for persons with 1000-2000 ppm exposure-years in the land-based cohort. When leukemia by cell type was examined among marine employees exposed to gasoline vapors, an elevated SMR of 132.9 (95% CI = 36.2-339.8; $n = 4$) was reported.

In the study of death certificates from New Hampshire by Schwartz *et al.*, elevated leukemia PMRs were observed for mechanics (PMR = 178, 95% CI = 81-392; $n = 6$), and leukemia PMRs were observed for both mechanics (PMR = 178, 95% CI = 81-392; $n = 6$) and service station employees (PMR = 328, 95% CI = 113-951; $n = 3$).[21] Lymphatic cancers were found to be elevated among mechanics (PMR = 200) and attendants (PMR = 116); however, these excesses were based on small numbers and were not statistically significant.

Two additional case-control or cancer-incidence studies have examined the relationship between gasoline exposure and leukemia,[30,31] (see TABLE 10). Jakobsson *et al.* (1993) linked occupational histories for persons through 64 years of age, obtained from the 1970 Swedish census, with incident cancer cases identified in the National Swedish Cancer Registry between 1971 and 1984, thus allowing the calculation of rates by occupation.[30] Petrol station workers were found to have an increased risk for acute myeloid leukemia (AML) (RR = 3.6, 95% CI = 1.7-6.6).

Lindquist *et al.* (1991) interviewed adult acute leukemia patients admitted to one of five hospitals participating in treatment studies organized by the Leukemia Group of Middle Sweden from September 1980 to May 1983.[31] Controls were taken from the population registry of the taxation authorities. An increased risk was observed (OR = 3.0, 95% CI = 1.1-9.2; $n = 18$) for professional drivers exposed to petroleum products. Professional drivers included persons driving cars, buses, and trucks, who refueled the vehicles and loaded and unloaded them.

DISCUSSION AND CONCLUSIONS

Kidney cancers, leukemias, and other cancers of the hematopoietic system are relatively rare; thus assessment of risk using the cohort mortality study design requires a sizable population with long-term follow-up in order to detect even moderate increases in risk with statistical significance. For example, in order for an SMR of 1.25 (i.e., 25% excess) to be statistically significant ($p < 0.05$), approximately 100 deaths due to the causes of concern must be observed. Further stratification by exposure requires a similar increase in population size and observed deaths. Case-control studies offer the possibility of increased statistical power and greater control over possible confounders, although exposure assessment in such studies may be problematic.

TABLE 10A. Case-Control Studies of Leukemia among Gasoline-Exposed Workers: Description of Studies

Author	Location	Minimum Employment	Examination Latency	Assessment by Length of Employment	Exposure
Jakobsson (1993)[30]	Sweden	—	No	No	Occupation information obtained from 1970 Swedish census. Surviving relatives of cases with elevated risk AML were interviewed about the cases work history.
Lindquist (1991)[31]	Sweden	—	Yes	Yes	Lifetime history was collected by interview of participants.

TABLE 10B. Case-Control Studies of Leukemia among Gasoline-Exposed Workers: Summary of Results

Author	Population Studied	No. of Cases	Location	Comparison Group	Ratio Cases: Controls	Results
Jakobsson (1993)[30]	AML cases from Swedish cancer registry 1971–1974	275	Sweden	—	—	RR = 3.6 for leukemia among patrol station attendant workers.
Lindquist (1991)[31]	Leukemia cases from 5 hospitals in Sweden 1980–1983	125	Sweden	Swedish population	1 : 1	OR = 3.0 for drivers exposed to petroleum products.

Several previous reviews of gasoline exposure and the risk of cancer have been published.[32–37] Cohort studies, taken as a whole, suggest an increased risk for kidney cancer among gasoline-exposed workers. Both Rushton and Schnatter were able to show an increased risk for kidney cancer in drivers where exposure was the highest. The study by Wong *et al.* is the exception; however, this study suffers from a major cohort selection bias and healthy worker effect, as previously discussed. The mixed and inconclusive results obtained by many cohort studies may be the result of insufficient statistical power and exposure misclassification. In contrast, case-control studies have provided stronger data concerning the association between kidney cancer and gasoline exposure. The study by Partanen is well conducted and demonstrates an increased risk, as well as an exposure response.

Animal data provide some evidence concerning biological plausibility of a causal association between gasoline exposure and kidney cancer. Inhalation studies exposing male rats to whole unleaded gasoline have demonstrated a dose-related increase in kidney cancer incidence.[38–40] Mechanistic studies have suggested a possible role of alpha-2-micro-globulin, found in male rats but not man, in the etiology of kidney cancers seen in the rat studies.[41–43] However, other researchers have proposed alternative mechanisms by which gasoline and other hydrocarbons could increase the risk of kidney cancer in man.[44] The propensity of many carcinogens to increase the risk of cancers at multiple sites suggests caution in the use of mechanistic data to discount strongly positive animal studies.[45]

Cohort studies by Rushton and Schnatter demonstrated elevated SMRs, although not statistically significant, for leukemia. As with the kidney cancer, the strongest evidence has been provided by case-control studies. Jakobsson *et al.* and Lindquist *et al.* found statistically elevated odds ratios for AML and all acute leukemias, respectively. The study by Schnatter demonstrated an elevated risk of multiple myeloma among marketing workers, with some suggestion of an exposure response. The biological plausibility of increased risk for cancers of the hematopoietic system due to exposure to gasoline has been clearly established by environmental studies that have shown exposure to benzene and 1,3 butadiene during gasoline handling. Additionally, genotoxic effects have been observed among gasoline-exposed workers. Gasoline pump mechanics exposed to an average of approximately 1 mg/m^3 have been shown to have increased frequencies and sizes of micronuclei in B-lymphocytes by Hogstedt *et al.*[46] Nilsson *et al.* (1996) observed genotoxic effects (single-strand breaks on DNA of leukocytes and urinary levels of the oxidative DNA adduct 8-hydroxydeoxyguanosine) in workers exposed to low levels of benzene (eight-hour TWA = 0.13 ppm) from gasoline,[13] and Lagorio *et al.* (1994) found increased urinary secretion of 8-hydroxydeoxyguanosine among filling station attendants in Italy.[47]

Risk assessments by OSHA estimated that benzene exposures of 1 ppm (3.2 mg/m^3) for a working lifetime (45 years) would result in 10 excess leukemia deaths per 1000 exposed workers (95% CI = 4-22).[48] This risk assessment, taken in conjunction with exposure data for workers handling gasoline throughout the distribution system, suggests an important cancer risk and the need for controls to further reduce exposure to gasoline. The findings of genotoxic effects at benzene exposure levels below 1 ppm provide additional support for control of exposure.

REFERENCES

1. MEHLMAN, M. A. 1990. Dangerous properties of petroleum-refining products: Carcinogenicity of motor fuels (gasoline). Teratog. Carcinog. Mutagen. **10:** 399-408.
2. KING, R. W. 1992. Automotive gasoline: Its composition and manufacture—past, present and future. J. Exposure Anal. Environ. Epidemiol. **2**(1): 9-22.
3. WIXTROM, R. N. & S. L. BROWN. 1992. Individual and population exposures to gasoline. J. Exposure Anal. Environ. Epidemiol. **2**(1): 23-78.
4. SAWYER, R. F. 1993. Trends in auto emissions and gasoline composition. Environ. Health Perspect. **101**(Suppl. 6): 5-12.
5. PAGE, N. P. & M. MEHLMAN. 1989. Health effects of gasoline refueling vapors and measured exposures at service stations. Toxicol. Ind. Health **5**(5): 869-891.
6. IARC. 1989. The Evaluation of Carcinogenic Risk to Humans: Occupational Exposures in Petroleum Refining; Crude Oil and Major Petroleum Fuels. IARC Monographs, Vol. 45. Lyon, France.
7. HARTLE, R. 1993. Exposure to methyl tert-butyl ether and benzene among service station attendants and operators. Environ. Health Perspect. **101**(Suppl. 6): 23-26.
8. ACGIH. 1995. Threshold limit values (TLVs) for chemical substances and physical agents. American Conference of Governmental Industrial Hygienists. Cincinnati, OH.
9. NATIONAL INSTITUTE FOR OCCUPATIONAL SAFETY AND HEALTH. 1994. Pocket Guide to Chemical Hazards. DHHS (NIOSH) Publication No. 94-116. National Institute for Occupational Safety and Health, Centers for Disease Control and Prevention. Cincinnati, OH.
10. NATIONAL TOXICOLOGY PROGRAM. 1994. Seventh Annual Report of Carcinogens. Vol. 1: 70-79. U.S. Department of Health & Human Services, National Institute of Environmental Health Sciences. Research Triangle Park, NC.
11. VIRMA, D. K., J. A. JULIAN, G. BEEBEE, W. K. CHENG, K. HOLBORN & L. SHAW. 1992. Hydrocarbon exposures at petroleum bulk terminals and agencies. Am. Ind. Assoc. J. **53**(10): 645-656.
12. RAPPAPORT, S. A., S. SELVIN & M. A. WATERS. 1987. Exposures to hydrocarbon components of gasoline in the petroleum industry. Appl. Ind. Hyg. **2**(4): 148-154.
13. NILSSON, R. I., R. G. NORDLINDER, C. TAGESSON, S. WALLES & B. G. JARVHOLM. 1996. Genotoxic effects in workers exposed to low levels of benzene from gasoline. Am. J. Ind. Med. **30:** 317-324.
14. MOWNINO, D. M. *et al.* 1995. Human exposure to volatile organic compounds: A comparison of organic vapor badge levels with blood levels. Int. Arch. Occup. Environ. Health **67:** 59-64.
15. SAVITZ, D. A. & R. MOORE. 1984. Cancer risk among oil refinery workers. J. Occup. Med. **26**(9): 662-670.
16. WONG, O. & G. K. RAABE. 1989. Critical review of cancer epidemiology in petroleum industry employees, with a quantitative meta-analysis by cancer site. Am. J. Ind. Med. **15:** 283-310.
17. SCHNATTER, A. R., A. M. KATZ, M. J. NICOLICH & G. THERIAULT. 1993. A retrospective mortality study among Canadian petroleum marketing and distribution workers. Environ. Health Perspect. **101**(Suppl. 6): 85-99.
18. RUSHTON, L. 1993. A 39-year follow-up of the U.K. oil refinery and distribution center studies: Results for kidney cancer and leukemia. Environ. Health Perspect. **101**(Suppl. 6): 77-84.
19. MCLAUGHLIN, J. K. 1993. Renal cell cancer and exposure to gasoline: A review. Environ. Health Perspect. **101**(Suppl. 6): 111-114.
20. WONG, O., F. HARRIS & T. J. SMITH. 1993. Health effects of gasoline exposure. II. Mortality patterns of distribution workers in the United States. Environ. Health Perspect. **101**(Suppl. 6): 63-76.
21. SCHWARTZ, E. 1987. Proportionate mortality ratio analysis of automobile mechanics and gasoline service station workers in New Hampshire. Am. J. Ind. Med. **12:** 91-99.

22. Lagorio, S., F. Forastiere, I. Iavarone *et al.* 1994. Mortality of filling station attendants. Scand. J. Work Environ. Health **20:** 331-338.
23. Lagorio, S., F. Forastiere, I. Iavarone *et al.* 1993. Exposure assessment in a historical cohort of filling station attendants. Intl. J. Epidemiol. **22;** No. 6 (Suppl. 2): S51-S56.
24. Kadamani, S., N. R. Asal & R. V. Nelson. 1989. Occupational hydrocarbon exposure and risk of renal cell carcinoma. Am. J. Ind. Med. **15:** 131-141.
25. Partanen, T., P. Heikkila, S. Hernberg *et al.* 1991. Renal cell cancer and occupational exposure to chemical agents. Scand. J. Work Environ. Health **17:** 231-239.
26. Domiano, S. F., J. E. Vena & M. K. Swanson. 1985. Gasoline exposure, smoking, and kidney cancer. J. Occup. Med. **27**(6): 398-399.
27. Poole, C., N. A. Dreyer, M. H. Satterfield *et al.* 1993. Kidney cancer and hydrocarbon exposures among petroleum refinery workers. Environ. Health Perspect. **101**(Suppl. 6): 53-62.
28. Steineck, G., N. Plato, M. Gerhardsson *et al.* 1990. Increased risk of urothelial cancer in Stockholm during 1985-87 after exposure to benzene and exhausts. Int. J. Cancer **45:** 1012-1017.
29. Gamble, J. F., E. D. Pearlman & M. J. Nicolich. 1996. A nested case-control study of kidney cancer among refinery/petrochemical workers. Environ. Health Perspect. **104:** 642-650.
30. Jakobsson, R., A. Ahlbom, T. Bellander & I. Lundberg. 1993. Acute myeloid leukemia among petrol station attendants. Arch. Environ. Health **48**(4): 255-259.
31. Lindquist, R., B. Nilsson, G. Eklund & G. Gahrton. 1991. Acute leukemia in professional drivers exposed to gasoline and diesel. Eur. J. Haematol. **47:** 98-103.
32. Enterline, P. E. & J. Viren. 1985. Epidemiologic evidence for an association between gasoline and kidney cancer. Environ. Health Perspect. **62:** 303-312.
33. Enterline, P. E. 1993. Review of new evidence regarding the relationship of gasoline exposure to kidney cancer and leukemia. Environ. Health Perspect. **101**(Suppl. 6): 101-103.
34. Raabe, G. K. 1993. Review of the carcinogenic potential of gasoline. Environ. Health Perspect. **101**(Suppl. 6): 35-38.
35. Harrington, J. M. 1987. Health experience of workers in the petroleum manufacturing and distribution industry: A review of the literature. Am. J. Ind. Med. **12:** 475-497.
36. Mehlman, M. A. 1992. Dangerous and cancer-causing properties of products and chemicals in the oil refining and petrochemical industry. VIII. Health effects of motor fuels: Carcinogenicity of gasoline—Scientific update. Environ. Res. **59:** 238-249.
37. Infante, P. F. 1993. State of the science on the carcinogenicity of gasoline with particular reference to cohort mortality study results. Environ. Health Perspect. **101**(Suppl 6): 105-109.
38. MacFarland, H. N., E. E. Ulrich & C. E. Holdsworth. 1984. A chronic inhalation study with unleaded gasoline vapor. J. Am. Coll. Toxicol. **3:** 231-248.
39. Kitchen, D. N. 1984. Neoplastic renal effects of unleaded gasoline in Fischer 344 rats: Renal effects of petroleum hydrocarbons. Adv. Mod. Environ. Toxicol. **7:** 65-72.
40. Short, B. G., J. A. Steinhagen & J. A. Swanberg. 1989. Promoting effects of unleaded gasoline and 2,2,4-trimethylpentane on the development of typical cell foci and renal tumors in rats exposed to N-ethyl-N-hydroxyethyl nitrosamine. Cancer Res. **49:** 6369-6378.
41. Borghoff, S. J., B. G. Short & J. A. Swenberg. 1990. Biochemical mechanisms and pathobiology of alpha-2-microglobulin nephropathy. Ann. Rev. Pharmacol. Toxicol. **30:** 349-367.
42. Hurd, G. C., J. S. Rodgers, K. P. Baeteke *et al.* 1993. Hazard evaluation of chemicals that cause accumulation of alpha-2-microglobulin, hylin droplet nephropathy and tubule neoplasia in the kidneys of male rats. Environ. Health Perspect. **99:** 343-349.
43. Swenberg, J. A., B. Short, S. J. Borghoff. *et al.* 1989. The comparative pathobiology of alpha-2-microglobulin nephropathy. Toxicol. Appl. Pharmacol. **97:** 35-46.

44. MELNICK, R. L. 1992. An alternative hypothesis on the role of chemically induced protein droplet (alpha-2-microglobulin) nephropathy in renal carcinogenesis. Regul. Toxicol. Pharmacol. **16:** 111-125.
45. HUFF, J. 1992. Applicability to humans of rodent-specific sites of chemical carcinogenicity: Tumors of the forestomach and of the Hardian, preputial and Zymbal glands induced by benzene. J. Occup. Med. & Toxicol. **1**(2): 109-141.
46. HOGSTEDT, B., A. HOLMEN, A. KARLSSON *et al.* 1991. Gasoline pump mechanics had increased frequencies and sizes of micronuclei in lymphocytes stimulated by pokeweed mitogen. Mutat. Res. **263:** 51-5.
47. LAGORIO, S., C. TAGESSON, C. FORASTIERE *et al.* 1994. Exposure to benzene and urinary concentration of 8-hydrooxydeoxyguanosine, biological marker of oxidative damage to DNA. Occup. Environ. Med. **51:** 739-743.
48. OCCUPATIONAL SAFETY AND HEALTH ADMINISTRATION. 1987. Occupational Exposure to Benzene, Final Rule. Federal Register **52**(176): 34460-34578.
49. PARKINSON, G. S. 1971. Benzene in motor gasoline—An investigation into possible health hazards in and around filling stations and in normal transport operations. Ann. Occup. Hyg. **14:** 145-153.
50. KEARNEY, C. A. & D. B. DUNHAM. 1986. Gasoline vapor exposures at a high volume service station. Am. Indus. Hyg. Assoc. J. **47**(8): 535-539.
51. MCDERMOTT, J. J. & G. A. VOS. 1979. Service station attendants exposure to benzene and gasoline vapors. Am. Ind. Hyg. Assoc. J. **40**(4): 315-321.
52. HADLER, C. A., G. S. VAN GORP, N. S. HATOUM & T. M. WARNE. 1986. Gasoline vapor exposure. Part I. Characterization of workplace exposures. Am. Ind. Hyg. Assoc. J. **47**(3): 164-172.
53. ELLIS, K. & R. OBENDORFER. 1984. Survey of Benzene Concentrations in Ambient Air. Air Management Services, Philadelphia Department of Public Health. Philadelphia.
54. TIRONI, G., G. J. NEBEL & R. L. WILLIAMS. 1986. Measurement of Vapor Exposure during Gasoline Refueling. General Motors Research Laboratories, Environmental Science Department. Warren, MI.
55. BOND, A. E., V. L. THOMPSON *et al.* 1986. Self-service Station Vehicle Refueling Exposure Study. U.S. Environmental Protection Agency. Research Triangle Park, NC.
56. CLAYTON ENVIRONMENTAL CONSULTANTS. 1983. Gasoline exposure study for the American Petroleum Institute. CEC Job No. 18629. Washington, DC.
57. MOEN, B. E., B. E. HOLLUND, M. BERSTEN *et al.* 1995. Exposure of the deck crew to carcinogenic agents on oil product tankers. Ann. Occup. Hyg. **39**(3): 347-361.
58. NORDLINDER, R. & O. RAMNAS. 1987. Exposure to benzene at different work places in Sweden. Ann. Occup. Hyg. **31**(3): 345-355.
59. IRVING, W. S. & T. A. GRUMBLES. 1979. Benzene exposures during gasoline loading at bulk marketing terminals. Am. Ind. Hyg. Assoc. J. **40**(6): 468-473.

Results of Long-term Experimental Studies on the Carcinogenicity of Methyl *tert*-Butyl Ether

FIORELLA BELPOGGI,[a] MORANDO SOFFRITTI,[b] FEDERICA FILIPPINI,[b] AND CESARE MALTONI[b]

[a]*Cancer Research Center*
European Ramazzini Foundation
of Oncology and Environmental Sciences
Bentivoglio Castle
40010 Bentivoglio (BO), Italy

[b]*European B. Ramazzini Foundation of Oncology and*
Environmental Sciences
Bologna, Italy

INTRODUCTION

In 1975, a broad project of experimental studies on the carcinogenicity of leaded and unleaded gasolines, diesel oil, kerosene, various aromatic hydrocarbons (benzene, toluene, xylenes, ethylbenzene), trimethylpentane (TMP), oxygenated additives, and products of gasoline combustion was started at the Cancer Research Center of the European Ramazzini Foundation of Oncology and Environmental Sciences. Within this project, all the six presently proposed gasoline oxygenated additives, alone or blended with gasoline, have been submitted to long-term carcinogenicity bioassays (TABLES 1 and 2).

The present report deals with the results of the bioassays on the presently most widely used oxygenated additive: methyl *tert*-butyl ether (MTBE). Partial results on MTBE have been already made public in several instances.[1]

MATERIALS AND METHODS

MTBE was supplied by a United States gasoline company; its purity was higher than 99%. During the experiments, the compound was stored at a temperature of 4°C.

Male (M) and female (F) Sprague-Dawley rats of the colony of the Bentivoglio (BT) Cancer Research Center (CRC) of the European Ramazzini Foundation were used. This colony of rats has been employed for various experiments in the BT Laboratory for nearly 25 years. Historical data are available on more than 10,000 historical controls, kept under observation for life-span and submitted to systematic necropsies and standardized histopathological examinations. Therefore, data on the expected incidence of the different types of tumors in control animals and on its fluctuations are available.

After weaning, at 4-5 weeks of age, the experimental animals were identified by ear punch, randomized in order to have not more than one male and one female

TABLE 1. BT Project of Experimental Bioassays on the Carcinogenicity of Gasoline Oxygenated Additives: Plan of Experiments

Materials		Type of Exposure (Route)	Animal System		
Category	Specific Materials		Species	Strain	Sex
Oxygenated additives	Methyl alcohol	Drinking water	Rat	Sprague-Dawley	M, F
		Gavage in olive oil	Rat	Sprague-Dawley	M, F
	Ethyl alcohol	Drinking water	Rat	Sprague-Dawley	M, F
		Gavage in olive oil	Rat	Sprague-Dawley	M, F
	Methyl-ter-butyl-ether (MTBE)	Gavage in olive oil	Rat	Sprague-Dawley	M, F
	Ethyl-ter-butyl-ether (ETBE)	Gavage in olive oil	Rat	Sprague-Dawley	M, F
	Di-isopropyl-ether (DIPE)	Gavage in olive oil	Rat	Sprague-Dawley	M, F
	Tert-amyl-methyl-ether (TAME)	Gavage in olive oil	Rat	Sprague-Dawley	M, F

TABLE 2. BT Project of Experimental Bioassays on the Carcinogenicity of Mixtures of Gasoline and Some Oxygenated Additives: Plan of Experiments

Materials		Type of Exposure	Animal System		
Category	Specific Materials	(Route)	Species	Strain	Sex
Mixtures	Gasoline + methyl alcohol	Gavage in olive oil	Rat	Sprague-Dawley	M, F
	Gasoline + ethyl alcohol	Gavage in olive oil	Rat	Sprague-Dawley	M, F
	Gasoline + MTBE	Gavage in olive oil	Rat	Sprague-Dawley	M, F
	Gasoline + ETBE	Gavage in olive oil	Rat	Sprague-Dawley	M, F

TABLE 3. Long-term Carcinogenicity Bioassays on Methyl-Tertiary-Butyl-Ether (MTBE), Administered by Stomach Tube to Sprague-Dawley Rats (Experiment BT 958): Plan of the Experiment

Group	Daily Dose (mg/kg b.w. in Olive Oil)	Animals	
		Sex	No.
I	1000	M	60
		F	60
		M + F	120
II	250	M	60
		F	60
		M + F	120
III	0[a]	M	60
		F	60
		M + F	120

[a] Olive oil alone.

of each litter in the same group, and housed 5 per cage. The animals were 8 weeks old at the start of the experiment.

The plan of the experiment is shown in TABLE 3.

The experiment on MTBE was started in September 1988.

Every single dose of MTBE was administered by gavage as 1 mL of extra virgin olive oil solution, once daily, 4 days weekly (Monday and Tuesday, Thursday and Friday), for 104 weeks. Administration of the compound at the highest dose (5-6 days weekly) would not have been tolerated by the rats. The solutions were prepared weekly and maintained at 4°C. Control animals were given 1 mL of extra virgin olive oil alone.

The animals were kept under observation until natural death, under highly standardized housing, diet, and experimental conduct conditions, identical to those used in the BT Laboratory over the last 25 years. In the experiments performed at the BT Cancer Research Center, the animals are usually allowed to live until natural death. By doing so, it is possible to allow the development of all the neoplastic potentialities. Mean daily feed and drinking water consumption were determined once weekly for the first 13 weeks from the start of the experiment, then every 2 weeks, until 112 weeks of age. Individual animal weight was measured once weekly from 8 weeks of age for the first 13 weeks, and then every 2 weeks until 112 weeks of age, and every 8 weeks until the end of the experiments. In order to detect and register all gross lesions, the animals were examined every week for the first 13 weeks, and then every 2 weeks until the end of the experiment.

The biophase of the experiment terminated after 166 weeks, with the death of the last animal at the age of 174 weeks.

Upon death, the animals were submitted to systematic necropsy. Histopathology was routinely performed on skin and subcutaneous tissue, the brain, pituitary gland,

Zymbal glands, salivary glands, Harderian glands, cranium (with oral and nasal cavities and external and internal ear ducts, 5 levels), tongue, thyroid and parathyroid, pharynx, larynx, thymus and mediastinal lymph nodes, trachea, lung and mainstem bronchi, heart, diaphragm, liver, spleen, pancreas, kidneys and adrenal glands, esophagus, stomach (fore and glandular), intestine (4 levels), bladder, prostate, uterus, gonads, interscapular fat pad, subcutaneous and mesenteric lymph nodes, and any other organ or tissue with pathological lesions.

All organs and tissues were preserved in 70% ethyl alcohol, except bones, which were fixed in 10% formalin and then decalcified with 10% formaldehyde and 20% formic acid in water solution. The normal specimens were trimmed, following the standard procedures of the BT Laboratory: i.e., parenchymal organs were dissected through the hilus to expose the widest surface, and hollow organs were sectioned across the greatest diameter(s). The pathological tissue was trimmed through the largest surface, including normal adjacent tissues. The trimmed specimens were processed as paraffin blocks, and 3-5 micron sections of every specimen were obtained. Sections were routinely stained with hematoxylin-eosine. Specific stainings were performed when needed. All slides were examined microscopically by the same group of pathologists; a senior pathologist reviewed all the tumors and any other lesion of oncological interest. All pathologists followed the same criteria of histopathological evaluation and classification.

Two statistical methods were used for the analysis of tumor incidence. The first method is a prevalence analysis for nonlethal tumors and is described in Hoel and Walburg.[2] The Leydig cell testicular tumors given in TABLE 8 were considered nonlethal. The second method assumes lethality of the tumors; the statistical method is a log-ranked test described in Mantel[3] and Cox.[4] This was used for the lymphomas/leukemias in TABLE 9.

RESULTS

Mean Daily Water and Feed Consumption. There were no differences in water and feed consumption among the animals of the treated and control groups of both sexes (FIGS. 1-4).

Body Weight. There were no relevant differences in the mean body weight of treated and control group male and female rats (FIGS. 5, 6).

Survival. The survival was the same among male rats of the treated and control groups up to 88 weeks of age (80 weeks from the start of the treatment); then there was a higher survival of the males treated at the higher dose (FIG. 7). A dose-related decrease in survival was observed among female rats from 24 weeks of age (16 weeks from the start of the treatment) (FIG. 8).

Nononcological Changes. No evident behavioral changes were observed in MTBE-treated animals. No treatment-related nononcological pathological changes were detected by gross inspection and histological examination.

Tumors and Other Oncological Changes. The occurrence of benign and malignant tumors of different site or type observed among male and female rats of all treated groups are listed in TABLES 4 and 5. Multiple tumors of the same site (monolateral and bilateral organs) and type were plotted only once, apart from mammary tumors of the same type, whose multiplicity was taken into account.

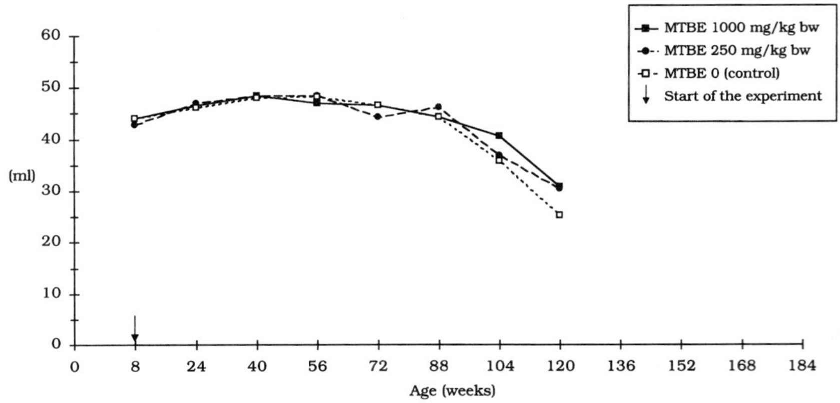

FIGURE 1. Mean daily water consumption in male rats.

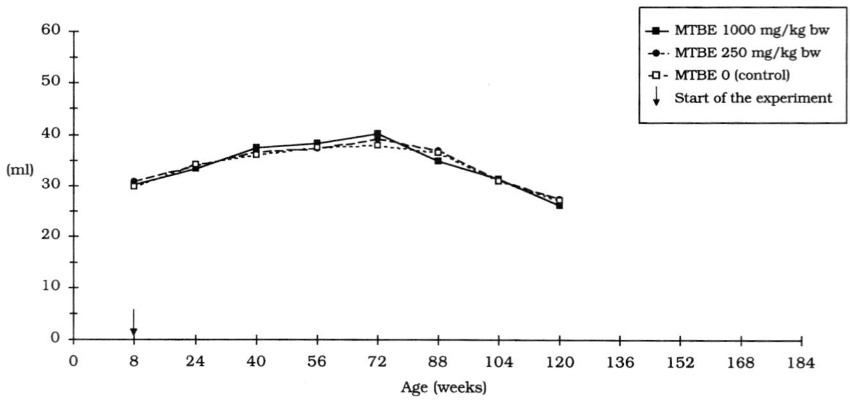

FIGURE 2. Mean daily water consumption in female rats.

The incidence of total benign and total malignant tumors is given in TABLES 6 and 7. There is a decrease in the incidence of benign tumors among females of the two treated groups (dose-related), and of malignant tumors among females treated at the higher dose. Such a decrease appears to be related to the higher mortality in the treated groups.

The incidence of testicular Leydig cell tumors increases sharply in rats treated with the higher dose TABLE 8. The increase was statistically significant at the $p <$ 0.05 level.

MTBE causes a dose-related increase in lymphomas and leukemias among female rats (TABLE 9). The fluctuation in the expected incidence of these neoplasias among female Sprague-Dawley rats in our historical controls is currently in a range below

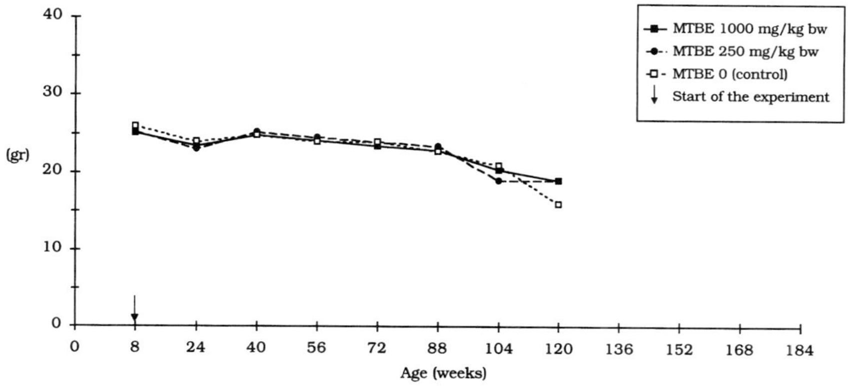

FIGURE 3. Mean daily feed consumption in male rats.

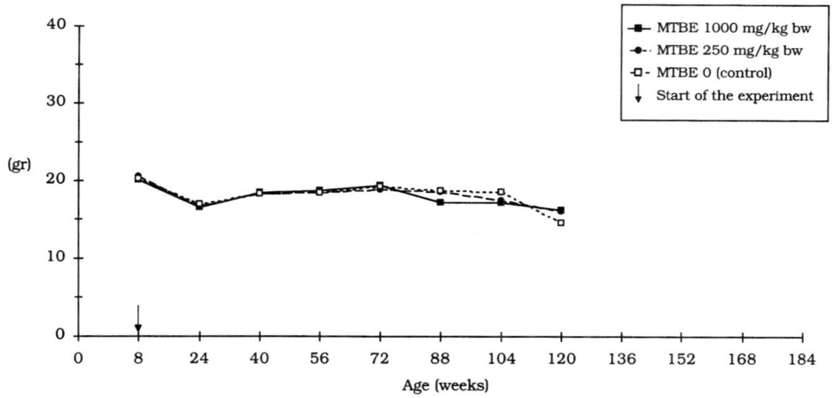

FIGURE 4. Mean daily feed consumption in female rats.

10%. The incidence of lymphomas and leukemias in male Sprague-Dawley rats, which is slightly lower among animals exposed to the higher dose of MTBE, is within the range of the expected fluctuations in the historical controls. The increase in the females was highly significant ($p < 0.01$) at the higher dose level and marginally significant ($p < 0.1$) at the mid-dose level.

An increase in dysplastic proliferation of lymphoreticular tissue was found in female rats treated with MTBE at both doses (TABLE 10). The term *dysplastic proliferation of lymphoreticular tissue* defines a hyperplastic lymphoid tissue, at various sites, in which atypical lymphoid cells (usually lymphoimmunoblasts), isolated and/or aggregated in small clusters, are observed. The incidence of this type of change is higher among animals treated at the lower dose. This apparently paradoxical effect

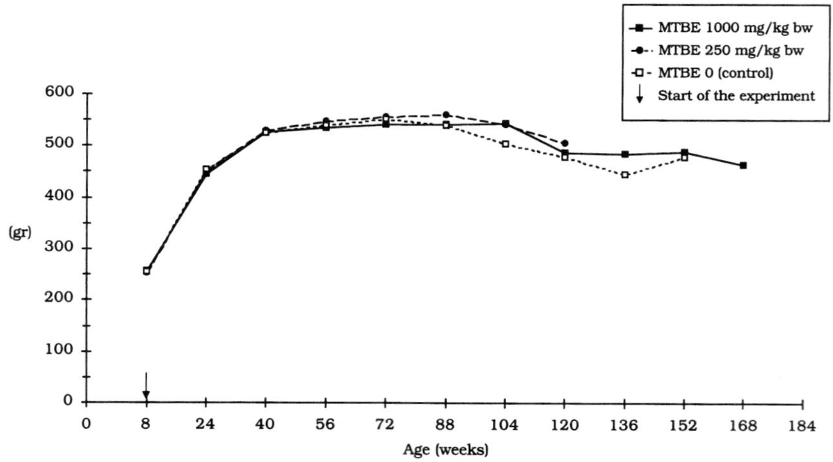

FIGURE 5. Mean body weight in male rats.

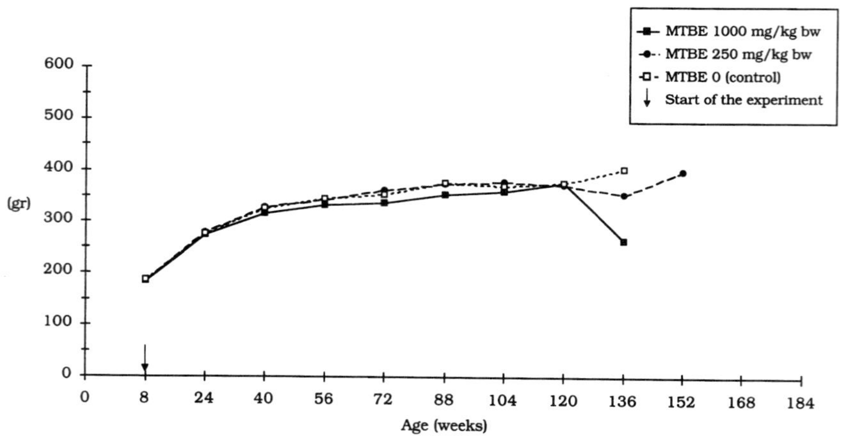

FIGURE 6. Mean body weight in female rats.

is probably due to the fact that most of these dysplastic proliferations might have developed into lymphomas and leukemias among female rats treated at the higher dose.

An increased incidence of uterine sarcomas was observed in female rats exposed to the lower dose.

The incidence of all the other tumors at various sites was in the range of the expected fluctuations. A dose-related decrease in mammary fibromas and fibroadenomas, and in pituitary adenomas and tumors of adrenal glands was observed in treated female animals; this effect may be due to the increased dose-related early mortality

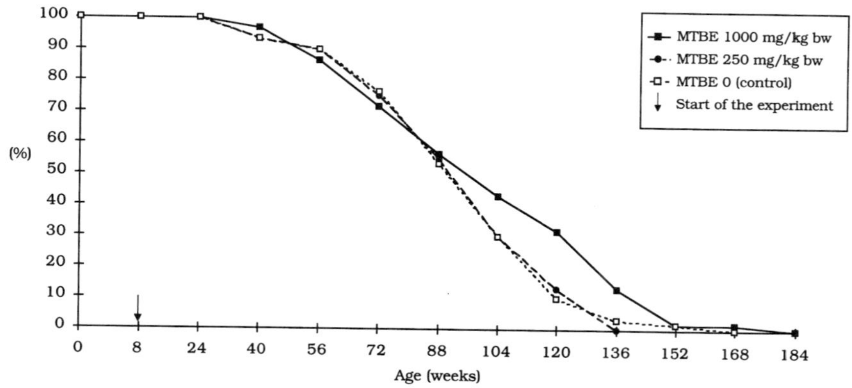

FIGURE 7. Survival of male rats.

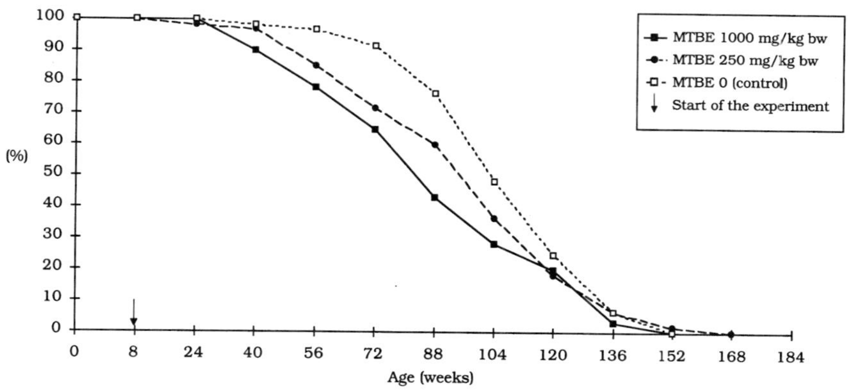

FIGURE 8. Survival of female rats.

caused by the treatment with MTBE, since the incidence of these tumors is age-dependent in our colony of Sprague-Dawley rats.

CONCLUSIONS

On the basis of the presented data, and with reference to the tested conditions, one must conclude:

(1) MTBE causes in males an increased incidence of Leydig cell testicular tumors, and in females an increased incidence of leukemias and related

TABLE 4. Long-term Carcinogenicity Bioassays on Methyl-Tertiary-Butyl-Ether (MTBE), Administered by Stomach Tube to Sprague-Dawley Rats (Experiment BT 958): Number and Percentage of Male Sprague-Dawley Rats Bearing Various Types of Benign and Malignant Tumors

		Groups					
		I: 1000 mg/kg b.w.		II: 250 mg/kg b.w.		III: 0 [a] (control)	
Site	Histotype	No.	%	No.	%	No.	%
Subcutaneous tissue	Fibroma	1	1.7	0	-	1	1.7
	Lipoma	1	1.7	0	-	0	-
	Liposarcoma	1	1.7	0	-	0	-
Mammary gland	Fibroma	3	5.0	2	3.3	1	1.7
	Fibrolipoma	0	-	1	1.7	0	-
	Lipoma	0	-	0	-	1	1.7
	Adenocarcinoma	1	1.7	1	1.7	1	1.7
	Liposarcoma	0	-	0	-	1	1.7
Zymbal glands	Carcinoma	2	3.3	1	1.7	3	5.0
Ear ducts	Carcinoma	3	5.0	3	5.0	2	3.3
Nasal cavities	Olfactory neuroblastoma	0	-	0	-	1	1.7
Oral cavity, lips, and tongue	Carcinoma	2	3.3	1	1.7	0	-
Larynx	Squamous cell carcinoma	0	-	1	1.7	0	-
Lung	Fibroangioma	0	-	0	-	1	1.7
	Adenocarcinoma	0	-	0	-	1	1.7
Liver	Fibroangioma	0	-	1	1.7	0	-
	Hepatocarcinoma	1	1.7	2	3.3	0	-
Pancreas	Islet cell adenoma	5	8.3	2	3.3	4	6.7
	Exocrine adenocarcinoma	1	1.7	0	-	0	-
Kidneys	Adenoma	2	3.3	1	1.7	1	1.7
Prostate	Adenocarcinoma	0	-	1	1.7	0	-
Testes[b]	Leydig cell tumor	11	18.3	2	3.3	2	3.3
Pituitary gland	Adenoma	10	16.7	9	15.0	11	18.3

TABLE 4. Long-term Carcinogenicity Bioassays on Methyl-Tertiary-Butyl-Ether (MTBE), Administered by Stomach Tube to Sprague-Dawley Rats (Experiment BT 958): Number and Percentage of Male Sprague-Dawley Rats Bearing Various Types of Benign and Malignant Tumors (*Continued*)

		Groups					
		I: 1000 mg/kg b.w.		II: 250 mg/kg b.w.		III: 0 [a] (control)	
Site	Histotype	No.	%	No.	%	No.	%
Thyroid gland	C-cell adenoma	1	1.7	2	3.3	4	6.7
	C-cell carcinoma	1	1.7	0	-	0	-
Adrenal glands	Cortical adenoma	0	-	1	1.7	1	1.7
	Pheochromocytoma	20	33.3	13	21.7	13	21.7
	Pheochromoblastoma	1	1.7	1	1.7	0	-
Central nervous system							
Brain	Oligodendroglioma	3	5.0	2	3.3	3	5.0
	Neuroblastoma	0	-	1	1.7	0	-
Meninges	Meningioma	0	-	1	1.7	0	-
Bones							
Cranium	Osteosarcoma	1	1.7	2	3.3	3	5.0
Soft tissues	Liposarcoma	0	-	1	1.7	0	-
Heart	Malignant Schwannoma	0	-	0	-	1	1.7
Subcutaneous lymph nodes	Fibroangioma	0	-	1	1.7	0	-
Hemolymphoreticular tissues[c,d]	Lymphomas and leukemias	7	11.7	9	15.0	10	16.7

[a] Olive oil alone.
[b] See TABLE 8.
[c] Including subcutaneous lymph nodes.
[d] See TABLE 9.

TABLE 5. Long-term Carcinogenicity Bioassays on Methyl-Tertiary-Butyl-Ether (MTBE), Administered by Stomach Tube to Sprague-Dawley Rats (Experiment BT 958): Number and Percentage of Female Sprague-Dawley Rats Bearing Various Types of Benign and Malignant Tumors[a]

		Groups					
		I: 1000 mg/kg b.w.		II: 250 mg/kg b.w.		III: 0 [b] (Control)	
Site	Histotype	No.	%	No.	%	No.	%
Skin	Dermatofibroma	0	–	1	1.7	1	1.7
	Squamous cell carcinoma	0	–	0	–	1	1.7
Subcutaneous tissue	Lipoma	1	1.7	0	–	0	–
Mammary gland	Fibroma and fibroadenoma	14 (16)	23.3	20 (27)	33.3	25 (41)	41.7
	Fibrolipoma	1	1.7	0	–	0	–
	Adenocarcinoma	2	3.3	4 (6)	6.7	4	6.7
	Carcinosarcoma	0	–	1	1.7	0	–
Zymbal glands	Carcinoma	2	3.3	0	–	2	3.3
Ear ducts	Acanthoma	1	1.7	0	–	0	–
	Carcinoma	0	–	0	–	4	6.7
Oral cavity, lips and tongue	Acanthoma	1	1.7	0	–	2	3.3
	Odontoma	0	–	0	–	1	1.7
	Carcinoma	0	–	2	3.3	1	1.7
Larynx	Squamous cell carcinoma	0	–	1	1.7	0	–
Pharynx	Squamous cell carcinoma	1	1.7	0	–	0	–
Lung	Fibroangioma	0	–	1	1.7	0	–
Stomach							
Forestomach	Acanthoma	3	5.0	2	3.3	1	1.7
Liver	Cholangiofibroma	0	–	1	1.7	0	–
Pancreas	Exocrine adenoma	1	1.7	2	3.3	1	1.7
	Islet cell adenoma	2	3.3	1	1.7	1	1.7
Kidneys	Lipoma	0	–	0	–	1	1.7
Ovaries	Granulosa cell tumor	1	1.7	3	5.0	0	–
	Granulosa and theca cell tumor	0	–	0	–	1	1.7
	Fibroma	1	1.7	0	–	0	–

TABLE 5. Long-term Carcinogenicity Bioassays on Methyl-Tertiary-Butyl-Ether (MTBE), Administered by Stomach Tube to Sprague-Dawley Rats (Experiment BT 958): Number and Percentage of Female Sprague-Dawley Rats Bearing Various Types of Benign and Malignant Tumors[a] (*Continued*)

		Groups					
		I: 1000 mg/kg b.w.		II: 250 mg/kg b.w.		III: 0 [b] (control)	
Site	Histotype	No.	%	No.	%	No.	%
Uterus	Polyp	12	20.0	12	20.0	13	21.7
	Fibroma	0	—	2	3.3	1	1.7
	Fibroangioma	1	1.7	0	—	0	—
	Granular cell tumor (Abrikossoff's tumor)	0	—	2	3.3	0	—
	Sarcoma	0	—	5	8.3	1	1.7
Uterus and vagina	Sarcoma	0	—	0	—	1	1.7[c]
Peritoneum	Lipoma	0	—	0	—	3	5.0
Pituitary gland	Adenoma	13	21.6	16	26.7	22	36.7
Thyroid gland	Follicular cell adenoma	2	3.3	0	—	0	—
	C-cell adenoma	3	5.0	10	16.7	5	8.3
Adrenal glands	Cortical adenoma	3	5.0	6	10.0	5	8.3
	Pheochromocytoma	10	16.7	11	18.3	18	30.0
	Cortical adenocarcinoma	0	—	4	6.7	3	5.0
	Pheochromoblastoma	0	—	0	—	2	3.3
Central nervous system							
Brain	Oligodendroglioma	0	—	0	—	1	1.7
Meninges	Meningioma	0	—	1	1.7	0	—
Bones							
Cranium	Osteosarcoma	1	1.7	0	—	1	1.7
Mesenteric lymph nodes	Fibroangioma	0	—	1	1.7	0	—
Hemolymphoreticular tissues[d,e]	Lymphoma and leukemias	12	20.0	6	10.0	2	3.3

[a] The numbers in parentheses are the numbers of tumors (one animal can bear more than one tumor).

[b] Olive oil alone.

[c] This sarcoma involved both uterus and vagina.

[d] Including mesenteric lymph nodes.

[e] See TABLES 9 and 10.

TABLE 6. Results of Long-term Carcinogenicity Bioassays on Methyl-Tertiary-Butyl-Ether (MTBE), Administered by Stomach Tube to Sprague-Dawley Rats (Experiment BT 958): Total Benign Tumors

				Benign Tumors			
		Animals		Animals Bearing Tumors		Tumors	
Group No.	Dose (mg/kg b.w. in Olive Oil)	Sex	No.	No.	%	No.	Per 100 Animals
I	000	M	60	34	56.7	54	90.0
		F	60	40	66.7	72	120.0
		M + F	120	74	61.7	126	105.0
II	250	M	60	26	43.3	36	60.0
		F	60	43	71.7	99	165.0
		M + F	120	69	57.5	135	112.5
III	0[a]	M	60	26	43.3	40	66.7
		F	60	49	81.7	117	195.0
		M + F	120	75	62.5	157	130.8

[a] Olive oil alone.

TABLE 7. Results of Long-term Carcinogenicity Bioassays on Methyl-Tertiary-Butyl-Ether (MTBE), Administered by Stomach Tube to Sprague-Dawley Rats (Experiment BT 958): Total Malignant Tumors

Group No.	Dose (mg/kg b.w. in Olive Oil)	Animals		Malignant Tumors			
				Animals Bearing Tumors		Tumors	
		Sex	No.	No.	%	No.	Per 100 Animals
I	1000	M	60	20	33.3	24	40.0
		F	60	16	26.7	18	30.0
		M + F	120	36	30.0	42	35.0
II	250	M	60	23	38.3	26	43.3
		F	60	19	31.7	25	41.7
		M + F	120	42	35.0	51	43.0
III	0[a]	M	60	25	43.3	26	43.3
		F	60	22	36.7	23	38.3
		M + F	120	47	39.2	49	40.8

[a] Olive oil alone.

TABLE 8. Results of Long-term Carcinogenicity Bioassays on Methyl-Tertiary-Butyl-Ether (MTBE), Administered by Stomach Tube to Sprague-Dawley Rats (Experiment BT 958): Leydig Cell Testicular Tumors

Group No.	Dose (mg/kg b.w. in Olive Oil)	No. at Start	Corrected Number[a]	Animals Bearing Leydig Cell Tumors		
				No.	%[b]	%[c]
I	1000	60	32	11	18.3	34.4[d]
II	250	60	25	2	3.3	8.0
III	0[e]	60	26	2	3.3	7.7

[a] Alive male rats at 96 weeks of age, when the first Leydig cell tumor was observed.
[b] Percentages are of the number at start.
[c] Percentages are of the corrected number.
[d] $p < 0.05$.
[e] Olive oil alone.

TABLE 9. Results of Long-term Carcinogenicity Bioassays on Methyl-Tertiary-Butyl-Ether (MTBE), Administered by Stomach Tube to Sprague-Dawley Rats (Experiment BT 958): Lymphomas and Leukemias

		Male					Female				
				Animals Bearing Lymphomas and Leukemias					Animals Bearing Lymphomas and Leukemias		
Group No.	Dose (mg/kg b.w. in Olive Oil)	No. at Start	Corrected Number[a]	No.	%[c]	%[d]	No. at Start	Corrected Number[b]	No.	%[c]	%[d]
I	1000	60	58	7	11.7	12.0	60	47	12	20.0	25.5[e]
II	250	60	59	9	15.0	15.3	60	51	6	10.0	11.8[f]
III	0[g]	60	59	10	16.7	16.9	60	58	2	3.3	3.4

[a] Alive male rats at 32 weeks of age, when the first leukemia was observed.
[b] Alive female rats at 56 weeks of age, when the first leukemia was observed.
[c] Percentages are of the number at start.
[d] Percentages are of the corrected number.
[e] $p < 0.01$.
[f] $p < 0.1$.
[g] Olive oil alone.

TABLE 10. Results of Long-term Carcinogenicity Bioassays on Methyl-Tertiary-Butyl-Ether (MTBE), Administered by Stomach Tube to Sprague-Dawley Rats (Experiment BT 958): Dysplastic Proliferation of Lymphoreticular Tissues (DPLT) at Various Sites

Group No.	Dose (mg/kg b.w. in Olive Oil)	Animals: Sex	Animals: No. at Start	Animals: Corrected Number[a]	Animals Bearing DPLT: No.	Animals Bearing DPLT: %[b]	Animals Bearing DPLT: %[c]
I	1000	F	60	59	9	15.0	15.3
II	250	F	60	59	15	25.0	25.4
III	0[d]	F	60	60	1	1.7	1.7

[a] Alive female rats at 26 weeks of age, when the first DPLT was observed.
[b] Percentages are of the number at start.
[c] Percentages are of the corrected number.
[d] Olive oil alone.

changes, and also an increase of uterine sarcomas (observed only at the lower tested dose);

(2) MTBE must therefore be considered carcinogenic in experimental animals.

On the basis of our data, further scientific information on the carcinogenicity of this industrially and commercially important compound are needed. The result of the ongoing research of the experimental project of the Cancer Research Center of our Foundation will provide supplementary data. In our opinion, however, as of now, MTBE must be considered potentially carcinogenic for humans.

SUMMARY

Methyl-*tert*-butyl ether (MTBE) was submitted to long-term carcinogenicity bioassays on Sprague-Dawley rats. The test compound was delivered in olive oil by stomach tube (gavage), at the doses of 1000, 250, and 0 mg/kg b.w. to groups of 60 males and 60 females, once daily, 4 times weekly, for 104 weeks. All animals were kept under control until spontaneous death.

MTBE was found to cause in males an increased incidence of Leydig cell testicular tumors in the group treated with the higher dose, and in females a dose-related increase of leukemias, an increase of dysplastic proliferations of lymphoreticular tissues, and also an increase of uterine sarcomas at the lower tested dose.

On the basis of the presented data, MTBE must be considered a potential carcinogen.

REFERENCES

1. BELPOGGI, F., M. SOFFRITTI & C. MALTONI. 1995. Methyl-tertiary-butyl ether (MTBE). A gasoline additive causes testicular and lymphohematopoietic cancers in rats. Toxicol. Ind. Health **11:** 119–149.
2. HOEL, D. G. & H. E. WALBURG. 1972. Statistical analysis of survival experiments. J. Natl. Cancer Inst. **49:** 361–372.
3. MANTEL, N. 1966. Evaluation of survival data on two new rank order statistics arising in its consideration. Cancer Chemother. Rep. **50:** 163–170.
4. COX, D. R. 1972. Regression models and life-tables (with discussion). J. R. Stat. Soc. B. **24:** 187–220.

Methyl Tertiary-Butyl Ether Antibodies among Gasoline Service Station Attendants

ARISTO VOJDANI,[a,b,c] GALAL NAMATALLA,[c] AND NACHMAN BRAUTBAR[d]

[b]*Immunosciences Lab., Inc.*
Beverly Hills, California 90211

[c]*Division of Dermatology*
Department of Medicine
Drew University School of Medicine and Science
Los Angeles, California 90059

[d]*Department of Medicine*
University of Southern California School of Medicine
Los Angeles, California 90059

INTRODUCTION

Methyl tertiary-butyl ether (MTBE) $(CH_3)_3C\text{-}O\text{-}CH_3$ is currently being used in many areas of the United States as an oxygenated additive in gasoline. This compound, along with other oxygenates such as methanol and ethanol, is being used to replace aromatics for reducing carbon monoxide and reactive evaporative and exhaust emissions, which lead to the formation of ozone in urban atmospheres.[1] MTBE is removed in the atmosphere by reaction with OH through a very complex mechanism. Through this complex mechanism t-butyl formate (TBF), formaldehyde, and 2-methoxy-2-methyl propanol (MMP) are produced.[2] The atmospheric oxidation of MTBE can be summarized in the following formulas:

$$\underset{\text{MTBE}}{CH3OC\ (CH_3)_3}+NO+OH \longrightarrow \underset{\text{TBF}}{HCOOC\ (CH_3)_3}+\underset{\text{MMP}}{CH3OC\ (CH_3)_2\ CHO}+H2O+NO2$$

$$CH_3OC\ (CH_3)_2\ CHO+OH+2NO \longrightarrow \underset{\text{FORMALDEHYDE}}{H_2CO} + \underset{\text{ACETONE}}{(CH_3)_2\ CO} + H2O+2NO2$$

In general, 60-70% of MTBE is converted to unreactive TBF, while the remaining 30-40% produces highly reactive MMP.[1,3] Other products such as formaldehyde acetone and methylacetate were detected.[4] TBF, which is a major degradation product in the urban setting, is considered to be inert; therefore, the mechanism of its atmo-

[a]Address for correspondence: Aristo Vojdani, Ph.D., M.T., Immunosciences Lab., Inc., 8730 Wilshire Boulevard, Suite 305, Beverly Hills, California 90211. Phone: 310/657-1077; fax: 310/657-1053.

spheric oxidation has been suggested to be unimportant.[1,2] While TBF and other degradation products in the urban setting are considered inert, immunologically these products may be reactive.

For example, TBF $CH_3\text{-}C(CH_3)_2\text{-}O\text{-}C(=O)\text{-}H$ as a hapten via the aldehyde group may bind to carrier protein(s) and induce antibody production against the haptenic group and the carrier proteins. The increased life of MTBE was associated with symptomatology of sinus congestion, headaches, skin rashes, and in some cases shortness of breath.[5,6] The mechanism for the induced symptomatology is not clear. Recently, Hutcheon *et al.*[7] suggested that repeated low-level exposures to MTBE may cause adverse health effects as a result of the intracellular release of its metabolites. Some of these metabolites, such as formaldehyde, have been shown to cause allergic reactions, skin rashes, shortness of breath, and immunological activation in the form of formaldehyde antibodies.[8] Pharmacokinetic studies[7] and clinical observations[5,6] suggest a possible common denominator in the immune system. Therefore, this study was undertaken to examine the effects of MTBE exposure on the immunological mechanisms in individuals exposed to MTBE or its degradation products in gasoline stations.

MATERIAL AND METHODS

The study population included two groups. Group one consisted of 24 subjects (6 females and 18 males ranging in age from 21 to 58 years) who were employed for more than two years in gasoline service stations and were exposed to gasoline vapor and motor vehicle emissions. Group two consisted of healthy controls (4 females and 8 males 24–60 years of age) with no history of exposure to gasoline other than once a week pumping gasoline into vehicles. The normal controls were examined by a physician and were in good health; all their laboratory results were within the normal range. Informed consent was obtained from the subjects after explanation of the blood drawing procedure.

MTBE ANTIBODY ASSAY

An enzyme immunoassay was developed for evaluation of antibodies against MTBE by preparation and coating of plates with two different conjugates.

Preparation of MTBE-Protein Conjugates

MTBE-protein conjugates were prepared from trimethylacetic anhydride.[5] Trimethylacetic anhydride was prepared by mixing 40 g of trimethylacetic acid with 31.4 g of acetic anhydride and was refluxed gently for 2 hours. The mixture was distilled off under reduced pressure of .05 mm Hg at a temperature below 40°C, and another 30 g of acetic anhydride was added, with refluxing continued for two additional hours. Distillation under reduced pressure was repeated until no more distillate came off below 40°C. The remaining material in the distillation flask was transferred to an Erlenmeyer flask, and 50 ml of anhydrous diethyl ether was added. This was allowed to stand at 5°C overnight for precipitation. The precipitate was collected by filtration and washed with a small amount of an anhydrous solution of benzene-hexane (1 : 2 by volume).

The trimethylacetic anhydride (55 mg) was dissolved in 7 ml of absolute ethanol and was added slowly, over 15 minutes, to a 20-ml solution of BSA or HSA (120 mg) in 0.1 M PBS. The pH was maintained between 7 and 8 by the addition by drop of 0.5 M sodium hydroxide. This mixture was stored overnight at 5°C and then dialyzed in the cold 0.05-M sodium hydroxide and finally extensively against distilled water. After being freeze-dried, the conjugate was analyzed for trimethylacetic acid contents.[6] The MTBE-BSA conjugate contained 18 trimethylacetic acid residues per molecule of BSA, and MTBE-HSA contained 14 haptenic residues per molecule of HSA protein.

Duplicate wells of microplate (costar) either were coated with 100 μl of 100-μg/ml of BSA, HSA alone, or MTBE-BSA and MTBE-HSA dissolved in 0.1 M PBS pH 7.2. After 2 hours' incubation at 25°C and overnight at 4°C plates were washed, and nonspecific bonds were blocked by an addition of 200 μl of 2% BSA. The washing step was repeated, and plates were dried and kept at 4°C until used for the determination of antibody levels.

Serum was diluted 1:200 in 0.1 M PBS pH 7.2 containing 0.05% Tween 20 and 1% BSA or 1% HSA for determination of anti-MTBE-BSA or anti-MTBE-HSA conjugates, respectively. For each antibody 100 μl of diluted specimen was added to duplicate wells coated either with the protein alone or with MTBE-protein conjugate. After one hour incubation at room temperature, plates were washed four times with PBS-tween, then incubated for one hour with affinity-purified goat anti-human IgG, IgA, IgM, and IgE, conjugated with alkaline phosphatase. The wells were then washed four times with PBS-tween, and 100 μl of para-nitrophenyl phosphate (1 mg/ml) was added to each well. The color development was allowed to proceed for 45 minutes at room temperature and then stopped by the addition of 3 n NaOH. The intensity of the color was measured by microtiter reader at 405 nM, and results were expressed by optical densities (OD).

Specificity and Cross-Inhibition Studies

For determination of MTBE antibody specificity, a cross-inhibition study was undertaken. Five different sera with elevated antibodies against MTBE-BSA or MTBE-HSA were selected. Each serum (3 ml), diluted 1 : 10 in serum diluent buffer, was divided into three different tubes. To tube number one, 1 mg of BSA; to tube number two, 1 mg of MTBE-BSA; and to tube number three, 1 mg MTBE-HSA in 100 μl of 0.1-M PBS was added and incubated for 2 hours at 37°C and thereafter overnight at 4°C. After removal of precipitate by centrifugation and a final dilution of 1 : 200, the samples from before and after cross-inhibition were then placed on plates coated with MTBE-BSA or MTBE-HSA. The subsequent steps followed were as described above in the ELISA assay.

TABLE 1. Antibody Levels to Hapten MTBE in Sera of Patients Exposed to Gasoline Vapor Expressed by Optical Densities

Group I	MTBE-BSA				MTBE-HSA			
Samples	IgG	IgM	IgA	IgE	IgG	IgM	IgA	IgE
1	0.13	0.12	0.11	0.07	0.14	0.13	0.12	0.09
2	0.68	0.85	0.10	0.09	0.53	0.71	0.14	0.11
3	0.12	0.11	0.12	0.06	0.16	0.12	0.11	0.08
4	0.18	0.16	0.11	0.08	0.13	0.18	0.13	0.12
5	0.14	0.19	0.13	0.07	0.12	0.15	0.18	0.06
6	0.64	0.98	0.12	0.07	0.57	0.82	0.16	0.09
7	0.11	0.16	0.10	0.08	0.15	0.14	0.12	0.12
8	0.16	0.15	0.11	0.09	0.11	0.11	0.15	0.11
9	0.12	0.19	0.14	0.12	0.18	0.22	0.19	0.05
10	0.17	0.18	0.12	0.11	0.15	0.20	0.11	0.08
11	0.11	0.17	0.09	0.05	0.12	0.13	0.11	0.07
12	0.56	1.18	0.09	0.06	0.43	0.97	0.12	0.13
13	0.14	0.23	0.16	0.09	0.12	0.18	0.18	0.06
14	0.46	0.65	0.13	0.11	0.35	0.47	0.11	0.05
15	0.10	0.13	0.11	0.13	0.11	0.16	0.17	0.08
16	0.47	0.39	0.12	0.11	0.32	0.31	0.14	0.14
17	1.56	2.27	0.10	0.12	1.24	1.85	0.15	0.11
18	0.18	0.16	0.14	0.09	0.16	0.12	0.12	0.09
19	0.13	0.11	0.17	0.08	0.12	0.14	0.13	0.08
20	0.1	0.15	0.16	0.06	0.13	0.12	0.14	0.06
21	0.19	0.24	0.15	0.11	0.17	0.20	0.12	0.09
22	1.87	2.68	0.19	0.09	1.38	2.43	0.11	0.12
23	0.13	0.17	0.12	0.06	0.12	0.15	0.13	0.14
24	0.15	0.19	0.11	0.05	0.13	0.14	0.16	0.11

RESULTS

Different levels of anti-MTBE antibodies (IgG and IgM) were detected in 36 different specimens used in this study. Results of nonspecific binding against BSA or HSA were negligible since they were very close to optical densities of negative antibody samples (0.05-0.15). In group one, which consisted of 24 subjects with a history of exposure to gasoline vapor and motor vehicle emissions, seven individuals (samples 2, 6, 12, 14, 16, 17, and 22) exhibited 3-15-fold elevation in antibody levels against MTBE-BSA or MTBE-HSA. These antibodies were elevated only for IgG and IgM but not for IgA or IgE (TABLE 1). Samples that were found to be positive for IgG and IgM against MTBE-BSA were also positive against MTBE-HSA. The IgG or IgM antibodies against MTBE-BSA or MTBE-HSA were not detected in blood samples of 12 healthy controls (group 2), as shown in TABLE 2. Only in one sample (sample #33) were optical densities as high as 0.45 detected against MTBE-BSA.

An independent *t*-test was employed to examine the differences between levels of anti-MTBE antibodies for the control and patient groups. When exposed patients

TABLE 2. Antibody Levels to Hapten, MTBE in Sera of Healthy Controls Expressed by Optical Densities

Group 2	MTBE-BSA				MTBE-HSA			
Samples	IgG	IgM	IgA	IgE	IgG	IgM	IgA	IgE
25	0.11	0.14	0.08	0.05	0.12	0.11	0.09	0.11
26	0.13	0.09	0.07	0.09	0.11	0.16	0.11	0.12
27	0.24	0.28	0.11	0.10	0.26	0.29	0.12	0.13
28	0.09	0.15	0.12	0.11	0.16	0.15	0.11	0.10
29	0.16	0.13	0.11	0.07	0.17	0.14	0.10	0.08
30	0.16	0.12	0.10	0.09	0.14	0.15	0.09	0.11
31	0.13	0.11	0.08	0.07	0.13	0.12	0.08	0.09
32	0.08	0.07	0.09	0.05	0.11	0.14	0.12	0.10
33	0.45	0.42	0.12	0.14	0.39	0.36	0.07	0.09
34	0.11	0.14	0.11	0.12	0.16	0.14	0.15	0.08
35	0.16	0.12	0.13	0.10	0.18	0.15	0.13	0.11
36	0.10	0.11	0.08	0.07	0.12	0.11	0.09	0.07

were compared with the control, we showed a statistically significant difference between each mean group, indicating that patients are more likely to have higher levels of IgG and IgM anti-MTBE than their control counterparts ($p < 0.001$).

In addition to this test, a nonparametric test was also employed to reanalyze the data. All optical density results were recorded by grouping those subjects who had OD's higher than 0.3 against their counterparts with OD values of less than 0.3. Then using χ^2 we compared patients with control groups. Similar results were detected. In each χ^2 test, we found that patients were more likely than the control group to have OD's higher than 0.3.

Demonstration of Specificity of the Antibodies

Five different sera from the gasoline-exposed group were absorbed with high concentrations of either BSA, HSA, MTBE-BSA, or MTBE-HSA. The results depicted in FIGURE 1 show that absorption with MTBE-HSA was able to reduce the OD's against MTBE-BSA by more than 65% in all tested sera. This cross-inhibition was similar for both IgG and IgM values. When absorption was performed with MTBE-BSA and checked for IgG or IgM anti-MTBE-HSA, the results were similar to those presented in FIGURE 1. More than 65% inhibition of OD's was observed; BSA or HSA alone was unable to reduce the antibody levels of these sera.

Association between Anti-MTBE Levels of Antibodies and the Presence of Health Symptoms

In general, the 24 individuals in group one who worked in service stations as gasoline or car repair attendants presented one or more symptoms previously described

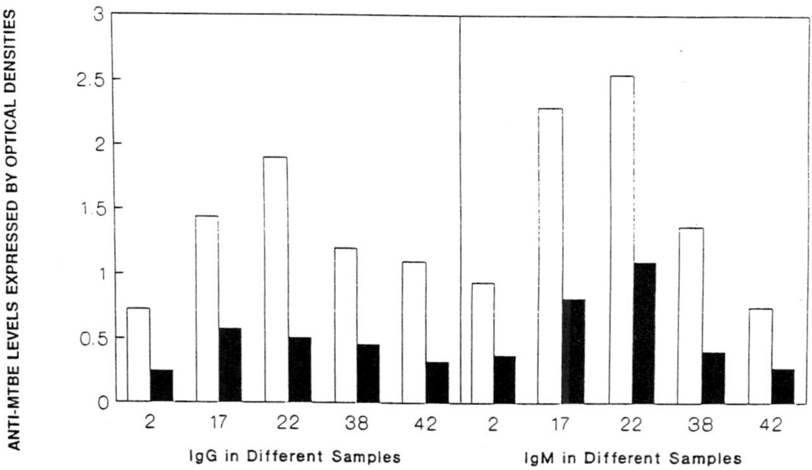

FIGURE 1. IgG or IgM anti-MTBE-BSA levels before ☐ and after ■ absorption with MTBE-HSA.

in MTBE-exposed patients[12,16] headaches; shortness of breath; burning eyes, nose, and throat; muscle weakness; fatigue; memory loss; and difficulty concentrating. However, antibody levels did not correlate with the number and severity of the reported symptomatologies. These antibodies were detected in both males and females with almost similar distribution.

DISCUSSION

Currently, a large research effort within the petroleum industry is devoted to developing new, more ''environment-friendly'' fuel formulations. A number of oxygen-containing compounds, such as alcohols and ethers, have been proposed as fuel additives. MTBA, a highly branched ether, is already used as a component of such formulations. Addition of MTBE to gasoline reduces the CO emissions. In addition to MTBE, ethyl *tert*-butyl ether (ETBE), diisopropyl ether (DIPE), and *tert*-amyl methyl ether (TAME) have been proposed for exploration. All these compounds have a comparatively high volatility, which makes their possible use as automotive fuel additives a potential source of emissions to the atmosphere. In 1993, MTBE was among the top 10 chemicals produced in the United States, with an annual production of 24,053 million pounds.[9]

While MTBE, ETBE, DIPE, and TAME and their decomposed products have been considered inert in atmosphere,[1,2] they may not be inert immunologically. Several studies have shown symptomatology suggestive of an immunological mechanism in these patients exposed to MTBE in gasoline.[5,6]

In 1993, state health officials in Connecticut invited the Centers for Disease Control (CDC) to assist in an investigation of exposure to MTBE in oxygenated gasoline.[6] Blood samples from 44 commuters and workers in the vicinity of traffic or automobiles were analyzed for the level of MTBE and other volatile organic compounds.[10–12] MTBE blood levels strongly correlated with personal breathing-zone and blood levels of other volatile organic compounds, such as benzene.[6,10]

Due to exposure to MTBE and its degraded products, a significant percentage of gasoline station employees, especially those who pump gas or work in a repair station, develop a variety of symptoms, including: skin irritation, severe headache, shortness of breath, chest pain, burning eyes, muscle weakness, fatigue, memory loss, difficulty in concentration, sleep disturbances, nausea, and intestinal disturbances. The mechanism mediating the symptomatology in those individuals exposed to MTBE and gasoline has not previously been studied.

Our study here of 24 individuals in group one with a history of exposure to gasoline vapor and motor vehicle emission show symptomatology previously described in MTBE-exposed patients.[5,6,10,11] Similar health complaints were reported by CDC in December 1992. Investigations in Fairbanks, Alaska suggested that the use of MTBE in oxygenated gasoline might be associated with such health complaints as headaches, eye irritation, and burning of the nose and throat.[5,13] Based on these observations and our results here, it is reasonable to propose the following chain of events: individuals with certain genetic makeup, after daily exposure to gasoline additives and their breakdown products, may develop some of the above symptomatologies and activation of the immune system, which in turn is associated with production of MTBE antibodies. Seven out of 24 subjects produced significant levels of IgG and IgM against MTBE (TABLE 1), while only 1 out of 12 in the control group produced some levels of MTBE antibodies.

The data presented in TABLE 1 and FIGURE 1 indicate that these antibodies are produced against the methyl or *tert* butyl group of MTBE $CH_3\text{-}\overset{\displaystyle CH_3}{\underset{\displaystyle CH_3}{\overset{|}{\underset{|}{C}}}}\text{-O-}CH_3$. Our data further suggests that anhydride of MTBE $(CH3)_3$ C-CO, after binding to the amino group of BSA or HSA, gave identical levels of antibodies whether the chemical group was bound to BSA or HSA (TABLE 1), further indicating the specificity to the methyl part of the molecule. The observation that MTBE-BSA absorption of positive sera was able to remove anti-MTBE-HSA antibodies and vice versa (FIG. 1) indicates a specificity to the methyl group of MTBE. These data indicate that MTBE exposure is associated with specific antibody response, which is probably mediated via the methyl group.

The role of antibody response to MTBE in any disease process requires additional studies. The documentation of specific antibody response to MTBE is one additional indicator of exposure and immune response. The observation that only 7 out of 24 exposed patients developed antibodies requires additional explanation. A reasonable explanation is that there may be a genetic predisposition that makes some individuals more susceptible than others. Indeed, genetic predisposition to xenobiotics has been described with other chemical exposures.[14] Future studies are required to address this question.

In conclusion our study shows that:

1. Individuals exposed to MTBE develop specific antibodies.
2. This response is specific to MTBE and is mediated via its methyl group.
3. Antibody response indicates exposure and activation of the immune system in individuals who may be more susceptible than others.
4. Antibody response to MTBE does not correlate with symptomatology.

SUMMARY

Occupational exposure to petroleum products (gasoline) and elevated blood levels of MTBE have been demonstrated among gasoline station attendants. While MTBE and its metabolites have been considered environmentally inert, immunologically these materials could be reactive.

This study was conducted to assess the immunological reactivity of humans to MTBE. Blood samples from 24 gasoline station attendants and 12 healthy controls were examined for levels of IgG, IgM, IgA, and IgE against MTBE by ELISA. In the gasoline-exposed group 7 out of 24 exhibited optical densities or antibody levels of 3-15-fold (OD 0.6-2.68) of the levels detected in controls (OD < 0.2).

The detected antibodies both against MTBE-BSA or MTBE-HSA were of IgG and IgM but not IgA or IgE isotypes. These antibodies at much lower levels (OD of 0.45) were detected in only 1 of the 12 healthy control groups. The specificity of these antibodies was evidenced by absorption of MTBE antibodies in different sera using the same haptenic group bound to a different carrier. These results indicate that immune reactions to MTBE do occur through hapten carrier reactions which, in some individuals, end with specific IgG and IgM production.

ACKNOWLEDGMENT

The authors wish to thank Ms. S. I. Haskins for her help in all aspects of transcription, editing, and structure.

REFERENCES

1. SMITH, D. F., T. E. KLEINDIENST, E. E. HUDGENS, C. D. MEIVER & J. J. BUFALINI. 1991. Photooxidation of methyl tertiary butyl ether. Int. J. Chem. Kinet. **23:** 907-924.
2. JAPAR, S. M., T. J. WALLINGTON, J. F. O. RICHERT & J. C. BALL. 1990. The atmospheric chemistry of oxygenated fuel additives: T-butyl alcohol, dimethyl ether, and methyl t-butyl ether. Int. J. Chem. Kinet. **22:** 1257-1269.
3. LANGER, S. & E. LJUNGSTROM. 1994. Reaction of the nitrate radical with some potential automotive fuel additives: A kinetic and mechanistic study. J. Phys. Chem. **98:** 5906-5912.
4. TUAZON, E. C., W. P. L. CARTER, S. M. ASCHMANN & R. ATKINSON. 1991. Products of the gas-phase reaction of methyl tert-butyl ether with the on radical in the presence of No_x. Int. J. Chem. Kinet. **23:** 1003-1015.

5. MOOLENAR, R. L., B. J. HEFFLIN, D. L. ASHLEY, J. P. MIDDAUGH & R. A. ETZEL. 1994. Methyl tertiary butyl ether in human blood after exposure to oxygenated fuel in Fairbanks, Alaska. Arch. Environ. Health **49:** 402-409.
6. WHITE, M. C., C. A. JOHNSON, D. L. ASHLEY, T. M. BUCHTA & D. J. PELLETIER. 1995. Exposure to methyl tertiary-butyl ether from oxygenated gasoline in Stamford, Connecticut. Arch Environ. Health **50:** 183-189.
7. HUTCHEON, D. E., J. D. ARNOLD, W. TEN HOVE & J. BOYLE III. 1996. Disposition, metabolism and toxicity of methyl tertiary-butyl ether: An oxygenate for reformulated gasoline. J. Toxicol. Environ. Health **47:** 453-464.
8. THRASHER, J. D., A. VOJDANI, G. CHEUNG & G. HEYER. 1987. Evidence of formaldehyde antibodies and altered cellular immunity in subjects exposed to formaldehyde in mobile homes. Arch. Environ. Health **42:** 347-350.
9. REISCH M. S. 1994. Top 50 chemicals production rose modestly last year. Chem. Eng. News **72:** 12-15.
10. NATIONAL INSTITUTE FOR OCCUPATIONAL SAFETY AND HEALTH. 1993. Health hazard evaluation report. National Center for Environmental Health, Stamford, Connecticut. HETA 93-802-2338. Centers for Disease Control and Prevention. Cincinnati, OH.
11. PALASSIS, J., R. W. HARTLE & J. L. HOLTZ. 1993. A method for determination of methyl tertiary-butyl ether in gasoline vapors and liquid gasoline samples. Appl. Occup. Environ. Hyg. **8:** 964-969.
12. ASHLEY, D. L., M. A. BONIN, F. L. CARDINALI *et al.* 1992. Determining volatile organic compounds in human blood from a large sample population by using purge and trap gas chromatography/mass spectrometry. Anal. Chem. **64:** 1021-1029.
13. ALASKA DEPARTMENT OF HEALTH AND SOCIAL SERVICES. 1992. Evaluation of health effects from exposure to oxygenated fuel in Fairbanks, Alaska. St. Alaska Epidemiol. Bull. No. 28. Fairbanks, AK.
14. DALY, A. K., S. CHOLERTON, M. ARMSTRONG & J. R. IDLE. 1994. Phenotyping for polymorphism in xenobiotic metabolism as a predictor of disease susceptibility. Environ. Health Perspect. Suppl. **9:** 55-61.

Scientific Update on Benzene[a]

URVASHI RANGAN[b] AND ROBERT SNYDER

Environmental Occupational Health Science Institute
681 Frelinghuysen Road
Piscataway, New Jersey 08855

INTRODUCTION

Benzene has been used in industrial applications since the 1800s. The first toxicity studies were described by Santesson[1] and Selling[2,3] as disrupting normal hematopoiesis in humans and animals. There have been several reports documenting bone-marrow hypoplasia and aplasia produced by benzene exposure.[4] Several reports of benzene-induced leukemia were made as early as the 1920s,[5,6] but characterizing the specific mechanism of toxicity will remain a challenge for the next century. Problems with exposure measurements in epidemiology studies and the lack of an animal model of benzene-induced leukemogenesis have prevented an accurate, dose-response assessment of toxicity. However, the advent of novel molecular biology techniques, improved analytical detection, biomarker identification, and stratification of clinical endpoints have greatly reduced the uncertainty regarding benzene-induced leukemia.

OVERVIEW OF BENZENE TOXICITY/LEUKEMOGENESIS

Over the past century, the chronic disease end points of benzene have typically been described as aplastic anemia or acute myeloid leukemia (AML). The progression of benzene toxicity was first observed in the workplace. The first signs of hematotoxicity, such as leucopenia, were reversible upon cessation of benzene exposure. However, prolonged exposure to high doses led to irreversible bone-marrow damage. Workers exposed to benzene solvent showed a range of hematotoxic effects including anemia, leucopenia, and thrombocytopenia.[4] Each of these is associated with the depression of one type of blood cell. In some cases, a depression in all types of blood cells results in pancytopenia, which is commonly associated with irreversible bone-marrow aplasia or aplastic anemia.

Benzene-induced AML is frequently, if not always, preceded by functional abnormalities in the bone marrow and in the growth of blood precursor cells well before the onset of leukemia. These abnormalities are heterogeneous but have been collectively described as a preleukemic syndrome[7] or myelodysplastic syndrome[8] (MDS). MDS is characterized by anemia, leukopenia, and thrombocytopenia in various combinations.

[a]This work was supported in part by the National Institute of Environmental Health Sciences under Grant ES-07148.

[b]Corresponding author. Phone: 908/445-3720; fax: 908/445-0119; e-mail: rangan@eohsi.rutgers.edu

It has been further suggested that MDS and AML represent a continuum of blood dyscrasias and should not be regarded as disparate disease endpoints,[7] whereas aplastic anemia and MDS display qualitatively distinct endpoints and appear to differ in origin.[9] In both cases, the bone marrow is ineffective in releasing mature white cells into the blood stream. In aplastic anemia, however, cells that are released from the bone marrow are normal in morphology. On the other hand, MDS patients display abnormal white cells in the bloodstream. In cases where the bone marrow does not undergo aplasia, the patient will frequently develop MDS. In almost every case of benzene-induced AML, a preleukemic (or MDS) state appears to precede the onset of overt leukemia.[10] This suggests that benzene-induced aplastic anemia may proceed to AML via an MDS phase.

Recent findings indicate that chromosomal abnormalities are most often associated with MDS and an increase in the *number* of chromosomal abnormalities is correlated with poorer prognosis and more rapid progression to AML.[11,12] There is evidence that aplastic anemia can be ''converted'' to MDS in patients undergoing intense immunosuppressive therapy.[13] Moreover, this change is frequently associated with the initiation of chromosomal abnormalities that are seen in MDS patients. There is no animal model of MDS, and therefore an understanding of the steps that link bone-marrow depression with leukemia must be established through mechanistic studies.

BENZENE METABOLISM AND TOXICITY

The weight of the evidence suggests that metabolism of benzene is critical for consequent toxicity.[4,14] The inhibition of benzene metabolism by toluene, a competitive inhibitor, results in a decrease of benzene metabolism and benzene-induced toxicity.[15] A decrease in liver metabolism by partial hepatectomy also reduces consequent toxicity, suggesting that primary benzene metabolism is important to toxicity.[16] In addition to hepatic metabolism, secondary metabolism of benzene metabolites can occur in bone marrow and exert tissue-specific toxicity that is associated with bone-marrow depression and damage.[17–22] Therefore, an understanding of the metabolic pathway of benzene is critical to fully understand a mechanism of toxicity.

Metabolic Pathway for Biotransformation

FIGURE 1 represents the Phase I metabolism of benzene in the liver. Benzene is oxidized by cytochrome P450 2E1 (CYP 2E1) to form a benzene oxide (which is in equilibrium with its oxepin form). This intermediate can be hydrated to form the dihydrodiol, leading to the formation of catechol. Alternatively, the benzene oxide can undergo rearrangement to form phenol. Phenol can then be hydroxylated to hydroquinone, which can then produce benzoquinone or 1,2,4-trihydroxybenzene (THB). Phenol can be hydroxylated to catechol, which can also form *o*-benzoquinone. In humans, THB appears to be formed primarily from hydroquinone.[23] All of these metabolites can undergo Phase II metabolism, which generally leads to excretion.[24] Metabolite-derived compounds measured in urine include glucuronide and sulfate conjugates, mercapturic acids, ring-opened metabolites, and DNA adducts.[24,25] Many of these have been investigated for use in monitoring workers exposed to benzene

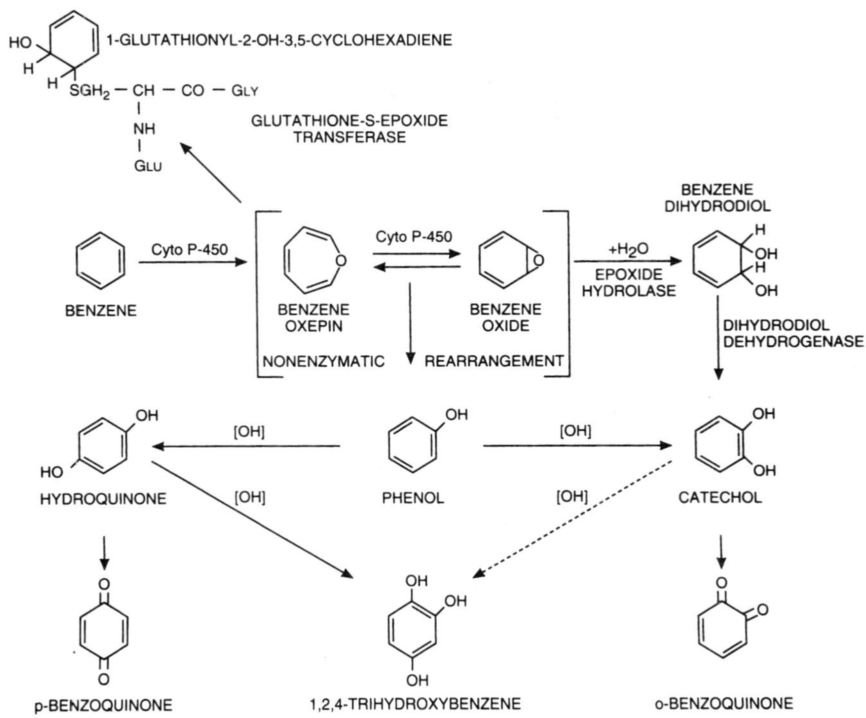

FIGURE 1. Phase I metabolism of benzene in the liver.

and are referred to as markers of exposure. However, liver perfusion studies from our laboratory suggest that some metabolites may escape Phase II metabolism, resulting in the release of free metabolites from the liver into the circulation.[26] Thus, free benzene metabolites may enter the bone marrow where the specific site of benzene toxicity is believed to occur. All of these metabolites continue to be studied for toxic potential and mechanism of action.

Benzene toxicity, which involves bone-marrow depression and leukemogenesis appears to be mediated through the metabolites of benzene. The targets of these metabolites are probably localized to the bone marrow to effect several cell types and a variety of functions. The relative potencies of each metabolite were described in a series of studies observing dose-related effects in mice on iron uptake by red blood cells as a measure of erythropoiesis[27] (TABLE 1). The numbers are not absolute values, but are indicative of the range of doses at which erythropoiesis may be significantly depressed. It is evident that although most of these metabolites are individually toxic, the synergy noted between metabolites is a likely explanation for the toxicity of benzene. Although THB was clearly ineffective in this study, it has tested positive in other benzene toxicity studies such as apoptosis in a human promyelocytic cell line (HL-60) and in human bone-marrow progenitor cells

TABLE 1. Relative Potencies of Benzene and Benzene Metabolites in Short-term Tests of Erythropoiesis[a]

Compound	Dose (mg/kg) (3 doses, 2 days)
Benzene	1000
Phenol	—
Hydroquinone sulfate	300
Hydroquinone	100
Catechol	100
6-OH-*t,t*-2, 4-hexadienal (CHO-M-OH)	20
Hydroquinone + phenol	10
Catechol + phenol	10
1,2,3-Benzenetriol	—
p-Benzoquinone	1
Muconaldehyde	1
Muconaldehyde + hydroquinone	0.05–0.01[b]

[a] Measured using the [^{59}Fe] uptake assay.
[b] Estimated value.

(CD34+).[28] THB has also been shown to cause DNA-adduct formation in murine bone marrow, *in vivo.*[29] In addition, it has been demonstrated to be a microsomal metabolite of benzene in the isolated mouse but not in rat hepatocytes.[15] This may contribute to the explanation of susceptibility variation to benzene toxicity in different species.

Many studies have looked at the potential toxicity mechanisms of these metabolites in the bone marrow. Irons and coworkers[13,30] suggested that covalent binding of hydroquinone to spindle-fiber protein could explain inhibition of cell replication by benzene. Consequent DNA damage could result in bone-marrow depression, leading to aplastic anemia, MDS, and AML.[31]

Oxidative stress or covalent binding (resulting in DNA alkylation) have been studied as two possible mechanistic explanations for benzene-induced MDS. Previous results from our laboratory suggest that hydroquinone (HQ) and trihydroxybenzene (THB) both cause depression in retinoic acid-induced differentiation of HL-60 cells, *in vitro.*[32] However, when levels of metabolite covalently bound to DNA were measured, the results showed that HQ-DNA adducts were found while THB-DNA adducts were not. On the other hand, both metabolites demonstrated modulation of oxidative stress levels in HL-60 cells. These data suggest that there may be at least two different pathways by which benzene exposure may lead to disease. One pathway involves the metabolic activation of benzene to species that covalently bind to DNA and produce mutagenicity expressed as leukemia. The second mechanism pertains to the production of metabolites that cause oxidative stress, which can damage DNA and lead to a mutagenic event with similar consequences.

Bone Marrow Targets of Benzene Metabolites

There are many stages in bone-marrow cell differentiation, maturation, and proliferation, including a number of functions unique to the stromal cells that provide targets for attack by benzene and its metabolites. These stages are regulated by various cytokines such as granulocyte/macrophage colony-stimulating factor (GM-CSF), granulocyte-colony stimulating factor (G-CSF), specific interleukins (IL), and leukotrienes (LT) that are involved in cell-signal transduction. The following studies have investigated the impact of benzene metabolites on specific cytokine-mediated pathways in hematopoiesis.

In one *in vitro* study, murine bone-marrow cells were pretreated with hydroquinone and subsequently stimulated with GM-CSF.[33] In normal bone marrow, GM-CSF will induce differentiation and maturation of specific myeloid progenitor cells to granulocyte/macrophage colony-forming units (CFU-GM). However, in this cell line, HQ and GM-CSF acted synergistically in forming CFU-GM, suggesting that progenitor cells previously unresponsive to GM-CSF were being recruited for differentiation to CFU-GM.

Kalf *et al.*[34–38] have conducted several *in vitro* studies investigating the disruption of cytokine-mediated pathways, by benzene and its metabolites, in a murine myeloid (32D) and HL-60 cell lines. The 32D myeloblasts were IL-3 dependent and G-CSF inducible for granulocytic differentiation. It was previously shown that short-term exposure of mice to benzene led to an increase in the total number of granulocyte progenitor cells and circulating granulocytes.[39]

In vitro studies in HL-60 and 32D cells indicated that this differentiation was mediated by the upregulation of LTD_4,[35] which mediates G-CSF in the terminal differentiation of granulocytes. In one study, HQ and *p*-BQ also upregulated granulocytic differentiation in normal murine myeloblasts.[34] Further characterization of this induction demonstrated that HQ could be oxidized to the more reactive *p*-BQ (most likely by bone marrow myeloperoxidase), and both can competitively bind to the LTD_4 receptor. In fact, *p*-BQ is capable of replacing LTD_4 induction of terminal granulocytic differentiation, whereas HQ seems to induce limited differentiation arresting at the myelocyte stage. Since the overproduction of bone-marrow cells is characteristic of MDS and AML, the potential role of apoptosis in benzene toxicity was investigated. Staurosporin, a protein kinase C (PKC) inhibitor, is typically used as a potent inducer of apoptosis *in vitro.* Stauroporin-induced apoptosis in myeloblast cells was inhibited with hydroquinone,[36] *in vitro,* which could explain the increase in the number of progenitor cells, *in vivo,* seen in mice exposed to benzene.[39]

Disruption of other cytokine pathways by benzene and its metabolites has also been investigated in stromal macrophages (another cell target of benzene toxicity) *in vitro.*[37] In murine and human stromal macrophage models, HQ by the oxidation to *p*-BQ has no effect on the translation or transcription of IL-1α nor IL-1β. However, there is significant inhibition of the proteolytic conversion of pre-IL-1α or pre-IL-1β to their respective active cytokine. Hydroquinone inhibits the calpain-mediated proteolytic conversion of pre-IL-1α to IL-1α in murine and human bone-marrow cells and also inhibits the IL-1β converting enzyme (ICE) in human marrow cells. The ability of these metabolites to bind to cytokine receptors and ultimately alter the fate of progenitor cells may play a role in the irreversible toxicity of benzene.[40]

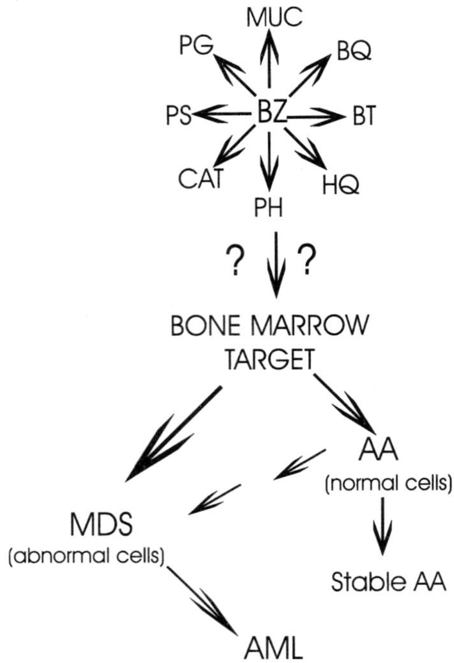

FIGURE 2. Generalized pathways for benzene toxicity.

Progression of Disease in Benzene Toxicity

FIGURE 2 depicts the generalized pathways for benzene toxicity. It is evident that benzene metabolites are most toxic to the bone marrow. Bone-marrow toxicity is an early sign of benzene toxicity that can manifest in aplastic anemia or myelodyplastic syndrome. Aplastic anemia can be, but is not always, associated with disease progression to MDS and AML. The association is related to the incidence of chromosomal abnormalities in hematopoietic cells. However, aplastic anemia may also remain stable without evidence of chromosomal anomalies.[41] When discussing benzene-initiated diseases, aplastic anemia must be separated from MDS and AML. The initiating event appears to be different for aplastic anemia, but not for MDS. These may be competing physiologic events that occur from the array of benzene metabolites. Exposed individuals with varied susceptibilities (including enzymatic and genetic) may also account for the difference seen in benzene-initiated disease.

The alteration of cytokines and other mediating pathways is likely to contribute to AA and MDS. The presence of chromosomal anomalies seems to be related to benzene-related MDS and AML and with progression of AA to MDS. Translocations may occur through inappropriate DNA maintenance. DNA topoisomerase II (topo II) is a sulfhydryl-dependent endonuclease required for DNA maintenance, including replication, recombination, chromosomal segregation, and chromosomal structure. *In vitro* studies of human placental topoisomerase II indicate that *p*-BQ interacts with sulfhydryl groups of topoisomerase II, thereby inhibiting enzymatic activity.[38]

There have also been studies looking at other putative benzene metabolites such as muconaldehyde (MUC) and its metabolic derivative, *trans-trans*-muconic acid. In CD-1 mice administered MUC for 16 days, similar bone-marrow depression effects were observed, such as hypocellularity and decreases in the number of red blood cells, lymphocytes, and significant increases in white blood cells mainly due to granulocyte proliferation.[42] These effects were comparable to those seen in benzene treated mice.

The potential pathways of benzene-induced toxicity multiplied by a variety of specific tissue, cell, protein, and DNA targets leads to a complicated dissemination and analysis of what metabolites are responsible for which potential endpoints that lead to the onset of AA, MDS, and AML. Bone-marrow toxicity is a common precursor of all three dysfunctions, but the lack of chromosomal aberrations seen in AA in contrast to MDS and AML suggest that more than one mechanism is responsible for the progression to disease. In addition, it is known that the bone marrow releases normal cells in AA and dysfunctional cells in MDS. Chromosomal translocations, cross-linking, and deletions seem associated with the MDS pathway and an abnormal bone-marrow cell production. If this is the case, what are the mechanisms responsible for benzene-induced aplastic anemia, where the marrow is severely depressed but the cells produced are normal? What causes some AA to convert to MDS while others remain stable? The degree of chromosomal damage seems to be associated with disease progression and poorer prognosis, but what initiates this cascade? The competing array of metabolites, variety of adverse bone-marrow effects, and susceptibility issues lie at the heart of characterizing benzene-related AA, MDS, and AML.

SUMMARY

The mechanism of benzene toxicity has been extremely difficult to fully characterize. Much progress has been made in assessing the relative potency of benzene metabolites but specific pathways to leukemia remain to be determined. Metabolite and mechanistic studies will have to focus on aplastic anemia and MDS and separate endpoints. This may serve to clarify the array of metabolite effects and consequent disparate effects. Biomarker research can contribute to the understanding of the toxicity process. The significance of understanding benzene toxicity will also lead to better clinical treatment of aplastic anemia and therapy-related MDS and AML, detection of populations particularly susceptible to benzene toxicity, screening of populations with suspected or unknown exposures, and determination of meaningful values for occupational and individual health risk while effectively monitoring ongoing exposures for early signs of toxicity.

REFERENCES

1. Santesson, C. G. 1897. Uber chronische vergiftung mit Steinkohlen-teerbenzin, vier Todesfalle. Arch. Hyg. Berlin **31:** 336.
2. Selling, L. 1910. A preliminary report of some cases of purpura haemorrhagica due to benzol poisoning. Bull. Johns Hopkins Hosp. **21:** 33.

3. Selling, L. 1916. Benzol as a leukotoxin. Studies on degeneration and regeneration of blood and hematopoietic organs. Bull. Johns Hopkins Hosp. **17:** 83.
4. Snyder, R. & J. J. Kocsis. 1975. Current concepts of chronic benzene toxicity. Crit. Rev. Toxicol. **3:** 265.
5. Mallory, T. B., E. A. Gall & W. J. Brickley. 1939. Chronic exposure to benzene (benzol). III. The pathogenic results. J. Ind. Hyg. Toxicol. **21:** 355.
6. Lignac, G. O. E. 1932. Benzene induced leukemia in humans and white mice. Klin. Wochenschr. **12:** 109.
7. Bagby, G. C., Jr. 1986. The concept of preleukemia: Clinical and laboratory studies. Crit. Rev. Oncol. Hematol. **4:** 203.
8. Tricot, G. J. K. 1991. The myelodysplastic syndromes. *In* Hematology, Basic Principles and Practice. R. Hoffman, E. J. Benz, Jr., S. J. Shatti, *et al.,* Eds.: 805. Churchill Livingstone. New York.
9. LeBeau, M. M. & R. A. Larson. 1991. Cytogenetics and neoplasia. *In* Hematology, Basic Principles and Practice. R. Hoffman, E. J. Benz, Jr., S. J. Shatti *et al.,* Eds.: 638. Churchill Livingstone. New York.
10. Irons, R. D. 1988. Studies on the mechanisms of chemically induced leukemia/lymphoma. Chem. Ind. Inst. Act. **8:** 1.
11. Oshaka, A., Y. Sugahara, Y. Imai, *et al.* 1995. Evolution of severe aplastic anemia to myelodysplasia with monosomy 7 following granulocytic colony-stimulating factor, erythropoietin and high-dose methylprednisolone combination therapy. Int. Med. **34**(9): 892.
12. Gonzalez-Barca, E., A. Domingo, A. Fernandez De Sevilla, *et al.* 1995. Clinical course of severe acquired aplastic anemia to myelodysplastic syndrome and acute leukosis. Med. Clin. **105**(6): 224.
13. Irons, R. D. & D. A. Neptun. 1980. Effects of principle hydroxy-metabolites of benzene on microtubule polymerization. Arch. Toxicol. **45:** 297.
14. Snyder, R., G. Witz & B. D. Goldstein. 1993. The toxicology of benzene. Environ. Health Perspect. **100:** 293.
15. Andrews, L. S., E. W. Lee, C. M. Witmer, *et al.* 1977. Effects of toluene on the metabolism, disposition, and hematopoietic toxicity of ^{3}H benzene. Biochem. Pharmacol. **26:** 293.
16. Sammett, D., E. W. Lee, J. J. Kocsis, *et al.* 1979. Partial hepatectomy reduces both metabolism and toxicity of benzene. J. Toxicol. Environ. Health **5:** 785.
17. Andrews, L. S., H. A. Sasame & J. R. Gilette. 1979. ^{3}H Benzene metabolism in rabbit bone marrow. Life Sci. **25:** 567.
18. Irons, R., J. Dent, T. Baker, *et al.* 1980. Benzene is metabolized and covalently bound in bone marrow *in situ.* Chem. Biol. Interact. **30:** 241.
19. Post, G., R. Snyder & G. F. Kalf. 1986. Metabolism of benzene and phenol in macrophages *in vitro* and inhibition of RNA synthesis by benzene metabolites. Cell Biol. Toxicol. **2:** 231.
20. Schlosser, M. J. & G. F. Kalf. 1989. Metabolic activation of hydroquinone by macrophage peroxidase. Chem. Biol. Interact. **72:** 191.
21. Subrahmanyam, V. V., P. Doane-Setzer, K. L. Steinmetz, *et al.* 1990. Phenol-induced stimulation of hydroquinone bioactivation in mouse bone marrow *in vivo:* Possible implications in benzene myelotoxicity. Toxicology **62:** 107.
22. Subrahmanyam, V. V., P. Kolanchana & M. T. Smith. 1991. Hydroxylation of phenol to hydroquinone catalyzed by a human myeloperoxidase-superoxide complex: Possible implications in benzene myelotoxicity. Free Radical Res. Commun. **15:** 285.
23. Inoue, O., K. Seiji, H. Nakatsuka, *et al.* 1989. Excretion of 1,2,4-benzenetriol in the urine of workers exposed to benzene. Br. J. Ind. Med. **46:** 559.
24. Snyder, R. & C. C. Hedli. 1996. An overview of benzene metabolism. Environ. Health Perspect. **104**(Suppl 6): 1165.

25. WITZ, G., Z. ZHANG & B. D. GOLDSTEIN. 1996. Reactive ring-opened aldehyde metabolites in benzene hematotoxicity. Environ. Health Perspect. **104**(Suppl 6): 1195.
26. HEDLI, C. C., M. J. HOFFMAN, S. JI, *et al.* 1997. Benzene metabolism in the isolated perfused mouse liver. Toxicol. Appl. Pharmacol. **146:** 60.
27. LEE, E. W., J. J. KOCSIS & R. SNYDER. 1981. The use of ferrokinetics in the study of experimental anemia. Environ. Health Perspect. **39:** 29.
28. MORAN, J. L., D. SIEGEL, X. M. SUN, *et al.* 1996. Induction of apoptosis by benzene metabolites in HL-60 and CD34+ human bone marrow progenitor cells. Mol. Pharmacol. **50**(3): 610.
29. PATHAK, D. N., G. LEVAY & W. J. BODELL. 1995. DNA adduct formation in the bone marrow of B6C3F1 mice treated with benzene. Carcinogenesis **16**(8): 1803.
30. PFEIFFER, R. W. & R. D. IRONS. 1983. Alteration of lymphocyte function by quinones through sulfhydril-dependent disruption of microtubule assembly. Int. J. Immunopharmacol. **5:** 463.
31. SNYDER, R. & G. F. KALF. 1994. A perspective on benzene leukemogenesis. Crit. Rev. Toxicol. **24**(3): 177.
32. HEDLI, C. C., N. R. RAO, K. R. REUHL, *et al.* 1996. Effects of benzene metabolite treatment on granulocyte differentiation and DNA adduct formation in HL60 cells. Arch. Toxicol. **70:** 135.
33. IRONS, R. D., W. S. STILLMAN, D. B. COLAGIOVANNI, *et al.* 1992. Synergistic action of the benzene metabolite hydroquinone on myelopoietic stimulating activity of granulocyte/macrophage colony-stimulating factor *in vitro.* Proc. Natl. Acad. Sci. USA **89:** 3691.
34. HAZEL, B. A. & G. F. KALF. 1996. Induction of granulocytic differentiation in myeloblasts by hydroquinone, a metabolite of benzene, involves the leukotriene D_4 receptor. Recept. Signal Transduc. **6:** 1.
35. HAZEL B. A., A. O'CONNOR, R. NICULESCU, *et al.* 1995. Benzene and its metabolite hydroquinone induce granulocytic differentiation in myeloblasts by interacting with cellular signaling pathways activated by granulocyte colony stimulating factor. Stern Cells **13:** 295.
36. HAZEL, B. A., C. BAUM & G. F. KALF. 1996. Hydroquinone, a bioreactive metabolite of benzene, inhibits apoptosis in myeloblasts. Stern Cells **14:** 730.
37. KALF, G. F., J. F. RENZ & R. NICULESCU. 1996. p-Benzoquinone, a reactive metabolite of benzene, prevents the processing of pre-interleukins-1α and -1β to active cytokines by inhibition of the processing enzymes, calpain, and interleukin-1β converting enzyme, Environ. Health Perspect. **104**(Suppl. 6): 1251.
38. HUTT, A. M. & G. F. KALF. Inhibition of human topoisomerase II by hydroquinone and p-benzoquinone, reactive metabolites of benzene. environ. Health Perspect. **104**(Suppl. 6): 1265.
39. DEMPSTER, A. M. & C. A. SNYDER. 1990. Short-term benzene exposure provides a growth advantage for granulocyte progenitor cells. Arch. Toxicol. **64:** 539.
40. IRONS, R. D. & W. S. STILLMAN. 1993. Cell proliferation and differentiation in chemical leukemogenesis. Stem Cells **11:** 235.
41. WHITE, J. R., K. M. JOSTEN, R. CHOPRA, *et al.* 1995. Absence of N-RAS point mutations in peripheral blood cells of patients with aplastic anemia and paroxysmal nocturnal haemoglobinurea. Br. J. Haematol. **91**(4): 921.
42. WITZ, G. W., G. RAO & B. D. GOLDSTEIN. 1985. Short-term toxicity of *trans-trans*-muconaldehyde. Toxicol. Appl. Pharmacol. **80:** 511.

Validation of Benzene Exposure Assessment

M. DOSEMECI,[a,c] N. ROTHMAN,[a] S.-N. YIN,[b] G.-L. LI,[b]
M. LINET,[a] S. WACHOLDER,[a] W.-H. CHOW,[a] AND
R. B. HAYES [a]

[a]*Division of Cancer Epidemiology and Genetics*
National Cancer Institute
Bethesda, Maryland 20892

[b]*Institute of Occupational Medicine*
Chinese Academy of Preventive Medicine
Beijing, China

INTRODUCTION

Benzene exposure has been related in numerous occupational studies to increased risk of acute myeloid leukemia (AML) and, in some reports, to other lymphohematopoietic malignancies.[1] Since 1987, the U.S. National Cancer Institute (NCI) has collaborated with the Chinese Academy of Preventive Medicine (CAPM) to study the health effects of benzene exposure in a large cohort of industrial workers in 12 cities in China. The study design and the extensive efforts to estimate historical exposures have been reported elsewhere.[2,3]

A relationship between benzene exposure and hematotoxicity has been recognized since 1862.[4] Benzene poisoning is a compensable condition in China,[5] and it provided the opportunity to examine the relationship between historical benzene exposure and the reported occurrence of benzene poisoning. We used these data and the strong association between benzene exposure and poisoning as an indirect means to validate the historical exposure-assessment procedure.

The validity of an exposure-assessment method used in an epidemiologic study is always a concern of investigators in the field.[6] Few studies have been carried out to validate assessment methods for specific exposures.[7–9] Usually, validation of an assessment method is carried out by comparing the estimated results with the results of actual monitoring data. Unfortunately, in retrospective exposure-assessment studies, we are not always able to validate historical estimates directly because of the lack of historical monitoring data. One way of solving this problem is to estimate current levels of exposure, using available information for selected settings,[6] and monitoring the current level of exposure for the same settings. An alternative approach is to use a well-established association between an exposure and an effect to validate

[c]Address for correspondence: Mustafa Dosemeci, Ph.D., Occupational Epidemiology Branch, Epidemiology and Biostatistics Program, National Cancer Institute, 6130 Executive Boulevard, Room 418, Rockville, Maryland 20852. Phone: 301/496-9093; fax: 301/402-1819; e-mail: DosemecM@EP-NDCE.NCI.NIH.GOV

the exposure-assessment method used in the study.[9,10] If a strong dose-response relationship is observed between the exposure and the disease, confidence in the exposure-assessment method increases.

This report presents the results of a validation study for a retrospective assessment procedure to evaluate historical benzene exposures that we used in a follow-up study of workers exposed to benzene in China.[8,9] The association between a clinical diagnosis of chronic benzene poisoning[5] and estimated historical benzene exposures[9] was used to evaluate the accuracy of the estimates developed from the assessment method.

METHODS

Exposure-Assessment Method Used in the Cohort Study

The general characteristics of the cohort are described elsewhere.[2] Historical estimates of benzene exposure since 1949 were developed for 74,828 workers employed in 672 benzene-exposed factories.[3] Exposure estimates were made for 18,435 factory/work unit (department)/job title/calendar-year time period combinations. Under the direction of the principal investigators at the CAPM and NCI, the field center directors and other senior collaborating occupational health personnel from each of the 12 field centers (Shanghai, Tianjin, Chengdu, Chongqing, Harbin, Shenyang, Jinzhou, Zhengzhou, Luoyang, Guangzhou, Nanchang, and Kaifeng) supervised all data-collection activities. Exposure data from factories and work history information on study subjects were collected from factory records by 370 abstractors in the 12 cities. Abstractors worked closely with work-unit supervisors, industrial hygienists, safety officers, and other long-term factory employees to identify the relevant historical exposure information.

The exposure assessment procedures included several steps: a study-specific standardized job-title dictionary focusing on the benzene-specific industries and occupations was developed for use in the collection of the work histories and historical exposure information. The large number of job titles of workers in Chinese benzene-producing or -using factories was classified into 60 benzene exposure-specific job-title categories in 11 major activity groups. The individual work history information abstracted from written factory records included the names of study factories, work units (department), and job titles held by subject, with starting and ending dates of each job. A job-title code was assigned to each job based upon the job-title dictionary. Historical exposure information was collected at each factory, using the following three forms: (1) *nonexposed factory form:* to collect information on exposure to other potential occupational risk factors for hematopoietic disorders in control factories with no benzene exposure; (2) *exposed factory form:* to collect factory-level exposure information in facilities where benzene was used or produced, including 8477 benzene measurements available since the 1950s; and (3) *exposed job-title form:* to collect exposure information at the job-title level for a total of 18,435 factory/work-unit/job-title/calendar-year combinations in seven time periods (1949-1959; 1960-1964; 1965-1969; 1970-1974; 1975-1979; 1980-1984; and 1985-1987). A factory exposure-assessment team consisting of industrial hygienists, safety officers, supervisors, and long-term employees used these data to develop a summary estimate of benzene exposure for each factory/work-unit/job-title/calendar-year combination. The estimate of benzene exposure level was developed in six concentration ranges (<1 ppm; 1-5 ppm; 6-10 ppm; 11-25 ppm; 26-50 ppm; and >50 ppm). A concentration range was assigned to each factory/work-unit/job-title/calendar-period combination.

We used the following strategies in estimating exposure to benzene: if benzene-monitoring data were consistent with the other descriptive exposure information, then the estimate was derived from the mean of the measurements after adjustment for the frequency of exposure to benzene. If there were no monitoring information for the specific work unit/job title/calendar period or if the measurement results were not consistent with the other exposure information, then monitoring results for similar job combinations were used after task-description comparisons and historical changes were considered. If there were no monitoring data for the similar job combination in the same calendar period, monitoring data for the same work-unit/job combination in other calendar periods were used, after adjustments for historical changes and exposure frequency. If none of the preceding sources were available for the given combination, the field center team used all available exposure information and their professional judgment to estimate the exposure level.

Following data collection and exposure assignment, all forms were sent to the data-editing and -processing center in Beijing. Machine editing, including logic and range checks, was carried out. Data were reviewed to resolve discrepancies between benzene exposure estimates and abstracted exposure information. Discrepancies between the completed work history forms and exposure data-collection forms were resolved by further data retrieval from the field centers. Various exposure indices were developed for each study subject by merging the work histories and the exposure information files, including the duration of exposure, intensity of exposure, and cumulative exposure.

Validation Study

The association between benzene exposure and clinical diagnosis of benzene poisoning has been used as an indirect validation of the exposure-assessment method. Duration of exposure, intensity of exposure, and cumulative exposure to benzene were the exposure variables and the diagnosis of benzene poisoning (BP) was the outcome variable. We abstracted historical information on benzene toxicity among benzene-exposed cohort members. Workers were screened for evidence of benzene-associated poisoning in factory clinics. Cases of BP were identified from factory records. Diagnosis required (1) white blood cell (WBC) count <4000 per mm^3 blood or WBC count between 4000 and 4500 per mm^3 blood and platelet count <80,000 per mm^3 blood, demonstrated in repeated blood tests performed over several months; (2) having worked in a factory with documented benzene exposure for at least six months; and (3) other causes of abnormal blood counts excluded.[11]

In the statistical analysis, subjects employed less than six months or those hired before 1949 were excluded. In addition, subjects from one city were excluded from the analyses, because we were unable to distinguish subjects with suspected benzene poisoning from subjects with chronic benzene poisoning. Person-years were accumulated after a 1.5-year lag from January 1, 1972 or from the first date of a benzene-

TABLE 1. Characteristics of the Validation Study Subjects by Gender

Characteristics	Men	Women	Total
Number of benzene poisoning subjects	171	241	412
Number of exposed subjects	32,055	30,179	62,234
Number of person-years	324,388	290,121	614,509

exposed job, whichever was later. Relative risks (RR) estimates, adjusted for age and sex, were obtained by Poisson regression analyses,[12] using EPICURE statistical analysis software.[13]

RESULTS

In total, there were 18,435 benzene exposure estimates, 38% based on monitoring data, primarily collected after 1975. The overall exposure levels for the seven time periods was 16.7 ppm, ranging from 20.4 ppm in the first period to 11.5 ppm in the last period, while the percentage of benzene in raw materials or products declined over the periods 1949–1959 to 1985–1987 from 40% to 28%.

Benzene exposure level varied by industry and occupation. The highest level of exposure to benzene was in the rubber–plastic industry (mean = 31 ppm), whereas the glass-products industry had the lowest exposure to benzene (mean = 6 ppm). The leather, chemical, and machinery industries showed similar exposure patterns (mean = 16 ppm, 14 ppm, and 15 ppm, respectively).

Like the findings for major industries, the highest benzene exposure was observed among rubber workers, especially among rubber glue applicators and vulcanizers with an average estimated exposure level of 53 and 41 ppm, respectively. Painters (spray, electrostatic, drip painters, and paint mixers), the largest occupational group in the cohort, had consistent exposure levels of about 20 ppm in the early years and 15 ppm in recent years. Chemical manufacturing workers (organic, insecticide, and benzene-production workers) showed variable exposure levels over the seven calendar-year periods, ranging between 38 ppm and 17 ppm.

Characteristics of the validation study are presented in TABLE 1. There were 412 benzene-poisoning cases among 62,234 exposed subjects (614,509 person-years) in 11 cities in China. TABLE 2 presents the results of the relative-risk analyses by various exposure indices. Relative risks of benzene poisoning increased with increasing duration of benzene exposure. Relative risks of benzene poisoning by duration of exposure are 1.3 (95%CI = 1.0–1.8), 1.6 (95%CI = 1.2–2.1), and 2.7 (95%CI = 1.9–3.9) for periods of 5–9 years, 10–19 years, and 20 and more years, respectively, compared to subjects who have less than five years of exposure to benzene. When we examined relative risks of BP by intensity of exposure at one and a half years prior to the diagnosis of benzene poisoning, compared to subjects who had less than 5 ppm exposure at that time, we obtained relative risks of 2.2 (95%CI = 1.7–2.9), 4.7 (95%CI = 3.4–6.5), and 7.2 (95%CI = 5.3–9.8) for intensity of 5–19 ppm, 20–

TABLE 2. Relative Risks of Benzene Poisoning by Duration of Exposure, Intensity of Exposure, and Cumulative Exposure

Duration of Exposure	<5 years	5-9 years	10-19 years	20 + years
Relative risk [*n*] (95% CI)	1.0 [92] —	1.3 [91] (1.0-1.8)	1.6 [148] (1.2-2.1)	2.7 [80] (1.9-3.9)
Intensity of Exposure[a]	<5 ppm	5-19 ppm	20-39 ppm	40 + ppm
Relative risk [*n*] (95% CI)	1.0 [109] —	2.2 [140] (1.7-2.9)	4.7 [58] (3.4-6.5)	7.2 [64] (5.3-9.8)
Cumulative Exposure	<40 ppm-years	40-99 ppm-years	100-399 ppm-years	400 + ppm-years
Relative risk [*n*] (95% CI)	1.0 [109]	1.7 [74] (1.3-2.3)	2.0 [128] (1.5-2.6)	2.4 [100] (1.8-3.2)

[a] Recent intensity of exposure (ppm) at 1.5 years prior to the diagnosis.

39 ppm, and 40 and more ppm categories. Relative risks of benzene poisoning by cumulative exposure to benzene are 1.7 (95% CI = 1.3-2.3), 2.0 (95% CI = 1.5-2.6), and 2.4 (95% CI = 1.8-3.2) for cumulative exposure of 40-99 ppm-years, 100-399 ppm-years, and 400 and more ppm-years, respectively, compared to subjects with cumulative exposure of less than 40 ppm-year.

DISCUSSION

We present a validation study for the retrospective exposure-assessment method that we used in a follow-up study of workers exposed to benzene in China. We were able to detect a very strong relationship between benzene and benzene poisoning using the assessment method that we used in the cohort mortality study. This suggests that our estimated exposure values are valid enough to detect the association between benzene exposure and hematotoxicity, and are reasonable measures to use in the evaluation of the relationship between benzene exposure and cancer risk. We observed higher relative risk with recent intensity than any other measure of exposure, suggesting that the level of recent exposure to benzene has more effect on risk of benzene poisoning than duration of exposure and cumulative exposure.

There are various advantages in conducting an occupational epidemiologic investigation in China, including the large number of study subjects, fewer jobs held per subject, fewer exposures per subject, easier access to factory records, standardized methods of recordkeeping utilized nationally, and administrative systems for tracing and follow-up. The average number of jobs held by a subject in the present study was 1.4, in contrast with 5-10 in most occupational studies in the United States.[14] Because Chinese workers hold fewer jobs than workers in western industrialized countries, the potential for confounding by other hazardous substances is reduced.

One of the limitations of the exposure assessment method used in this study was the lack of walk-through surveys by a single industrial hygiene coordinator. Clearly, this approach was impractical given the large number ($N = 672$) of study factories. Nevertheless, a standardized approach was developed and intensive training undertaken to use the experience of the individual factory industrial hygienists and safety officers. Another limitation was the lack of personal sampling for air monitoring. Nearly all of the benzene measurements were based on short-term area sampling. Although multicenter decision making may lead to differences in interpretation of the historical exposure information, every effort was made to standardize the assignment of exposure, including central training of the field center directors and centralized review procedures carried out at the CAPM and at NCI. Because of these limitations and the historical nature of the retrospective exposure assessment, exposure ranges were used rather than quantitative point estimates.

Several studies have compared the results of exposure estimates used by various investigators.[9,10,15–23] These comparisons were carried out to measure the agreement between raters,[15–17] between assessment methods,[18,19] between information sources,[20,21] or between exposure measures.[22,23] Most of these comparisons were carried out on estimates of exposures rather than their effects on risk estimates. Few investigators[9,10,22,23] have used relative risks of an outcome in the comparison process as we did in the present presentation.

In conclusion, the strong association observed between benzene exposure and benzene poisoning provides confidence in the validity of the method that we developed for the assessment of retrospective exposure to benzene in the cohort study of workers exposed to benzene in China.

SUMMARY

We conducted a methodologic study to validate a quantitative retrospective exposure assessment method used in a follow-up study of workers exposed to benzene. Assessment of exposure to benzene was carried out in 672 factories in 12 cities in China. Historical exposure data were collected for 3179 unique job titles. The basic unit for exposure assessment was a factory/work-unit/job-title combination over seven periods between 1949 and 1987. A total of 18,435 exposure estimates was developed, using all available historical information, including 8477 monitoring data. Overall, 38% of the estimates were based on benzene monitoring data. The highest time-weighted average exposures occurred in the rubber industry (30.7 ppm), particularly for rubber glue applicators (52.6 ppm). Because of its recognized link with benzene exposure, the association between a clinical diagnosis of benzene poisoning (hematotoxicity) and benzene exposure was evaluated (412 cases and 614,509 person-years) to validate the exposure-assessment method. Relative risks of benzene hematotoxicity increased very sharply with increasing estimated intensity of benzene exposure. Odds ratios were 2.2 (95% CI: 1.7-2.9), 4.7 (95% CI: 3.4-6.5), and 7.2 (95% CI: 5.3-9.8) for the intensity levels of less than 5 ppm, 5-19 ppm, 20-39 ppm, and 40 and more ppm, respectively. This sharp trend between benzene hematotoxicity and estimated exposure to benzene indicated that the exposure-estimation method used in this cancer epidemiology study is reliable.

REFERENCES

1. AKSOY, M. 1988. Benzene carcinogenicity. *In* Benzene Carcinogenicity, M. Aksoy, Ed.: 113-152. CRC Press. Boca Raton, FL.
2. YIN, S.-N., M. S. LINET, R. B. HAYES, G.-L. LI, M. DOSEMECI, Y.-Z. WANG, W.-H. CHOW, Z.-L. JIANG, S. WACHOLDER, W.-U. ZHANG, T.-R. DAI, X.-J. CHAO, X.-J. ZHANG, P.-Z. YE, Q.-R. KOU, J.-F. MENG, J.-S. ZHO, X.-F. LIN, C.-Y. DING, B. KNELLER & W. J. BLOT. 1994. A cohort study of benzene exposed workers in China: I. Method and resources. Am. J. Ind. Med. **26:** 383-400.
3. DOSEMECI, M., S.-N. YIN, R. HAYES, G. LI, M. LINET, R. KNELLER, W. H. CHOW, Z.-L. JIANG, S. WACHOLDER, W.-U. ZHANG, T.-R. DAI, X.-J. CHAO, X.-J. ZHANG, P.-Z. YE, Q.-R. KOU, J.-F. MENG, J.-S. ZHO, X.-F. LIN, C.-Y. DING, B. KNELLER & W. J. BLOT. 1994. A cohort study of benzene exposed workers in China. II: Exposure assessment. Am. J. Ind. Med. **26:** 401-411.
4. AKSOY, M. 1988. Benzene hematotoxicity. *In* Benzene Carcinogenicity, M. Aksoy, Ed.: 59-112. CRC Press. Boca Raton, FL.
5. YIN, S.-N., Q. LI, F. TIAN, C. DU & C. JIN. 1987. Occupational exposure to benzene in China. Br. J. Ind. Med. **44:** 192-195.
6. ULFVARSON, U. 1992. Validation of exposure information in occupational epidemiology. Am. J. Ind. Med. **21:** 125-132.
7. HERTZMAN, C., K. TESCHKE, H. DIMICH-WARD & A. OSTRY. 1988. Validity and reliability of a method for retrospective evaluation of chlorophenate exposure in the lumber industry. Am. J. Ind. Med. **14:** 703-713.
8. JOFFE, M. 1992. Validity of exposure data derived from a structured questionnaire. Am. J. Epidemiol. **135:** 564-570.
9. KIPEN, H. M., R. P. CODY & B. D. GOLDSTEIN. 1989. Use of longitudinal analysis of peripheral blood counts to validate historical reconstructions of benzene exposure. Environ. Health Perspect. **82:** 199-206.
10. DOSEMECI, M., J. K. MCLAUGHLIN, J.-Q. CHEN, Z. WU, F. HEARL, M. MCCAWLEY & W. BLOT. 1994. Indirect validation of a retrospective exposure assessment method used in a nested case-control study of lung cancer and silica exposure. Occup. Environ. Med. **51:** 136-138.
11. MINISTRY OF PUBLIC HEALTH IN CHINA. 1994. Diagnostic criteria and principles of management of occupational benzene poisoning. *In* Toxicological and Epidemiological Studies on Benzene in China, S.-N. Yin and G.-L. Li, Eds.: 198-201. Beijing.
12. BRESLOW, N. E. & N. E. DAY. 1987. Statistical Methods in Cancer Research. Vol. II. The Design and Analyses of Cohort Studies. International Agency for Research on Cancer. Lyon, France.
13. PRESTON, D. L., J. H. LUBIN, D. A. PIERCE & M. E. MCCONNEY. 1993. Epicure User's Guide. Hirosoft International Corporation. Seattle, WA.
14. STEWART, A. P., A. BLAIR, D. CUBIT, E. BALES, S. A. KAPLAN, J. WARD, W. GAFFEY, M. T. O'BERG & J. WALRATH. 1986. Estimating historical exposures to formaldehyde in a retrospective mortality study. Appl. Ind. Hygiene. **1:** 34-41.
15. GOLDBERG, M. S., J. SIEMIATYCKI & M. GERIN. 1986. Inter-rater agreement in assessing occupational exposure in a case-control study. Br. J. Ind. Med. **43:** 667-676.
16. KROMHOUT, H., Y. OOSTENDORP, D. HEEDERIK & J. S. M. BOLEIJ. 1987. Agreement between qualitative exposure estimates and quantitative exposure measurements. Am. J. Ind. Med. **12:** 551-562.
17. TESCHKE, K., C. HERTZMAN, H. DIMICH-WARD, A. OSTRY, J. BLAIR & R. HERSHLER. 1989. A comparison of exposure estimates by worker raters and industrial hygienists. Scand. J. Work Environ. Health **15:** 424-429.
18. DOSEMECI, M., P. A. STEWART & A. BLAIR. 1989. Evaluating occupation and industry separately to assess exposure in case-control studies. Appl. Ind. Hygiene **4:** 256-259.

19. SIEMIATYCKI, J., R. DEWAR & L. RICHARDSON. 1989. Cost and statistical power associated with five methods of collecting occupation exposure information for population-based case-control studies. Am. J. Epidemiol. **130:** 1236-1246.
20. COGGON, D., E. C. PIPPARD & E. D. ACHESON. 1985. Accuracy of occupational histories obtained from wives. Br. J. Ind. Med. **42:** 563-564.
21. ROSENBERG, C. R., M. N. MULVIHILL, A. FICHBEIN & S. BLUM. 1987. An analysis of the validity of self reported occupational histories using a cohort of workers exposed to PCBs. Br. J. Ind. Med. **44:** 702-710.
22. BLAIR, A. & P. A. STEWART. 1992. Do quantitative exposure assessment improve risk estimates in occupational studies of cancer? Am. J. Ind. Med. **21:** 53-63.
23. DOSEMECI, M., P. COCCO, M. GOMEZ, P. A. STEWART & E. F. HEINEMEN. 1994. Effects of three features of a job exposure matrix on risk estimates. Epidemiology **5:** 124-127.

Immune Function in n-Hexane–Exposed Workers

A. KARAKAYA,[a,b] B. YÜCESOY,[b] S. BURGAZ,[c] AND A. E. KARAKAYA[c]

[b]*Department of Toxicology*
Faculty of Pharmacy
Ankara University
06100, Tandoğan, Ankara

[c]*Department of Toxicology*
Faculty of Pharmacy
Gazi University
06330, Hipodrom, Ankara, Turkey

n-Hexane is commonly used as a solvent in various industries. It is produced during the cracking and fractional distillation of crude oil and is used in such applications as printing of laminated products; vegetable oil extraction; as a solvent in glues, paints, varnishes, and inks; as a diluent in the production of plastics and rubber; and as a minor component of gasoline. The National Institute for Occupational Safety and Health (NIOSH) estimates that approximately 2.5 million workers in the United States are potentially exposed to hexane annually.[1] Until recently, n-hexane and the other industrial hexacarbon solvents were thought to have little potential for hazard since their acute toxicity is quite low. Vapor concentrations of many hundreds of parts per million are tolerated for several minutes without causing discomfort among workers.[2] It is now recognized that the hexacarbons are capable of inducing polyneuropathy in both experimental animals and humans.

The neurotoxic effects of n-hexane, described in persons occupationally exposed to this solvent, have been associated with its principal metabolite 2,5-hexandione (2,5-Hxdn). 2,5-Hxdn is considered to be the ultimate neurotoxic agent. In addition to 2,5-Hxdn, other metabolites—5-hydroxy-2-hexanone, 2,5-hexanediol (2,5-Hxdl)—which are further biotransformed to 2,5-Hxdn, have been shown to possess relatively more neurotoxic potential than the parent compound.[3,4] The neurotoxic syndrome is the best described as a sensorimotor or motor polyneuropathy. The first cases of n-hexane polyneuropathy were reported in 1964 in Japan, then in Italy, Morocco, France, and the United States in the laminating process or in furniture or shoe factories, where workers were exposed for months, throughout the working day, to n-hexane levels in excess of 500 ppm.[5]

There is a close dynamic relationship between the nervous and immune systems, and there is also increasing evidence to show that the central nervous system controls

[a] Address for correspondence: Prof. Dr. Asuman Karakaya, Department of Toxicology, Faculty of Pharmacy, Ankara University, 06100, Tandoğan, Ankara, Turkey. Phone: 90-312/212-6805; fax: 90-312/213-1081; e-mail: karakaya@io.pharmacy.ankara.edu.tr

the activities of the immune system;[6] but very little information is available on the immunological effects of n-hexane and its metabolites in animals. Any indication of immunological impairment following chronic exposure to organic solvents is of great importance to occupational health. It has been suggested that organic solvents and their metabolites may be particularly important in this regard, since they may affect certain immunological parameters. Immunological effects of n-hexane and its metabolites have previously been reported in laboratory animals, but no evidence has been found about the immunological effects of occupational exposure to n-hexane in humans. The rodent studies indicated that 2,5-Hxdn and 2,5-Hxdl exposure can result in suppression of a variety of immune functions at different dose levels. Singh *et al.*[7] reported prominent atrophy of the thymus in rats given 2,5-Hxdl; and Kannan *et al.*[8] found that 2,5-Hxdl exposure caused impairment of immunocompetence affecting cell-mediated, humoral-mediated, and indirect immune responses in mice. 2,5-Hxdn also caused a severe dose-dependent thymic atrophy in rats following a single dose. In addition to thymic alterations induced by 2,5-Hxdn, a significant decline in the cellular population of spleen and mesenteric lymph node was encountered in rats exposed either to single or repeated doses.[9] Upreti and Shanker[10] also suggested that 2,5-Hxdn treatment caused profound impairment of immunity and altered host resistance in mice even before the onset of peripheral neuropathy.

n-Hexane is one of the most commonly used solvents in various leather and shoe-making industries in Turkey. The numbers of polyneuropathy cases caused by occupational exposure to n-hexane are still of concern in our country. In 1987 the diagnosis of polyneuropathy was reported in 20 workers; and in 1992 this diagnosis was reported in 25 workers in the manufacture of leather products (unpublished data). However, to our knowledge, the urinary 2,5-Hxdn levels of Turkish shoemakers potentially exposed to n-hexane have not been previously reported. At this point, we investigated time-weighted average (TWA) concentrations of the n-hexane in the breathing-zone air of some small shoe factories, total urinary 2,5-Hxdn concentrations of workers, and the chronic effects of n-hexane on white blood cell counts and serum immunoglobulin levels of the workers who are exposed occupationally to this solvent.[11] We studied a population of 35 workers employed in 7 small factories, where the jobs included use of glues and adhesives containing n-hexane. A total of 23 control samples were collected from age-matched subjects with no history of n-hexane exposure. We observed that the working conditions are unhealthy, with poor ventilation allowing exposure to occur through both inhalation and skin absorption. The TWA intensity of exposure to n-hexane at seven shoe factories ranged between 23–215 ppm (mean value 123 ppm). In another study of this group,[12] the mean TWA concentration of n-hexane in 12 shoe workshops was 126.1 ppm. A significant, but low, correlation ($r = 0.40$; $p < 0.001$) between TWA intensity of environmental exposure to n-hexane and the concentration of 2,5-Hxdn in urine was found. The value detected in the workplace does not exceed the threshold limit value in Turkey (500 ppm), which is rather high when compared to the limit values for other countries[13] (TABLE 1). The urinary 2,5-Hxdn levels appeared significantly higher in the exposed group than in the control group (mean values 2.39 vs. 0.41 $\mu g\ g^{-1}$ creatinine; $p < 0.001$).[11] There was no significant difference between the white blood cell counts in the two groups. Conversely, we observed a significant reduction in total serum IgG,

TABLE 1. Limits of Occupational Exposure to n-Hexane (IRPTC-1990)

Country	Exposure limit	Value	Effective Date
Belgium	TLV-TWA	50 ppm	1989
Finland	MPC-TWA	50 ppm	1989
Germany	MAC-TWA	50 ppm	1989
Italy	TLV-TWA	100 ppm	1985
Japan	MAC-TWA	40 ppm	1985
Romania	MPC-TWA	340 ppm	1975
United States	TLV-TWA	50 ppm	1990
Turkey	TLV-TWA	500 ppm	1973

NOTE: TLV = threshold limit value; TWA = time-weighted average.

IgM and IgA concentrations in n-hexane exposed workers, suggesting that chronic exposure of workers to n-hexane is associated with immunological changes.

In conclusion, available data from animal studies of short-term exposure to n-hexane are not sufficient to make a proper judgment of risk, because of the differences in dose, duration of exposure, and species. However, our findings do provide further evidence that n-hexane toxicity is not limited to the nervous system, but that it can also effect the immune system in humans. Further investigation of the exposed population would better define the nature and mechanism of the effect.

REFERENCES

1. LADOU, J. 1990. Occupational Medicine. Prentice Hall. Englewood Cliffs, NJ.
2. AMDUR, M. O., J. DOULL & C. D. KLAASSEN. 1991. Casarett and Doull's Toxicology. Pergamon Press. New York.
3. KRASAVAGE, W. J., J. L. O'DONOGHUE, G. D. DIVENCENZO, *et al.* 1980. The relative neurotoxicity of methyl n-butyl ketone, n-hexane and their metabolites. Toxicol. Appl. Pharmacol. **52:** 433-441.
4. SPENCER, P. S., H. H. SCHAMBURG, M. F. SABRI, *et al.* 1980. The enlarging view of hexacarbon neuropathy. Crit. Rev. Toxicol. **7:** 279-356.
5. GRAHAM, D. G., V. AMARNATH, W. M. VALENTINE, *et al.* 1995. Pathogenetic Studies of Hexane and Carbon Disulfide Neurotoxicity. Crit. Rev. Toxicol. **25:** 91-112.
6. MILLER, K., J. TURK & S. NICKLIN. 1992. Principles and Practice of Immunotoxicology. Blackwell Scientific Publications. London.
7. SINGH, K. P., K. KANNAN, S. K. GOEL, *et al.* 1983. 2,5-Hexanediol induced thymic atrophy and lymphocytotoxicity in rat. Ind. Health. **21:** 235-242.
8. KANNAN, K., K. P. SINGH, S. K. GOEL, *et al.* 1985. Effect of 2,5-hexanediol on immunocompetence of mice. Environ. Res. **36:** 14-25.
9. UPRETI, R. K., K. P. SINGH, A. K. SAXENA, *et al.* 1986. Effect of 2,5-hexanedione on lymphoid organs of rats: A preliminary report. Environ. Res. **39:** 188-198.
10. UPRETI, R. K. & R. SHANKER. 1987. 2,5-Hexanedione-induced immunomodulatory effect in mice. Environ. Res. **43:** 48-59.

11. Karakaya, A., B. Yücesoy, S. Burgaz *et al.* 1996. Some immunological parameters in workers occupationally exposed to n-hexane. Hum. Exp. Toxicol. **15:** 56–58.
12. Burgaz, S., İ. Çok, L. Ulusoy, *et al.* 1997. Biological monitoring of n-hexane exposure in shoe workers. Biomarkers. **2:** 25–28.
13. IPCS International Programme on Chemical Safety. 1991. n-Hexane. EHC 122. WHO. Geneva.

Industrial Contamination with Glycol Ethers Resulting in Teratogenic Damage

DOLORES SAAVEDRA,[a,b] MANUEL ARTEAGA,[c] AND MARTHA TENA[a]

[a]*Research Division*
Dr. Manuel Gea González General Hospital
México 14000, D.F., México

[c]*Faculty of Medicine*
University Nacional Autónoma de México
and
School of Medicine
Panamerican University
México, D.F., México

INTRODUCTION

There is no doubt that this century has witnessed great technological innovations and a great deal of industrial progress, all of which has modified in an important manner life on this planet. This progress has brought many great benefits; on the other hand, there have been some changes in our environment that are harmful to our health in both the short and long run. In order to reduce these problems, some programs have been started all around the world.

At the labor level, this industrial progress has increased worker exposure to different chemical and physical agents, some of which have a known noxious effect. Generally, knowledge of these harmful actions and the consequences of exposure to these industrial agents has been acquired only after serious accidents in the workplace that have exposed the problem and are the basis for the preventative measures that have to be taken to keep new cases from occurring.

Nevertheless, no matter how conscientiously we try to make the environment healthy, in only a very few cases is the fetus considered to be susceptible to pollution. Some environmental agents are capable of crossing the placental barrier and entering the embryo, causing structural, functional, or biochemical abnormalities that will result in congenital malformations and/or psychomotor retardation. All the agents capable of modifying intrauterine development are known as teratogens.

The purpose of this paper is to report a case of worker contamination that took place about 20 years ago in the city of Matamoros in the state of Tamaulipas, Mexico,

[b] Address for correspondence: Dra. Dolores Saavedra Ontiveros, Subdirección de Investigación, Hospital General "Dr. Manuel Gea González," Calzada de Tlalpan 4800, México 14000, D.F., México. Phone: 666-6021; fax: 528-1747; e-mail: schavira@mail.internet.com.mx

which up to now has not been reported, that describes a new human teratogenic syndrome, which has been confirmed by animal experimentation.

MATERIALS AND METHODS

A protocol was undertaken in three consecutive stages: (1) epidemiological; (2) clinical; and (3) experimental.

Epidemiological Trial

A field study was carried out on patients of the Municipal Medical Service of Matamoros, Tamaulipas, Mexico, to determine the characteristics of the affected population and to discover their hygienic-dietetic habits, working history, and medical records. A possible source of environmental pollution was studied in an effort to determine if it was implicated as a risk factor or etiological agent in producing the mental and physical damage in the study group.[1]

A "case-and-control" study was done to determine if there was any strong association between the supposed factors involved and the subject phenotype. Finally, the affected families were studied to determine the teratogenic behavior of the agents involved.[2–4]

Clinical Study

A clinical study was performed by a multidisciplinary group at the Dr. Manuel Gea Gonzalez General Hospital in Mexico City. The affected families were transferred to the hospital where they could be examined by the hospital specialists and the various laboratory tests needed to evaluate the damage and to profile the syndrome were done free of charge for the patients and their mothers.

Experimental Study

The experimental study was a controlled blind study[3,4] using 90 pregnant Wistar rats, which were divided into two groups: (1) control, and (2) experimental. When the rats reached their twenty-first day of gestation, the fetuses were delivered by cesarean section to evaluate their weight, size, and external and internal morphology. The fetuses were then decapitated and prepared in paraffin for the central nervous system histopathological study; 4-μm incisions were made and dyed with hematoxilin-eosin, bodian, and fast blue.

Control Group

The control group was subdivided into two subgroups:

A_1 (n = 20), which were administered 0.5 mL of saline solution every 24 h from the eighth to the twentieth day of gestation. The saline solution was administer orally (n = 10) and intraperitoneally (n = 10).

A_2 (n = 10), for which no procedures were done.

Experimental Group

The experimental group was also divided into two subgroups:

B_1 *(n = 30),* which were administered 0.5 mL of methyl cellosolve (MC) diluted at 5%, 10%, or 20% in the two different ways: oral (n = 15) or intraperitoneal (n = 15).

B_2 *(n = 30),* which were also administered 0.5 mL of ethylene glycol (EG) diluted at 5%, 10%, or 20% in the oral (n = 15) or intraperitoneal (n = 15) ways.

RESULTS

Epidemiological Trials

In the municipal medical service of Matamoros there were 134 patients who were followed up because they manifested some congenital malformations with or without mental retardation. Among them, 44 youngsters of both sexes were found to have certain peculiar facial features that resembled those of others in the group more than they did family members, they also exhibited varying degrees of mental retardation.

All 44 patients studied were born locally between April 1971 and September 1977, and they were all offspring of working mothers who were employed by an American company located in the town since 1970 and that operated continuously until it closed in April 1977. The company produced radio and television capacitors.

These factory workers were in constant direct contact with two organic solvents: methyl cellosolve (HO-CH_2-CH_2-O-CH_3) and ethylene glycol (HO-CH_2-CH_2-OH),[5,6] through cutaneous, oral, and respiratory routes, because during workdays the workers kept their hands in the liquid solvents without the protection of gloves or masks. This was in the "wet assembling department," where the containers holding the concentrated solvents were kept open, and the fumes were inhaled because there was no ventilation and no extractors in the factory (FIG. 1). In addition, the solvents could have been ingested when the workers had their meals with their hands still wet from the solvents because they did not wash them. These conditions existed even while they were pregnant.

The workers sometimes suffered to varying degrees from symptoms of intoxication,[7,8] from strong headaches or cutaneous rash to repeated vomiting with dehidratation, temporal loss of conciousness and coma; in the severe cases, intrahospital treatment was needed. However, the medical community did not detect the problem at that time because the affected workers were given care in several medical centers in nearby cities. A significant increase in the number of abortions or stillborns was also not detected.

Several other kinds of contamination, such as radiation, heavy metals, or pesticides, were discharged.

A case-control study was started, dividing the affected patients at the municipal medical center into two subgroups: all the patients with peculiar facies, and as a "control," the patients with any other kind of congenital malformation or mental retardation. We considered as "exposed" all the mothers who were in direct contact during their pregnancy with EG and MC in their work, and as " nonexposed" the

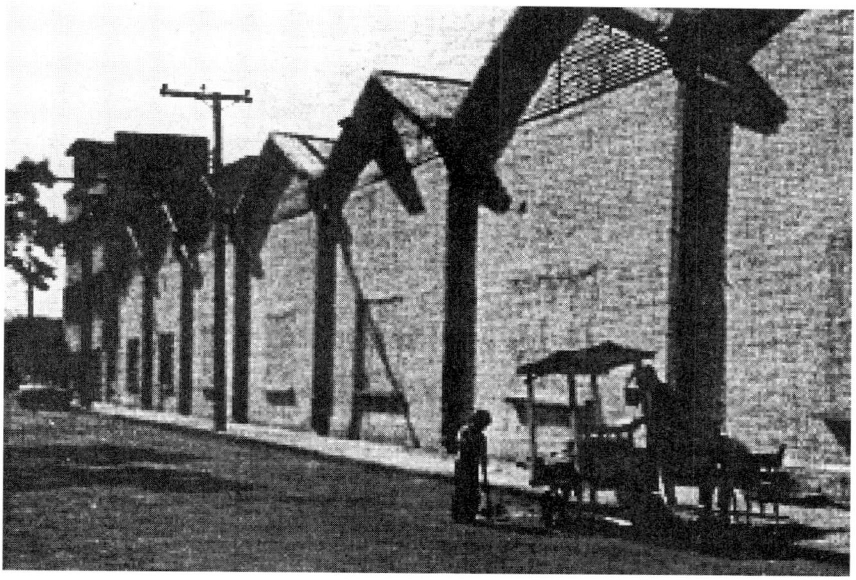

FIGURE 1. External view of the factory, where lack of ventilation or extracts was noted. This picture was taken with an Instamatic camera and given to us by an exworker.

mothers working in the nearby factories, but who were not in direct contact with any such organic solvents during their pregnancy.

We found in this group that the "exposed" mothers had affected children, and that all patients with the peculiar facies were offspring of mothers who had been exposed. On the other hand, the opposite situation was not found. All this suggests a causal relation more than a risk factor.

Of the 44 patients described, 32 were the only ones affected in their families, the remaining 12 came from 5 families, 4 of which accounted for 2 siblings each, and one of which had the remaining 4 siblings.

The clinicoepidemilogical study of the affected families proved that the solvents EG and MC involved in this incident had a teratogenical outcome, because: (a) the patients had a similar nondescribed phenotype (they resembled each other more than they did their own families); (b) there was a relation between the length of exposure during the pregnancy and the different degrees of fetal affection; (c) there was a relation between the mothers' susceptibility (determined by the symptoms caused by exposure to the solvent, with or without pregnancy) and the degree to which their children were affected (the severity of their physical and mental damage); and (d) a metabolic tolerance was observed in those workers who had more than one pregnancy during the time they worked in the factory (the first pregnancy resulted in a child with a more pronounced illness than did the subsequent pregnancies, even though the time of exposure was the same).

Clinical Study

Of the 44 patients, 22 were males and 22 were females, born between 1971 and 1977. Except in the five families that had more than one affected member, none of the patients had congenital malformations or similar phenotypes in their family backgrounds. The personal medical histories revealed different degrees of psychomotor and language retardation in all of the cases, and most of them had lachrymal duct obstruction and/or a history of repetitive medial otitis.

Clinical and Paraclinical Findings

Twenty-two patients, chosen at random from the 44 detected, were sent to Mexico City by the municipal authorities in order to be studied by specialists at the Dr. Manuel Gea González General Hospital.

During the general examination varying degrees of mental retardation were noted, as well as the peculiar facies. Numerous musculoskeletal abnormalities were found in all cases. Although height was normal in all cases, the weight/mass ratio was abnormal in two cases: one suffering from second-degree malnutrition, and the other from obesity. The routine laboratory tests including liver function, thyroid function, electrocardiogram, chest X rays, and ultrasonographic scanning, were normal, except for a megacolon in one case. The chromosomal study done by the GTG banding technique was normal in all patients.

The craniofacial genetic evaluation confirmed the following abnormalities: low or abnormal hair line implantation in the forehead, palpebral fissures with mongoloid obliquity; epicanthus, telecanthus, and hypertelorism; retrusion of the middle third of the face; and mandibular prognathism, but the most significant feature was a wide nose, mainly at the base. Also noted, though less frequently, arched or clefted palate and small or displasic ears were observed (FIG. 2a and 2b).

In orthopedics, a ligamentary hyperlaxity, vertebral malposition, static foot alterations, and structural malformations of the bone structures of the hand, hip, and spine were found in all cases, and with less frequency head antepulsion, short neck with mobility limitation, esternocleidomatoid hypertrophy, and limb shortening. Only two patients had severe muscular atrophy. The different X rays confirmed the structural abnormalities in the spine, hips, hands, and foot (FIG. 2c and 2d).

The Ophthalmology Department found ametropya in the great majority of patients as well as ocular motility alterations, and with less frequency corneal pathology of the iris and conjunctival illness.

The otorrhynolaryngology exam showed mild to moderate clinical hypoacusia, narrow external canal (<4 mm), impacted earwax, perforated tympanic membrane, and, with less frequency, cholesteatoma. Tonal audiometry showed hearing loss in the canal, and this was confirmed in 50% of the patients. The impedanciometry was also abnormal in half of the cases. On the other hand, the evoked auditory potentials were normal in all cases. The ear CT scan confirmed the clinically observed stenosis of the external canal and showed an enlarged jugular vein in those patients.

In orthodontics, the anterior wide bite was confirmed in all patients. The AP and lateral cephalometry confirmed the growth pattern alterations, resulting in craniofacial

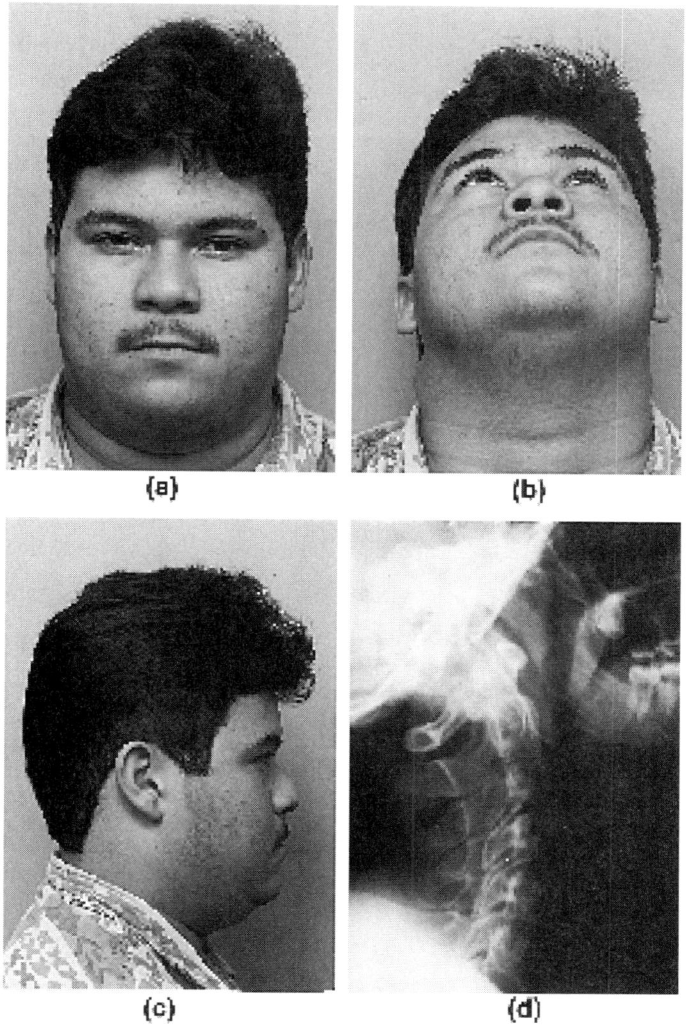

FIGURE 2. Clinical findings. **(a)(b)(c)** Affected patient showing the typical facial appearance; a wide nose and short and retruded middle third of the face are noted, as well as mandibular gonial angles and short neck. **(d)** X ray of cervical spine showing vertebral fussion.

disproportions. The orthopantomography showed abnormal dental structures in the great majority of the patients.

The phoniatry evaluation reported in the majority of cases multiple dyslalias and deficient compensatory abilities, and less frequently severe language retardation and compensatory articulation.

In the psychological sphere, all patients showed simple perpetual interpersonal dysfunctions, such as maternal dependency, shyness, and insecurity.

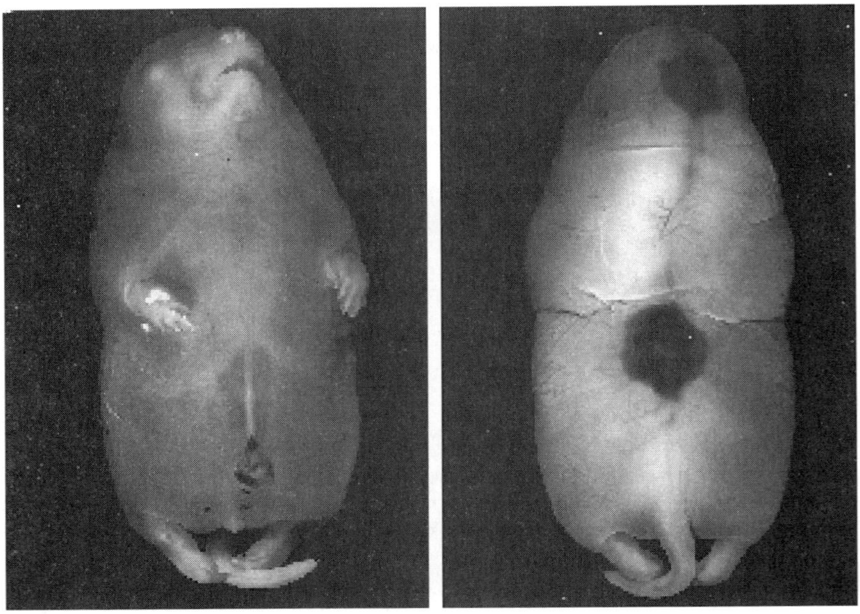

FIGURE 3. Rat fetus treated with EG showing small rounded cranial shape, ocular fibrosis, dysplastic ears, short nose, short mandible, macroglosia, pseudoterigium coli, cutis aplasia, and oligodactily.

The Neurology Department demonstrated alterations in the higher mental functioning in all patients. Some experienced diminished muscular tone and strength and alterations in the cerebellum. The neurophysiologic exams diagnosed abnormal visual conditions in half of the patients. Brain mapping showed a low voltage with hemispherical asymmetry and paroxystical focal activation in 25% of patients; the CT brain scan confirmed various degrees of cerebral atrophy associated with abnormalities in the circumvolutions in such patients, and in two cases, the callosum agenesis.

Concerning the genitourinary system penile hipospadia was detected in two males, and one of them had unilateral cryptorchidism. Two females had bilateral ovarian cysts and one of them an isolated mammary cyst.

The other areas examined were reported as normal.

Treatment

Medical, surgical, and rehabilitation support was given to all of the examined 22 patients without charge to them.

All the mothers received a routine clinical checkings, and a GTG Kariotype, chest X rays, papanicolau stain, and liver function tests, all of which were considered normal; in only six mothers were bilirrubin and liver enzymes increased; in those cases the results must be reevaluated for diagnosis of permanent liver damage due to chronic exposure to the toxic solvents.

Experimental Study Findings

Control Group

There were no significant differences between the two subgroups in any of the variables studied. The average weight was 4.838 g (SD = 0.287) and the average height was 38.87 mm (SD = 1.018), and no malformations were detected.

Experimental Group

Subgroup B_1 (MC). In 33% of the rats a complete reabsorption of the fetuses was observed, which corresponds to the highest dose concentration administered (20%). Of the other treated rats, live fetuses were obtained; of them, 54.6% were considered normal, 13% showed growth retardation, and, in addition to retarded growth, 32.3% of the fetuses were malformed. The three different categories of fetus coexisted in the different rat litters. There were no differences found in the proportions whether the solvent was administered orally or intraperitoneally, but they were in relation to the dose: at 5% dilution, 30.4% of the fetuses were abnormal; at 10% dilution, 60.4% were abnormal; and, finally, at 20% dilution, all of the fetuses obtained were abnormal and in three rats all of the fetuses were reabsorbed.

The external malformations observed are, in order of frequency: abnormal craniofacial shape, limb shortening, generalized edema, cutis aplasia, tail reduction abnormalities, omphalocele, posterior limb atrophy, wide and short neck (pseudoterigium coli), and caudal implantation of the anterior limbs. There were no malformations detected in the thoracoabdominal organs.

Subgroup B_2 (EG). No reabsorptions were observed like those in the previous subgroup, so live fetuses were obtained from all treated rats; of these, 56% were normal fetuses, 32.4% showed growth retardation, and in 11.6% the growth retardation appeared in conjunction with some external malformations. Coexistence of the three categories of fetus was observed in the same litters. The intraperitoneal route was the most effective one for the solvent teratogenicity. There was also a relationship between the dosage administered and the frequency of abnormal fetuses: at 5% dilution, 64.1% were abnormal, 59.2% with growth retardation and 4.9% malformed; at 10% dilution, 47.4% were abnormal, but only 20.6% had growth retardation and 16.6% were malformed; finally, at 20% dilution, 22.2% were abnormal, 7.4% with growth retardation and 14.8% malformed, but the malformations were more severe.

The external malformations were, in order of frequency: generalized edema, abnormal craniofacial shape, oligodactily and limb shortening, cutis aplasia, wide and short neck (pseudoteririum colli), and a caudal implantation of the anterior limbs (FIG. 3). No abnormalities were detected in the thoraco-abdominal organs.

In both groups, the craniofacial malformations detected were an abnormally rounded small head, eyelid coloboma, ocular fibrosis, and shortening of the nasal and mandibular length. In some cases, facial asymmetry and prognatism of different degrees were also noted.

In both subgroups of treated rats, the central nervous system showed an increase in vascularity, diminishment in the mielinogenesis and dendritogenesis, and the presence of areas of devastation. All of these abnormalities were more severe in the EG subgroup.

DISCUSSION

As was shown in the three stages of this study, MC and EG were teratogenic. These industrial-use organic solvents were capable of affecting a population group, causing not only a transitory toxic effects but also permanently modifying the embryonic development of those who were exposed by accident in the prenatal stage. These substances are not found in the list of verified teratogenic action agents;[9–11] nevertheless, their toxic effects have been thoroughly studied. It is recognized that both solvents can be absorbed cutaneously, orally, or through breathing.[12]

In the course of the study it was discovered that a group of female Mexican workers periodically inhaled the vapor of the solvents and were constantly absorbing it through the skin, though in lower concentrations. It seems possible that the solvents were also ingested, because some of it remained on their hands at meal time.

It was impossible to determine the amounts absorbed, because contact had occurred more than 20 years previous and occurred over the subjects' entire working lives. During that period, there were cases of intoxication that varied from slight to severe[7,8] that were caused by individual susceptibility and the period of employment in the Wet Assembling Department where contact was greatest. On the other hand, the factory did not have any ventilation systems, so the vapors spread throughout the work area. Thus, we can conclude that in this group the exposure was chronic and the dosage low.

The ''case-and-control'' study evidentiates the fact that the prenatal contact with MC and EG acted not as risk factor for malformations, but rather as the causal agent.[4] A case-and-control study was made by Holmberg,[13] in which he compared 118 women exposed to 14 different organic solvents during their first trimester of pregnancy, who gave birth to children with congenital abnormalities at highly significant statistical frequency in relation to the control group. However, he did relate particular phenotypes to any of the solvents studied. Some of the malformations were similar to those we found. Also, a European collaborative case-control study[14] showed that women exposed to glycol ethers were at high risk of having abortions and giving birth to malformed children, mainly with oral clefts, heart defects, and musculoskeletal anomalies, as well as spermatic damage in exposed males.

Our clinicoepidemiological study corroborated the behavior of MC and EG as teratogens, because enough supporting evidence was collected to classify them as such.[2] These findings imply that similar effects would occur in other cases, since the clinical findings were similar in all the patients. A dose-effect relation was also observed, since the phenotypic variability could be related to the duration of exposure (their length of stay in the Wet Assembling Department) and the period of pregnancy (first, second, or third trimester); such clinical variation could also be explained by maternal susceptibility, which is related to the individual's detoxification capacity, so if the mother had a low enzymatic capacity, the fetus received a higher quantity of the solvents. This detoxification capacity was demonstrated when enzymes were introduced, which explains why, with a similar time-dosage exposure during a second pregnancy, the offspring manifested fewer malformations. This has also been described in the fetal alcohol syndrome.

The clinical study allowed us to describe this new syndrome, which we named "the Saavedra Syndrome"; it shares some clinical characteristics with the fetal alcoholic syndrome, which is a similar model, but other, distinctive data exist that allow us to differentiate the two syndromes.[15–21] Most of the manifestations were in the craniofacial, musculoskeletal, and central nervous systems, in both syndromes; but in fetal alcoholic syndrome, hypertricosis and hypoplasia of the thenar and hypothenar eminencies are evident, while they were not observed in any of our cases. On the other hand, the prominent mandible and the gonial angles have never been described in fetal alcoholic syndrome, but are constant features in our cases. Nevertheless, the wide nose is the most characteristic finding and could constitute the differential diagnostic key. Head antepulsion and esternocleidomastoid hypertrophy were observed in a high proportion of our cases, but these are not described in fetal alcoholic syndrome; nor are polydactily and bone structural alterations. On the other hand, our patients did not show any thoracoabdominal organ malformations, as occur in fetal alcoholic syndrome.

Ethyl alcohol is also an organic solvent, with a similar chemical structure to MC and EG; for that reason a relative resemblance between both clinical pictures could be expected, perhaps secondary to a similar pathogenic mechanism.

Finally, the experimental study showed, that MC and EG are undoubtedly teratogenic agents. Variations in the frequency and size of the malformations could be explained by individual susceptibility, because we did not use an isogenic strain in the experiment; this variation is commonly observed in human beings. In spite of the small number of published studies on glycol ether, the teratogenicity of organic solvents has not been well established, until now there being more written about MC than EG at the same dosage.[22,23]

In addition, another way to alter the morphogenesis of both solvents is to causing severe intrauterine growth retardation. The fact that no significant differences in weight and size were found between the control subgroups implies that animal handling was adequate, causing no important stress, a factor that should be discarded as a cause of the intrauterine growth retardation, meaning that this retardation could be explained by the direct effect of the solvents. This growth retardation was observed in both experimental groups, though greater after low doses of EG, although it has not been found in humans, which were exposed to both solvents simultaneously. We also observed reproductive damage in experimental animals, but only in MC at 20%, which caused 100% fetal reabsorptions. This effect was not observed in our experiment with EG, in spite of fact that Lamb has described it.[10] The difference could be in the dosage used, which could also be the reason we do not detect this type of damage in human beings. When it did manifest, as an increased abortion rate, in our studied group, it was because of chronic exposure and a low dosage.

In relation to the frequency of total abnormal manifestations, there was a significant difference between the two experimental groups. There were more frequent and severe malformations caused by MC, which suggests that it has a greater teratogenic power.

In relation to the method of administration, the frequency of exposure to MC made no difference, but EG was more effective when administered intraperitoneal, suggesting that it is not absorbed well when administered orally to our strain of Wistar rats, even though it had been cited as being effective.

Concerning the dosage, it was clear that there is a correlation between the number of doses and the magnitude of the effect. In relation to the type of malformation found in both groups, the craniofacial area and the limbs were the most frequently affected. These malformations also occur in the fetal alcohol syndrome in rats, but in human beings there are distinctive features that allow us to make a proper diagnosis.

The generalized edema, such as cutis aplasia, was not detected in any human being, so this could be considered a species-specific abnormality. The pseudopterigium coli observed in rats could correspond to the esternocleidomastoid hypertrophy, and/or secondary neck shortening with vertebral malformations in humans; however, skeletal abnormalities are difficult to pinpoint in rat fetuses. The central nervous system findings could correlate with the CT brain scan, explaining the mental retardation and behavior alterations seen among affected human beings.

It is very important to note that each of the three areas of research in this study—epidemiological, clinical, and experimental—arrived at the same conclusion: methyl cellosolve and ethylene glycol are teratogenic agents in human beings and experimental animals. Dissemination of this knowledge could help prevent the development of new cases in similar situations, and reinforce the idea of work protection for pregnant women as one of the most essential human rights.

REFERENCES

1. Vega Franco, L. & H. Garcia Manzanedo. 1987. Bases Esenciales de la Salud Pública, Chaps. 1, 3, and 4: 1-9, 23-54, 59-63. La Prensa Médica Mexicana. México.
2. Warkany, J. 1975. Congenital Malformations, 2nd edit, Chap. I. Teratogenesis: 3-49. Chicago Year Book Medical Publisher. Chicago.
3. Moreno Altamirano, L. & F. Cano Valle. 1988. Epidemilogía Clínica. Facultad de Medicina, Ed.: 18-19, 109-112. National Autonomous University of Mexico. Mexico City.
4. Fletcher, R., S. Fletcher & E. Wagner. 1988. Epidemilogía Clínica, 2nd edit.: 1-18, 91-104. Consulta. Barcelona.
5. Heaton, D. 1991. An Introduction of Industrial Chemistry, 2nd edit.: 22-41. Blackie. Glasgow, Scotland.
6. De Bussy, J. H. 1972. Materials and Technology, Vol. IV, Petroleum and Organic Chemicals: 745-765. Landgman. Chicago.
7. Gosselin, T. R. 1976. Clinical Toxicology of Commercial Products, 4th ed. 668, 1211. Williams and Wilkins. Baltimore, MD.
8. Merck Index. 1989. An Encyclopedia of Chemicals Drugs and Biologicals, 11th edit. Susan Budavari, Ed.: 599, 951-952. Merck. Rahway, NJ.
9. Sheikh, J. 1979. Teratogenic effects on organic solvents. Lancet **3:** 963.
10. Lamb, J. C., R. R. Maronpot, D. K. Gulati, *et al.* 1985. Reproductive and developmental toxicity of ethylene glycol in the mouse. Toxicol. Appl. Pharmacol. **81:** 100.
11. Shepard, T. H. 1989. Catalog of Teratogenic Agents, 6th ed.: 262-263, 411-412. The Johns Hopkins Press. Baltimore, MD.

12. IRVING, S. & L. RICHARD. 1989. Dangerous Properties of Industrial Materials: 1-9, 2215-2216. Van Nostrand Reinhold. New York.
13. HOLMBERG, R. 1979. Central nervous system defects in children born to mothers exposed to organic solvents during pregnancy. Lancet **28:** 177.
14. HA, M. C., S. CORDIER, B. DANANCHE, A. BERGERET, L. MANDEREAU & F. BRUNO. 1996. Congenital malformations and occupational exposure to glycol ethers: A European collaborative case-control study. *In* Occupational Hygiene, Vol. 2: 417-421. Gordon & Breach. Amsterdam.
15. LANIC, H. W. 1971. Fish phenotype in a offspring of an alcoholic mother. Exp. Zool. **177:** 51.
16. JONES, K. L., S. W. SMITH, C. N. VILELAND & A. P. STRESBUTH. 1973. Pattern of malformation in offspring of chronic alcoholic woman. Lancet **1:** 1267.
17. BARNES, D. E. & D. W. WALKER. 1981. Prenatal ethanol esposure permanently reduces the number of pyramidal neurons in rat hippocampus. Dev. Brain Res. **1:** 330.
18. ABEL, E. L. 1983. In utero alcohol exposure functional and structural brain damage. Neuro. Toxicol. Teratol. **5:** 363.
19. SAMSON, H. H. & K. A. GRANT. 1983. Ethanol induced microcephaly in the neonatal rat: Relation of dose. Alcohol Clin. Exp. Res. **7:** 120.
20. JONES, K. L. 1988. Smith's Recognizable Patterns of Human Malformations. 4th edit.: 491-494, 630-640. Saunders. Philadelphia.
21. GORLIN, R., M. M. COHEN & L. S. LEVIN. 1990. Syndromes of the Head and Neck, 3rd edit.: 16-20. Oxford. New York.
22. NELSON, B. K., J. V. SETZEDR, W. S. BRIGHTWELL, *et al.* 1982. Comparative inhalation teratogenicity of four industrial glycol ether solvents in rats. Teratology **25:** 64A.
23. PRICE, C. J., C. A. KIMMEL, R. W. TYL & M. C. MARR. 1985. The developmental toxicity of ethylene glycol in rats and mice. Toxicol. Appl. Pharmacol. **81:** 113.

Mortality of Power Workers Exposed to Phenoxy Herbicides and Polychlorinated Biphenyls in Waste Transformer Oil

ALASTAIR HAY [a,b] AND JOHN TARREL [c]

[a]*Pathological Sciences*
School of Medicine
Old Medical School
Leeds LS2 9JT, England

[c]*Tarrel Consulting Services, Ltd.*
217 George Street
Fredericton, New Brunswick
Canada E3B 1J4

INTRODUCTION

Most of the electricity supplied to the Canadian province of New Brunswick is delivered by overhead power lines. Many of the lines cover vast distances across rural areas that are sparsely populated. Terrain in these areas is often rough, and the growth of vegetation under the lines delays the access of engineers carrying out repairs or routine maintenance work.

The control of vegetation under the power lines presents a continual problem for the power companies. In New Brunswick, up until 1950, most of the vegetation (including trees) under the power lines was cut down by hand. However, the increasing cost of manual labor led to the examination of other methods for vegetation control. In 1950, the New Brunswick Power Commission (NB Power) began to experiment with the use of the herbicides. Initial trials were successful, and NB Power used increasing amounts of herbicide on ''rights-of-way'' (or ''rows'') under the power lines. The most efficient of the herbicides tested was a one-to-one combination of two well-known phenoxy compounds: 2,4-dichlorophenoxyacetic acid (2,4-D), and 2,4,5-trichlorophenoxyacetic acid (2,4,5-T). NB Power purchased this combination from suppliers, who included Naugatuck Chemicals, Chipman Chemicals, and Dow Canada.

In the mid 1980s, sprayers in Canada became concerned about evidence that suggested that use of phenoxy herbicides presented health risks. Case control studies had linked the herbicide 2,4,5-T with an increased risk of development of soft tissue sarcoma.[1,2] An association had also been found between exposure to phenoxy herbicides and/or chlorophenols, and the development of malignant lymphoma.[3] In addition, an increased incidence of gastrointestinal cancer was discovered among

[b]Phone: 44-113/233-5682; fax: 44-113/233-5672; e-mail: patawmh@south-01.novell.leeds.ac.uk

workers who had been exposed, following an industrial accident in 1953, to 2,4,5-trichlorophenol and the contaminant 2,3,7,8-tetrachlorodibenzodioxin (dioxin).[4] The dioxin is produced during the manufacture of 2,4,5-trichlorophenol. Trichlorophenol is used to make the herbicide 2,4,5-T in a procedure that leads to the contamination of the formulations with dioxin.

Some former employees of NB Power who had been involved in the spraying procedures were members of a group called SODA (Sprayers of Dioxin Association). SODA arranged for a preliminary mortality analysis to be carried out in 1984. The analysis suggested a high mortality rate for the cohort. However, problems were encountered when NB Power (the former employer) proved unwilling to assist SODA with the identification process. The company stated in addition that no employment records were available to confirm or deny identification of participants in its spray program at the time in question.

In 1991, however, NB Power agreed to cooperate with SODA and assist the group financially in its legal action against the chemical companies who had supplied the phenoxy herbicides. SODA representatives were granted complete access to all NB Power documents (including employment records) relating to the spray program (FIG. 1a,b).

The cooperation between NB Power and SODA enabled a more complete identification of the cohort to be made, and for a detailed analysis of mortality to be conducted. This paper describes the results of this analysis.

Investigation of NB Power records revealed that there were occasions when waste oils were added to the herbicide mixture. This use of oil was considered to increase the length of time herbicides were in contact with foliage. Plants absorb the herbicides through the leaves. Water-based herbicides are frequently washed off by rainfall. The addition of oil increases the persistence of the chemicals. In 1958, NB Power experimented with the addition of waste oils (including waste transformer oil) to herbicide mixtures. The analysis we report also attempts, therefore, to assess mortality for the period before transformer oil was introduced, and for the period after this procedure was followed (FIG. 2).

COHORT

The cohort that is the subject of the mortality analysis was made up of individuals who participated in the spray programs operated by NB Power, and who met all the following criteria: (i) employed by NB Power (full-time, part-time, seasonal, or casual); (ii) took part in the spray program between June 1950 and June 1966; (iii) participated for a period of at least 30 days consecutively and for at least one spray season; (iv) were employed in one or more of the categories of spray crew member, spray crew supervisor, foreman, truck driver supplying herbicides to the spray site.

IDENTIFICATION OF COHORT

A professional independent investigator was retained to assist in the identification of the cohort. Using a provisional list, made up of approximately 200 named individu-

Please Return To
CENTRAL FILES
By

Form No. 17

THE NEW BRUNSWICK ELECTRIC POWER COMMISSION

APPLICATION FOR EMPLOYMENT

Note:- Carefully state all pertinent information

File: 4-110

1. Full Name G [redacted] T H [redacted] Date MAY 17/65 R
(Print name and address in block letters)
Address 22 [redacted] AVE Tel. No. [redacted] 2448
B [redacted] Unempl. Ins. No. [redacted] 016 [redacted]

2. Type of work desired .... When could you begin? ....
Wage or salary expected .... May we refer to your present or past employer? ....
Present or last wage or salary ....

3. State name of relatives employed in Provincial Government service: ....
Type of work and location of their work ....
Were you previously employed with N.B.E.P.C.? Yes........ No........ When ....

4. Sex M. ALE Height 6 FT. Marital status: Number of Dependents:
F. Weight 175 LBS Married YES Children 2
Date of Birth 16 [redacted] 1927 Single .... Others ....
Next of Kin WIFE [redacted] AS ABOVE [redacted] 2448
Relationship Name Address Tel. No.

5. Are you a Canadian citizen? Yes ✓ No........ If not, state nationality ....
Place of Birth BARKERS PT. N.B.
Languages: Spoken ENGLISH Written ENGLISH
Physical condition (mention any defects) ....

FIGURE 1a. Application for employment with New Brunswick Electric Power Commission. Some personal details have been obscured for the photograph.

N.B.E.P.C. EMPLOYEE DATA

1. ENTERED SERVICE 2. PROMOTED 3. DEMOTED 4. TRANSFERRED 5. RATE CHANGE 6. OCCUPATIONAL CHANGE 7. LAY OFF 8. RESIGNED 9. DISCHARGED 10. PENSIONED

DATE EFFECTIVE	CHANGE	DEPT.	POSITION	CLASS	LOCATION	RATE HR. DY. MO.	REMARKS
4-May/59	1	Distribu.	Machine Oper.		Oromocto	1.47	
3-Nov/59	4	Constru.	"		Highline	1.47	
		"	Truck Driver		"	1.70, 1.72	
1-May/65		"	"		"	294.50	; 306.50
1-Jan/66	5	"	"		"	319.	
1-Jan/67	5	"	"	II	"	$332.	; 360.
1-Jan/68	5	"	"	"	"	385.	acting Truck Oper.
1-Jan/69	5	"	"	"	"	432.	at 391, 1/9/68-3/1
1-Jan/70	5	"	"	"	"	411.69	Equiv. (446.00/M.)
1-Jan/71	5	"	Truck Operator II		"	436.62	Equiv. (473.00/M.)
1-Sept/71	5	"	"	"	"	462.46	Equiv. (501.00/M.)
1-May/72	5	"	"	"	"	508.62	Equiv. (551.00/M.
1-Jan/73	5	"	"	"	"	543.69	Equiv. (589.00/M.
1-Jan/74	5	" Appointed	" Warehouse Helper,	"	Confirmed 7/7/74	587.08	" (636.00/M.)
7-Jan/74	2,4,5,6	Purchasing	& Truck Driver		Service Centre	648.00	" (702.00/M.)
1-Jan/75	5	"	"		"	847.38	" (918.00/M.
3-Mar/75	2,5,6	"	Warehouseman		"	924.92	" (1002.00/M
1-Jan/76	5	"	"		"	998.77	Eq. (1082/M)
1/1/77	5	"	"		"	1058.77	Eq. (1147/M)
1/1/78	5	"	"		"	1101.23	Eq. (1193/M)

RECORD OF SUSPENSION

DATE	DATE	DATE	REASON

FIGURE 1b. New Brunswick Electric Power Commission. Summary data on employment history.

Waste Oil

Waste oil is well worth saving for the chemical control operation. It is recommended that people who have waste oil to dispose of should pick up empty drums from the pile marked "CONTAMINATED DRUMS" to collect it. Arrangements could be made with the store's personnel to have any waste oil transported to this site.

Waste oil for this purpose may include:-

(1) Transformer oil which is not considered worth filtering.

(2) Residual cleaning fluids such as varsol, etc.

(3) Oil engine lubrication oil.

Deteriorated transformer oil which can be filtered should not be brought to this site, but must be kept in some other location until reconditioned by the filter press operator.

J. E. [illegible],
Transmission Maintenance Engineer.

JEG/mm

c.c. P. C. Levesque — M. Grandy
L. K. Hargavel — R. [illegible]urington
C. J. McKinley — [illegible]. Trask
G. Lawlor — D. Knight
R. Thomas

FIGURE 2. Internal memo of New Brunswick Electric Power Commission.[6] First paragraph reads "waste oil is well worth saving for the chemical control operation." Indent reads "waste oil for this purpose may include:- (1) Transformer oil which is not considered worth saving."

als included in the 1984 analysis, the investigator examined NB Power documents for the names of additional former company employees. The list was then checked to ascertain that individuals met the entry criteria. Length of participation in the spray program was established. Some survivors, who had been involved in the spraying program some 25–40 years earlier, had difficulty in recalling how long they participated. Difficulties also arose where relatives were asked to complete data sheets for sprayers who had since died. Information on the first year of spraying was important for this analysis in order to calculate person years of exposure to herbicides for each individual. This information was also required for those individuals who had died, to compare actual versus expected deaths, according to the duration of exposure.

In cases where there was some doubt about the years of participation in the spray program, other sources were checked for confirmation, as follows: (I) NB Power records documenting years of spraying; (II) where no relevant NB Power documents existed, survivors' recollections were used, together with any employment records and documentary evidence they had retained; (III) where a former sprayer was deceased, details were obtained from relatives and fellow crew members; (IV) where no documentary evidence was available and the steps in (II) and (III) above could not be followed, the following procedure was adopted: (a) where the year, or a range of years, was indicated, then either the first year mentioned or the earliest year in the range was recorded to be the first year of involvement with spraying; (b) if no year was indicated, the year of first spraying was recorded as 1950. (Only one member of the cohort was categorized using procedure b. This individual is now deceased). Category IV above is likely to result in the person years of exposure and expected deaths being slightly overstated, and the standardized mortality ratio (SMR) understated.

As a result of the identification process, a cohort of 225 individuals was assembled, of whom 127 were still surviving and 98 had died by 31 May 1992, which was the date selected as the end point of the study. Of those individuals provisionally identified as sprayers, some were included and some excluded from the cohort.

INCLUSIONS

1. Six deceased individuals who were identified as sprayers by relatives, but for whom there is no documentary evidence, were included in the cohort. All but one sprayed during the first five years of the program. No surviving sprayer confirmed that these six individuals were sprayers. It is possible that there were no surviving sprayers from the crews with whom these individuals had worked.

2. Five surviving sprayers for whom there is no documentary evidence, and no recall by any other surviving sprayer, were included in the cohort. Four of these five individuals sprayed for one year only.

EXCLUSIONS

1. Seven individuals who could not be traced were excluded from the cohort. No personal details (e.g., birth date) could be discovered for them. Population migration rates from New Brunswick are very low. It is possible that these individuals have died.

2. Fourteen individuals who were identified as sprayers were excluded from the program because they were not employees of NB Power. These individuals were either subcontracted to the company as sprayers; or they sprayed on behalf of other organizations.

3. One further individual (deceased) was excluded because his widow reported that he had first sprayed in 1967.

4. One individual was excluded who sprayed for only three weeks in one year; and one was excluded who was employed only in the inspection of transmission lines for one day per week.

EXPOSURE TO CHEMICALS

When NB Power began its herbicide program, sprayers used equipment that they carried in a knapsack on their back. The herbicide was sprayed from a lance. Sprayers have reported that when the lance was raised to increase the distance the spray would travel, liquid spray ran down the nozzle onto their arms. Chemicals also leaked from backpacks, soaking clothing.

Backpack spraying was not a practical solution for spraying miles of lines. In 1955, NB Power began to use an ex-military half-track vehicle known as "Muskeg." This was ideally suited to the negotiation of rough terrain. Crew members included a vehicle operator, a foreman, four sprayers, and a driver for the truck supplying the Muskeg with chemicals. Two sprayers stood to either side of the Muskeg, spraying vegetation. On steep hills, sprayers usually walked behind the Muskeg, spraying as they walked. Workdays were typically 9–9.5 hours over a period of 4 months each year, from mid-May until mid-September.

Spray crews had no protective clothing or equipment. In the intense summer heat, many stripped to the waist. Instructions issued to the chemical crew foremen in 1958 as well as in 1962[5] stated that ". . . concentrates of 2,4-D and 2,4,5-T are non-poisonous and non-toxic to humans, animals or fishes. That means that no ill effect will result if placed in contact with the body, or if taken internally." This reassuring message reinforced the poor hygiene already present. Conditions for the crews were primitive, with no facilities for washing. Hands were rarely washed before eating, even if a stream was nearby. Many crew members reported that they did not change work clothes from one day to the next.

Prior to 1958, spray crews mixed approximately one gallon of herbicide concentrate with 100 gallons of water in a 300-gallon tank on the Muskeg. Application rates were approximately 60 gallons of dilute herbicide per acre. Empty Muskeg tanks were refilled with herbicides and water from the accompanying truck. In rough terrain, the Muskeg carried its own chemical concentrate to mix with water taken from local streams.

In 1958, NB Power decided to increase the contact time of the herbicide on plants by the addition of oil to the diluent. In successful small-scale experiments, 4 pounds of active herbicide was mixed with 10 gallons of waste transformer oil and 90 gallons of water. In 1959, the addition of transformer oil became routine. The Power Commission arranged to collect and store oil that was too contaminated to reuse in the transformers from which it was drained.[6]

NB Power's three herbicide suppliers all recommended the use of this type of oil, either in correspondence with the Power Commission or in their promotional literature[7–9] (FIGURE 3a–c). It is not clear where the idea to use transformer oil originated. Chemical companies are known to have recommended the use of fuel oil, diesel oil, or kerosene instead of water in certain herbicide applications. Oil-based mixtures penetrated the bark or stumps of trees more easily than water-based solutions. The recommendation to use waste transformer oil appears to have been specifically targeted at power companies.

The composition of the waste transformer oil used by the NB Power company sprayers is not known. It is therefore not possible to estimate the quantity of the constituent chemicals (polychlorinated biphenyls and polychlorinated dibenzofurans) to which sprayers would have been exposed.

Attempts have been made to assess exposures to dioxins, to 2,4,5-T, and to 2,4-D.[10] Soil samples from sprayed rows have been assayed for their dioxin content, and the results were compared with samples from unsprayed rows. NB Power records

Naugatuck Chemicals

Division of Dominion Rubber Company Limited

June 29 1951

[illegible]

Attention of Mr. [illegible]

Gentlemen:

Thank you for [illegible] letter of [illegible] the use of brush control Herbicides.

In [illegible] letter you ask for information [illegible] materials [illegible] used when [illegible] with oil as a carrier. This will depend [illegible] coverage that you can obtain from [illegible] equipped. I believe we mentioned in an earlier letter that [illegible] Water & Power, when using waste transformer oil [illegible] coverage with 10 gallons per acre of brush. However, [illegible] fuel oil, the same nozzle [illegible] gallons of [illegible] mixture per acre of brush.

FIGURE 3a. Letter from Naugatuck chemicals,[7] advising New Brunswick Electric Power Commission about the use of oil as a carrier for the herbicides. 6th line, 2nd paragraph reads "... when using waste transformer oil. ..."

were used to collect information on sprayed areas. 2,3,7,8-Tetrachlorodibenzodioxin is a contaminant of 2,4,5-T that degrades slowly in the environment.[10] The soil data was used to calculate the dioxin content of the 2,4,5-T. The use of exposure models to assess inhalation and dermal absorption of herbicides and dioxin exposure does not give precise answers. The calculations indicate that the dioxin exposure could range over four orders of magnitude, while the estimates of the exposure to the herbicides indicated that exposures could vary by at least tenfold.[10]

DATA HANDLING AND ANALYSIS

The mortality of the cohort was assessed by comparing the actual deaths among sprayers with deaths that would have been expected, based on age-specific mortality rates for the Province of New Brunswick.

Expected deaths at a given age are the product of total person years exposure to risk of death (at that age) and the population mortality rate (for that age). Total expected deaths are obtained by summing the expected deaths at each age. To determine person years exposed to risk of death for a particular spray, the starting point was 1 June of the year first sprayed, and the end point for survivors was 31

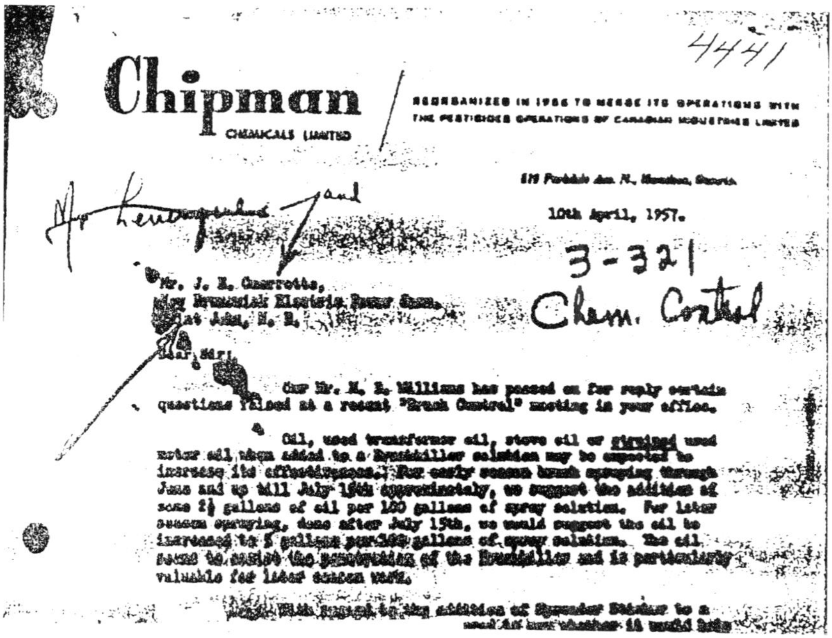
Chipman
CHEMICALS LIMITED
REORGANIZED IN 1956 TO MERGE ITS OPERATIONS WITH THE PESTICIDES OPERATIONS OF CANADIAN INDUSTRIES LIMITED

10th April, 1957.

Our Mr. M. E. Williams has passed on for reply certain questions raised at a recent "Brush Control" meeting in your office.

Oil, used transformer oil, stove oil or ... used motor oil when added to a Brushkiller solution may be expected to increase its effectiveness. For early season brush spraying through June and up till July 15th approximately, we suggest the addition of some 2½ gallons of oil per 100 gallons of spray solution. For later season spraying, done after July 15th, we would suggest the oil be increased to 5 gallons per 100 gallons of spray solution. The oil seems to assist the penetration of the Brushkiller and is particularly valuable for later season work.

FIGURE 3b. Letter from Chipman Chemicals,[8] advising New Brunswick Electric Power Commission about addition of oil to herbicide formulations to increase effectiveness. 1st line, 2nd paragraph reads "Oil, used transformer oil. . . ."

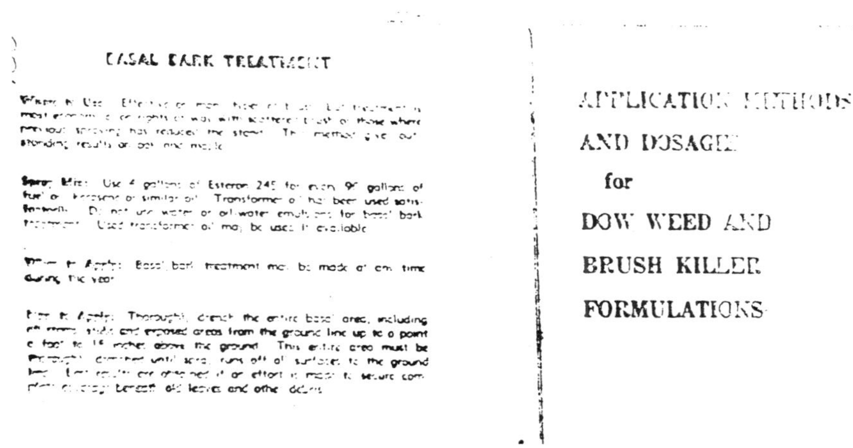

FIGURE 3c. Promotional brochure of Dow Canada.[9] Treatment of bark with Dow Weed and Brush Killer Formulations. 2nd paragraph reads "**Spray Mix:** Use 4 gallons of Esteron 245 for every 90 [or 96?] gallons of fuel oil, kerosene or similar oil. Transformer oil has been used satisfactorily."

May 1992. The end point for sprayers who had died was 31 May following the date of death.

As population mortality rates vary over time, person years were recorded by both ages and calendar years.

Age-specific and calendar year-specific rates for mortality for New Brunswick males for the years 1950–1989 inclusive were developed by Statistics Canada (at our request) for all causes of death combined and for some selective causes. The mortality rates for males were used to determine expected deaths. The 1989 rates were used for the years 1989–1991 inclusive, since final data for 1990 and 1991 were not available for use by Statistics Canada at the time.

Actual deaths included in the analyses were those that occurred before 1 June 1992. Deaths that have occurred subsequently have not been considered. Standardized mortality ratios were determined by dividing actual by expected deaths. Confidence intervals (CIs) of 95% were obtained based on the Poisson distribution. Results were considered significant at $p < 0.05$ when the CI did not include 100.

SMRs were calculated for the entire cohort over the whole period under analysis, and also for the specific durations, age groups, and subgroups. SMRs were also calculated for individuals who first sprayed before 1958 and for those who sprayed between 1959 and 1966. Most SMRs were obtained for all causes of death combined. Some supplementary analyses were carried out for selected causes of death. Coding for these was based on ICD-9 (Ninth Revision of the International Classification of Diseases Adapted for use in the United States, 1975). Death certificates (principally those written in New Brunswick) were used to record the cause of death. The New Brunswick Registrar of Vital Statistics provided ICD coding for all New Brunswick death certificates. For jurisdictions other than New Brunswick, and for those cases where ICD codes were not included on death certificates, the cause of death was coded using the ICD-9 manual. Only four death certificates needed to be treated in this way.

RESULTS

The total person years for the entire cohort for the period under study was 6,525. Results for all causes of death combined (i.e., total mortality) for the total cohort by duration since first exposure are shown in TABLE 1, and by ranges of attained ages are shown in TABLE 2. The SMR for the total cohort for all durations since first exposure to the herbicide is 154% (CI 126%–188%) based on 98 actual deaths versus 63.55 expected deaths. Statistically significant excess mortality ($p < 0.05$) was observed for all causes of death for the following years since first exposure: 20–24; 25–29; 20–29; 15 and over; 20 and over; 25 and over (TABLE 1)

Statistically significant mortality ($p < 0.05$) was observed for the following attained age ranges: 30–39; 50–59; 30–49; 30–59; 40–59 (TABLE 2).

Separate analyses were carried out for two subgroups of the total cohort, namely those who first sprayed in 1958 or earlier (YFS 50–58) and those who first sprayed in 1959 or later (YFS 59–66). Statistically significant excess deaths were recorded for those who sprayed between 1950 and 1958, and where the years since first exposure were either 10 and over or all durations (TABLE 3). For the individuals who

TABLE 1. Actual and Expected Deaths for Total Cohort by Duration since First Exposure

Duration (Years)	Deaths		SMR (%)	CI (%)
	Actual	Expected		
0-4	6	4.47	134	49-292
5-9	8	5.95	134	58-264
10-14	12	7.91	152	79-266
15-19	14	9.95	141	77-237
20-24	19	11.09	171	103-267[a]
25-29	25	10.32	242	157-358[a]
0-9	14	10.42	134	73-225
10-19	26	17.86	146	95-215
20-29	44	21.41	206	150-277[a]
30 and over	14	13.86	101	55-170
25 and over	39	24.18	161	114-220[a]
20 and over	58	35.27	164	125-214[a]
15 and over	72	45.22	159	125-201[a]
All durations	98	63.55	154	126-188

[a] $p < 0.05$.

TABLE 2. Actual and Expected Deaths for Total Cohort by Ranges of Attained Ages

Attained Age Range	Deaths		SMR (%)	CI (%)
	Actual	Expected		
Less than 30	1	1.87	53	1-295
30-39	11	3.11	354	177-634[a]
40-49	9	7.54	119	55-226
50-59	29	13.80	210	141-302[a]
60-69	20	17.76	113	69-174
70-79	22	14.66	150	94-227
80 and over	6	4.81	125	46-273
30-49	20	10.65	188	115-289[a]
30-59	49	24.45	200	148-265[a]
40-59	38	21.34	178	126-244[a]
60-79	42	32.42	130	94-176
All ages	98	63.55	154	126-188[a]

[a] $p < 0.05$.

TABLE 3. Actual and Expected Deaths for Subgroups YFS 50-58 and YFS 59-66 by Duration since First Exposure

Duration (Years)	Deaths		SMR (%)	CI (%)
	Actual	Expected		
YFS 50-58				
Less than 20	28	21.84	128	85-186
20 and over	48	30.18	159	117-211[a]
All durations	76	52.02	146	116-184[a]
YFS 59-66				
Less than 20	12	6.44	186	96-326
20 and over	10	5.09	196	94-361
All durations	22	11.53	191	120-288[a]

[a] $p < 0.05$.

sprayed between 1959 and 1966, a significant excess of deaths among the sprayers was only observed when all years since first exposure were combined.

The results for the subgroups should be interpreted with caution for the following reasons. Documentary evidence of the first year of spraying is not available for all individuals. In addition, the year in which spraying first took place is not certain for those individuals who had died; and for those where information on the first year of spraying was gathered from relatives. This has no material effect on the analysis for the total cohort, but it could have an effect on the analysis for the subgroups segregated by "years first sprayed." Some individuals who first sprayed in 1958 or earlier are also known to have sprayed in 1959 or later. They may therefore have been subjected to both types of exposure (i.e., herbicides only and herbicides plus transformer oil).

Results for selected causes of death are shown in TABLE 4. The results are grouped into six summary causes of death. TABLE 4 records the actual and expected deaths by selected summary of causes of death for the total cohort and for the two subcohorts. For the total cohort, a statistically significant excess in mortality was observed for "all heart disease"; and for "all accidents, suicides and homicides." There was a substantial excess mortality for "all malignant neoplasms" (SMR 139%; CI 86%-213%), but this was not statistically significant.

For the subcohort "YFS 1958 and earlier" there was a statistically significant excess mortality for "all heart disease" and " all accidents, suicides and homicides." Once again, there was an excess mortality for "all malignant neoplasms," but this was not statistically significant. For the subcohort "YFS 1959 and later" a statistically significant excess mortality was observed for "all heart disease."

The various causes of death are broken down according to duration since first exposure and attained age ranges in TABLES 5-8. Results in TABLE 5 record the SMRs for the total cohort for two selected causes of death—"all malignant neoplasms" and "all heart disease." Statistically significant excess mortality for "all malignant neoplasms" was observed for subgroups where the years since first exposure were

TABLE 4. Actual and Expected Deaths by Selected Summary Causes of Death for Total Cohort and Two Subcohorts

Cohort and Summary Cause	Deaths		SMR (%)	CI (%)
	Actual	Expected		
Total Cohort				
All malignant neoplasms	21	15.08	139	86-213
All heart disease	44	24.37	181	131-243[a]
All respiratory disease	2	4.11	49	6-177
Chronic liver disease	2	0.99	202	24-729
All accidents, suicides, homicides	17	7.56	225	131-360[a]
All other causes	12	11.44	105	54-184
All causes	98	63.55	154	126-188[a]
Subcohort YFS 1958 and earlier				
All malignant neoplasms	18	12.30	146	87-231
All heart disease	34	20.23	168	116-235[a]
All respiratory disease	1	3.37	30	1-167
Chronic liver disease	2	0.80	250	30-903
All accidents, suicides, homicides	13	5.80	224	119-383[a]
All others causes	8	9.52	84	36-165[a]
All causes	76	52.02	146	116-184[a]
Subcohort YFS 1959 and later				
All malignant neoplasms	3	2.78	108	22-315
All heart disease	10	4.14	213	102-392[a]
All respiratory disease	1	0.74	135	3-752
Chronic liver disease	0	0.19	0	N/A
All accidents, suicides, homicides	4	1.76	227	62-581
All other causes	4	1.92	208	57-532
All causes	22	11.53	191	120-288[a]

[a] $p < 0.05$.

20 and over, or 20-29. For "all heart disease," statistically significant excesses were observed for the following years since first exposure: 20-29, 20 and over, and 25 and over.

TABLE 6 provides a breakdown by attained age ranges for the same categories as in TABLE 5. A significant excess SMR for "all heart disease" was observed for those aged 30-39, 30-49, 50-69, and all durations.

The actual and expected deaths for "all respiratory disease," "chronic liver disease," and "all other causes" were too few to permit any meaningful breakdown for either duration since first exposure or age ranges. However, detailed analysis for the category "all accidents, suicides and homicides" is shown in TABLE 7. The results for the total cohort indicate a statistically significant excess for the following years since first exposure: 20 and over, 25 and over, and all durations. A statistically significant excess SMR was observed for the age ranges 30-39, 50-59, and all ages.

TABLE 8 provides a detailed breakdown of actual and expected deaths for the category "all other causes." All other causes are those deaths not included in the

TABLE 5. Actual and Expected Deaths by Duration since First Exposure, for Total Cohort for Summary Causes of Death "All Malignant Neoplasms" and "All Heart Disease"

	Deaths			
Duration (Years)	Actual	Expected	SMR (%)	CI (%)
All malignant neoplasms				
0-09	4	5.26	76	21-195
20-29	12	5.62	214	111-375[a]
30 and over	5	4.20	119	39-277
25 and over	11	7.16	154	7-276
20 and over	17	9.82	173	101-277[a]
All durations	21	15.08	139	86-231
All heart disease				
0-9	7	3.69	190	76-391
10-19	11	7.25	152	76-272
20-29	19	8.30	229	138-357[a]
30 and over	7	5.13	136	55-280
25 and over	17	9.07	187	109-299[a]
20 and over	26	13.43	194	127-285[a]
All durations	44	24.37	181	131-243

[a] $p < 0.05$.

TABLE 6. Actual and Expected Deaths by Attained Age Ranges for Summary Causes of Death "All Malignant Neoplasms" and "All Heart Disease"

	Deaths			
Duration (Years)	Actual	Expected	SMR (%)	CI (%)
All malignant neoplasms				
Under 30	0	0.11	0	N/A
30-49	1	1.72	58	1-323
50-69	14	8.61	163	89-274
70 and over	6	4.64	129	47-281
All ages	21	15.08	139	86-213
All heart disease				
Under 30	0	0.09	0	N/A
30-39[a]	5	0.54	926	300-2158[b]
30-49	8	3.09	259	112-510[b]
50-69	22	13.30	165	103-249[b]
70 and over	14	7.89	177	97-297
All durations	44	24.37	181	131-243[b]

[a] Identified separately because of very high SMR.
[b] $p < 0.05$.

TABLE 7. Actual and Expected Deaths by Duration since First Exposure and Attained Age Ranges for Total Cohort for Summary Cause of Death "All Accidents, Suicides, Homicides"

	Deaths			
Duration and Age Range	Expected	Actual	SMR (%)	CI (%)
Duration				
0-19	5.06	10	198	95-364
20-29	1.87	5	267	87-622
30 and over	0.63	2	317	38-1144
25 and over	1.41	5	355	115-827[a]
20 and over	2.50	7	280	112-577[a]
All durations	7.56	17	225	131-360[a]
Age range				
Under 30	1.38	1	72	2-401
30-39	1.57	5	318	103-741[a]
40-49	1.90	4	211	57-540
50-59	1.42	7	493	198-1016[a]
60 and over	1.29	0	0	N/A
All ages	7.56	17	225	131-360[a]

[a] $p < 0.05$.

TABLE 8. Actual and Expected Deaths by Duration since First Exposure and Attained Age Ranges for Total Cohort for Summary Cause of Death "All Other Causes"

	Deaths			
Duration and Age Range	Expected	Actual	SMR (%)	CI (%)
Duration				
0-9	1.92	1	52	1-290
10-19	3.26	5	153	50-356
20-29	3.67	6	163	60-355
30 and over	2.59	0	0	N/A
All durations	11.44	12	105	54-184
Age ranges				
Under 50	1.88	1	53	1-295
50-69	5.07	3	59	12-172
70 and over	44.9	8	178	77-351
All ages	11.44	12	105	54-184

TABLE 9. Malignant Neoplasms Recorded as Cause of Death

Carcinoma of the lung	8
Oat cell carcinoma of the lung	1
Carcinoma of the stomach	3
Prostate cancer	2
Seminoma right testicle (leading to metastatic carcinoma)	1
Primary tumor of the liver	1
Metastatic cancer of thyroid	1
Carcinomatosis, primary, in pancreas	1
Bronchogenic carcinoma	1
Metastatic cancer	1
Total malignant neoplasms	21

five selected summary causes that were chosen for analysis. No statistically significant differences were noted in the observed and expected deaths for "all other causes."

Details concerning the individual causes of death are not shown, as they are too numerous. However, the details of different neoplasms recorded as the cause of death will be of more interest, and they are recorded in TABLE 9. Carcinoma of the lung accounted for some 40% of all neoplasms.

DISCUSSION

The findings of our investigation of exposure to the phenoxy herbicides in the spraying program conducted by NB Power surprised us. Most other investigations of workers exposed to phenoxy herbicides report no overall increase in the mortality of the workers.[11] On the contrary, there has often been a decrease noted in the overall mortality, which is accounted for by the "healthy worker" effect. Individuals who are able to work are generally healthier than is the population at large. Therefore, any study that investigates the mortality of a group of working individuals is likely to show a lower mortality rate for those in employment than for the population as a whole. Investigations carried out on workers occupationally exposed to polychlorinated biphenyls have also not registered an increase in the mortality rate.[12–14] For some of those studies where the mortality analysis was carried out on PCB-exposed workers, the number of deaths noted was smaller than in our cohort.[12,13,15]

Various mortality studies have been conducted involving an analysis of more deaths than occurred in our cohort, and investigation of these studies[14] indicates that they, too, find no increase in the mortality of workers occupationally exposed to PCBs. One factor in particular has to be considered with regard to our subcohort, which was exposed to both phenoxy herbicides and to PCBs. These individuals were subjected to significant concentrations of both these agents. We know (from interviews with those individuals still living at the time our study was conducted) that none had been given any instructions concerning the need to observe hygienic measures when spraying herbicides. In consequence, individuals suffered repeated and heavy skin exposure to herbicides. Some referred to occasions when workers sprayed one another with the herbicide mixtures as a means of keeping cool on the hot summer days. In consequence, our subcohort (YFS 59 and later) would have been exposed to significant quantities of herbicides and PCBs.

From the evidence that we have been able to obtain, the likely concentrations of PCBs in the herbicide formulation used was 10%. This information was obtained from a number of internal memos of NB Power. These communications also indicated that the transformer oil that was to be used in the herbicide spray program was waste oil obtained from old transformers. Any transformer oil that could be recycled was used again in new transformers, but older and dirtier oil was kept for the herbicide spraying program. This waste transformer oil, which was used in the spraying program, would have contained other contaminants, such as polychlorinated dibenzofurans. It is possible that it also contained additional polychlorinated dibenzodioxins from the chlorinated benzenes that would have been present in the waste transformer oils. PCBs were commonly mixed with chlorinated benzenes (generally in a mix of 30% to 40% by volume) for use in large-capacity transformers and capacitors.[14]

It was not possible for us to calculate the concentration of any of the constituents of the oil added to the herbicide spray mixture. The waste oil was obtained from capacitors and transformers where arcing would have taken place. This process is likely to have increased the concentration of polychlorinated dibenzofurans present in the oil. It is possible, therefore, that our cohort was exposed to higher concentrations of polychlorinated dibenzofurans than other individuals occupationally exposed to PCBs, and the subject of analyses by other investigators. Some large cohorts of individuals known to have experienced exposure in the course of the manufacture of capacitors and transformers are likely to have been exposed to lower concentrations of the polychlorinated dibenzofurans than our cohort.[4] Workers in the capacitor producing industry would have been handling cleaner transformer oil.[14]

Two metaanalyses of workers exposed either to chlorophenoxy herbicides and chlorophenols, or to 2,3,7,8-tetrachlorodibenzodioxin were published a number of years ago.[11,16] The first of these analyses, a historical cohort study of mortality, was conducted using an international register of 18,910 production workers or sprayers from 10 countries. Exposure was reconstructed from questionnaires, factory or spraying records, and job histories. Cause-specific national death rates were used as a reference. The study reported no excess in all causes of mortality, no excess for all neoplasms, and no excess for the most common epithelial cancers, or for lymphomas. However, a statistically nonsignificant twofold excess risk, based on four observed deaths, was noted for soft tissue sarcoma.[11] Unlike our study, this metaanalysis additionally reported no excess for deaths due to accident, suicide, or homicide.[11]

No soft tissue sarcomas were observed in our cohort. The metaanalysis of those workers exposed to phenoxy-herbicides[11] appeared to indicate an increased SMR for cancers of the testicle (SMR 225, 7 cases, 499 total cancers); thyroid (SMR 367, 4 cases); other endocrine glands (SMR 462, 3 cases); and of the nose and nasal cavity (SMR 291, 3 cases). These calculations were based on a small number of deaths. In our cohort, 21 deaths were due to cancer. We documented single cases of testicular, thyroid, and pancreatic cancer. There were also three cases of prostatic cancer, and one of these individuals also had carcinoma of the lung. There were too few deaths from malignancy in our cohort to enable us to perform any meaningful statistical analysis of individual causes of death.

A retrospective cohort study of mortality of 5,172 workers who were employed at 12 chemical plants in the United States producing chemicals contaminated with dioxin was reported in 1991.[16] Of the workers in this cohort, 1,052 had died by 31 December 1987. The overall rate of mortality in this group was not elevated when compared with national rates for all causes of death in the United States.[16] Mortality from heart disease was also similar to national rates (SMR 96).[16]

In a subcohort of 1,520 workers with more than one year of exposure to dioxin and more than 20 years since first exposure, the mortality was significantly increased for soft tissue sarcoma (3 deaths, SMR 952) and for cancers of the respiratory system (SMR 142). Mortality for all cancers combined was slightly but significantly elevated in the overall cohort of 5,172 workers.[16] In our cohort there were eight deaths from carcinoma of the lung; one death from an oat-cell carcinoma of the lung; one from carcinoma of the prostate and of the lung; and one from carcinoma of the bronchus. There are too few carcinomas of the respiratory tract in our cohort for any subdivision to be made, but if we exclude the one individual with carcinoma of the prostate as well as of the lung, there were 10 deaths in our cohort due to cancers of the respiratory tract. In other words, some 48% of all cancers in our cohort were due to cancer of the respiratory tract. In the cohort of 5,172 workers exposed to dioxin there were 265 deaths recorded as due to cancer, with some 89 due to cancers of the trachea, bronchus, and lung. This represented some 34% of all cancers.[16] Smoking was not assessed for the mortality study of workers exposed to dioxin, nor were we able to assess it for our mortality study. We have no evidence to suggest that the smoking history of the sprayers was in any way different from that of the population of New Brunswick as a whole.

The most significant difference between the deaths recorded in our cohort and those recorded in other cohorts of workers exposed to phenoxy herbicides or exposed to dioxin is the number of deaths in our cohort due to heart disease. Most of the deaths we recorded were due to heart disease. We have no explanation for this excess of mortality, other than the possible differences in the nature of the exposure sustained by the spray team members in our cohort. We consider their exposure to have been substantial.

The mortality rate for the sprayers in our cohort who sprayed before 1958 was significantly greater than expected. The individuals who participated in the spraying program in this period would have been exposed to phenoxy herbicides. For those individuals who sprayed in 1959 and up until the summer of 1966, there would have been additional contact with waste transformer oil present in the phenoxy herbicide mixture. The mortality rate for individuals who sprayed in the latter period was even greater than that for those who were exposed to phenoxy herbicides alone. However, we feel that it is important to point out that some of those individuals who first sprayed in 1958 or earlier also sprayed after 1959. In consequence of this, they were subjected to both types of exposure—namely, to herbicides alone, and to herbicides plus transformer oil. Thus the mortality rate for workers who first sprayed in 1958 or earlier may have been increased because some individuals were also exposed to waste transformer oil.

We can find no evidence that other investigators have documented the use of waste transformer oil in phenoxy herbicide spray formulations. It was only as the result of a court action against the chemicals companies who provided the herbicides to NB Power that documents were uncovered that advised the power company to use waste transformer oil. These documents were either specific letters addressed to members of NB Power or, as in the case of Dow Canada, in the promotional literature that was distributed by the chemical company. In view of the evidence that electric power companies were advised to use transformer oil in this manner, it is possible that other cohorts of workers exposed to phenoxy herbicides may also have been exposed to polychlorinated biphenyls and polychlorinated dibenzofurans in the waste transformer oil. It may be necessary, therefore, to reevaluate other cohorts if they include sprayers who worked for electric power corporations to assess if there was also exposure to transformer oil.

RECORDS

All of the records and the documents accumulated by the Sprayers of Dioxin Association have been deposited in the New Brunswick Provincial Archives.

SUMMARY

Herbicide spray crews employed by a Canadian power company between 1950 and 1967 had a higher than expected death rate, with a standardized mortality ratio of 157% (CI 130%-194%). In 1991, the cohort consisted of 225 former sprayers of whom 127 were still alive and 98 had died. Eligibility for inclusion in the cohort was based on employer records; and a history of spraying for 30 days or more in at least one spray season.

Deaths expected were based on age-specific population mortality rates for New Brunswick. The all-age SMR for the total cohort was 159%. After 1958, however, waste transformer oil was added to the phenoxy-herbicide spray mixture, the oil representing 10% of the final mixture. Spray crews wore no protective clothing. Subdividing the cohort into spray years 1950-1958 and 1959-1967 yielded SMRs of 146% (CI 115%-184%); and 215% (CI 139%-318%), respectively. The transformer oil was used during the period 1959-1967. Most excess deaths were due to cardiovascular disease.

ACKNOWLEDGMENT

We wish to thank Mr. J. White of the Sprayers of Dioxin Association for his help with this work.

REFERENCES

1. Hardell, L. & A. Sandstrom. 1979. Case-control study: Soft-tissue sarcoma and exposure to phenoxy acetic acids or chlorophenols. Br. J. Cancer **39:** 711-717.

2. ERIKSSON, M., L. HARDELL, N. BERG, T. MOLLER & O. AXELSON. 1981. Soft-tissue sarcomas and exposure to chemical substances: A case-referent study. Br. J. Ind. Med. **38:** 27-33.
3. HARDELL, L., M. ERIKSSON, P. LENNER & E. LUNDGREN. 1981. Malignant lymphoma and exposure to chemicals especially organic solvents, chlorophenols and phenoxy acids: A case-control study. Brit. J. Cancer **43:** 169-176.
4. THIESS, A. M., R. FRENTZEL-BEYME & R. LINK. 1982. Mortality study of persons exposed to dioxin in a trichlorophenol-process accident that occurred in the BASF AG on November 17, 1953. Am. J. Ind. Med. **3:** 179-189.
5. NEW BRUNSWICK ELECTRIC POWER COMMISSION. 1958. Transmission line R-o-w maintenance. Chemical control operation. Instruction to foreman (Fill 3-321 Chemical Control).
6. Internal New Brunswick Power Commission memo from J. E. Guerrette to G. Gagnon, 28 October 1959.
7. Letter from J. A. Cruikshank, Sales Manager, Eastern Division, Naugatuck Chemicals; to P. C. Levesque, New Brunswick Electric Power Commission. 29 June 1951.
8. Letter from J. A. Stearman, Chipman Chemicals, Ltd.; to J. E. Guerrette, New Brunswick Electric Power Commission. 10 April 1957.
9. Dow Vegetation Killers. Promotion brochure for Dow Canada. Date uncertain (likely to be mid-1950s).
10. ECO LOGIC. Estimation of worker exposure to chemicals and herbicide spray. Eli Eco Logic Int. Inc., Rockwood, Ontario. 13 May 1992.
11. SARACCI, R., M. KOGEVINAIS, P. A. BERTAZZI, B. H. B. MESQUITA, D. COGGAN, L. M. GREEN, T. KAUPPINEN, K. A. L'ABBE, M. LITTORIN, E. LYNGE, J. D. MATHEWS, M. NEUBERGER, J. OSMAN, N. PEARCE & R. WINKELMANN. 1991. Cancer mortality in workers exposed to chlorophenoxy herbicides and chlorophenols Lancet **338:** 1027-1032.
12. GUSTAVSSON, P., C. HOGSTED & C. RAPPE. 1986. Short-term mortality and cancer incidence in capacitor manufacturing workers exposed to polychlorinated biphenyls (PCBs) Am. J. Ind. Med. **10:** 341-344.
13. BROWN, D. P. & M. JONES. 1981. Mortality and industrial hygiene study of workers exposed to polychlorinated biphenyls. Arch. Environ. Health **36:** 120-129.
14. JAMES, R. C., H. BUSCH, C. H. TAMBURRO, S. M. ROBERTS, J. D. SCHELL & R. D. HARBISON. 1993. Polychlorinated biphenyl exposure and human disease. J. Occup. Med. **35:** 136-148.
15. BERTAZZI, P. A., L. RIBOLDI, A. PESATORI, L. RADICI & C. ZOCCHETTI. 1987. Cancer mortality of capacitor manufacturing workers. Am. J. Ind. Med. **11:** 76.
16. FINGERHUT, M. A., W. E. HALPERIN, D. A. MARLOW, L. A. PIACITELLI, P. A. HONCHAR, M. H. SWEENEY, A. L. GRIEFE, P. A. DILL, K. STEENLAND & A. J. SURUDA. 1991. Cancer mortality in workers exposed to 2,3,7,8-tetrachlorodibenzo-p-dioxin. N. Engl. J. Med. **324:** 212-218.

Lymphohematopoietic Cancers and Butadiene and Styrene Exposure in Synthetic Rubber Manufacture[a]

G. MATANOSKI,[b,c] E. ELLIOTT,[c] X. TAO,[c]
M. FRANCIS,[d] A. CORREA-VILLASENOR,[c] AND
C. SANTOS-BURGOA[e]

[c]*Department of Epidemiology*
Johns Hopkins University
School of Hygiene and Public Health
615 North Wolfe Street
Baltimore, Maryland 21205

[d]*Battelle*
2101 Wilson Boulevard, Suite 800
Arlington, Virginia 22201

[e]*Escuela de Salud Publica de México*
Av. Universidad No. 655
Col. Santa Maria Ahuacatitla
C.P. 62508
Cuernavaca, Morelos, México

Styrene and 1,3-butadiene are two chemicals that form the bases of common types of synthetic rubber. Both chemicals are carcinogenic in animals. Styrene oxide as a metabolite of styrene causes stomach cancers in species given the chemical by gavage.[1] Data from human studies are limited, and any observed effects often cannot be tied specifically to styrene, which raises questions regarding its carcinogenicity for humans.[2] Butadiene exposure limits had been set on the basis of fire and explosion hazards. However, in the early eighties, toxicology studies indicated that this chemical caused cancer at multiple sites in animals, including the lymphohematopoietic system, lung, heart, brain, and other sites.[3] Several studies in human populations exposed to butadiene have shown increased risks of cancers, especially in the lymphohematopoietic system.[4] Some have questioned the findings of these studies because the type of cancer was not the same for workers in primary butadiene production as compared to end-use industries such as rubber manufacture.[5] Specifically, studies of butadiene production workers showed risks of lymphosarcoma,[6–8] and studies in synthetic rubber production showed leukemia risks.[9–12]

The population for analysis in this paper is from the Matanoski *et al.* cohort, and the study examines exposures of the cases of lymphohematopoietic cancers and

[a]This research was supported in part by National Institutes of Health Grant No. OH-02730 and Environmental Protection Agency Contract No. CR817613.

[b]Phone: 410/955-8183; fax: 410/276-0290.

controls from that cohort as reported in the Santos-Burgoa *et al.* study.[10,11,13,14] That study of lymphohematopoietic cancers had shown a very high risk of leukemia from estimated exposures to butadiene based on a ranking scheme developed with the help of industry representatives (O.R. = 7.4 95% CI 1.3–41.3).[11] The purpose of the current paper is to determine the risks of these cancers in relation to both styrene and butadiene using measured monitoring data from most of the synthetic rubber production plants included in the original study. Use of measured levels of chemicals for each job may provide further clarification of the risks associated not only with butadiene but also with styrene.

PREVIOUS STUDIES OF POPULATION

The original cohort of 12,110 workers with one or more years of employment from seven United States and one Canadian plant had demonstrated low all-cause mortality.[13] However, production workers had an increased risk of deaths from "other lymphatic cancers" (ICD-9 202 and 203), and black production workers had an increased risk of leukemia. Industry representatives were asked to score each job for both styrene and butadiene exposures on a scale of 1 to 10. Jobs were given the same scores for seven of the eight plants in the study with some slight modification of scores of only one plant because of variation in production practices. For each worker in the nested case-control study of all lymphohematopoietic cancers, the job score for each job was multiplied by the number of months spent in that job, and these job-specific cumulative scores, summed over all jobs, provided a total cumulative score for an individual. The analysis indicated that butadiene cumulative scores and selected work areas (labor, laboratory, and support services) were associated with an increased odds ratio for leukemia.[11] Subsequently, a review of industrial hygiene measurements of butadiene and styrene levels for seven of the eight study plants indicated that the monitored levels differed by plant.[10] This meant that the original study design, which matched cases and controls by plant and duration worked based on the presumption that exposures were similar across plants, may have overmatched for exposure and diluted the observed association with butadiene.

MATERIAL AND METHODS

The 59 lymphohematopoietic cancer cases included in the current study are the same as those from the Santos-Burgoa study. The cases generally had 10 or more years of employment and 20 years of follow-up.[10] The cases were selected based on the classification of lymphohematopoietic cancers (LHC) as they appeared on death certificates. For the current study, hospital records were reviewed to verify diagnosis for 55 of the 59 cases. Records were available for all but one leukemia case, and diagnoses were correct in all instances. Following review, all leukemias could be classified into subtype. Classification of non-Hodgkins lymphomas and lymphosarcomas on death certificates did not correspond to the hospital diagnoses based on specific ICD code. Of the 13 cases reviewed, however, all but two fell into the combined category of ICD 200 and 202. The two cases with incorrect death certificate diagnoses based on hospital records were omitted from this study, but one new case was added from the hospital record review of other cancers, resulting in 12 cases, 7 lymphosarcomas (ICD 200) and 5 non-Hodgkins lymphomas (ICD 202). The diagnoses of cases of multiple myeloma and Hodgkins disease were unchanged after hospital review. The new classifications resulted in 58 total cases; the case classifications based on hospital diagnoses were used to distinguish the specific cancer subgroups. For the four cases for which a complete hospital record could not be obtained, the death certificate diagnoses were used.

The 1242 controls included in this study are part of a larger case-control study of several cancer sites. These controls were selected to represent the frequency distribution of population sizes across the eight plants and are similar in age distribution to the cases. The controls represent one percent of the plant population. Since controls had to live as long as or longer than cases, their duration of employment and, thus, their exposure potential is slightly longer than that of the case group, leading to possible higher cumulative exposures. For that reason, all models using the cumulative exposures included the "duration worked" variable in the model.

EXPOSURE

A total of 3,952 butadiene and 3,649 styrene exposure measurements were gathered from seven of the eight plants and from NIOSH. Most measurements represented personal monitoring data, and these were the only values used to represent job exposures. Despite the large number of measurements, some jobs in some plants had no values. However, all jobs had a rank score from the previous exposure estimation done by industry representatives.

For the current analysis, the assumption is that the *relative* exposures of jobs are similar across plants, but the *actual* exposure values for a specific job will differ by plant. The z-score transformation was used to estimate exposure for all jobs with missing measurements for each plant. These estimations used the actual values from other plants to get the relative values by job and the measurements for the plant to calculate missing job exposures for that plant. Thus, after these calculations, every job had an exposure level that was unique by plant and was based on monitoring data for that plant. The single plant with no industrial hygiene measurements was assigned values for jobs based on the values of a similar plant in the same geographic area. These job- and plant-specific exposure levels and the job histories of cases and controls were used to calculate both a cumulated exposure in parts per million times number of months exposed (ppm-months) and a time-weighted average exposure in parts per million (ppm) based on total cumulated exposure in ppm-months divided by the total time employed for both styrene and butadiene for each individual.

ANALYSIS

Unconditional logistic regression analysis was done using SPSS with beta values calculated using a continuous variable for ln-transformed chemical exposure measures.[15] These beta values also were converted into corresponding odds ratios for a time-weighted average exposure to each chemical at 1 ppm. Multivariate models included birth year, year of hire before or after 1950, hire age, race, and duration worked. The variables were tested for their contribution to the model using step-down modeling. Although butadiene and styrene levels are correlated, the correlation did not interfere with the use of both variables in the model.

RESULTS

The associations between specific categories of lymphohematopoietic cancers and the chemicals clearly differ by type of cancer. Leukemias and Hodgkins disease are associated with time-weighted average butadiene exposure. The other cancers in this ICD-9 group 200–209, except for non-Hodgkins lymphomas (ICD-9 202), have significant associations with exposure to styrene (TABLE 1). Although none of the demographic variables are significant in the model, leukemia cases are more likely to be younger and to have been hired after 1950 compared to controls. The observed association suggests that there is a significant increase in the risk of leukemia for each unit increase in the average measured levels of butadiene. Based on the leukemia model, as shown in TABLE 1, the odds ratio calculated for exposure to butadiene at the low average working lifetime level of 1 ppm is 1.5 (95% CI 1.1, 2.1). The odds ratio for Hodgkin's disease associated with a similar butadiene exposure at 1 ppm is 1.7 (95% CI 1.0, 3.0). The associations between the continuous measure of styrene exposure and all LHC, all lymphomas, lymphosarcomas, and multiple myeloma are also highly significant. The odds ratio for multiple myeloma associated with low-level styrene exposure at 1 ppm is 3.0 (95% CI 1.3, 7.0). The risk of lymphosarcoma is significantly associated with increasing styrene exposure, and the odds ratio at 1 ppm exposure is 3.9 (95% CI 1.6, 9.6). The association between all lymphomas and styrene is represented by an odds ratio at 1 ppm of 2.7 (95% CI 1.2, 5.8).

TABLE 2 represents use of a cumulative dose to assess associations between these two chemicals and lymphohematopoietic cancers. In all but the models for multiple myeloma, a term for duration worked contributes significantly to the model. This term usually is negative and suggests the risk is higher for those reaching a cumulative dose in a shorter time period, that is, those with a higher-intensity dose. For workers with a long duration worked and a long latency for some of these diseases, this may also represent early exposure periods in their work history. The associations of leukemia and Hodgkins disease with butadiene are still present when using the cumulative exposure measure, but for leukemia styrene exposure also plays a role. In most cases, the use of a cumulative measure does not present any different conclusions than that of time-weighted exposure variables. Only in the combined category of lymphomas (ICD-9 200 and 202) did the best model include demographic variables. The odds ratios for these cancers increased the earlier the birth year and the older the age at first hire of the subjects.

The review of hospital records allowed classification of leukemias into the major types, lymphoid and myeloid, but further subclassification into acute and chronic categories resulted in insufficient numbers for modeling. It should be noted that among the lymphoid leukemias 5 out of 10 were classified as acute. This ratio is in marked contrast to that reported by the national cancer registries, in which only eight

TABLE 1. Associations between Lymphohematopoietic Cancers[a] and Exposure to Average Time-Weighted Butadiene [ln(ppm + 1)] and Styrene [ln(ppm + 1)] Levels as Continuous Variables

		Butadiene			Styrene			Final Model[c]	
Cause[a] (ICD - 9 No.)	No. of Cases	Beta	*p*	OR at 1 ppm[b] (95% CI)	Beta	*p*	OR at 1 ppm[b] (95% CI)	Variables	Model *p*
LHC (200–209)	58				1.140	0.000	2.20 (1.46, 3.33)	STY only	0.001
Lymphomas (200 & 202)	12				1.415	0.014	2.67 (1.22, 5.84)	STY only BY, agehire	0.020
Lymphosarcoma (200)	7				1.956	0.003	3.88 (1.57, 9.59)	STY only	0.011
Lymphoma (202)	5						2.62 (0.40, 17.15)	None	>0.050
Hodgkins[d] (201)	8	0.787	0.056	1.73 (0.99, 3.02)				BD only	0.077
Myeloma (203)	10				1.604	0.009	3.04 (1.33, 6.96)	STY only	0.021
Leukemia (204–207)	26	0.588	0.018	1.50 (1.07, 2.10)				BD only	0.026

[a] Cause as diagnosed from hospital records. LHC = all lymphohematopoietic cancers.

[b] Odds ratio for exposure at 1 ppm compared to 0 ppm: OR = exp[beta*ln(1 ppm + 1)]. 95% Cl = exp[(beta = 1.96SE)*ln(1 ppm + 1)]. Example LHC: OR = exp[1.14*ln(1 ppm + 1) = 2.20].

[c] Step-down unconditional logistic regression models included birth year (BY), age of hire (agehire), year of hire before 1950 (Hirebf50), race, duration, styrene [ln(ppm + 1)](STY), and butadiene [ln(ppm + 1)] (BD) as continuous variables. In all cases, the most parsimonious model included only a single chemical variable.

[d] The association between Hodgkins disease and butadiene is stronger if time and age variables are in the model, but the model is not significantly better.

TABLE 2. Associations between Lymphohematopoietic Cancers[a] as Related Cumulative Exposure to Butadiene and Styrene [ln(ppm months + 1)] as Continuous Variables

Cause[a] (ICD - 9 No.)	No. of Cases	Butadiene Beta	Butadiene *p*	Styrene Beta	Styrene *p*	Final Model[b] Variables	Final Model[b] Model *p*
LHC (200–209)	58			0.400	0.000	STY & duration	0.000
Lymphomas (200 & 202)	12					none	>0.050
Lymphosarcoma (200)	7					None	>0.050
Lymphomas (202)	5					None	>0.050
Hodgkins (201)	8	0.573	0.032			BD only, duration	0.042
Myeloma (203)	10			0.447	0.023	STY only	0.013
Leukemia (204–207)	26	0.240	0.054	0.481	0.006	BD, STY, duration	0.001

[a] Causes as diagnosed from hospital records. LHC = all lymphohematopoietic cancers.

[b] Step-down unconditional logistic multiple regression models included birth year (BY), age of hire (agehire), year of hire before 1950 (Hirebf50), race, duration, styrene [ln(ppm months + 1)](STY), and butadiene [ln(ppm months + 1)] (BD).

percent of adult lymphoid leukemia cases are listed as acute.[16] Because of the unusual distribution of lymphoid leukemias in this population, the subgroups have been examined separately in TABLE 3.

In addition, the previous study of lymphohematopoietic cancers in this cohort had reported an association between leukemia and longest job held for each individual in three work area categories: laboratory, service, and labor.[11] Service work is defined by jobs that support other activities in the plant, including special tank-cleaning teams. Laboratory work could include jobs in both chemical as well as physical labs. The latter labs test the physical strength of a product and would have lower exposures to butadiene and styrene. Research and development labs are also included here and have very diverse exposures. Chemical laboratory workers would have the highest butadiene and styrene exposures in this group. Each worker was classified to the work area where he had worked the longest. For this study, the same three work areas were combined into a single "job" variable (service, labor, or laboratory), which was compared to all other job groups as reference (process, utility, maintenance, warehouse, administration, pilot plant, and engineering).

The results shown in TABLE 3 indicate that the model for all leukemias with the job variable added still shows an association with exposure to butadiene similar to the model without job (TABLE 1); but the variable for work in service, labor, or laboratory areas also explains some of the difference between cases and controls.

TABLE 3. Associations between Leukemia and Major Subtypes and Exposures to Average Time-Weighted Butadiene [ln(ppm + 1)] and Styrene [ln(ppm + 1)] as Continuous Variables and Longest Job in Services, Labor, or Laboratory

		Butadiene			Job			Final Model[c]	
Cause[a] (ICD-9 No.)	# Cases	Beta	*p*	OR at 1 ppm[b] (95% CI)	Beta	*p*	OR (95% CI)	Variables	Model *p*
All Leukemias (204–207)	26	0.572	0.026	1.49 (1.05, 2.11)	0.973	0.015	2.64 (1.21, 5.30)	BD, job	0.005
Lymphoid (204)	10	0.757	0.042	1.69 (1.02, 2.80)				BD	0.060
Myeloid (205)	15				1.591	0.012	3.70 (1.33, 10.29)	Job	0.013

[a] Causes as diagnosed from hospital records.

[b] Odds ratio for exposure at 1 ppm compared to 0 ppm: OR = exp[beta*ln(1 ppm + 1)]. 95% Cl = exp[(beta = 1.96SE)*ln(1 ppm + 1)]. Example leukemia: OR = exp[0.572*ln(1 ppm + 1) = 1.49].

[c] Step-down unconditional logistic regression models included birth year (BY), age of hire (agehire), year of hire before 1950 (Hirebf50), race, duration, job, styrene [ln(ppm + 1)](STY), and butadiene [ln(ppm + 1)] (BD) as continuous variables. In all cases, the most parsimonious model included only a single chemical variable.

The model is much more significant than one with butadiene alone. Styrene is not associated with all leukemia or with either the lymphoid or myeloid subtypes. The odds ratio for exposure to butadiene at 1 ppm is 1.5 (95% CI 1.1, 2.1); and the odds ratio associated with holding a longest job in the service, labor, or laboratory areas is 2.6 (95% CI 1.2, 5.3).

The risks differ for the two leukemia cell types (TABLE 3). Lymphoid leukemia is associated with exposure to butadiene with an odds ratio of 1.7 (95% CI 1.0, 2.8) at average exposures of 1 ppm. There is no association of this leukemia with the work area variable. Myeloid leukemia is associated only with work area with an odds ratio of 3.7 (95% CI 1.3, 10.3). These data would suggest either that the risks from industrial exposures associated with the various leukemia cell types differ or that some jobs have not been correctly measured for exposure to the chemicals. The numbers of cases were too small to divide the cell types further into acute and chronic subsets.

DISCUSSION

The results of the analysis of lymphohematopoietic cancers and their subgroups of cancer indicate that, while all are associated with industrial exposures in synthetic rubber manufacture, the agents associated with the risks differ. Lymphosarcoma and myeloma cases are associated with styrene exposure, and Hodgkins disease and leukemia cases are associated with butadiene exposure. The analysis of risks is difficult because the population in this industry are exposed to two possible carcinogens, butadiene and styrene, and their uses are closely linked in the work environment. The use of actual measured data by job as in this study helped to distinguish the effects from the two exposures. The data suggest that each agent may be related to different cancers. In some cases, the differences are very clear. For example, the 10 myeloma cases show a strongly positive association with styrene and a negative but nonsignificant association with butadiene. A relationship between styrene and myeloma has appeared in previous reports describing risks in the styrene manufacturing industry, which strengthens the finding.[17,18] The recent international study in the polystyrene industry did not report the risks of styrene associated with subclasses of lymphohematopoietic cancers.[19]

The association between lymphosarcoma and styrene is represented with a high odds ratio similar to that seen with multiple myeloma, but the association is unexpected based on reports from butadiene production facility studies.[6–8] These previous reports indicated an association between butadiene exposure and the risk of lymphosarcoma identified from death certificates. In this current study, hospital records have been used to identify cases since death certificates have been shown to frequently misclassify lymphoma deaths, exchanging causes between the ICD 200 and ICD 202 categories. After using medical records to correctly diagnose cases, both cancers appear to be associated with styrene in this study. This finding does not rule out the possibility of a risk of lymphosarcoma from butadiene exposure. Styrene exposure is associated with a very high risk of lymphosarcoma, but styrene was not present in the butadiene production industry. If both agents are carcinogenic for the lymphatic system, it may be difficult to distinguish risks from exposure to each independently without more precise dose information. The risk associated with styrene exposure may have masked a risk associated with butadiene exposure.

The risks of leukemia and Hodgkins are significantly associated with butadiene exposure and not styrene in models where both chemicals are included and when the average time-weighted intensity of exposure is used. However, styrene usually remained as the last variable for withdrawal in a step-down model of leukemia but did not contribute significantly to the models. Since exposures to both chemicals are correlated and precise measures over 30 to 40 years are not available, distinguishing between the 2 chemicals is obviously difficult. The risk of leukemia is related not only to butadiene exposure but also to work area. Based on the odds ratio, the risk of leukemia is estimated to increase by 50% from exposure to as low as 1 ppm of butadiene on average over a working lifetime. The risk increases 160% from work in three selected areas, laboratory, labor, and service. Leukemia may represent multiple diseases with multiple risk factors. The risks from chemicals may differ by cell type, in which case combining all leukemias conceals and dilutes effects.

To examine the issue regarding homogeneity of risks by subtype, leukemia subgroups were examined. Although the number of cases by group were small, the data suggest that the risks differ by leukemia type. Lymphoid leukemias are associated with exposure to butadiene, and myeloid leukemias are associated with working in laboratory, labor, or service areas. These data may represent not true differences in risk by subtype but imprecisely measured exposures by job. The fact that myeloid leukemia did not demonstrate a significant association with either styrene or butadiene does not mean that one or both of the chemicals are not related to myeloid leukemia. In fact, if job is not considered and both chemicals are examined for their association with myeloid leukemia, butadiene is associated with a risk of myeloid leukemia but with a p value = 0.14. Based on that model, the data suggest that myeloid leukemia is associated with exposure to butadiene with an odds ratio similar to that reported for lymphoid leukemia. Therefore, these jobs need to be reexamined for the levels and patterns of exposure to butadiene.

The three work areas associated with a risk of leukemia are likely to have serious problems of underreporting of exposures. The service classification included tank cleanup crews, but few measurements were recorded for this group, which has the potential for high intermittent levels. The laboratories had very different measured exposures depending on the type, location, and responsibilities of the lab as well as the specific jobs the workers held in that work area. However, it is often difficult to distinguish the exact laboratory that is related to a measurement. The measured levels of recent years undoubtedly represented a lower exposure than would have been present in the past since various types of controls to reduce exposures have been introduced in the industry. These factors could have diluted differences in exposures according to the exact laboratory and its operations. For many laboratory workers in some plants, the personnel data did not permit a separation of jobs according to specific activities in specific laboratories, and therefore the data are diluted still further by using an average exposure level for all jobs across laboratories to calculate average weighted exposures of individuals in some plants. Limiting the analysis only to the plants where jobs could be specified as to exact laboratory work would reduce the already small number of cases for analysis. Similar problems exist for the ''labor'' classification. Thus, (1) inadequate measurements of exposures in these work areas, current and past, (2) adding together laboratory measurements from locations with major exposure differences into a single category, and (3) imprecision in defining exact work location and job from personnel records in work areas with marked variation in exposures by job make it difficult to distinguish the chemical exposures that are associated with these work areas. The association between the job category and leukemia indicates that specific jobs within these areas need better definition of exposures in order to determine why this association between work area and leukemia exists.

The use of a cumulative exposure measure resulted in only minor differences in overall conclusions regarding risks but did demonstrate a tendency to emphasize risks associated with styrene. A possible explanation for this finding is that intensity of exposure is a more important measure of risk associated with butadiene exposure than is total cumulative dose. This hypothesis is supported by experiments in animals that indicated that exposure intensity is more important in carcinogenicity than is exposure duration.[20] In this study, an association with intensity of exposure is suggested by the fact that models using cumulative dose are improved with the addition of a variable for duration, which usually is negative. This indicates that the longer the worker is employed to reach the observed cumulative dose, the lower that worker's risk. Use of a cumulative exposure measure dilutes the effect of high-intensity exposures. However, exposure measures used in this study have not emphasized "intensity" as a variable. The exposure measures themselves are subject to repeated averaging. The exposures by job have been averaged over a workday, over many individual measures, over many jobs included in a single common job class and even over similar jobs across the industry, and, perhaps most importantly, over long time periods. Thus, any high exposure levels are diluted. Some jobs have exposure to both chemicals, and cumulative exposures to both styrene and butadiene will then be multiplied by a constant number of months in the job. That increases the levels for both chemicals. However, unlike butadiene exposure, styrene has low exposures for *most* industry jobs, which adds to the cumulative exposure for styrene and not butadiene. Thus, low-level styrene exposure tends to dominate cumulative measures.

The major strength of the data derived from this study is that the associations are based on measured values for each job of individual workers in each plant. While there are many obvious drawbacks to such data, the foremost being the fact that the measures represent more recent exposures in the industry, the fact that they are actual values removes possible biases that can arise from professional estimates of exposure that reflect individual beliefs about what exposures should be assigned to what jobs. The use of the data to assign exposures to each individual is based on two assumptions: that the relative exposures by jobs are constant across plants and time and that exposure levels for all jobs differ by plant. The latter assumption appears to be correct when measurements by plant weighted by jobs are examined. A review of relative exposures by jobs across plants suggests similar constant relationships, which would support the first assumption. However, the data cannot be used to examine changes in relationships over time since the measurements cover only the recent 15 to 20 years of plant operations and are sparse. Further modeling could be done using estimates of differences in exposures by job over time. If the relative exposure differences for specific jobs have changed greatly over time, this would be an important correction, which could influence the associations, especially for the jobs with the highest exposures in the past. Further work is needed to correct for these differences over time.

Work in the synthetic rubber manufacturing industry is clearly associated with a risk of leukemia. Not only has our examination of this cohort identified the risk, but also the study of Delzell *et al.*, which independently investigated a population that included a high proportion of the present cohort, identified a similar risk.[12,21] Using a different approach from the one in this study and estimating chemical exposures for jobs based on interviews and using cumulative exposure-years to determine risk ratios, Macaluso *et al.* has reported a stronger association between butadiene and leukemia than with styrene in the Delzell cohort.[21] The data from the current analysis using measured values indicates the same association between leukemia and butadiene. The fact that this association does not hold for other lymphohematopoietic cancers except for Hodgkins strengthens the probability that the associations between the specific chemicals and cancers are real. The positive association between styrene and myeloma in models where there is a negative association with butadiene would indicate that these measured values can distinguish the differences in risk for the two chemicals. Despite the small number of cases of lymphosarcoma in this population, there is a significant association between this cancer and styrene but not butadiene. These findings indicate that both chemicals appear to be possible carcinogens for lymphohematopoietic cancers in this population. The combined presence of both chemicals in many jobs may actually conceal some of the risks from each agent alone. Further efforts will be needed to separate these effects.

SUMMARY

The described nested case-control study of lymphohematopoietic cancers occurring in a cohort of synthetic rubber production workers was conducted to determine the associations of these cancers with exposure to butadiene and styrene. Cases have been confirmed through hospital record review of 95 percent of the cancers. Exposures are based on measured values of the two chemicals from personal monitoring data in seven of the eight plants under study.

The results indicate that the risk of leukemia increases with exposure to a time-weighted average butadiene measure. The odds ratio at only 1 ppm average butadiene exposure is 1.50 (95% CI 1.07, 2.10). Work in specific areas also contributes to the risk, possibly because these areas have not been completely characterized for differences in butadiene exposure. Hodgkins disease is also associated with butadiene exposure. Multiple myeloma, lymphosarcoma, and all lymphomas are associated with exposure to styrene. Since workers in this industry are apparently exposed to two carcinogenic agents, further effort must be made to distinguish the exposures to each chemical over time and to characterize their interrelationship with the risk of cancers of the lymphohematopoietic system.

ACKNOWLEDGMENTS

The authors wish to thank the participating rubber companies, the International Institute of Synthetic Rubber Products, and the National Institute of Occupational Safety and Health for providing the monitoring data that was used in the analysis.

REFERENCES

1. McConnell, E. E. & J. A. Swenberg. 1993. Styrene and styrene oxide: Results of studies on carcinogenicity in experimental animals. *In* Butadiene and Styrene: Assessment of Health Hazards: 323-334. IARC Scientific Publication No. 127. Lyon.
2. International Agency for Research on Cancer. 1994. Styrene. *In* IARC Monographs on the Evaluation of Carcinogenic Risks to Humans. Vol 60: Some Industrial Chemicals: 233-320. IARC. Lyon.
3. Melnick, R. L. & J. E. Huff. 1993. 1,3-Butadiene induces cancer in experimental animals at all concentrations from 6.25 to 8000 parts per million. *In* Butadiene and Styrene: Assessment of Health Hazards: 309-322. IARC Scientific Publication No. 127. Lyon.
4. Landrigan, P. J. 1993. Critical assessment of epidemiologic studies on the carcinogenicity of 1,3-butadiene and styrene. *In* Butadiene and Styrene: Assessment of Health Hazards: 375-388. IARC Scientific Publication No. 127. Lyon.
5. Acquavella, J. F. 1996. Butadiene epidemiology: A summary of results and outstanding issues. Toxicology **113:** 148-156.
6. Downs, T. D., M. M. Crane & K. W. Kim. 1987. Mortality among workers at a butadiene facility. Am. J. Ind. Med. **12:** 311-329.
7. Divine, B. J., J. K. Wendt & C. M. Hartman. 1993. Cancer mortality among workers at a butadiene production facility. *In* Butadiene and Styrene: Assessment of Health Hazards: 345-362. IARC Scientific Publication No. 127. Lyon.
8. Ward, E. M., J. M. Fajen, A. M. Ruder, R. A. Rinsky, W. E. Halperin & C. A. Fessler-Flesch. 1996. Mortality study of workers employed in 1,3-butadiene production units identified from a large chemical workers cohort. Toxicology **113:** 157-168.
9. Meinhardt, T. J., R. A. Lemen, M. S. Crandall & R. J. Young. 1982. Environmental epidemiologic investigations of the styrene-butadiene rubber industry. Scand. J. Work Environ. Health **8:** 250-259.
10. Matanoski, G. M., M. Francis, A. Correa-Villasenor, E. Elliott, C. Santos-Burgoa & L. Schwartz. 1993. Cancer epidemiology among styrene-butadiene rubber workers. *In* Butadiene and Styrene: Assessment of Health Hazards: 363-374. IARC Scientific Publication No. 127. Lyon.
11. Santos-Burgoa, C., G. M. Matanoski, S. Zeger & L. Schwartz. 1992. Lymphohematopoietic cancer in styrene-butadiene polymerization workers. Am. J. Epidemiol. **136:** 843-854.
12. Delzell, E., N. Sathiakumar, M. Macaluso, M. Hovinga, R. Larson, F. Barbone, C. Beall & P. A. Cole. 1996. A follow-up study of synthetic rubber workers. Toxicology **113:** 182-189.
13. Matanoski, G. M., C. Santos-Burgoa & L. Schwartz. 1990. Mortality of a cohort of workers in styrene-butadiene polymer manufacturing industry (1943-1982). Environ. Health Perspect. **86:** 107-117.
14. Matanoski, G. M. & C. Santos-Burgoa. 1994. Butadiene and lymphatic and hematopoietic cancer (letter to editor). Epidemiology **5:** 261-262.
15. SPSS Inc. 1990. SPSS/PC+. Version 4.0.1. Chicago.
16. SEER Registries 1991, 1994. SEER Cancer Statistics Review, 1973-1991: Tables and Graphs, National Cancer Institute. L. A. G. Ries, B. A. Miller, B. F. Hankey, C. L. Kosary, A. Harras & B. K. Edwards, Eds. NIH Pub. No. 94-2789. Bethesda, MD.
17. Ott, M. G., R. C. Kolesar, H. C. Scharnweber, E. J. Schneider & J. R. Venable. 1980. A mortality survey of employees engaged in the development or manufacture of styrene-based products. J. Occup. Med. **22:** 445-460.
18. Bond, G., K. M. Bodner, G. W. Olsen & R. R. Cook. 1992. Mortality among workers engaged in the development or manufacture of styrene-based products—An update. Scand. J. Work Environ. Health **18:** 145-154.
19. Kogevinas, M., G. Ferro, R. Saracci, A. Andersen, M. Biocca, D. Coggon, V. Gennaro, S. Hutchings, H. Kolstad, I. Lungberg, E. Lynge & T. Paryanen. 1993. Cancer mortality in a international cohort of workers exposed to styrene. *In*

Butadiene and Styrene: Assessment of Health Hazards: 289-300. IARC Scientific Publication No. 127. Lyon.

20. Melnick, R. L., J. Huff, B. J. Chou & R. A. Miller. 1990. Carcinogenicity of 1, 3-butadiene in C57B1/6 × C 3HF1 mice at low exposure concentrations. Cancer Res. **50:** 6592.

21. Macaluso, M., R. Larson, E. Delzell, N. Sathiakumar, M. Hovinga, J. Hulian, D. Muir, P. Cole. 1996. Leukemia and cumulative exposure to butadiene, styrene and benzene among workers in the synthetic rubber industry. Toxicology **113:** 190-202.

Underestimating Risk for Three Important Human Carcinogens: Vinyl Chloride, Benzene, and Butadiene

MARVIN S. LEGATOR[a]

Division of Environmental Toxicology
Department of Preventive Medicine and Community Health
University of Texas Medical Branch
Galveston, Texas 77555

INTRODUCTION

The last 10 years has seen an unprecedented development of procedures, including biomarkers of effect such as chromosome painting, DNA repair evaluations, and somatic cell mutation assays, that can be applied to monitoring individuals exposed to toxic substances.[1] These new procedures, as well as older conventional ones, are being underutilized in human monitoring studies.[2]

In establishing priorities for testing chemicals, one has to question the wisdom of continuing to allocate sparse resources to test chemicals that are well characterized as human carcinogens. Spending time and money conducting further studies on well-characterized human chemical carcinogens will be of little value to the victims of chemical exposure. The pressing need is to clean up the known hazardous chemical pollutants.

Chemicals already identified as animal carcinogens (IARC 2A or 2B) and where significant human exposure to them exists should receive our immediate attention for application of these new and relevant genetic screening procedures. The need to reevaluate this group of chemicals is especially critical given the existing data, which suggests that current risk assessment, based on extrapolation from high-dose animal studies to low-dose chronic exposure in humans, underestimates the true risk of chemical exposure.

In this paper I will (a) review data that indicates that extrapolation from high-dose animal experiments to low-dose human exposure may underestimate the true genotoxic (carcinogenic) risk for human exposure to vinyl chloride, benzene, and butadiene; (b) indicate how *in vitro* and *in vivo* mechanistic and toxicokinetic studies with butadiene were misinterpreted and led to faulty conclusions as to the true risk of human exposure; and (c) discuss the need to utilize existing biomarkers of effect to characterize populations exposed to known animal carcinogens.

[a] This paper was previously published in the *Journal of Clean Technology, Environmental Toxicology, and Occupational Medicine,* Volume 5, Number 3, 1994. It is reprinted with permission.

EXTRAPOLATING FROM HIGH-LEVEL ANIMAL EXPERIMENTS TO LOW-LEVEL HUMAN EXPOSURE UNDERESTIMATES TRUE RISK

In traditional lifetime cancer bioassays in laboratory animals, chemicals are usually tested at the maximum tolerated doses (MTD) and fractions of the MTD. The rational for using high levels, upon which to base human exposure at low chronic levels, is the belief that this approach maximizes the detection of carcinogenic chemicals. This procedure is usually viewed as, and in theory should provide, a means to prevent human exposure to even weak mutagens (carcinogens). Several investigators have criticized this approach as being overconservative, unrealistic, and capable of producing false positive results.[3] There are several examples with important industrial chemicals, however, that indicate that extrapolation from high-dose animal experiments to the more typical low-level human exposure is not conservative but significantly underestimates the true risk to humans.

Vinyl Chloride

Bialar *et al.*,[4] evaluating a series of chemicals, reported on the incidence of liver angiosarcoma in female rats after exposure to vinyl chloride. The measured dose-response curve for angiosarcoma induced by vinyl chloride indicated a 10-fold underestimate of risk when high-level exposure (3,000–6,000 ppm) was compared to doses in the 1–50 ppm range. The authors concluded that: ". . . in a high percentage of animal bioassays, the one-hit formula is not conservative when applied in the usual way to animal data. It remains possible that the one-hit formula may indeed by conservative at sufficiently low doses (below the observational range), but the usual procedure applied to the usual dose range, can be non conservative in estimating the slope of the formula at such low doses. Risk assessments for regulation of carcinogens should incorporate some measure of additional uncertainty." The authors suggest a number of reasons for this underestimation including saturation of enzymes at high doses.

Vinyl chloride can be considered a prototype of a group of carcinogens where there is a degree of similarity in regard to the drug-metabolizing enzymes including phase I and phase II enzymes responsible for both activation and detoxification. If we address those chemicals where P450 is one of the major phase I biotransforming enzymes, we could include a wide number of xenobiotics.[5] Since a variety of different enzymes or metabolic systems are involved in bioactivation reactions, which include both phase I and phase II enzymatic systems, any concentration-dependent alteration in either activation or detoxification would have a significant effect on mutation and cancer formation. These concentration-dependent differences would then be translated into different quantitative conclusions in estimating risk from animals to man.

Benzene

Benzene is known to interact with pluripotent stem cells to induce hematopoietic neoplasms.[6] In mice exposed to benzene for 22 hours per day/7 days per week/for

6 weeks at 40, 100, and 1,000 ppb, an increase in somatic cell mutations was detected with the autoradiographic *hprt* mutant lymphocyte assay.[7] At all three doses, a significant increase in mutant frequency over the controls was observed. At the highest dose, however, there was a significant decrease in mutant frequency from the values obtained at the medium-dose level. Additionally, in a study to determine chromosome damage in lymphocytes (mixed chemical exposure including benzene), mice exposed for six weeks were evaluated. Chromosome breakage increased at the low and medium concentrations when compared to controls, but not at the high concentration. This lack of response at the high concentration appeared to correlate with a significant induction of glutathione S-transferase (GST) enzymes in the liver. The authors concluded that, since GST is part of a detoxification pathway, induction of this enzyme system by the higher doses of benzene may have detoxified the benzene to less mutagenic or nonmutagenic metabolites.[8]

In a series of papers[9–12] using both data from *in vivo* studies with mice, rats, and monkeys and a physiological model, both activation and detoxification pathways were investigated. At high benzene concentration in mice (600 ppm), phenyl conjugates are the predominate urinary metabolites. At low concentrations (25 ppm and lower), the level to which humans might be exposed, the predominate toxic metabolites are hydroquinone conjugates and muconic acid. A major conclusion of these studies is that in three different animal species (mice, rats, and monkeys), the metabolic pathways leading to production of the putative toxic metabolites appear to be low-capacity, high-affinity pathways that are saturated at relatively low-exposure concentrations. The detoxification pathways are predominately high-capacity, low-affinity pathways, and they increase at higher concentrations. The authors conclude, ''If the total formation of the putative toxic metabolites is predictive of the toxicity of benzene, then the animal studies suggest that calculations of the risk associated with low-dose exposures based on the results of animal studies conducted at [high] doses would underestimate the toxicity of benzene.''

1.3-Butadiene

In a review article that suffered from unfortunate timing, Bond *et al.* concluded that butadiene is not genotoxic in occupationally exposed workers, and that the preponderance of evidence suggest that butadiene will not be carcinogenic to humans at current occupational or environmental exposure levels.[13] Shortly after this report, Dezell and Cole confirmed that butadiene should be classified as a human carcinogen.[14] Just prior to the Bond *et al.* report, Legator *et al.* and Ward *et al.*[15,16] reported that in workers exposed to only 1–3 ppm of butadiene, there was a significant increase in mutant frequencies when evaluated by the autoradiograhic *hprt* mutant lymphocyte assay.[14] Additionally, Au *et al.* reported increased levels of chromosome damage in a DNA repair assay in the same group of workers.[17]

Major reasons for misinterpreting and indeed being misled by mechanistic and pharmacokinetic studies with butadiene may be due to the fact that nonrelevant *in vitro* data and acute high-level exposure animal data formed the basis for many of the inferences on potential butadiene effects with chronic low-level human exposure. In the study by Himmelstein[18] inferences about the presence of the butadiene mono-

or diepoxide in blood were made only after a 6-hour exposure using 62.5 ppm of butadiene as the lowest concentration, with the maximum concentration being 8,000 ppm. *In vitro* data formed the bases leading to the conclusion concerning differences in tissue metabolism, activation/detoxification kinetics, and potency of both the mono- and diepoxide. Valid conclusions should be based, primarily, on chronic low-level animal exposure and human monitoring data.

An example of the proper use of animal studies is the analysis of hemoglobin adducts in rats and mice.[19] In the adduct formation studies similar frequencies in adduct formation were found at low concentrations. Species divergence occurred only at high concentrations. It is also significant that hemoglobin adducts from butadiene exposure were found in a population of workers exposed to only 1–3 ppm. One of the major conclusions by Bond, that any cancer risk assessment for butadiene should use *in vitro* human tissue metabolic data, has proved to be incorrect.

The overall findings with butadiene indicate that species may vary quantitatively but not qualitatively as to butadiene metabolites, and that extrapolation from high-level acute studies may not be significant in terms of low-dose chronic human exposure. Given the nature of the metabolic activation pathways and the detoxification pathways, it is probable that a shift in metabolism and detoxification also occurs at high doses. This suggests that, like benzene and vinyl chloride, extrapolation from high-dose animal studies to low-dose human exposure may underestimate the risk of this chemical. Butadiene is a prime example of how one can be misled by inappropriate mechanistic and pharmacokinetic studies.

FUTURE DIRECTIONS AND MONITORING NEEDS

In the future there will be numerous opportunities for genetic monitoring in the workplace and in communities exposed to toxic substances. Given the difficulties in identifying populations and scarce resources for conducting genetic monitoring, we must prioritize as to the types of chemical exposures and the nature of the exposed populations to be studied. The lowest priority should be given to those populations that are known to be exposed to high concentrations of mutagens and carcinogens. Clearly, if a population is exposed to high levels of known toxins (such as carcinogenic polyaromatic hydrocarbons, benzene, and vinyl chloride), there is little benefit to be derived from doing yet another study. Exposure to known toxins should require reducing or eliminating exposure. The highest priority should be give to those chemicals where there is substantial exposure, and where animal, or perhaps limited human, studies indicate that the chemical is a carcinogen, an IARC 2A or 2B chemical. It is in this category of chemicals that we have most likely incorrectly estimated risk by extrapolating from high-dose animal studies to low-level human exposure. If vinyl chloride, benzene, and butadiene represent a more general phenomena, we have probably underestimated the risk of several carcinogens. Human monitoring will allow us to more accurately determine the risk for individuals exposed to these agents.

In addition to prioritizing IARC 2 chemicals, we should also consider occupational and population exposure to *low* levels of known toxins. These studies may permit more accurate regulatory decisions.

The argument for continually testing high levels of substances known to be genotoxic is usually based on the need for method development and validation.

Unfortunately, the history of the field of genetic toxicology is that of continually evaluating methods that are seldom applied to what should be our immediate goal: eliminating or modifying human exposure to carcinogenic and mutagenic substances. Clearly, we have underutilized the methods that are already validated and currently available for human monitoring studies. Method development and validation is critical, but we should keep in mind that the reason we are developing and validating methods is to apply these techniques to identifying and characterizing genotoxic substances. Given the fact that we are dealing with our target species, humans, and that we are usually evaluating critical genetic events, we should be able to move quickly in the application of these techniques. There is every reason for using our newly developed cytogenetic techniques (such as chromosome painting), new DNA repair evaluations, and somatic cell mutation assays for evaluating populations exposed to known carcinogenic solvents such as trichloroethylene or perchloroethylene. Similarly, we should also move out of the workplace and look at communities exposed chronically to low levels of carcinogenic and mutagenic agents. Although we can be proud of the contributions to human welfare made by genetic toxicologists, these accomplishments are minor compared to what can be accomplished in the near future. Major contributions will be made if we immediately utilize human monitoring to fill in the large information gaps that are present for most of the chemicals in our environment. The potential underestimation of risk when using animal data, as in the cancer bioassay program, makes it even more urgent to utilize genetic monitoring in industrial and community populations exposed to carcinogens.

REFERENCES

1. Au, W. W. 1993. Abnormal chromosome repair and risk of developing cancer. Environ. Health Perspect. **101**(Suppl. 3): 303-308.
2. Legator, M. S. 1994. Genetic Toxicology: Lessons from the past, directions for the future. Environ. Mol. Mutagen. **23**(Suppl. 24): 3-6.
3. McClain, R. M. 1994. Mechanistic considerations in the regulation and classification of chemical carcinogens. *In* Nutritional Toxicology. F. N. Kotsonis, M. Mackey & J. Hijele, Eds.: 273-304. Raven Press. New York.
4. Bailar III, J. C., A. Edmund, C. Crouch, R. Shaikh & D. Spiegelman. 1988. One-hit models of carcinogenesis: Conservative or not? Risk Anal. **8:** 485-497.
5. Halpert, J. R., F. P. Guengerich, J. R. Bend & M. A. Correia. 1994. Contemporary issues in toxicology: Selective inhibitors of cytochromes P450. Toxicol. Appl. Pharmacol. **125:** 163-175.
6. Kalf, G. F. 1987. Recent advances in the metabolism and toxicity of benzene. CRC Crit. Rev. Toxicol. **18**(2): 141-159.
7. Ward, Jr., J. B., M. M. Ammenheuser, V. M. S. Ramanujam, D. L. Morris, E. B. Whorton, Jr. & M. S. Legator. 1992. The mutagenic effects of low level subacute inhalation exposure to benzene in CD-1 mice. Mutat. Res. **268:** 49-57.
8. Au, W. W., J. B. Ward, Jr., V. M. S. Ramanujam, B. L. Harper, M. T. Moslen & M. S. Legator. 1988. Genotoxic effects of a sub-acute low-level inhalation exposure to a mixture of carcinogenic chemicals. Mutat. Res. **203:** 103-115.
9. Medinsky, M. A., P. J. Sabourin, G. Lucier, L. S. Birnbaum & R. F. Henderson. 1989. A physiological model for simulation of benzene metabolism by rats and mice. Toxicol. Appl. Pharmacol. **99:** 193-206.
10. Medinsky, M. A., P. J. Sabourin, R. F. Henderson, G. Lucier & L. S. Birnbaum. 1989. Differences in the pathways for metabolism of benzene in rats and mice simulated by a physiological model. Environ. Health Perspect. **82:** 43-49.

11. HENDERSON, R. F., P. J. SABOURIN, W. E. BECHTOLD, W. C. GRIFFITH, M. A. MEDINSKY, L. S. BIRNBAUM & G. W. LUCIER. 1989. The effect of dose, dose rate, route of administration, and species on tissue and blood levels of benzene metabolites. Environ. Health Perspect. **82:** 9-17.
12. HENDERSON, R. F., P. J. SABOURIN, M. A. MEDINSKY, L. S. BIRNBAUM & G. L. LUCIER. 1992. Benzene dosimetry in experimental animals: Relevance for risk assessment. Prog. Clin. Biol. Res. **374:** 93-105.
13. BOND, J. A., L. RECIO & D. ANDJELKOVICH. 1995. Epidemiological and mechanistic data suggest that 1,3-butadiene will not be carcinogenic to humans at exposures likely to be encountered in the environment or workplace. Carcinogenesis **16**(2): 165-171.
14. DELZELL, E., N. SATHIAKUMAR, M. HOVINGA, M. MACALUSO, J. JULIAN, R. LARSON & P. COLE. 1996. A follow-up study of synthetic rubber workers. Toxicology **113**(1-3): 182-189.
15. LEGATOR, M. S., W. W. AU, M. AMMENHEUSER & J. B. WARD, JR. 1993. Elevated somatic cell mutant frequencies and altered DNA repair responses in nonsmoking workers exposed to 1,3-butadiene. Butadiene and Styrene: Assessment of Health Hazards. IARC Scientific Publications No. 127. M. Sorsa, K. Peltonen, H. Vainio & K. Hemminki, Eds.: 253-263. International Agency for Research on Cancer. Lyon.
16. WARD, JR., J. B., M. M. AMMENHEUSER, W. E. BECHTOLD, E. B. WHORTON, JR. & M. S. LEGATOR. 1994. *hprt* mutant lymphocyte frequencies in workers at a 1,3-butadiene production plant. Environ. Health Perspect. **102**(Suppl. 9): 79-85.
17. AU, W. W., W. E. BECHTOLD, E. B. WHORTON, JR., M. S. LEGATOR. 1995. Chromosome aberrations and response to γ-ray challenge in lymphocytes of workers exposed to 1,3-butadiene. Mutat. Res. **334:** 125-130.
18. HIMMELSTEIN, M. W., M. J. TURNER, B. ASGHARIAN & J. A. BOND. 1994. Comparison of blood concentrations of 1,3-butadiene and butadiene epoxides in mice and rats exposed to 1,3-butadiene by inhalation. Carcinogenesis **15:** 1479-1486.
19. OSTERMAN-GOLKAR, S. M., J. A. BOND, J. B. WARD, JR., M. S. LEGATOR. 1993. Use of haemoglobin adducts for biomonitoring exposure to 1,3-butadiene. Butadiene and Styrene: Assessment of Health Hazards. IARC Scientific Publications 127. M. Sorsa, K. Peltonen, H. Vainio & K. Hemminki, Eds.: 127-134. International Agency for Research on Cancer. Lyon.

Living in a Chemical World

Health Impact of 1,3-Butadiene Carcinogenesis

CARLOS SANTOS-BURGOA,[a,b]
ROCÍO ALATORRE EDEN-WYNTER,[a]
HORACIO RIOJAS-RODRÍGUEZ,[a] AND
GENEVIEVE M. MATANOSKI[c]

[a]*Work, Environment, and Health Institute*
Cerrada del Convento 48-A, Oficinia D-H
Col. Santa Ursula Xitla
Delegación Tlalpan
México, D.F. 14420, México

[c]*Johns Hopkins School of Hygiene and Public Health*
615 North Wolfe Street
Baltimore, Maryland 21205

INTRODUCTION

1,3-Butadiene is an alkene of four carbon and six oxygen atoms (C_4H_6). A colorless, noncorrosive gas, it is volatile, having a low boiling point (–4.4°C), low odor threshold, and high vapor pressure (1840 mm Hg at 21°C), making it flammable and explosive. Given its two double bonds (CH_2=CH-CH=CH_2), it is so reactive that it easily polymerizes and forms different compounds, a reaction accelerated in the atmosphere by photooxidation processes. Butadiene is within the top 20 chemicals produced in the United States.[1]

1,3-Butadiene is produced at the end of the monomer production facilities. Such monomers are polymerized to produce rubber. It can be found in the recycling industry and in tire production plants. Worldwide these industries employ more than 250,000 workers. It is found in food from packaging contamination. Butadiene is also detected in nonindustrial environments, such as in houses with biomass burning, as exists in most developing countries and in nonurban houses in developed nations.[2] As a by-product of cigarette smoking, it is detectable in smokers' homes. A significant amount of butadiene is generated from the combustion of gasoline in cities with heavy traffic (TABLE 1). For example, we estimate that in Mexico City about 10,000 pounds of butadiene is emitted into the atmosphere by mobile sources (authors' estimate). Butadiene may affect a quarter of a million industrial workers and potentially more than 500 million inhabitants worldwide.

[b]Phone: 52-5/573-6929; fax: 52-5/513-3151; e-mail: rtn0523@rtn.net.mx

TABLE 1. Potential Human Exposure to 1,3-Butadiene

Source	Concentration Range (ppm)	Estimated Exposed Population	
		U.S.A.	Worldwide
Industry			
Monomer[16]	0–142	5,000	20,000
Polymer[17]	0.03–374	52,000	210,000
Burning of plastic/rubber[17]	?	?	?
Tires[17]	small	?	?
Food[17]	5–6,600 μ/kg^{-1}	?	?
Indoor Environment			
Biomass burning[2]	17 g/cooked meal	?	?
One cigarette[17]	0.14	40,000,000	6,000,000,000
		?	?
Smoker's home[17]	0.0045–0.01	?	?
Gas stove[2]	0.05 g/cooked meal		
General environment[18]			
Urban (population > 1 million)	0.001–0.15	21,000,000	461,000,000
Within 50-km radius of butadiene plant	0.3–2	52,000,000	100,000,000
Rural	0.00002	?	?

RESEARCH TRENDS

The first toxicological data about butadiene came during the Second World War, when butadiene was used as a strategic chemical. Its epoxide was identified as a potential animal carcinogen in 1957.[3] More toxicological research followed the first rubber tire and synthetic rubber epidemiologic studies showing a carcinogenic risk; however, a key industry-sponsored rat study finished in the late 1970s was not published until 1987. After the epi studies further confirmed the risk, the growth of toxicological research has been exponential.

FIGURE 1 shows that epidemiological research has developed slowly, and exposure assessment studies more slowly still. Besides the IARC and other institutional reviews more than 30 reviews have been done. In June 1995, an industry- and government-sponsored symposium Evaluation of Butadiene Health Risks was held at Blaine, Washington.[4]

Of the existing reviews there are at least nine risk assessments, most of them occupational, the others general or specialized reviews (TABLE 2). In this article we will not undertake another review, but we intend to put to rest some of the controversies that arise in them. For an overview of the research and the insight on the controversies, we invite you to read the paper by Melnick[5] and its opposing review by Bond,[6] both published in *Carcinogenesis.*

Malignant neoplasms of ectodermic and mesodermic origin have been reported in rodent studies. The frequency of rare sarcomas in exposed animals are of interest.

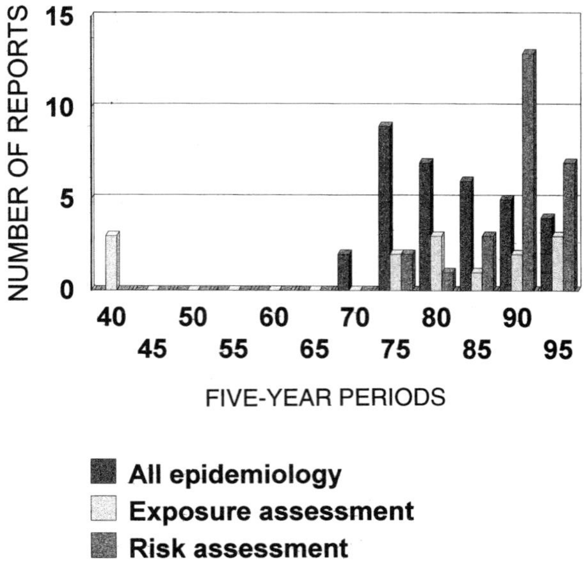

FIGURE 1. Trends in 1,3-butadiene-related research.

TABLE 2. 1,3-Butadiene Reviews/Risk Assessments

Review	Date	Risk Assessment	Date
Turnbull *et al.*	1990	EPA-Carcinogen Assessment Group	1985
Grossman *et al.*	1990	EPA-Office of Toxic Substances	1985
Acquavella	1990	ICF/Clement (OSHA)	1986
Landrigan	1990	Environ Chemical Manufacturers' Association	1986
Cote & Bayard	1990	OSHA	1990
Abelson	1992	NIOSH	1991
Dankovic *et al.*	1992	California Air Resources Board	1991
Landrigan	1992	Shell Oil Company	1990
IARC	1992	Fielder	1995
Melnick & Huff	1992		
Cole	1993		
Park	1993		
Hesse	1994		
Melnick & Kohn	1995		
Bond *et al.*	1995		
Schwarze	1995[a]		
Cageen *et al.* [a]	1995		

[a] Unpublished.

These tumors are dose dependent and are more frequent on mice, intensity being a better predictor of risk than cumulative exposure. An issue that has been raised is that rats appear to be more resistant to butadiene, or, from another point of view, mice appear to be more susceptible.

Other, nonneoplastic effects that are relevant for the younger population throughout the world, and not so extensively studied, are hematological, neurological, and reproductive effects. Of the latter, both defects and developmental problems have been identified.

What can be agreed from the toxicology is that butadiene is a transspecies carcinogen, affecting mice, rats, primates, and humans, with multiple organ targets. It is metabolized to mutagenic and carcinogenic epoxides, having different toxicokinetic patterns. Furthermore, it appears to behave with less severity, although through similar pathways, in humans, as identified by its genotoxic patterns.

Excessive emphasis has been put on interspecies differentials, given the susceptibility in mice and the lack of site specificity. Rarely had such emphasis been given before for other toxic agents; such differentials exist in other type 1 carcinogens, such as benzene, as heterogeneity is well known. Toxicology researchers are not addressing the issue of whether butadiene is a carcinogen, but are accumulating evidence to favor a more conservative, or less stringent, exposure limit when the quantitative dose-response curves are to be developed. Before further discussing the pertinence of such analyses, I would like to address some epidemiological issues.

LACK OF CONSISTENCY IN EPIDEMIOLOGIC RESEARCH?

The imbalance in the study of the different sources of human exposure to 1,3-butadiene is striking (TABLE 3). Industrial populations have been the object of epi studies of this chemical, as with many carcinogen. General and indoor environment studies, where most of the potentially exposed population are, have so far not been addressed. Detractors of the epidemiologic studies that have been done constantly mention the lack of consistency between studies.[7]

Some of this apparent inconsistency comes from a lack of understanding by these detractors that the studies differ in the production processes they address: in monomer production, butadiene is found as a final product of ethanol + acetaldehyde and of the olefin cracking processes. It is a downstream product. In polymer production it is detected in the whole process, even as a residual monomer after polymerization. Of these, the biggest cohort studies come from the study of the eight North American plants; these studies have been updated twice.[8,9] In the industrial polymer users studies, butadiene is not found as a monomer, since it is either polymerized or trapped in bubbles within rubber. Therefore, not all rubber studies show butadiene exposure equally, nor do all butadiene studies show workers exposed to this chemical.

Further confusion is produced by the improved epidemiological study design and exposure assessment (TABLE 4). The initial studies were crude in their exposure classification: to have ever worked at an area or plant was considered sufficient. Later authors used other work status designations that indirectly indicated working conditions. Then, the areas longest or last worked at were used. The latest studies have detailed individual work histories, even qualitatively and quantitatively estimating

TABLE 3. Classification of 1,3-Butadiene Epidemiological Studies

Site	Author
Industrial setting	Divine/Downs
	Ward
Monomer production (butatiene at end)	NIOSH
Polymer production (butatiene throughout entire process)	Meinhardt
	Matanoski/Santos Burgoa
	Delzell/Macaluzo
Polymer user—tires (butadiene polymerized—solid)	Ward/Ruder
	Spiritas/Taulbee/McMichael/Andjelkovich
General environment	
Urban	none
Within 50-km radius of butadiene plant	none
Rural	none
Indoor	
Biomass burning	Smith
Other	

exposure to butadiene and other chemicals. When the Hopkins cohort update[9] was initiated, styrene was suspected for carcinogenesis; benzene could also be involved, and butadiene had to be accounted for. Our exposure assessors were never biased by the butadiene hypothesis; such a "virginal" privilege will never happen again.

In the scatterplots of FIGURE 2 show the significant point risk estimates of different monomer and polymer studies. Twelve of thirteen leukemia estimates are above the double risk for leukemias and have the strongest effect; lymphomas appear less frequently. Gastrointestinal cancers are shown as relevant at least twice. Other diseases, such as cardiovascular mortality, appear with less potency.

In spite of these findings several authors have published letters or reviews remarking that the epidemiology is inconclusive because of lack of consistency. A *Science* editorial[10] seeks to downplay what is called the "exaggerated carcinogenicity" of butadiene. To put to rest this perception, let us focus on the cohort studies of the eight styrene-butadiene rubber plants.

These studies are industry-sponsored research that has been updated twice (TABLE 5). The second update, which extended the follow-up into 1991, was completely redone by researchers at the University of Alabama,[11] independently from the Hopkins group, who received no further support; their first results were reported this year at the public symposium in Blaine, Washington. In the first Hopkins study by Dr. Matanoski, exposure was estimated by last-worked area. The cohort update extended follow-up and considered the longest job held, accounting for most of the exposure probability. Both cohort studies used only the underlying cause of death. For the nested case-control study[12] we ascertained cases by the basic, the underlying, or the contributing cause of death listed in the death certificate, obtaining increased case identification; we developed a new job dictionary and distinct work area classification.

TABLE 4. Exposure Assessment and Design of Various Industry-Based 1,3-Butadiene Studies

Author	Design	Type	Exposure Assessment
North Carolina	Historical cohort	Tire	Ever at work area during employment
Meinhardt	Historical cohort	SBR	Near plant
Downs/Divine	Historical cohort nested case-control	Butadiene	Low routine Nonroutine Unknown During employment
Ward/Ruder	Historical cohort	SBR	Ever at plant during employment
Matanoski/Santos-Burgoa	Historical cohort nested case-control	SBR	Last and longest work period at plant area (cohort) Exposure matrix and individual job histories (case-control) Cumulative and lagged
Delzell/Macaluzo/Cole	Historical cohort nested case-control	SBR	Exposure matrix and job histories Estimated butadiene concentration Cumulative

NOTE: SBR = styrene-butadiene rubber.

It took a year just to generate the exposure matrix. We then gathered the study cancers and their tightly matched controls, and reformulated their job histories, obtaining a semiquantitative cumulative exposure estimate. In the second update the Alabama researchers improved the exposure estimation, doing detailed job histories in all cohort members, and quantifying butadiene concentrations at work areas.[11]

FIGURE 3 shows the leukemia butadiene risk ratios. Perhaps the point ratios differ somewhat, but their ranges are close. As expected, larger study sizes give smaller confidence intervals; the cohort studies have smaller confidence intervals than the case control study. Also, the longer the follow-up, the higher the risk estimate, as each update increases the strength of the association and reduces the healthy worker bias. The cohort studies (1, 2, and 4) have shown leukemia risks up to fourfold; the case-control studies show a sevenfold risk, with the best models having an odds ratio of 13. Certainly the first cohort update and the corresponding nested case-control study do not have the same risk estimate. Why would it be so?

TABLE 6 summarizes the rationale to develop a nested case-control study, its advantages and differences from a cohort study. The exposure estimates are different, as are the population sizes and the cases ascertained. In the cohort study we compared the cohort with the external total population of the United States; in the case-control study we asked whether leukemia workers differed from matched control workers

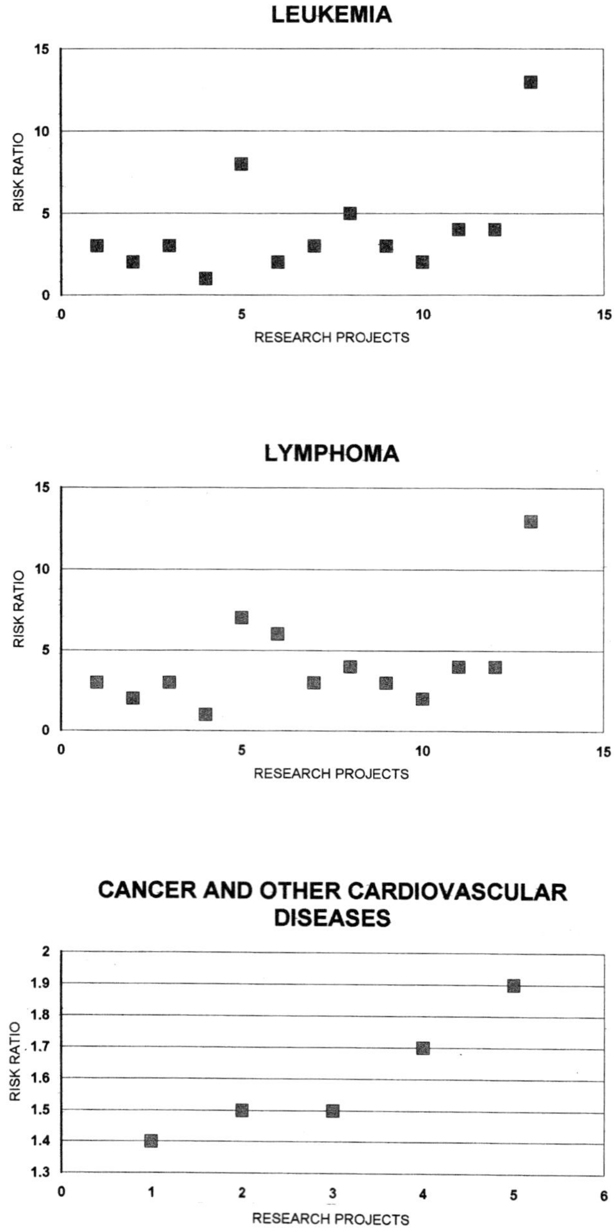

FIGURE 2. 1,3-Butadiene monomer and polymer epidemiology significant point risk ratios.

TABLE 5. Study Design Improvements in the Eight North American Styrene-Butadiene Rubber Plants

I	Original cohort	1943-1977	Area-based exposure
II	First cohort update	1943-1982	Area-based exposure
III	Case-control within Cohort II	1943-1982	Individually cumulative exposure to butadiene and/or styrene
IV	Second cohort update	1943-1991	Area based
V	Case-control within Cohort IV	1943-1991	Individually cumulative exposure to butadiene and/or styrene

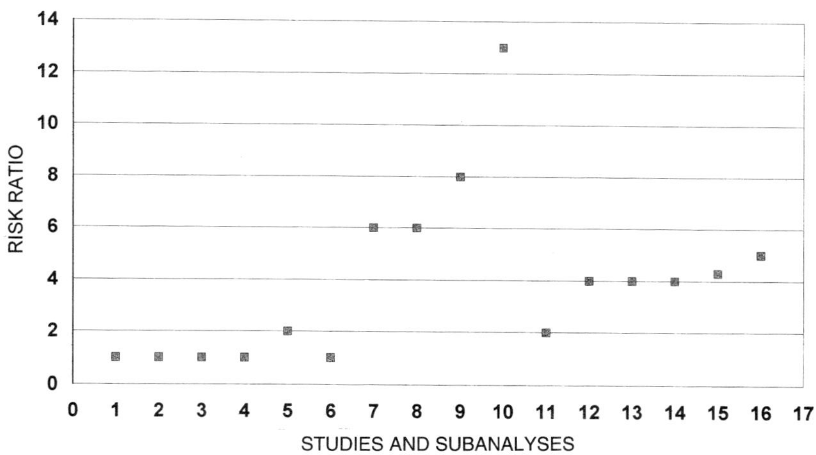

FIGURE 3. Leukemia butadiene point risk ratios in North American styrene-butadiene rubber plant studies. Studies 1-3, Matanoski & Schwartz, 1987;[8] studies 4-7, Matanoski *et al.,* 1989;[9] studies 8-10, Santos-Burgoa *et al.,* 1992;[12] studies 11-16, Delzell *et al.,* 1995.[11]

in regard to butadiene exposure. That is a different question and a different comparison. The study population in the case-control study did not represent the whole cohort but the subset that developed leukemia. The detail and quality of exposure estimation were enhanced in the case-control study, with less opportunity for missclassification of exposure. To look for consistency in ratios[7] demonstrates ignorance of epidemiologic methods or willingness to confuse the audience anyway, the risk ratios lay within the same range.

CAUSALITY ON BUTADIENE CARCINOGENICITY

It is pertinent to take a position on the causality of butadiene carcinogenicity. We believe that there is a strong biological basis to support the hypothesis. From the studies' designs themselves it is clear that exposure occurred before disease was

TABLE 6. Why to Do a Nested Case-Control Study

	Concurrent Cohort (Experimental)	Historical Cohort	Nested Case-Control within Cohort
Population	Large	Largest	Small
Comparison population	External	External	Internal
When exposure is measured	Before start and during study (prospective)	Before of after (retrospective)	After (retrospective)
Precedence of exposure	Precedent	Precedent	Precedent
Number of confouders measured	Many	Small	Intermediate
Cost	Very high	High	Low
Detail of exposure measurement	Intermediate	Poor or very crude	Very detailed
Quality of exposure	Correct	Poor	Best yield
Confidence intervals	Narrowest	Narrow	Wide
Misclassification of subjects' exposure	Lowest	Highest	Low
Risk ratio	Precise	Underestimated	Better estimate

identified; a latency period of 5 to 10 years was found. Butadiene targets mesodermic cancers, mainly those originating from the lymphohemopoietic tissues, with a very strong leukemia effect. Toxicological studies consistently show that butadiene is carcinogenic to Swiss mice without the murine leukemia virus and to Sprague-Dawley rats in spite of metabolic and pharmacokinetic differences. Effects are found in Wistar rats and $B6C3F_1$ mice. All epidemiological studies show the same tendency and strength of association. The effect of butadiene is dose dependent in animals and humans. The risk is strong, up to fourfold in cohort analysis and 5-13-fold in nested case-control studies. During the panel discussion at the Blaine meeting, the epidemiologists who conducted the studies independently of Hopkins, explicitly characterized 1,3-butadiene as a type 1 human carcinogen. At this meeting, industry epidemiologists also admitted that butadiene is human leukemogen.

SCOPE FOR NEW RESEARCH

In what direction should science go in order to support interventions to protect the people's health, which is our essential responsibility? We need to combine toxicology and epidemiology as equal partners in environmental and occupational health. Both scientific disciplines are better off integrating efforts, rather than speaking in different languages. It is necessary to understand their theoretical bases, and the advantages and limitations of their methodologies, setting aside obsolete visions of bench-versus field-based science. Such an approach has greatly affected the development of butadiene carcinogenicity prevention, and the Collegium Ramazinni should make an effort in this direction.

Toxicological studies are underway in preparation for the bargaining that will unfold around the exposure limits; epidemiological research needs to develop in order to better understand the diverse issues of actual human exposure, disease process, effect of exposure intensity, and other issues relevant for prevention. Is it true that "mechanistic studies are getting in the way of what's important, that is people," as was once mentioned by Richard Monson?

We have to be aware that whatever risk assessment we perform, the population's risk characterization will be limited by the lack of understanding of various nonoccupational human population groups and environments. We should be concerned about workers exposed with greater intensity in industry; but consideration should also be given to other sources of butadiene and to the worldwide population exposed to them, mainly from nonfixed sources, especially gasoline combustion.

There are many priorities for research (TABLE 7). The 1995 Health Effects Institute review[13] identified areas of priority for research, again emphasizing species differences in pharmacokinetics, as well as susceptibility biomarkers. I think toxicologists should advance science by working out the optimal detoxification pathways when biological systems confront real chemical mixtures. Similarly, their research should better simulate real exposure patterns, as opposed to working rhythms or general exposure patterns, as was recently done by Melnick.[14] Toxicology could greatly enlighten health research by addressing noncancer end points – the neurological and reproductive effects of butadiene, its role in atherogenesis. Finally, to provide inexpensive biomarkers should be a goal for tight collaboration with epidemiologists.

Exposure assessment should be emphasized both at high and/or intense exposures as well as at low and/or intermittent general environment concentrations. We have to build human exposure models in industry and nonindustry settings in order to better predict effective interventions, especially for cancer prevention.

Finally, epidemiology should analyze pathology-validated cancer diagnoses, considering the immunological characterization of lymphohemopoietic cancers, as well as mesodermic cancers. Epidemiologists should work with toxicologists on the available urinary biomarkers as well as on other, noncancer diseases.

CONCLUSION

We want to close with a cry for cancer prevention. We have been putting off taking a stand for decades. We epidemiologists and toxicologists are losing ground when we do not give effective recommendations. Publication of research has been delayed; agencies and analysts have inappropriately ignored available knowledge. When is the IARC again going to assemble a working group and take a position? Are we going to have an occupational protective standard next year? How long will worldwide sources continue to say that 1000 ppm is the accepted limit? (On November 4, 1996, after the presentation of this paper, the United States Occupational Safety and Health Administration published the Final Rule on Occupational Exposure, setting it at 1 ppm.[15]) When are we going to have an air quality standard for butadiene? It is my opinion that research has to be targeted at the prevention of risk in human populations, and that it is time to take well-supported action.

TABLE 7. Knowledge of 1,3-Butadiene Needed for Prevention of Excessive Exposure

Health Effects Institute (1995)	Santos-Burgoa
In vivo and *in vitro* pharmacokinetic species differences	Toxicology
Development and validation of physiologically based 1,3-butadiene dosimetry model	
	Real Mixtures
	Real exposure patterns
	Noncancer endpoints
	Inexpensive biomarkers
Frequency of mutational spectra in relevant tissues	Exposure assessment
Identification of cancer-related DNA adducts produced by butadiene	
	Personal exposure monitoring
	industry
	general population
Model of tumor development taking account of species differences in tumor types	
	Ambient monitoring
	industry
	outdoor
	indoor
Epidemiology studies of new populations at higher exposures	
	Exposure biomarkers
	for highly exposed
	for low exposures
	in general population
	Epidemiology
	Validated histopathology
	Cellular origin of cancer
	T-cell leukemia/lymphoma
	Sarcomas (mesodermic)
	Other diseases
	Arteriosclerosis
	Reproductive
	Neurological
	Validated useful biomarkers
	Morbidity studies

REFERENCES

1. PEDERSON, D. H., R. O. YOUNG & D. S. SUNDEN. 1983. Model for the Identification of High Risk Occupational Groups using RTECS (Register of Toxic Effects of Chemical Substances) and NOHS (National Occupational Hazards Survey) Data. NIOSH Publication 117. Washington, DC.
2. ZHANG, J. & K. R. SMITH. 1996. Hydrocarbon emissions and health risks from cookstoves in developing countries. J. Exposure Anal. Environ. Epidemiol. **6**(2): 147-161.
3. MCCAMMAN, C. J., P. KOTIN & H. L. FALK. 1957. The carcinogenic potency of certain epoxides. Proc. Am. Assoc. Cancer Res. **2:** 229-230.
4. INTERNATIONAL INSTITUTE OF SYNTHETIC RUBBER PRODUCERS. 1995. International Symposium on Health Effects from 1,3 Butadiene. Blaine, Washington, June 28-29, 1995.

5. Melnick, R. L. & M. C. Kohn. 1995. Mechanistic data indicate than 1,3-butadiene is a human carcinogen. Carcinogenesis **16**(2): 157-163.
6. Bond, J. A., L. Recio & D. Andjelkovich. 1995. Epidemiological and mechanistic data suggest than 1,3-butadiene will not be carcinogenic to humans at exposures likely to be encountered in the environment or workplace. Carcinogenesis **16**(2): 165-171.
7. Acquavella, J. F. & S. R. Cowles. 1993. Re: ''Lymphohematopoietic cancer in styrene-butadiene polymerization workers.'' Am. J. Epidemiol. **138**(9): 765-766.
8. Matanoski, G. M. & L. Schwartz. 1987. Mortality of workers in styrene-butadiene polymer production. J. Occup. Med. **29** (8): 675-680.
9. Matanoski, G. M., C. Santos-Burgoa, S. L. Zeger & L. Schwartz. 1989. Epidemiologic data related to health effects of 1,3-butadiene. *In* Assessment of Inhalation Hazards. ILSI Monographs. Springer-Verlag, New York.
10. Abelson, A. 1993. Cancer phobia: Exaggerated carcinogenicity of 1,3-butadiene. Science **237:** 473.
11. Delzell, E. *et al.* 1995. A follow-up study of synthetic rubber workers. Presented at the International Symposium: Evaluation of Butadiene and Isoprene Health Risks. Satellite Symposium to the International Congress of Toxicology. Blaine, Washington. June 27-29, 1995.
12. Santos-Burgoa, C., G. M. Matanoski, S. Zeger & L. Schwartz. 1992. Lymphohematopoietic cancer in styrene-butadiene polymerization workers. Am. J. Public Health **136**(7): 848-854.
13. Health Effects Institute (HEI). 1995. Program Summary. Research on Benzene and 1,3-Butadiene. Health Effects Institute. Boston.
14. Melnick, R. *et al.* 1995. Inhalation Toxicity and Carcinogenicity of Isoprene in Rats and Mice: Comparisons with 1,3-Butadiene. National Institute of Environmental Health Sciences. Research Triangle Park, NC.
15. Federal Register. 1996. Part II. Department of Labor. Occupational Safety and Health Administration 29 CFR Part 1910 *et al.* Occupational Exposure to 1,3-Butadiene Final Rule. Vol. 61, No. 214.
16. Divine, B. J. 1990. An update on mortality among workers at 1,3-butadiene facility. Preliminary results. Environ. Health Perspect. **86:** 119-128.
17. International Agency for Research on Cancer. 1993. Scientific Publication No. 127. World Health Organization. Lyon.
18. Rhoad, M. J. 1982. Industry position paper on 1,3-butadiene. International Institute of Synthetic Rubber Producers Memorandum, October, 1982. Houston, TX.
19. Turnbull, D. *et al.* 1990. Assessment of the potential risk to workers from exposure to 1,3-butadiene. Environ. Health Perspect. **86:** 159-171.
20. Grossman, E. A. & J. Martonik. 1990. OSHA's approach to risk assessment for setting a revised occupational exposure standard for 1,3-butadiene. Environ. Health Perspect. **86:** 155-158.
21. Acquavella, J. F. 1990. Future directions in epidemiology studies of 1,3-butadiene exposed workers. Environ. Health Perspect. **86:** 129-134.
22. Landrigan, P. J. 1990. Critical assessment of epidemiologic studies on the human carcinogenicity of 1,3-butadiene. Environ. Health Perspect. **86:** 143-148.
23. Cote, I. L. & S. Bayard. 1990. Cancer risk assessment of 1,3-butadiene. Environ. Health Perspect. **86:** 149-163.
24. Dankovic, D. A. *et al.* 1992. Carcinogenicity of butadiene. Health Perspect. **257:** 1330-1331.
25. Melnick, R. L. & J. Huff. 1992. 1,3-butadiene toxicity and carcinogenicity in laboratory animals and humans. Rev. Environ. Contam. Toxicol. **124:** 111-144.
26. Park, R. M. 1993. Butadiene epidemiology re-interpreted again. Epidemiology **3**(6): 559-560.
27. Hesse, J. M. 1995. The Dutch Programme for Existing Substances: The Case of 1,4-Butadiene. Presented at the International Symposium: Evaluation of Butadiene and

Isoprene Health Risks. Satellite Symposium to the International Congress of Toxicology. Blaine, Washington, June 27-29, 1995.
28. KOHN, M. & R. L. MELNICK. 1995. Effects of the Structure of a Toxicokinetics Model of Butadiene Inhalation Exposure on Computed Products. Presentation at the International Symposium: Evaluation of Butadiene and Isoprene Health Risks. Satellite Symposium to the International Congress of Toxicology. Blaine, Washington, June 27-29. 1995.
29. BOND, J. A. *et al.* 1995. Epidemiological and mechanistic data suggest that 1,3-butadiene will not be carcinogenic to humans. Carcinogenesis, **16**(2): 165-171.
30. FIELDER, R. J. 1995. Risk assessment of butadiene. Prospectives of the UK in the Non-Occupational Area. Presented at the International Symposium: Evaluation of Butadiene and Isoprene Health Risks. Satellite Symposium to the International Congress of Toxicology. Blaine, Washington, June 27-29, 1995.
31. DOWNS T. D. *et al.* 1987. Mortality among workers at a butadiene facility. Am. J. Ind. Med. **12:** 311-329.
32. WARD, E. M. *et al.* 1995. Mortality study of workers in 1,3-butadiene production units identified from a chemical cohort. Environ. Health Perspect. **6:** 598-603.
33. MEINHARDT, T. J. *et al.* 1982. Environmental epidemiologic investigation of the styrene-butadiene rubber industry. Scand. J. Work Environ. Health **4:** 250-259.
34. SPIRITAS, R. 1977. Mortality among rubber workers: Relationship to job with styrene-butadiene exposure. *In* Proceedings of NIOSH Styrene-Butadiene Briefings, Covington, Kentucky, April 30, 1976. J. W. Lloyd, Ed.: 9-18. NIOSH Publication 77-129. U.S. Government Printing Office. Washington, D.C.

Results of Long-term Carcinogenicity Studies of Chlorine in Rats

MORANDO SOFFRITTI,[a] FIORELLA BELPOGGI,[b]
ANGELA LENZI,[b] AND CESARE MALTONI [b]

[a]*Cancer Research Center*
European Ramazzini Foundation
of Oncology and Environmental Sciences
Bentivoglio Castle
40010 Bentivoglio (BO), Italy

[b]*European B. Ramazzini Foundation of Oncology and*
Environmental Sciences
Bologna, Italy

INTRODUCTION

The annual consumption of drinking water at world level has been estimated at 440 billions of cubic meters,[1,2] and is destined to grow in relation to the increase of the planet's population, and to the gradual emancipation of the emerging countries, which entails a growing per capita consumption of water.

Most drinking water is made such by the process of chlorination. The use of chlorine to reduce the level of bacteria in drinking water started at the beginning of this century,[3] and chlorination remains probably the major example of interventive disease prevention of the modern age. The chlorine products used for chlorination are the following: gaseous chlorine (Cl_2); chlorine dioxide (ClO_2); calcium hypochlorite ($CaOCl_2$); sodium hypochlorite (NaOCl); sodium chlorite ($NaClO_2$); chloramines (Cl_2 + NH_4) such as monochloramine (NH_2Cl), dichloroamine ($NHCl_2$) and trichloroamine (NCl_3).[4]

Sodium hypochlorite was the first compound to be used for the chlorination of drinking water, and is still today the material most commonly used for this purpose.

In spite of the diffusion of drinking water chlorination, studies to evaluate the possible carcinogenic risks of chlorination are scanty or inadequate. Such risks may be due to the compounds used for chlorination per se, or to their by-products formed in the water. Once in water, chlorine may in fact react and produce halogenated organic compounds of various types and, in particular, halomethanes.[4]

In two surveys on the presence of halomethanes in drinking water, performed in the United States at national level in the '70s, it was found that chloroform, bromodichloromethane, chlorodibromomethane, and bromoform are the halomethanes most frequently and abundantly present in chlorinated drinking waters.[5,6]

A review, performed by the International Agency for Research on Cancer in 1991,[4] of the available epidemiological studies on the relationship between malignant tumors and chlorinated water consumption, came to the conclusion that these studies were inadequate to provide definitive conclusions. A later review of the epidemiological studies (meta-analysis) suggested a positive association between the consumption of chlorinated water and an increase in bladder and rectum carcinomas.[7] Since chlorinated waters have a variable composition and contain a variety of halogenated compounds, it is difficult to identify the risk derived from specific chemical agents by means of epidemiological studies.

The relationship between the level of trihalomethanes in drinking water and the mortality rate for cancer in the community was studied by two epidemiological investigations: these studies found a relation between the level of trihalomethanes and the mortality rate from tumors of different sites, in particular of the bladder, but also of the colon-rectum, brain and kidney, and lymphomas.[8,9]

Long-term carcinogenicity bioassays on experimental animals represent an alternative approach to epidemiology, for identifying and quantifying the potential carcinogenic risks due to the products related to the chlorination of drinking water. The available experimental carcinogenicity studies deal partly with the chlorine compounds used for disinfection, and partly with the halomethanes produced in water. The experimental studies on the carcinogenicity of the chemical compounds used for chlorination, available since 1989, deal with chlorine, and sodium chlorite and hypochlorite, and were reviewed by the International Agency for Research on Cancer in 1991.[4] A preliminary study on chlorine performed on rats gave negative results.[10] Altogether, the experimental studies conducted on rats and mice on the carcinogenicity of sodium chlorite and hypochlorite provide inadequate evidence of the carcinogenicity of these compounds.[4] It must be pointed out, however, that these studies were insufficient to come to any definitive conclusion.

In 1991, the results of long-term carcinogenicity bioassays (104 weeks) on chlorine (in the form of sodium hypochlorite and monochloramine), administered in drinking water to rats and mice, were made available.[11] In this study, levels of chlorination of 0 (control), 70 (low dose), 140 (middle dose), and 275 (high dose) ppm were administered to Fischer 344/N rats and B6C3F$_1$ mice, male and female, 5-6 weeks old at the beginning of the experiment (50 animals/sex/dose). The results show an increase in the incidence of leukemias both in the female rats administered with chlorine (hypochlorite) (16% in the control group, 14% in the low-dose group, 37% in the middle-dose group, and 32% in the high-dose group), and in those administered with chloramine (16% in the control group, 22% in the low-dose group, 30% in the middle-dose group, 32% in the high-dose group).

Experimental studies on the carcinogenicity of the most common halomethanes have given positive results. Chloroform, administered by stomach tube, induces tumors of the liver and kidney in mice;[12,13] when administered by stomach tube or in drinking water to rats, it induces an increase in the incidence of tumors of the kidney[12,14] and thyroid,[12] and of neoplastic nodules in the liver.[15] Chlorodibromomethane, bromodichloromethane, and bromoform, administered by stomach tube to Fischer 344/N rats and to B6C3F$_1$ mice, male and female, cause liver tumors in mice, kidney tumors in mice and rats, and/or tumors of the colon and rectum in rats.[16–18]

In consideration of the importance of the problem of the potential carcinogenic risk of chlorination, due to the compounds used per se, and to their haloderivatives, a long-term carcinogenicity bioassay on sodium hypoclorite has been performed in the Laboratory of the Cancer Research Center (CRC) in the Castle of Bentivoglio

(BT) of the European Ramazzini Foundation. The results of this study are herein reported.

MATERIALS AND METHODS

The sodium hypochlorite used in the experiment was produced by Montedison (Italy), and supplied to the public agency for water distribution in Bologna (A.CO.SE.R.) as a standard solution with the following characteristics:

- yellow-green liquid, with a density of 1.2 ± 0.1;
- hypochlorite content corresponding to a concentration of active chlorine of 120 g/kg (12%);
- content of other compounds: NaCl 8 g/l (max), other chlorides 10 g/l (max), chlorates 3 g/l (max) and Na_2CO_3 6 g/l (max).

A.CO.SE.R. provided the CRC/BT with a basic solution of hypochlorite, corresponding to an active chlorine concentration of 50 g/kg (5%). During the whole period of treatment, a stock of basic solution was supplied every two months, and kept in the dark at a temperature of 4–5°C. The decrease in concentration of active chlorine, from the date of delivery to the end of every stockage period, was found to be below 0.03%. The levels of organic haloderivatives formed in the basic solution, detected by analyses performed at delivery and at the end of every stockage period, were the following:

- methylchloroform < 0.1 μg/l
- chloroform < 20.0 μg/l
- carbon tetrachloride < 0.2 μg/l
- bromodichloromethane < 0.1 μg/l
- chlorodibromomethane < 0.1 μg/l
- trichloroethylene < 0.1 μg/l
- tetrachloroethylene < 0.1 μg/l

Male and female Sprague-Dawley rats of the colony of the CRC/BT were used. This colony of rats has been used for various experiments in the BT laboratory for nearly 25 years. Data are available on more than 10,000 historical controls, kept under observation for life span and submitted to systematic necropsies and standardized histopathological examinations. Therefore, data on the expected incidence of the different types of tumors in control animals and on its fluctuations are available.

After weaning, at 4–5 weeks of age, the experimental animals were identified by ear punch, randomized in order to have no more than one male and one female of each litter in the same group, and housed 5 per cage. The animals were 12 weeks old at the start of the experiment.

TABLE 1. Long-term Carcinogenicity Bioassays on Sodium Hypochlorite, Administered in Drinking Water Supplied ad Libitum (Experiment BT 7003): Plan of the Experiment

Group	Concentration (mg/l)	Animals	
		Sex	No.
I	750	M	50
		F	50
		M + F	100
II	500	M	50
		F	50
		M + F	100
III	100	M	50
		F	50
		M + F	100
IV	0	M	50
		F	50
		M + F	100

The plan of the experiment is shown in TABLE 1.

Every morning fresh solutions of sodium hypochlorite at the required concentrations were prepared; the residual drinking water from the day before was removed, and the glass drinking bottles were washed and filled with fresh solution.

The animals were kept under observation until natural death, under highly standardized housing and diet conditions, the same used in the BT laboratory over the last 25 years. In the experiments performed at the CRC/BT, the animals are usually allowed to live until natural death. By doing so, it is possible to obtain the development of all neoplastic potentialities. Mean daily feed and drinking water consumption were determined once weekly for the first 13 weeks from the start of the experiment, and then every 2 weeks until 116 weeks of age. Individual animal weight was measured once weekly for the first 13 weeks of the experimental biophase, and then every 2 weeks until 116 weeks of age (104 weeks of biophase), and every 8 weeks until the end of the experiment. In order to detect and register all gross lesions, the animals were examined every week for the first 13 weeks, and then every 2 weeks until the end of the experiment.

The biophase of the experiment terminated after 139 weeks, with the death of the last animal at the age of 151 weeks.

Upon death, the animals were submitted to systematic necropsy. Histopathology was routinely performed on skin and subcutaneous tissue, the brain, pituitary gland, Zymbal glands, salivary glands, Harderian glands, cranium (with oral and nasal cavities and external and internal ear ducts) (5 levels), tongue, thyroid and parathyroid, pharynx, larynx, thymus and mediastinal lymph nodes, trachea, lung and mainstem bronchi, heart, diaphragm, liver, spleen, pancreas, kidneys and adrenal glands, esophagus, stomach (fore and glandular), intestine (4 levels), bladder, prostate, uterus,

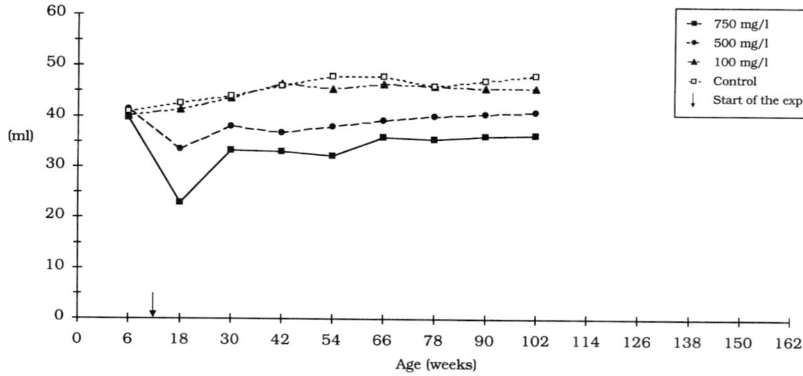

FIGURE 1. Mean daily water consumption in male rats.

gonads, interscapular fat pad, subcutaneous and mesenteric lymph nodes, and any other organ or tissue with pathological lesions.

All organs and tissues were preserved in 70% ethyl alcohol, except bones, which were fixed in 10% formalin and then decalcified with 10% formaldehyde and 20% formic acid in water solution. The normal specimens were trimmed, following the standard procedures of the BT laboratory: i.e., parenchymal organs were dissected through the hilus to expose the widest surface, and hollow organs were sectioned across the greatest diameter(s). The pathological tissue was trimmed through the largest surface, including normal adjacent tissues. The trimmed specimens were processed as paraffin blocks, and 3-5 micron sections of every specimen were obtained. Sections were routinely stained with hematoxylin-eosin. Specific stainings were performed when needed. All slides were examined microscopically by the same group of pathologists; a senior pathologist reviewed all the tumors and any other lesion of oncological interest. All pathologists followed the same criteria of histopathological evaluation and classification.

RESULTS

Mean Daily Water and Feed Consumption. A dose-related decrease of the mean daily water consumption was observed in animals treated with chlorine (FIGS. 1, 2). No significant differences were observed in feed consumption among the animals of either sex in the different groups (FIGS. 3, 4).

Body Weight. A slight decrease in mean body weight was observed in animals treated with the highest dose of chlorine; this was more evident in males (FIGS. 5, 6).

Survival. Survival was higher, from 78 weeks of age, in males treated with the lowest dose (FIGS. 7, 8).

Nononcological Changes. No evident behavioral changes were observed in treated animals. No treatment-related nononcological pathological changes were detected by gross inspection and routine histological examination.

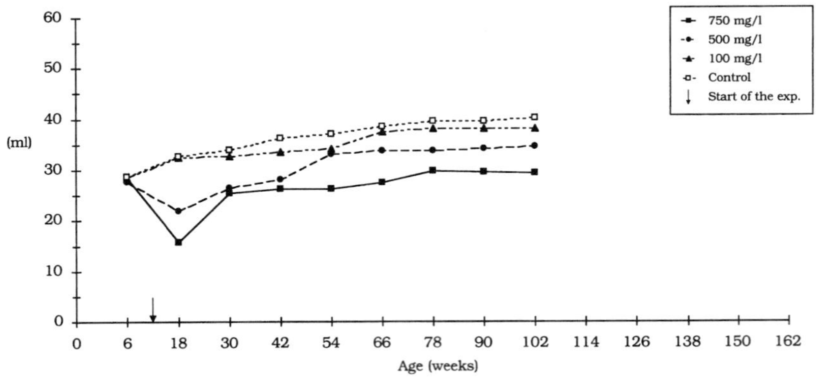

FIGURE 2. Mean daily water consumption in female rats.

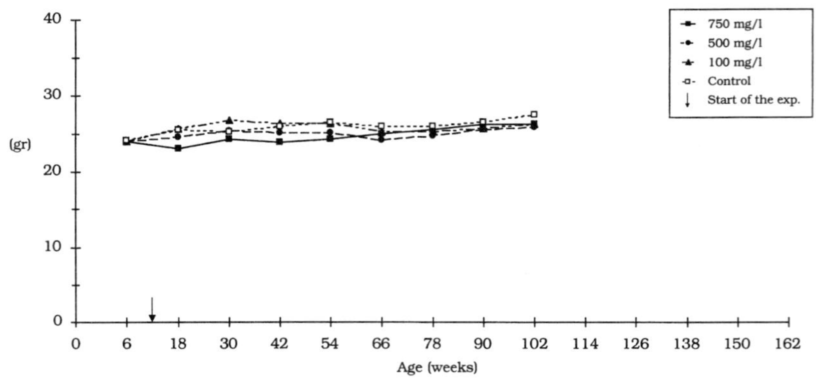

FIGURE 3. Mean daily feed consumption in male rats.

Tumors. The benign and malignant tumors observed among male and female rats of all groups are listed in TABLES 2 and 3. Multiple tumors of the same site (monolateral and bilateral organs) and type were plotted only once, apart from the mammary tumors of the same type, whose multiplicity has been taken into account.

As regards the incidence of total benign and malignant tumors (TABLES 4, 5), hypochlorite treatment seems to cause an increase in malignant tumors in male rats, at all doses, which is not dose related. The greater increase in the group treated with the lowest dose may be related partly to the longer survival of the animals.

In the female rats of the three treated groups, an increase of lymphomas and leukemias was observed (TABLE 6). An increase of tumors of the stomach was found in male rats exposed to the highest and to the lowest doses of sodium hypochlorite (TABLE 7). Among these tumors, a squamous cell carcinoma of the forestomach and two leiomyosarcomas of the stomach were detected.

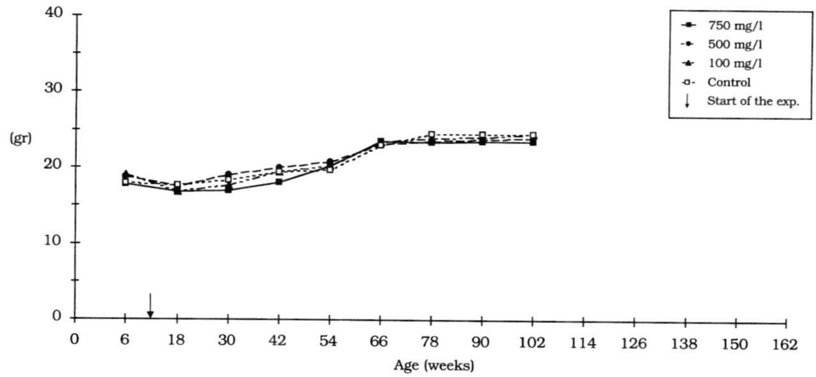

FIGURE 4. Mean daily feed consumption in female rats.

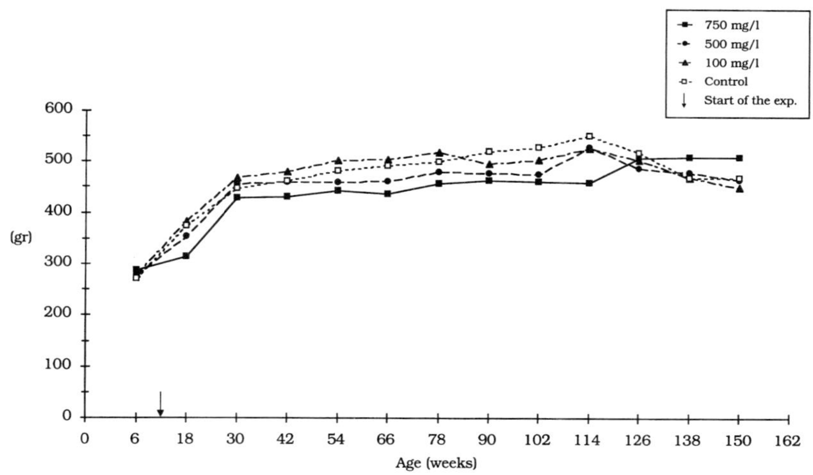

FIGURE 5. Mean body weight in male rats.

Three lung adenomas were observed in the group of females exposed to the lowest dose (TABLE 8).

CONCLUSIONS

The results of the study show that, under the tested experimental conditions, chlorine at high concentration may represent a carcinogenic risk.

This conclusion is based mainly on the increase of leukemias in female rats, not clearly dose related in the range of tested concentrations. In the control group, the

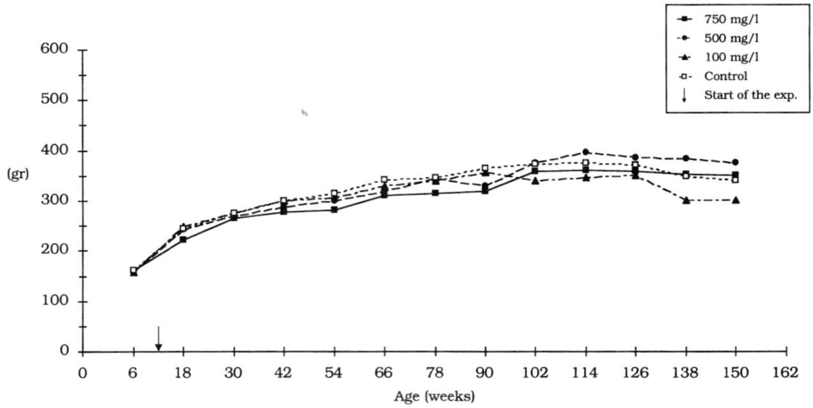

FIGURE 6. Mean body weight in female rats.

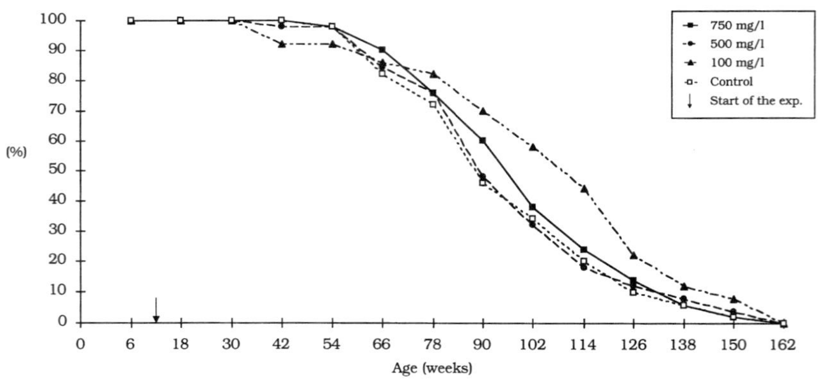

FIGURE 7. Survival in male rats.

incidence of leukemias in females is unusually low (0) with reference to other studied groups of historical controls, in which, however, the incidence of leukemias is usually contained between 0 and 10%. These results confirm the ones of the study of the National Toxicology Program (1991).[11]

Furthermore, one must consider the results on gastric and pulmonary tumors. As far as gastric tumors are concerned, beyond the increase of the total incidence on the groups treated with the highest and the lowest doses, the observation of one squamous cell carcinoma and two leiomyosarcomas deserve proper consideration, since these tumors are unusually rare in the BT colony of Sprague-Dawley rats. As far as pulmonary tumors are concerned, the observation of three adenomas among females treated with the lowest dose, in our opinion, cannot be considered casual,

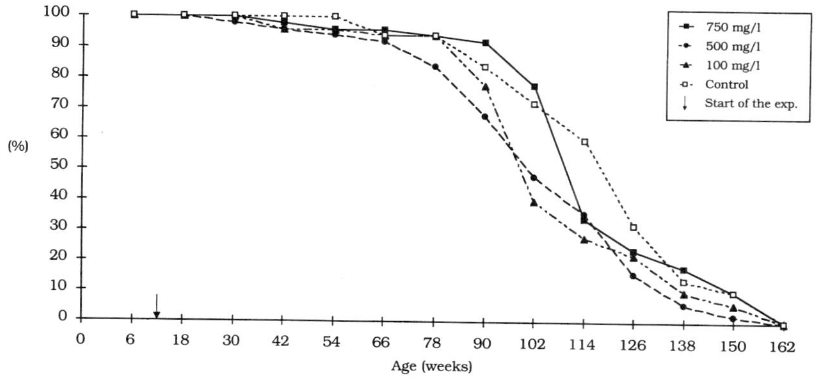

FIGURE 8. Survival in female rats.

in consideration of the fact that the incidence of this tumor is very low in our historical controls (≤0.1%).

The presented study does not permit the formulation of hypotheses regarding the mechanism of the carcinogenic action of chlorine.

The reported results and those of the study of the United States National Toxicology Program (1991)[11] converge in indicating the potential carcinogenic risk for humans of drinking water chlorination. The dimension of the problem is immense, since today it is chlorination that largely makes the supply of drinking water possible, and its substitution with alternative methods may present difficulties of no easy solution. However, the problem has been brought out into the open, and cannot be ignored. As of now, on the basis of the available knowledge, it appears necessary to start, with no further procrastination, on a program of studies that may allow an adequate quantitative assessment of the carcinogenicity of chlorination, on which regulations and strategies of public health should be based. A life span experiment for studying the effects of low doses of chlorine on large numbers of animals (megaexperiment), adequate to expose the carcinogenic effects of concentrations of chlorine lower than those which have been tested is, in our opinion, a most urgent step.

SUMMARY

Four groups, each of 50 male and 50 female Sprague-Dawley rats, of the colony used in the Cancer Research Center of Bentivoglio of the Ramazzini Foundation, 12 weeks old at the start of the study, received drinking water containing sodium hypochlorite, resulting in concentrations of active chlorine of 750, 500, and 100 mg/l (treated groups), and tap water (active chlorine <0.2 mg/l) (control group), respectively, for 104 weeks.

Among the female rats of the treated groups, an increased incidence of lymphomas and leukemias has been observed, although this is not clearly dose related. Moreover, sporadic cases of some tumors, the occurrence of which is extremely unusual among

TABLE 2. Long-term Carcinogenicity Bioassays on Sodium Hypochlorite, Administered in Drinking Water Supplied ad Libitum (Experiment BT 7003): Number and Percentage of Male Sprague-Dawley Rats Bearing Various Types of Benign and Malignant Tumors[a]

		Groups							
		I: 750 mg/l		II: 500 mg/l		III: 100 mg/l		IV: 0 (Control)	
Site	Histotype	No.	%	No.	%	No.	%	No.	%
Subcutaneous tissue	Fibroma	0	–	0	–	1	2.0	0	–
	Fibroliposarcoma	0	–	0	–	1	2.0	0	–
	Liposarcoma	0	–	0	–	0	–	1	2.0
Mammary gland	Fibroma	1	2.0	1 (2)	2.0	0	–	1	2.0
	Adenocarcinoma	0	–	1	2.0	0	–	0	–
	Fibrosarcoma	0	–	0	–	0	–	1	2.0
Zymbal glands	Adenoma	0	–	0	–	0	–	1	2.0
	Carcinoma	0	–	0	–	1	2.0	0	–
Ear ducts	Carcinoma	2	4.0	2	4.0	3	6.0	1	2.0
Nasal cavities	Carcinoma	1	2.0	1	2.0	0	–	1	2.0
Oral cavity, lips and tongue	Acanthoma	1	2.0	0	–	0	–	1	2.0
	Carcinoma	2	4.0	1	2.0	6	12.0	1	2.0
Stomach[b]									
Forestomach	Acanthoma	4	8.0	2	4.0	3	6.0	1	2.0
	Squamous cell carcinoma	0	–	0	–	1	2.0	0	–
Glandular stomach	Fibrosarcoma	0	–	0	–	1	2.0	0	–
	Leiomyosarcoma	1	2.0	0	–	0	–	0	–
Intestine	Adenomatous polyp	0	–	0	–	1	2.0	0	–
Liver	Cholangioma	0	–	1	2.0	0	–	0	–
	Hepatocarcinoma	0	–	1	2.0	0	–	1	2.0
Pancreas	Exocrine adenoma	0	–	0	–	0	–	1	2.0
	Islet cell adenoma	1	2.0	3	6.0	4	8.0	1	2.0
Seminal vesicles	Adenocarcinoma	0	–	1	2.0	0	–	1	2.0

Testes	Leydig cell tumor	2	4.0	0	—	2	4.0	2	4.0
Peritoneum	Mesothelioma	1	2.0	1	2.0	1	2.0	0	—
Pituitary gland	Adenoma	6	12.0	5	10.0	7	14.0	4	8.0
Thyroid gland	C-cell adenoma	0	—	1	2.0	1	2.0	0	—
	C-cell carcinoma	2	4.0	1	2.0	1	2.0	0	—
Parathyroid gland	Adenoma	1	2.0	0	—	0	—	1	2.0
Adrenal glands	Cortical adenoma	1	2.0	0	—	0	—	0	—
	Pheochromocytoma	22	44.0	19	38.0	28	56.0	18	36.0
	Pheochromoblastoma	2	4.0	3	6.0	2	4.0	0	—
Central nervous system									
Brain	Oligodendroglioma	0	—	0	—	1	2.0	0	—
Major peripheral nerves	Malignant Schwannoma	0	—	1	2.0	0	—	0	—
Bones									
Cranium	Osteosarcoma	0	—	1	2.0	4	8.0	2	4.0
Other	Chordoma	0	—	0	—	0	—	1	2.0
Spleen	Fibroangioma	0	—	1	2.0	0	—	0	—
Hemolymphoreticular tissues[c,d]	Lymphomas and leukemias	6	12.0	6	12.0	4	8.0	4	8.0

[a] Numbers in parentheses indicate the number of tumors (one animal can bear more than one tumor).
[b] See TABLE 7.
[c] Including spleen.
[d] See TABLE 6.

TABLE 3. Long-term Carcinogenicity Bioassays on Sodium Hypochlorite, Administered in Drinking Water Supplied ad Libitum (Experiment BT 7003): Number and Percentage of Female Sprague-Dawley Rats Bearing Various Types of Benign and Malignant Tumors[a]

		Groups							
		I: 750 mg/l		II: 500 mg/l		III: 100 mg/l		IV: 0 (Control)	
Site	Histotype	No.	%	No.	%	No.	%	No.	%
Subcutaneous tissue	Fibrosarcoma	1	2.0	0	—	0	—	0	—
	Liposarcoma	0	—	0	—	0	—	1	2.0
Mammary gland	Fibroadenoma and fibroma	20 (25)	40.0	15 (21)	30.0	17 (18)	34.0	20 (23)	40.0
	Fibrolipoma	0	—	1	2.0	0	—	0	—
	Adenocarcinoma	5 (6)	10.0	2	4.0	3	6.0	6	12.0
	Fibrosarcoma	0	—	0	—	0	—	1	2.0
	Liposarcoma	0	—	1	2.0	0	—	0	—
	Fibroistiocytosarcoma	3	6.0	1	2.0	0	—	0	—
	Carcinosarcoma	0	—	1	2.0	0	—	0	—
Zymbal glands	Carcinoma	0	—	1	2.0	0	—	0	—
Ear ducts	Carcinoma	0	—	4	8.0	3	6.0	2	4.0
Nasal cavities	Carcinoma	0	—	1	2.0	0	—	2	4.0
Oral cavity, lips and tongue	Carcinoma	1	2.0	1	2.0	4	8.0	2	4.0
Lung[b]	Adenoma	0	—	0	—	3	6.0	0	—
Stomach[c]									
Forestomach	Acanthoma	0	—	2	4.0	1	2.0	1	2.0
Salivary glands	Adenocarcinoma	1	2.0	0	—	0	—	0	—
Liver	Cholangioma	1	2.0	0	—	0	—	0	—
	Hepatocarcinoma	0	—	0	—	0	—	1	2.0
Pancreas	Exocrine adenoma	0	—	0	—	0	—	1	2.0
	Islet cell adenoma	1	2.0	0	—	1	2.0	2	4.0
	Islet cell adenocarcinoma	0	—	0	—	0	—	2	4.0
Kidneys	Adenocarcinoma	0	—	0	—	0	—	1	2.0
Pelvis and ureters	Transitional cell carcinoma	0	—	1	2.0	0	—	0	—

Ovaries	Sertoli cell tumor	0	—	0	—	2	4.0	2	4.0
	Granulosa and theca cell malignant tumor	0	—	0	—	0	—	2	4.0
Uterus	Polyp	3	6.0	7	14.0	3	6.0	3	6.0
	Leiomyoma	0	—	0	—	1	2.0	1	2.0
	Adenocarcinoma	0	—	1	2.0	2	4.0	2	4.0
	Squamous cell carcinoma	0	—	0	—	1	2.0	0	—
	Sarcoma	0	—	1	2.0	1	2.0	0	—
	Carcinosarcoma	0	—	0	—	0	—	1	2.0
Uterus and vagina	Sarcoma	1	2.0	0	—	0	—	1	2.0
Peritoneum	Mesothelioma	1	2.0	0	—	0	—	1	2.0
	Liposarcoma	0	—	0	—	0	—	1	2.0
Pituitary gland	Adenoma	17	34.0	15	30.0	19	38.0	15	30.0
Thyroid gland	C-cell adenoma	0	—	2	4.0	1	2.0	5	10.0
	Follicular adenocarcinoma	0	—	1	2.0	0	—	0	—
Adrenal glands	Cortical adenoma	0	—	1	2.0	0	—	4	8.0
	Pheochromocytoma	16	32.0	10	20.0	7	14.0	10	20.0
	Cortical adenocarcinoma	0	—	2	4.0	0	—	1	2.0
	Pheochromoblastoma	1	2.0	0	—	1	2.0	2	4.0
Central nervous system									
Brain	Oligodendroglioma	2	4.0	0	—	0	—	0	—
Meninges	Meningioma	0	—	2	4.0	0	—	0	—
Major peripheral nerves	Malignant Schwannoma	0	—	1	2.0	0	—	0	—
Bones									
Cranium	Osteosarcoma	0	—	4	8.0	1	2.0	0	—
	Pericytosarcoma	0	—	0	—	1	2.0	0	—
Heart	malignant Schwannoma	1	2.0	0	—	0	—	0	—
Spleen	fibroangioma	0	—	0	—	1	2.0	0	—
Mesenteric lymph nodes	fibroangioma	0	—	1	2.0	0	—	0	—
Hemolymphoreticular tissues[d,e]	lymphomas and leukemias	11	22.0	7	14.0	8	16.0	0	—

[a] Numbers in parentheses indicate the number of tumors (one animal can bear more than one tumor).

[b] See TABLE 8.

[c] See TABLE 7.

[d] Including spleen and mesenteric lymph nodes.

[e] See TABLE 6.

TABLE 4. Results of Long-term Carcinogenicity Bioassays on Sodium Hypochlorite, Administered in Drinking Water Supplied ad Libitum (Experiment BT 7003): Total Benign Tumors

				Benign Tumors			
		Animals		Animals Bearing Tumors		Tumors	
Group No.	Concentration (mg/l)	Sex	No.	No.	%	No.	Per 100 Animals
I	750	M	50	31	62.0	39	78.0
		F	50	34	68.0	63	126.0
		M + F	100	65	65.0	102	102.0
II	500	M	50	24	48.0	34	68.0
		F	50	32	64.0	62	124.0
		M + F	100	56	56.0	96	96.0
III	100	M	50	37	74.0	47	94.0
		F	50	35	70.0	57	114.0
		M + F	100	72	72.0	104	104.0
IV	0	M	50	25	50.0	31	62.0
		F	50	37	74.0	67	134.0
		M + F	100	62	62.0	98	98.0

TABLE 5. Results of Long-term Carcinogenicity Bioassays on Sodium Hypochlorite, Administered in Drinking Water Supplied ad Libitum (Experiment BT 7003): Total Malignant Tumors

Group No.	Concentration (mg/l)	Animals		Malignant Tumors			
				Animals Bearing Tumors		Tumors	
		Sex	No.	No.	%	No.	Per 100 Animals
I	750	M	50	16	32.0	17	34.0
		F	50	24	48.0	29	58.0
		M + F	100	40	40.0	46	46.0
II	500	M	50	16	32.0	20	40.0
		F	50	20	40.0	30	60.0
		M + F	100	36	36.0	50	50.0
III	100	M	50	17	34.0	26	52.0
		F	50	20	40.0	25	50.0
		M + F	100	37	37.0	51	51.0
IV	0	M	50	13	26.0	14	28.0
		F	50	21	42.0	29	58.0
		M + F	100	34	34.0	43	43.0

TABLE 6. Results of Long-term Carcinogenicity Bioassays on Sodium Hypochlorite, Administered in Drinking Water Supplied ad Libitum (Experiment BT 7003): Lymphomas and Leukemias

Group No.	Concentration (mg/l)	Animals		Animals Bearing Lymphomas and Leukemias		
		Sex	No.	No.	%	Latency[a] (weeks)
I	750	M	50	6	12.0	92.7
		F	50	11	22.0	112.5
		M + F	100	17	17.0	105.5
II	500	M	50	6	12.0	100.6
		F	50	7	14.0	107.7
		M + F	100	13	13.0	104.5
III	100	M	50	4	8.0	95.5
		F	50	8	16.0	115.6
		M + F	100	12	12.0	108.9
IV	0	M	50	4	8.0	106.5
		F	50	0	—	—
		M + F	100	4	4.0	106.5

[a] Age at death.

TABLE 7. Results of Long-term Carcinogenicity Bioassays on Sodium Hypochlorite, Administered in Drinking Water Supplied ad Libitum (Experiment BT 7003): Tumors of the Stomach

Group No.	Concentration (mg/l)	Animals		Animals Bearing Tumors of the Stomach							
				Acanthomas		Sq. Cell Carcinomas		Sarcomas		Total	
		Sex	No.	No.	%	No.	%	No.	%	No.	%
I	750	M	50	4	8.0	0	—	1	2.0	5	10.0
		F	50	0	—	0	—	0	—	0	—
		M + F	100	4	4.0	0	—	1	1.0	5	5.0
II	500	M	50	2	4.0	0	—	0	—	2	4.0
		F	50	2	4.0	0	—	0	—	2	4.0
		M + F	100	4	4.0	0	—	0	—	4	4.0
III	100	M	50	3	6.0	1	2.0	1	2.0	5	10.0
		F	50	1	2.0	0	—	0	—	1	2.0
		M + F	100	4	4.0	1	1.0	1	1.0	6	6.0
IV	0	M	50	1	2.0	0	—	0	—	1	2.0
		F	50	1	2.0	0	—	0	—	1	2.0
		M + F	100	2	2.0	0	—	0	—	2	2.0

TABLE 8. Results of Long-term Carcinogenicity Bioassays on Sodium Hypochlorite, Administered in Drinking Water Supplied ad Libitum (Experiment BT 7003): Adenomas of the Lung

Group No.	Concentration (mg/l)	Animals		Animals Bearing Adenomas of the Lung	
		Sex	No.	No.	%
I	750	M	50	0	—
		F	50	0	—
		M + F	100	0	—
II	500	M	50	0	—
		F	50	0	—
		M + F	100	0	—
III	100	M	50	0	—
		F	50	3	6.0
		M + F	100	3	3.0
IV	0	M	50	0	—
		F	50	0	—
		M + F	100	0	—

the untreated rats of the colony used (historical controls), were detected in chlorine-exposed animals.

The results of this study confirm the results of the experiment of the United States National Toxicology Program (1991), which showed an increase of leukemia among female Fischer 344/N rats following the administration of chlorine (in the form of sodium hypochlorite and chloramine) in their drinking water.

The data here presented call for further research aimed at quantifying the oncogenic risks related to the chlorination of drinking water, to be used as a basis for consequent public health measures.

REFERENCES

1. Organization for Economic Co-operation and Development. 1994. Italy. OECD Environmental Performance Review. Paris.
2. Ottavi, C. 1994. La gestione razionale del ciclo di utilizzazione antropica dell'acqua. *In* Atti del Convegno della Sezione Italiana Acque Sotterranee dell'Associazione Mineraria Subalpina e dell'Associazione Idrotecnica. Italiana Sez. Piemonte, Liguria, Valle d'Aosta, su: ''Gestione integrata delle risorse idriche.'' Lerici, Italy.
3. National Research Council. 1977. Drinking water and health. National Academy Press, Vol. 1. Washington.
4. International Agency for Research on Cancer. 1991. Monographs on the evaluation of carcinogenic risk to humans, Vol. 52. Chlorinated drinking water, chlorination by-products, some other halogenated compounds, cobalt and cobalt compounds. IARC. Lyon.
5. Symons, J. M., T. A. Bellar, J. K. Carswell *et al.* 1975. National organics reconaissance survey for halogenated organic. J. Am. Water Works Assoc. **67:** 634-646.
6. Brass, H. J., M. A. Feige, T. Halloran *et al.* 1977. The national organic monitoring survey: Sampling and analyses for purgeable organic compounds. *In* Drinking Water Quality Enhancement through Source Protection. R. Pojasek, Ed.: 393-416. Ann Arbor Sci. Publ. Ann Arbor, MI.
7. Morris, R. D., A. M. Audet, I. F. Angelillo *et al.* 1992. Chlorination, chlorination by-products, and cancer: A meta-analysis. Am. J. Public Health **82:** 955-963.
8. Cantor, H. P., R. Hoover, T. J. Mason *et al.* 1978. Associations of cancer mortality with halomethanes in drinking water. J. Natl. Cancer Inst. **61:** 979-985.
9. Hogan, M. D., P.-Y. Chi, D. G. Hoel *et al.* 1979. Association between chloroform levels in finished drinking water supplies and various site-specific cancer mortality rates. J. Environ. Pathol. Toxicol. **2:** 873-887.
10. Druckrey, H. 1968. Chlorinated drinking water toxicity tests, involving seven generations of rats. Food Cosmet. Toxicol. **6:** 147-154.
11. National Toxicology Program. 1991. Toxicology and carcinogenesis studies of chlorinated and chloraminated water (deionized and charcoal-filtered) in F344/N rats and $B6C3F_1$ mice. TR392. DHHS Publ. No. (NIH) 91-2847. National Institutes of Health. Bethesda, MD.
12. International Agency for Research on Cancer. 1979. Monographs on the evaluation of carcinogenic risk of chemicals to humans, Vol. 20. Some halogenated hydrocarbons. IARC. Lyon.
13. Roe, F. J. C., A. K. Palmer, A. N. Worden *et al.* 1979. Safety evaluation of toothpaste containing chloroform. I. Long-term studies in mice. J. Environ. Pathol. Toxicol. **2:** 799-819.
14. Jorgenson, T. A., E. F. Meierhenry, C. J. Rushbrook *et al.* 1985. Carcinogenicity of chloroform in drinking water to male Osborne-Mendel rats and female $B6C3F_1$ mice. Fundam. Appl. Toxicol. **5:** 760-769.

15. Tumasonis, C. F., D. N. McMartin & B. Bush. 1985. Lifetime toxicity of chloroform and bromodichloromethane when administered over a lifetime in rats. Ecotoxicol. Environ. Saf. **9:** 233–240.
16. National Toxicology Program. 1985. Toxicology and carcinogenesis studies of chlorodibromomethane in F344/N rats and $B6C3F_1$ mice. TR 282. DHHS Publ. No. (NIH) 85-2538. National Institutes of Health. Bethesda, MD.
17. National Toxicology Program. 1987. Toxicology and carcinogenesis studies of bromodichloromethane in F344/N rats and $B6C3F_1$ mice. TR 321. DHHS Publ. No. (NIH) 88-2537. National Institutes of Health. Bethesda, MD.
18. National Toxicology Program. 1989. Toxicology and carcinogenesis studies of bromoform in F344/N rats and $B6C3F_1$ mice. TR 350. DHHS Publ. No. (NIH) 89-2805. National Institutes of Health. Bethesda, MD.

Results of a Long-term Experimental Study on the Carcinogenicity of Vinyl Acetate Monomer in Mice

CESARE MALTONI,[a] ADRIANO CILIBERTI,[b] GIUSEPPE LEFEMINE,[b] AND MORANDO SOFFRITTI[b]

[a]*Cancer Research Center*
European Ramazzini Foundation
of Oncology and Environmental Sciences
Bentivoglio Castle
40010 Bentivoglio (BO), Italy

[b]*European B. Ramazzini Foundation of Oncology and*
Environmental Sciences
Bologna, Italy

INTRODUCTION

Vinyl acetate monomer (VAM) is an important monomer of the plastics industry. It is a colorless liquid, insoluble in water, soluble in ethanol, ether, acetone, benzene, chloroform, and carbon tetrachloride, with a vapor pressure of 115 mm Hg at 25°C. VAM was produced for the first time in 1912. It is produced commercially mainly by two processes: in one, used since 1920, acetylene and acetic acid are reacted in the vapor phase over a catalyst bed; in the other the ethylene is reacted with acetic acid in the presence of oxygen. Commercial production of VAM was first reported in the United States in 1928.[1,2]

VAM is produced in many countries: Japan (6 companies), China and the United States (5 companies), Germany and the Russian Federation (2 companies), and Brazil, Canada, France, Mexico, Poland, Romania, Spain, Thailand, the United Kingdom and Venezuela. The total world capacity of VAM production was about 1,000,000 tonnes in 1965. World production rose to 3,000,000 tonnes in 1982, but had decreased to 2,500,000 tonnes by 1988. In the United States, VAM ranks 40th among the 50 most highly produced (by volume) chemicals.[3]

VAM is used primarily to produce polyvinyl acetate emulsions and polyvinyl alcohol (these uses account for about 75% of the total VAM produced worldwide). It is also used for the production of polyvinyl-acetals, of ethylene-vinyl acetate copolymers, and polyvinyl-acetate chloride copolymers. The multiple uses of the various VAM products have been recently reviewed.[3]

Polyvinyl acetate is an intermediate in the conversion to polyvinyl alcohol and acetals. Its principal use is in adhesives for paper, wood, glass, metals, and porcelain. It is also used: in latex water paint; for paper coating, for textile and leather finishing; as a base for inks and lacquers, in heat-sealing films, in shatterproof photographic bulbs; as an emulsifying agent in cosmetics, pesticide formulations and pharmaceuticals; and as a food additive.

Polyvinyl acetate is used as a component in the production of chewing gum; the amount of the polymer used in chewing gum varies from country to country: in some European countries it is higher than average, while in the United States it seems to be lower (around 5% of the final product in the United States).

Polyvinyl alcohol is used in sizing for textile warp and yarn, in laminating adhesives, photosensitive films and cements, as a binder for cosmetics, ceramics, leather, nonwoven fabrics and paper, and as an emulsifying agent, thickener, and stabilizer. It is the most highly produced (by volume) synthetic water-soluble plastic in the world.

Polyvinyl acetals are produced by the condensation of polyvinyl alcohol with an aldehyde. Commonly used aldehydes are formaldehyde, acetaldehyde, and butyralhyde. Polyvinyl formal, polyvinyl acetal, and polyvinyl butyral are mainly used in adhesives, paints, lacquers, and films. Polyvinyl butyral is used in sheet form as an interlayer in safety glasses and as shatter-resistant acrylic protection in aircraft.

Ethylene-vinyl acetate copolymers improve the adhesive properties of hot-melt and pressure-sensitive adhesives. They are also used in medical tubing, milk packaging, and beer-dispensing equipment. Plastic containers with barrier layers of ethylene-vinyl alcohol copolymers are replacing many glass and metal containers for packaging food.

Polyvinyl chloride-acetate copolymers, compounded with plasticizers, are used for cable and wire coverings, in chemical plants, and in protective garments.

The occupational exposure limits for vinyl acetate in various industrial countries range from 10 to 70 mg/m^3.[3] Polyvinyl acetate, ethylene-vinyl acetate-vinyl alcohol copolymers, ethylene-vinyl acetate copolymers, vinyl acetate-vinyl chloride copolymers, and vinyl acetate-crotonic acid copolymers have been approved for use by the United States Food and Drug Administration[4] as components of surfaces in contact with food and beverages.

VAM has an irritative effect on the upper respiratory system in humans. After subchronic and chronic exposure by inhalation it causes, in experimental animals, hyperplasia, metaplasia of the respiratory epithelium, and bronchitis and bronchiolitis.[3]

Experimental studies on reproductive and prenatal effects have shown that VAM causes parental toxicity (including decreased fertility), developmental toxicity, and minor skeletal alterations.[3]

VAM shows genotoxic effects both in human and rodent cells.[3]

In vitro, VAM is metabolized, mainly by hydrolysis, to acetaldehyde and acetic acid.[5,6] Rats exposed to VAM exhaled acetaldehyde as a result of hydrolysis by esterase.[6,7] Acetaldehyde is known to be carcinogenic in experimental animals,[8] and its carcinogenic potential was clearly demonstrated by a recent research performed on rats in our laboratory.[9]

Although VAM has been commercially produced for more than 60 years and represents a major monomer of the plastics industry, the carcinogenicity studies on this monomer are, in our opinion, still inadequate.

To date, five experimental studies on VAM carcinogenicity are reported in the scientific literature. In a first experiment, performed in our laboratory in the early '70s, a group of 96 male and female Sprague-Dawley rats was exposed by inhalation for 4 hours per day, 5 days per week, for 52 weeks, to 2,500 ppm (maximum tolerated concentration) of VAM. Early mortality was high: only 49 animals survived for 26 or more weeks. No tumors related to VAM were reported during 135 weeks.[10–12] Because of the poor survival of the animals, this study was not adequate for exposing the carcinogenic potential of the monomer.

In a second experiment VAM was administered at the doses of 2500, 1000, and 0 mg/l in drinking water for 100 weeks, to groups of 20 male and 20 female Fischer F344 rats, 7 to 8 weeks of age, which were then kept under observation for the rest of their life span (130 weeks). An increase of liver neoplastic nodules, of uterine adenocarcinomas and polyps, and of thyroid C-cell adenomas was observed.[13] It must be noted that the number of the animals tested was small, and that the histopathological examination was limited to gross lesions and major organs only.

The results of three further carcinogenicity experiments, in which VAM was administered by inhalation to mice and rats, and by drinking water, *in utero,* to rats, were published in 1994.

In the inhalation experiment on mice, groups each of 60 male and 60 female Swiss mice, about 7 weeks of age, were exposed to 600, 200, 50, and 0 ppm vinyl acetate (purity >99%) for 6 hours per day, 5 days a week, for about 104 weeks. No treatment-related increase in tumor incidence was observed.[14]

In the inhalation experiment on rats, groups of 60 male and 60 female Sprague-Dawley rats, about 7 weeks of age, were exposed to 600, 200, 50, and 0 ppm vinyl acetate (purity >99%) for 6 hours per day, 5 days a week, for about 104 weeks. A slightly increased incidence of nasal cavity tumors (benign and malignant) was found in animals of each sex.[14]

In the *in utero* drinking water experiment on rats, a total of 72 male and 144 female Sprague-Dawley rats (age unspecified) were divided into 4 groups and received vinyl acetate (purity >99%) at 5000, 1000, 200, and 0 mg/l in the drinking water. Treatment commenced 10 weeks before mating; treatment of males was continued for an additional 4 weeks and that of females throughout mating, gestation, and lactation. Two males of the F_0 generation in each group were paired with one female from the same group for up to 15 days. After weaning, groups of 60 male and 60 female F_1 pups were selected and were administered 5000, 1000, 200, and 0 mg/l vinyl acetate in drinking water for 104 weeks. No treatment-related increase in tumor incidence was observed.[15]

One must note that in these last three experiments the biophase was truncated at 104 weeks, thus not allowing the animals to express to the possible maximum extent their neoplastic potentialities.

Two studies on the carcinogenicity of VAM were performed in humans. In a cohort study aimed at identifying the specific exposure associated with an excess of lung cancer risk in a United States synthetic chemical plant, 19 chemicals were considered, one of which was VAM: the subgroup with undifferentiated large-cell lung cancer had had slightly higher cumulative exposure to VAM.[16]

A nested case-control study was conducted in a cohort of 29,139 men, employed in two large chemical manufacturing facilities and a research and development center in the United States, who had died in 1940-78 with non-Hodgkin's lymphoma, multiple myeloma, lymphocytic leukemia, or nonlymphocytic leukemia as the underlying or contributing cause of death. Exposure to 21 chemicals was assessed on the basis of information about work activity, work area, and production over time. Potential exposure to vinyl acetate was reported for 7 of 52 men who had died with non-Hodgkin's lymphoma (odds ratio 1.2), 3 of 20 with multiple myeloma (odds ratio 1.6), 2 of 39 with nonlymphocytic leukemia (odds ratio 0.5), and 2 of 18 with lymphocytic leukemia (odd ratio 1.8).[17]

These two studies on workers do not allow any conclusions to be drawn on the carcinogenic potential of VAM.

The International Agency for Research on Cancer (IARC) Monograph of 1995[3] concludes that VAM is possibly carcinogenic to humans (Group 2B), on the basis of the available results both of carcinogenicity studies and of other information relevant to an evaluation of carcinogenicity of the monomer—namely, the evidence that: (1) VAM is biotransformed into acetaldehyde; (2) VAM and acetaldehyde are genotoxic in human and animal cells; (3) acetaldehyde is carcinogenic in experimental animals; and (4) VAM and acetaldehyde induce nasal tumors after administration by inhalation.

In the '80s we started a project of three long-term bioassays for assessing the carcinogenic potential of VAM. These studies were performed with a similar protocol on Sprague-Dawley rats, Wistar rats, and Swiss mice. This report deals with the results of the experiment on mice.

MATERIALS AND METHODS

VAM was supplied by an Italian chemical plant. The analyses of the sample of VAM supplied showed the following impurities:

- benzene 30-45 ppm
- methyl and ethyl acetate 50 ppm
- crotonaldehyde 6-16 ppm
- acetaldehyde 2-11 ppm
- acetone 330-500 ppm

Male and female Swiss mice were used.

VAM was administered in drinking water at two concentrations for 78 weeks. The experiment included breeders and offspring. The treatment of male and female breeders and of male and female offspring started when the female breeders were at the 12th day of pregnancy.

The plan of the experiment is shown in TABLE 1.

All animals were kept under control for their life span. The drinking water with or without the monomer was changed every morning. The solutions of VAM were prepared just before the daily water supply was provided.

The mice were submitted daily to observation and weighed periodically, weekly within the first 13 weeks of the experiment, every 2 weeks until the treatment was

TABLE 1. Long-term Carcinogenicity Bioassays on Vinyl acetate (VAM), Administered to Swiss Mice in Drinking Water Supplied ad Libitum (BT 52): Plan of the Experiment

Group No.	Concentration (ppm, v/v)	Animals		
		Age at Start (weeks)	Sex	No.
I	5,000	17 (breeders)	M	13
			F	37
			M + F	50
		Embryos (offspring)	M	49
			F	48
			M + F	97
II	1,000	17 (breeders)	M	13
			F	37
			M + F	50
		Embryos (offspring)	M	37
			F	44
			M + F	81
III	0[a]	17 (breeders)	M	14
			F	37
			M + F	51
		Embryos (offspring)	M	38
			F	48
			M + F	86

[a] Drinking water alone.

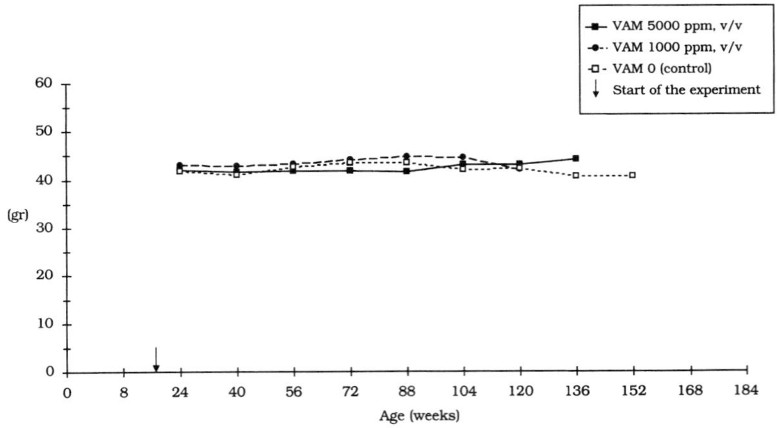

FIGURE 1. Mean body weight in male breeder mice.

stopped, and then every 8 weeks until the end of the experiment. In order to detect and register all gross lesions, the animals were examined every week for the first 13 weeks, and then every 2 weeks until the end of the experiment.

At death all animals were submitted to systemic necropsy. Specimens for histopathology include: brain, pituitary gland, Zymbal glands, salivary glands, Herderian glands, head (5 sections) (only in animals that survived more than 100 weeks), tongue, thyroid, thymus and mediastinal lymph nodes, lung, heart, diaphragm, liver, spleen, pancreas, kidneys and adrenal glands, esophagus, stomach, intestine (4 levels), bladder, prostate, uterus, gonads, interscapular fat pad, subcutaneous and mesenteric lymph nodes, and any other organs and tissues with pathological lesions. All organs and tissues were preserved in 70% ethyl alcohol, except bones, which were fixed in 10% formalin and then decalcified with a 10% formaldehyde and 20% formic acid in water solution. The normal specimens were trimmed, following the standard procedures of the Bentivoglio laboratory: i.e., parenchymal organs were dissected through the hilus to expose the widest surface, and hollow organs were sectioned across the greatest diameter(s). The pathological tissue was trimmed to allow for the largest surface, including normal adjacent tissues. The trimmed specimens were processed as paraffin blocks, and 3-5-micron sections of every specimen were obtained. Sections were routinely stained with hematoxylin-eosin. Specific stainings were performed when needed. All slides were examined microscopically by the same group of pathologists; a senior pathologist reviewed all the tumors and any other lesion of oncological interest. All pathologists followed the same criteria of histopathological evaluation and classification.

RESULTS

Body Weight. There were no differences in mean body weight in treated and control groups of male and female breeders (FIGS. 1, 2). In the treated offspring at

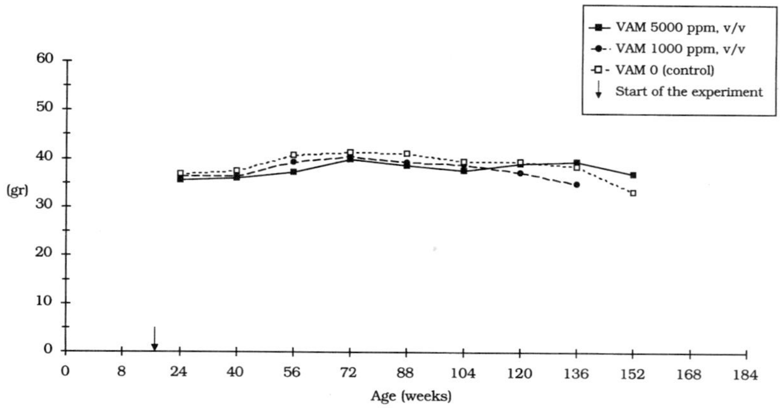

FIGURE 2. Mean body weight in female breeder mice.

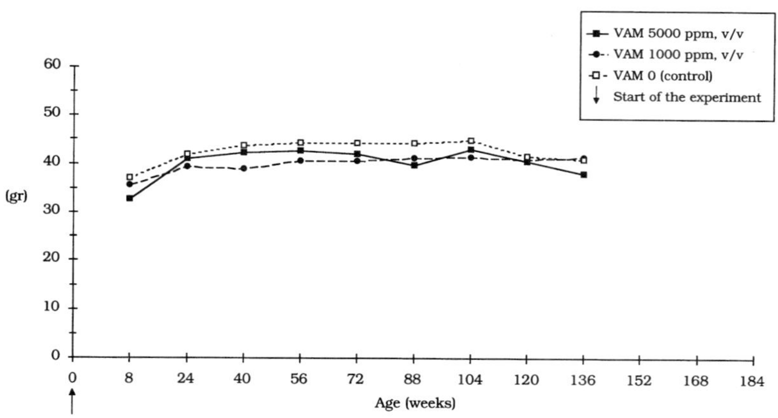

FIGURE 3. Mean body weight in male offspring mice.

both tested doses, there is a slight decrease in mean body weight in the animals of both sexes, more evident in females (FIGS. 3, 4).

Survival. In male breeders up to 72 weeks of age, there was a decrease in survival of treated animals at both doses; then from 72 to 120 weeks an increase of survival was observed among the animals treated with the higher dose (FIG. 5). The female breeders treated with the lower dose had a slight decrease in survival (FIG. 6). In male and female offspring treated with the higher dose an increase in survival was observed (FIGS. 7, 8).

Nononcological Changes. No evident behavioral changes were observed in VAM treated animals. No treatment-related nononcological pathological changes were detected by gross inspection and histological examination.

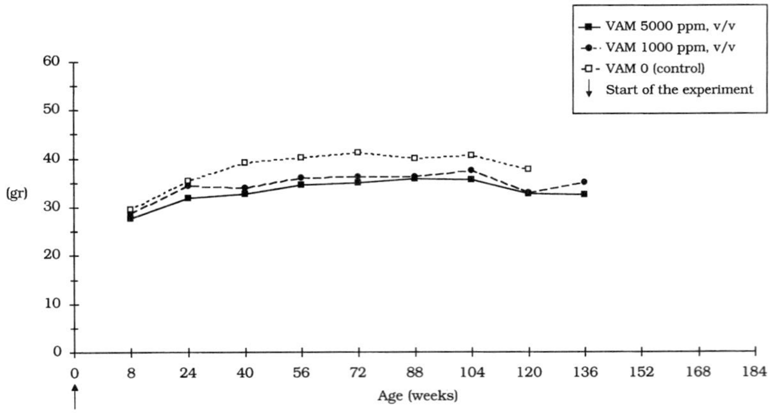

FIGURE 4. Mean body weight in female offspring mice.

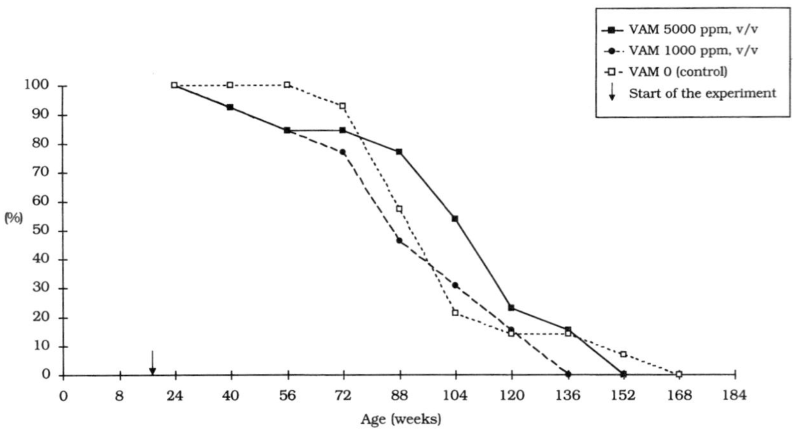

FIGURE 5. Survival in male breeder mice.

Tumors. The entire results are shown in TABLES 2 and 3. Multiple tumors of the same site (monolateral and bilateral organs) and type were plotted only once, apart from mammary and pulmonary tumors of the same type, whose multiplicity has been taken into account.

At the higher dose VAM increases the incidence of total benign tumors in female breeders and offspring (TABLE 4). An increase of total malignant tumors has been observed in male and female breeders and offspring treated with the higher dose (TABLE 5). Such increase was sharper among offspring.

Zymbal gland carcinomas were more numerous among female breeders treated with the higher dose, among female and male offspring treated with the higher dose,

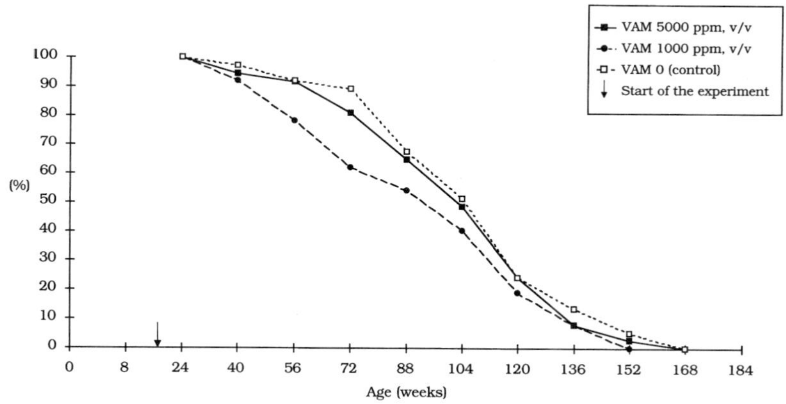

FIGURE 6. Survival in female breeder mice.

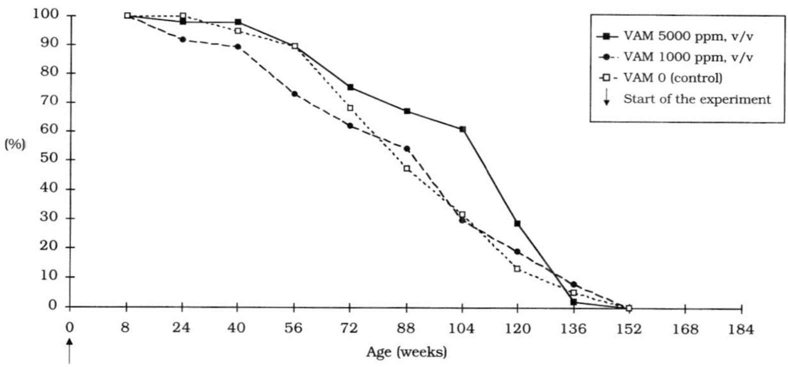

FIGURE 7. Survival in male offspring mice.

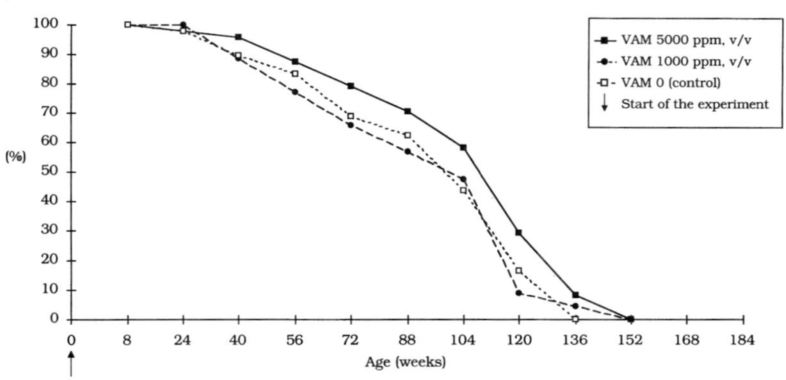

FIGURE 8. Survival in female offspring mice.

TABLE 2. Long-term Carcinogenicity Bioassays on Vinyl Acetate (VAM), Administered to Swiss Mice in Drinking Water Supplied ad Libitum (Experiment BT 52): Number and Percentage of Male Swiss Mice Bearing Various Types of Benign and Malignant Tumors[a]

		Groups											
		I: 5000 ppm				II: 1000 ppm				III: 0 (Control)			
		Breeders		Offspring		Breeders		Offspring		Breeders		Offspring	
Site	Histotype	No.	%	No.	%	No.	%	No.	%	No.	%	No.	%
Skin	Squamous cell carcinoma	0	—	0	—	0	—	0	—	0	—	1	2.6
Mammary gland[b]	Adenocarcinoma	0	—	0	—	0	—	1	2.7	0	—	0	—
Harderian glands	Adenoma	1	7.7	1	2.0	0	—	1	2.7	1	7.1	4	10.5
	Adenocarcinoma	0	—	1	2.0	0	—	0	—	0	—	0	—
Zymbal glands[c]	Carcinoma	0	—	2	4.1	0	—	0	—	0	—	0	—
Oral cavity[d]	Squamous cell carcinoma	1	7.7	10	20.4	0	—	0	—	0	—	0	—
Tongue[e]	Squamous cell carcinoma	1	7.7	7	14.3	0	—	0	—	0	—	1	2.6
Lung[f]	Adenoma	3 (4)	23.1	11 (19)	22.4	2	15.4	6 (9)	16.2	2 (3)	14.3	6 (7)	15.8
	Adenocarcinoma	2 (4)	15.4	2	4.1	2	15.4	0	—	2	14.3	1	2.6
Esophagus[g]	Squamous cell carcinoma	0	—	12	24.5	0	—	0	—	0	—	0	—
Stomach													
Forestomach[h]	Acanthoma	1	7.7	8	16.3	0	—	1	2.7	0	—	0	—
	Squamous cell carcinoma	0	—	2	4.1	0	—	0	—	0	—	0	—
Glandular	Adenomatous polyp	0	—	0	—	0	—	1	2.7	0	—	0	—
stomach[i]	Adenocarcinoma	1	7.7	0	—	0	—	0	—	0	—	1	2.6
Intestine	Adenocarcinoma	0	—	0	—	0	—	0	—	0	—	1	2.6
Liver[j]	Angioma and fibroangioma	1	7.7	0	—	0	—	0	—	1	7.1	1	2.6
	Hepatocarcinoma	2	15.4	17	34.7	4	30.7	8	21.6	3	21.4	10	26.3
	Angiosarcoma	1	7.7	2	4.1	0	—	0	—	0	—	2	5.3
Pancreas	Islet cell adenoma	1	7.7	0	—	0	—	0	—	1	7.1	1	2.6
Kidneys	Adenoma	0	—	0	—	0	—	0	—	0	—	1	2.6
	Adenocarcinoma	0	—	2	4.1	0	—	1	2.7	0	—	1	2.6

Seminal vesicles	Adenoma	0	—	0	—	0	—	0	—	0	—	2	5.3
	Adenocarcinoma	0	—	1	2.0	0	—	0	—	0	—	0	—
Testes	Leydig cell tumor	0	—	1	2.0	0	—	2	5.4	0	—	1	2.6
	Angioma	0	—	0	—	0	—	0	—	0	—	1	2.6
Peritoneum	Angiosarcoma	0	—	1	2.0	0	—	1	2.7	0	—	0	—
Thyroid gland	C-cell carcinoma	1	7.7	0	—	0	—	0	—	0	—	0	—
Adrenal glands	Cortical adenoma	0	—	0	—	0	—	1	2.7	0	—	0	—
	Pheochromocytoma	0	—	0	—	0	—	0	—	0	—	3	7.9
	Pheochromoblastoma	0	—	0	—	1	7.7	0	—	0	—	0	—
Bones													
Cranium	Osteosarcoma	0	—	1	2.0	0	—	0	—	0	—	0	—
Heart	Angiosarcoma	0	—	0	—	0	—	0	—	0	—	1	2.6
Mediastinum	Fibroangioma	0	—	0	—	0	—	0	—	1	7.1	0	—
Spleen	Angioma and fibroangioma	0	—	2	4.1	0	—	1	2.7	0	—	0	—
	Angiosarcoma	0	—	2	4.1	0	—	1	2.7	0	—	1	2.6
Mesenteric lymph nodes	Fibroangioma	0	—	0	—	1	7.7	0	—	0	—	0	—
Hemolymphoreticular tissues[k,l]	Lymphomas and leukemias	4	30.8	23	46.9	2	15.4	17	45.9	4	28.6	15	39.5

[a] The numbers in parentheses indicate the number of tumors (one animal can bear more than one tumor).
[b] See TABLE 15.
[c] See TABLE 6.
[d] See TABLE 7.
[e] See TABLE 8.
[f] See TABLE 12.
[g] See TABLE 9.
[h] See TABLE 10.
[i] See TABLE 11.
[j] See TABLE 13.
[k] See TABLE 16.
[l] Including spleen and mesenteric lymph nodes.

TABLE 3. Long-term Carcinogenicity Bioassays on Vinyl Acetate (VAM), Administered to Swiss Mice in Drinking Water Supplied ad Libitum (Experiment BT 52): Number and Percentage of Female Swiss Mice Bearing Various Types of Benign and Malignant Tumors[a]

		Groups											
		I: 5000 ppm				II: 1000 ppm				III: 0 (Control)			
		Breeders		Offspring		Breeders		Offspring		Breeders		Offspring	
Site	Histotype	No.	%	No.	%	No.	%	No.	%	No.	%	No.	%
Skin	Squamous cell carcinoma	0	–	1	2.1	0	–	0	–	0	–	0	–
Subcutaneous tissue	Angiosarcoma	0	–	0	–	0	–	1	2.3	0	–	1	2.1
Interscapular fat pad	Angiosarcoma	0	–	1	2.1	0	–	0	–	0	–	0	–
Mammary gland[b]	Adenocarcinoma	6	16.2	7	14.6	4	10.8	5	11.4	6 (7)	16.2	9 (10)	18.8
	Liposarcoma	0	–	3	6.3	1	2.7	0	–	0	–	0	–
	Angiosarcoma	0	–	0	–	0	–	2	4.5	0	–	0	–
Harderian glands	Adenoma	1	2.7	4	8.3	0	–	2	4.5	1	2.7	2	4.2
	Adenocarcinoma	0	–	1	2.1	0	–	1	2.3	0	–	0	–
Zymbal glands[c]	Carcinoma	1	2.7	4	8.3	0	–	2	4.5	0	–	0	–
Oral cavity[d]	Carcinoma	1	2.7	9	18.8	0	–	0	–	0	–	0	–
Tongue[e]	Carcinoma	3	8.1	12	25.0	1	2.7	0	–	0	–	0	–
Lung[f]	Adenoma	6 (10)	16.2	11 (21)	22.9	6 (8)	16.2	3	6.8	3	8.1	6 (7)	12.5
	Adenocarcinoma	1	2.7	3 (4)	6.3	1	2.7	1	2.3	0	–	0	–
Esophagus[g]	Acanthoma	1	2.7	3	6.3	0	–	0	–	0	–	0	–
	Squamous cell carcinoma	6	16.2	18	37.5	0	–	0	–	0	–	0	–
Stomach													
Forestomach[h]	Acanthoma	5	13.5	11	22.9	0	–	0	–	0	–	0	–
	Squamous cell carcinoma	3	8.1	7	14.6	0	–	0	–	0	–	0	–

Glandular stomach[i]	Adenocarcinoma	1	2.7	1	2.1	0	—	0	—	0	—	0	—
Intestine	Adenocarcinoma	0	—	1	2.1	0	—	0	—	0	—	0	—
Liver[d]	Cholangioma	1	2.7	4	8.3	0	—	1	2.3	0	—	1	2.1
	Angioma	1	2.7	0	—	0	—	1	2.3	0	—	1	2.1
	Hepatocarcinoma	0	—	2	4.2	0	—	0	—	0	—	1	2.1
	Angiosarcoma	0	—	1	2.1	0	—	0	—	1	2.7	1	2.1
Pancreas	Islet cell adenoma	1	2.7	2	4.2	1	2.7	3	6.8	2	5.4	0	—
Kidneys	Adenoma	0	—	0	—	1	2.7	0	—	0	—	0	—
Ovaries	Cystadenoma	0	—	3	6.2	1	2.7	2	4.5	0	—	3	6.2
	Granulosa cell tumor	0	—	0	—	0	—	1	2.3	0	—	1	2.1
	Theca cell tumor	0	—	0	—	0	—	0	—	0	—	1	2.1
	Sertoli cell tumor	0	—	1	2.1	0	—	1	2.3	0	—	0	—
	Angioma and fibroangioma	1	2.7	0	—	2	5.4	2	4.5	1	2.7	0	—
	Adenocarcinoma	1	2.7	1	2.1	0	—	1	2.3	0	—	0	—
	Granulosa cell malignant tumor	1	2.7	0	—	0	—	0	—	0	—	0	—
Uterus[k]	Polyp	3	8.1	7	14.6	2	5.4	4	9.1	5	13.5	5	10.4
	Leiomyoma	2	5.4	6	12.5	0	—	3	6.8	1	2.7	2	4.2
	Angioma and fibroangioma	0	—	1	2.1	1	2.7	2	4.5	1	2.7	2	4.2
	Squamous cell carcinoma	0	—	1	2.1	0	—	0	—	0	—	0	—
	Adenocarcinoma	6	16.2	7	14.6	2	5.4	6	13.6	1	2.7	5	10.4
	Leiomyosarcoma	2	5.4	4	8.3	0	—	2	4.5	1	2.7	0	—
	Angiosarcoma	0	—	0	—	0	—	1	2.3	0	—	0	—
Peritoneum	Mesothelioma	1	2.7	0	—	0	—	0	—	0	—	0	—
Pituitary gland	Adenoma	0	—	1	2.1	0	—	1	2.3	0	—	0	—
Thyroid gland	C-cell adenoma	0	—	0	—	0	—	0	—	0	—	1	2.1
Adrenal glands	Pheochromocytoma	0	—	2	4.2	0	—	1	2.3	0	—	0	—
Bones	Osteosarcoma	0	—	0	—	0	—	1	2.3	1	2.7	0	—

TABLE 3. Long-term Carcinogenicity Bioassays on Vinyl Acetate (VAM), Administered to Swiss Mice in Drinking Water Supplied ad Libitum (Experiment BT 52): Number and Percentage of Female Swiss Mice Bearing Various Types of Benign and Malignant Tumors[a] (*continued*)

		Groups											
		I: 5000 ppm				II: 1000 ppm				III: 0 (Control)			
		Breeders		Offspring		Breeders		Offspring		Breeders		Offspring	
Site	Histotype	No.	%	No.	%	No.	%	No.	%	No.	%	No.	%
Spleen	Angioma and fibroangioma	1	2.7	0	–	0	–	2	4.5	1	2.7	0	–
	Angiosarcoma	0	–	1	2.1	0	–	1	2.3	0	–	2	4.2
Mesenteric lymph nodes	Fibroangioma	1	2.7	0	–	0	–	0	–	0	–	0	–
Hemolymphoreticular tissues[l,m]	Lymphomas and leukemias	18	48.6	33	68.8	22	59.5	28	63.6	18	48.6	27	56.3

[a] The numbers in parentheses indicate the number of tumors (one animal can bear more than one tumor).
[b] See TABLE 15.
[c] See TABLE 6.
[d] See TABLE 7.
[e] See TABLE 8.
[f] See TABLE 12.
[g] See TABLE 9.
[h] See TABLE 10.
[i] See TABLE 11.
[j] See TABLE 13.
[k] See TABLE 14.
[l] See TABLE 16.
[m] Including spleen and mesenteric lymph nodes.

TABLE 4. Results of Long-term Carcinogenicity Bioassays on Vinyl Acetate (VAM), Administered to Swiss Mice in Drinking Water Supplied ad Libitum (BT 52): Total Benign Tumors

Group No.	Concentration (ppm, v/v)	Animals: Age at Start (weeks)	Animals: Sex	Animals: No.	Benign tumors: Animals Bearing Tumors: No.	Benign tumors: Animals Bearing Tumors: %	Benign tumors: Tumors: No.	Benign tumors: Tumors: Per 100 Animals
I	5,000	17	M	13	5	38.5	8	61.5
		(breeders)	F	37	20	54.1	28	75.7
			M + F	50	25	50.0	36	72.0
		Embryos	M	49	17	34.7	31	63.3
		(offspring)	F	48	29	60.4	66	137.5
			M + F	97	46	47.4	97	100.0
II	1,000	17	M	13	3	23.1	3	23.1
		(breeders)	F	37	10	27.0	16	43.2
			M + F	50	13	26.0	19	38.0
		Embryos	M	37	10	27.0	16	43.2
		(offspring)	F	44	16	36.4	29	65.9
			M + F	81	26	32.1	45	55.6
III	0[a]	17	M	14	5	35.7	7	50.0
		(breeders)	F	37	12	32.4	15	40.5
			M + F	51	17	33.3	22	43.1
		Embryos	M	38	14	36.8	21	55.3
		(offspring)	F	48	16	33.3	26	54.2
			M + F	86	30	34.9	47	54.7

[a] Drinking water alone.

TABLE 5. Results of Long-term Carcinogenicity Bioassays on Vinyl Acetate (VAM), Administered to Swiss Mice in Drinking Water Supplied ad Libitum (BT 52): Total Malignant Tumors

		Animals			Malignant Tumors			
					Animals Bearing Tumors		Tumors	
Group No.	Concentration (ppm, v/v)	Age at Start (weeks)	Sex	No.	No.	%	No.	Per 100 Animals
I	5,000	17 (breeders)	M	13	11	84.6	15	115.4
			F	37	26	70.3	51	137.8
			M + F	50	37	74.0	66	132.0
		Embryos (offspring)	M	49	41	83.7	85	173.5
			F	48	45	93.8	119	247.9
			M + F	97	86	87.7	204	210.3
II	1,000	17 (breeders)	M	13	6	46.2	9	69.2
			F	37	28	75.7	31	83.8
			M + F	50	34	68.0	40	80.0
		Embryos (offspring)	M	37	24	64.9	29	78.4
			F	44	33	75.0	52	118.2
			M + F	81	57	70.4	81	100.0
III	0[a]	17 (breeders)	M	14	7	50.0	9	64.3
			F	37	21	56.8	29	78.4
			M + F	51	28	54.9	38	74.5
		Embryos (offspring)	M	38	26	68.4	35	92.1
			F	48	30	62.5	47	97.9
			M + F	86	56	65.1	82	95.3

[a] Drinking water alone.

and among female offspring treated with the lower dose (TABLE 6). The incidence of the squamous cell dysplasia of the gland was higher among male and female breeders treated with the higher dose, among male and female offspring treated with the higher dose, and among female breeders treated with the lower dose (TABLE 6). Such increase was sharper among females.

At the higher dose, in male and female breeders and offspring, VAM causes squamous cell carcinomas of the oral cavity (TABLE 7).

The incidence of tongue carcinomas is increased among male and female breeders and offspring treated with the higher dose (TABLE 8). The incidence of squamous cell dysplasia also increased among female breeders and among male and female offspring treated with the higher dose (TABLE 8).

Squamous carcinomas and squamous cell dysplasia of the esophagus are increased among male and female breeders and offspring treated with the higher dose of VAM (TABLE 9). A marginal increase of acanthomas in this organ has been found among female breeders and offspring treated with the higher dose (TABLE 9).

Also the incidence of squamous cell carcinomas and acanthomas of the forestomach has been found enhanced among female breeders and male and female offspring treated with the higher dose (TABLE 10). The forestomach acanthomas are more numerous among male and female breeders and offspring treated with the higher dose (TABLE 10).

A borderline increase of oncological lesions of the stomach was found among all treated animals (TABLE 11).

The number of lung tumors per 100 animals was increased among male and female breeders and offspring treated with the higher dose and among female breeders treated with the lower dose (TABLE 12).

A slight increase of hepatocarcinomas was observed among male offspring treated with the higher dose (TABLE 13).

The incidence of malignant tumors (leiomyosarcomas and adenocarcinomas) of the uterus was found to be increased in treated groups: the increase was dose correlated (TABLE 14). Uterine leiomyomas were found to be enhanced in offspring treated with the higher dose (TABLE 14).

No correlation between the treatment with VAM and the incidence of mammary cancers (TABLE 15) and lymphomas and leukemias (TABLE 16) was found.

Altogether the results indicate that the neoplastic response to treatment was more pronounced among female animals and in offspring.

CONCLUSIONS

In the tested experimental conditions, VAM has been shown to cause tumors in several body sites: therefore it must be considered a multipotential carcinogen.

Of particular significance is the increase of squamous cell carcinomas of the oral cavity, tongue, esophagus, and forestomach, and of the tumors of the stomach. The sites of these tumors were the most directly exposed, since VAM was administered by oral route.

The results of our bioassays of VAM on Sprague-Dawley and Wistar rats are now been elaborated and will soon be published. However, already, on the basis of

TABLE 6. Results of Long-term Carcinogenicity Bioassays on Vinyl Acetate (VAM), Administered to Swiss Mice in Drinking Water Supplied ad Libitum (BT 52): Adenomas, Squamous Cell Dysplasias, and Carcinomas of the Zymbal Glands

		Animals			Animals Bearing Lesions of the Zymbal Glands					
					Adenomas		Squamous Cell Dysplasias		Carcinomas	
Group No.	Concentration (ppm, v/v)	Age at Start (weeks)	Sex	No.	No.	%	No.	%	No.	%
I	5,000	17 (breeders)	M	13	0	—	1[a]	7.7	0	—
			F	37	0	—	6[a]	16.2	1	2.7
			M + F	50	0	—	7	14.0	1	2.0
		Embryos (offspring)	M	49	0	—	4[a]	8.2	2	4.1
			F	48	0	—	11[b]	22.9	4	8.3
			M + F	97	0	—	15	15.5	6	6.2
II	1,000	17 (breeders)	M	13	0	—	0	—	0	—
			F	37	0	—	3[a]	8.1	0	—
			M + F	50	0	—	3	6.0	0	—
		Embryos (offspring)	M	37	0	—	0	—	0	—
			F	44	0	—	2	4.5	2[a]	4.5
			M + F	81	0	—	2	2.5	2	2.5
III	0[c]	17 (breeders)	M	14	0	—	0	—	0	—
			F	37	0	—	1	2.7	0	—
			M + F	51	0	—	1	2.0	0	—
		Embryos (offspring)	M	38	0	—	2	5.3	0	—
			F	48	0	—	3	6.3	0	—
			M + F	86	0	—	5	5.8	0	—

[a] One animal is bearing a bilateral tumor.
[b] Five animals are bearing bilateral tumors.
[c] Drinking water alone.

TABLE 7. Results of Long-term Carcinogenicity Bioassays on Vinyl Acetate (VAM), Administered to Swiss Mice in Drinking Water Supplied ad Libitum (BT 52): Acanthomas, Squamous Cell Dysplasias, and Squamous Cell Carcinomas of the Oral Cavity

		Animals			Animals Bearing Lesions of the Oral Cavity					
					Acanthomas		Squamous Cell Dysplasias		Squamous Cell Carcinomas	
Group No.	Concentration (ppm, v/v)	Age at Start (weeks)	Sex	No.	No.	%	No.	%	No.	%
I	5,000	17 (breeders)	M	13	0	—	0	—	1	7.7
			F	37	0	—	0	—	1	2.7
			M + F	50	0	—	0	—	2	4.0
		Embryos (offspring)	M	49	0	—	0	—	10	20.4
			F	48	0	—	0	—	9	18.8
			M + F	97	0	—	0	—	19	19.6
II	1,000	17 (breeders)	M	13	0	—	0	—	0	—
			F	37	0	—	0	—	0	—
			M + F	50	0	—	0	—	0	—
		Embryos (offspring)	M	37	0	—	0	—	0	—
			F	44	0	—	0	—	0	—
			M + F	81	0	—	0	—	0	—
III	0[a]	17 (breeders)	M	14	0	—	0	—	0	—
			F	37	0	—	0	—	0	—
			M + F	51	0	—	0	—	0	—
		Embryos (offspring)	M	38	0	—	0	—	0	—
			F	48	0	—	0	—	0	—
			M + F	86	0	—	0	—	0	—

[a] Drinking water alone.

TABLE 8. Results of Long-term Carcinogenicity Bioassays on Vinyl Acetate (VAM), Administered to Swiss Mice in Drinking Water Supplied ad Libitum (BT 52): Acanthomas, Squamous Cell Dysplasias, and Squamous Cell Carcinomas of the Tongue

		Animals			Animals Bearing Lesions of the Tongue					
					Acanthomas		Squamous Cell Dysplasias		Squamous Cell Carcinomas	
Group No.	Concentration (ppm, v/v)	Age at Start (weeks)	Sex	No.	No.	%	No.	%	No.	%
I	5,000	17 (breeders)	M	13	0	—	0	—	1	7.7
			F	37	0	—	3	8.1	3	8.1
			M + F	50	0	—	3	6.0	3	6.0
		Embryos (offspring)	M	49	0	—	4	8.2	7	14.3
			F	48	0	—	7	14.6	12	25.0
			M + F	97	0	—	11	11.3	19	19.6
II	1,000	17 (breeders)	M	13	0	—	0	—	0	—
			F	37	0	—	0	—	1	2.7
			M + F	50	0	—	0	—	1	2.0
		Embryos (offspring)	M	37	0	—	0	—	0	—
			F	44	0	—	1	2.3	0	—
			M + F	81	0	—	1	1.2	0	—
III	0[a]	17 (breeders)	M	14	0	—	0	—	0	—
			F	37	0	—	0	—	0	—
			M + F	51	0	—	0	—	0	—
		Embryos (offspring)	M	38	0	—	0	—	1	2.6
			F	48	0	—	0	—	0	—
			M + F	86	0	—	0	—	1	1.2

[a] Drinking water alone.

TABLE 9. Results of Long-term Carcinogenicity Bioassays on Vinyl Acetate (VAM), Administered to Swiss Mice in Drinking Water Supplied ad Libitum (BT 52): Acanthomas, Squamous Cell Dysplasias, and Squamous Cell Carcinomas of the Esophagus

Group No.	Concentration (ppm, v/v)	Animals: Age at Start (weeks)	Animals: Sex	Animals: No.	Acanthomas: No.	Acanthomas: %	Squamous Cell Dysplasias: No.	Squamous Cell Dysplasias: %	Squamous Cell Carcinomas: No.	Squamous Cell Carcinomas: %
I	5,000	17 (breeders)	M	13	0	—	4	30.8	0	—
			F	37	1	2.7	6	16.2	6	16.2
			M + F	50	1	2.0	10	20.0	6	12.0
		Embryos (offspring)	M	49	0	—	4	8.2	12	24.5
			F	48	3	6.3	7	14.6	18	37.5
			M + F	97	3	3.1	11	11.3	30	30.9
II	1,000	17 (breeders)	M	13	0	—	0	—	0	—
			F	37	0	—	0	—	0	—
			M + F	50	0	—	0	—	0	—
		Embryos (offspring)	M	37	0	—	0	—	0	—
			F	44	0	—	0	—	0	—
			M + F	81	0	—	0	—	0	—
III	0[a]	17 (breeders)	M	14	0	—	0	—	0	—
			F	37	0	—	0	—	0	—
			M + F	51	0	—	0	—	0	—
		Embryos (offspring)	M	38	0	—	0	—	0	—
			F	48	0	—	0	—	0	—
			M + F	86	0	—	0	—	0	—

[a] Drinking water alone.

TABLE 10. Results of Long-term Carcinogenicity Bioassays on Vinyl Acetate (VAM), Administered to Swiss Mice in Drinking Water Supplied ad Libitum (BT 52): Acanthomas, Squamous Cell Dysplasias, and Squamous Cell Carcinomas of the Forestomach

Group No.	Concentration (ppm, v/v)	Animals: Age at Start (weeks)	Animals: Sex	Animals: No.	Acanthomas: No.	Acanthomas: %	Squamous Cell Dysplasias: No.	Squamous Cell Dysplasias: %	Squamous Cell Carcinomas: No.	Squamous Cell Carcinomas: %
I	5,000	17 (breeders)	M	13	1	7.7	0	—	0	—
			F	37	5	13.5	0	—	3	8.1
			M + F	50	6	12.0	0	—	3	6.0
		Embryos (offspring)	M	49	8	16.3	1	2.0	2	4.1
			F	48	11	22.9	0	—	7	14.6
			M + F	97	19	19.6	1	1.0	9	9.3
II	1,000	17 (breeders)	M	13	0	—	0	—	0	—
			F	37	0	—	0	—	0	—
			M + F	50	0	—	0	—	0	—
		Embryos (offspring)	M	37	1	2.7	0	—	0	—
			F	44	0	—	0	—	0	—
			M + F	81	1	1.2	0	—	0	—
III	0[a]	17 (breeders)	M	14	0	—	0	—	0	—
			F	37	0	—	0	—	0	—
			M + F	51	0	—	0	—	0	—
		Embryos (offspring)	M	38	0	—	0	—	0	—
			F	48	0	—	0	—	0	—
			M + F	86	0	—	0	—	0	—

[a] Drinking water alone.

TABLE 11. Results of Long-term Carcinogenicity Bioassays on Vinyl Acetate (VAM), Administered to Swiss Mice in Drinking Water Supplied ad Libitum (BT 52): Adenomatous Polyps, Glandular Dysplasias, and Adenocarcinomas of the Stomach

Group No.	Concentration (ppm, v/v)	Animals: Age at Start (weeks)	Animals: Sex	Animals: No.	Adenomatous Polyps: No.	Adenomatous Polyps: %	Glandular Dysplasias: No.	Glandular Dysplasias: %	Adenocarcinomas: No.	Adenocarcinomas: %
I	5,000	17 (breeders)	M	13	0	–	0	–	1	7.7
			F	37	0	–	0	–	1	2.7
			M + F	50	0	–	0	–	2	4.0
		Embryos (offspring)	M	49	0	–	3	6.1	0	–
			F	48	0	–	0	–	1	2.1
			M + F	97	0	–	3	3.1	1	1.0
II	1,000	17 (breeders)	M	13	0	–	0	–	0	–
			F	37	0	–	0	–	0	–
			M + F	50	0	–	0	–	0	–
		Embryos (offspring)	M	37	1	2.7	0	–	0	–
			F	44	0	–	1	2.3	0	–
			M + F	81	1	1.2	1	1.2	0	–
III	0[a]	17 (breeders)	M	14	0	–	0	–	0	–
			F	37	0	–	0	–	0	–
			M + F	51	0	–	0	–	0	–
		Embryos (offspring)	M	38	0	–	0	–	1	2.6
			F	48	0	–	0	–	0	–
			M + F	86	0	–	0	–	1	1.2

[a] Drinking water alone.

TABLE 12. Results of Long-term Carcinogenicity Bioassays on Vinyl Acetate (VAM), Administered to Swiss Mice in Drinking Water Supplied ad Libitum (BT 52): Adenomas and Adenocarcinomas of the Lung

		Animals			Animals Bearing Tumors				Total Tumors			
					Adenomas		Adenocarcinomas		Animals Bearing Tumors		Tumors	
Group No.	Concentration (ppm, v/v)	Age at Start (weeks)	Sex	No.	No.	%	No.	%	No.	%	No.	Per 100 Animals
I	5,000	17 (breeders)	M	13	3	23.1	2	15.4	4	30.8	8	61.5
			F	37	6	16.2	1	2.7	7	18.9	11	29.7
			M + F	50	9	18.0	3	6.0	11	22.0	19	38.0
		Embryos (offspring)	M	49	11	22.4	2	4.1	13	26.5	21	42.9
			F	48	11	22.9	3	6.3	11	22.9	25	52.1
			M + F	97	22	22.7	5	5.2	24	24.7	46	47.4
II	1,000	17 (breeders)	M	13	2	15.4	2	15.4	4	30.8	4	30.8
			F	37	6	16.2	1	2.7	6	16.2	9	24.3
			M + F	50	8	16.0	3	6.0	10	20.0	13	26.0
		Embryos (offspring)	M	37	6	16.2	0	—	6	16.2	9	24.3
			F	44	3	6.8	1	2.3	4	9.1	4	9.1
			M + F	81	9	11.1	1	1.2	10	12.3	13	16.0
III	0[a]	17 (breeders)	M	14	2	14.3	2	14.3	4	28.6	5	35.7
			F	37	3	8.1	0	—	3	8.1	3	8.1
			M + F	51	5	9.8	2	3.9	7	13.7	8	15.7
		Embryos (offspring)	M	38	6	15.8	1	2.6	7	18.4	8	21.1
			F	48	6	12.5	0	—	6	12.5	7	14.6
			M + F	86	12	14.0	1	1.2	13	15.1	15	17.4

[a] Drinking water alone.

TABLE 13. Results of Long-term Carcinogenicity Bioassays on Vinyl Acetate (VAM), Administered to Swiss Mice in Drinking Water Supplied ad Libitum (BT 52): Hepatocarcinomas

		Animals			Animals Bearing Hepatocarcinomas	
Group No.	Concentration (ppm, v/v)	Age at Start (weeks)	Sex	No.	No.	%
I	5,000	17 (breeders)	M	13	2	15.4
			F	37	0	—
			M + F	50	2	4.0
		Embryos (offspring)	M	49	17	34.7
			F	48	2	4.2
			M + F	97	19	19.6
II	1,000	17 (breeders)	M	13	4	30.7
			F	37	0	—
			M + F	50	4	8.0
		Embryos (offspring)	M	37	8	21.6
			F	44	0	—
			M + F	81	8	9.9
III	0[a]	17 (breeders)	M	14	3	21.4
			F	37	0	—
			M + F	51	3	5.9
		Embryos (offspring)	M	38	10	26.3
			F	48	1	2.1
			M + F	86	11	12.8

[a] Drinking water alone.

TABLE 14. Results of Long-term Carcinogenicity Bioassays on Vinyl Acetate (VAM), Administered to Swiss Mice in Drinking Water Supplied ad Libitum (BT 52): Leiomyomas, Leiomyosarcomas, and Adenocarcinomas of the Uterus

		Animals			Animals Bearing Tumors							
					Leiomyomas		Leiomyosarcomas		Adenocarcinomas		Total Malignant Tumors	
Group No.	Concentration (ppm, v/v)	Age at Start (weeks)	Sex	No.	No.	%	No.	%	No.	%	No.	%
I	5,000	17 (breeders)	F	37	2	5.4	2	5.4	6	16.2	8	21.6
		Embryos (offspring)	F	48	6	12.5	4	8.3	8	16.7	12	25.0
II	1,000	17 (breeders)	F	37	0	—	0	—	2	5.4	2	5.4
		Embryos (offspring)	F	44	3	6.8	2	4.5	6	13.6	8	18.2
III	0[a]	17 (breeders)	F	37	1	2.7	1	2.7	1	2.7	1	2.7
		Embryos (offspring)	F	48	2	4.2	0	—	5	10.4	5	10.4

[a] Drinking water alone.

TABLE 15. Results of Long-term Carcinogenicity Bioassays on Vinyl Acetate (VAM), Administered to Swiss Mice in Drinking Water Supplied ad Libitum (BT 52): Mammary Cancers

Group No.	Concentration (ppm, v/v)	Animals: Age at Start (weeks)	Animals: Sex	Animals: No.	Animals Bearing Tumors: No.	Animals Bearing Tumors: %	Tumors: No.	Tumors: Per 100 animals
I	5,000	17	M	13	0	—	0	—
		(breeders)	F	37	6	16.2	6	16.2
			M + F	50	6	12.0	6	12.0
		Embryos	M	49	0	—	0	—
		(offspring)	F	48	10	20.8	10	20.8
			M + F	97	10	10.3	10	10.3
II	1,000	17	M	13	0	—	0	—
		(breeders)	F	37	5	13.5	5	13.5
			M + F	50	5	10.0	5	10.0
		Embryos	M	37	1	2.7	1	2.7
		(offspring)	F	44	7	15.9	7	15.9
			M + F	81	8	9.9	8	9.9
III	0[a]	17	M	14	0	—	0	—
		(breeders)	F	37	6	16.2	7	18.9
			M + F	51	6	11.8	7	13.7
		Embryos	M	38	0	—	0	—
		(offspring)	F	48	9	18.8	10	20.8
			M + F	86	9	10.5	10	11.6

[a] Drinking water alone.

TABLE 16. Results of Long-term Carcinogenicity Bioassays on Vinyl Acetate (VAM), Administered to Swiss Mice in Drinking Water Supplied ad Libitum (BT 52): Lymphomas and Leukemias

Group No.	Concentration (ppm, v/v)	Animals: Age at Start (weeks)	Animals: Sex	Animals: No.	Animals Bearing Lymphomas and Leukemias: No.	Animals Bearing Lymphomas and Leukemias: %
I	5,000	17 (breeders)	M	13	4	30.8
			F	37	18	48.6
			M + F	50	22	44.0
		Embryos (offspring)	M	49	23	46.9
			F	48	33	68.8
			M + F	97	56	57.7
II	1,000	17 (breeders)	M	13	2	15.4
			F	37	22	59.5
			M + F	50	24	48.0
		Embryos (offspring)	M	37	17	45.9
			F	44	28	63.6
			M + F	81	45	55.6
III	0[a]	17 (breeders)	M	14	4	28.6
			F	37	18	48.6
			M + F	51	22	43.1
		Embryos (offspring)	M	38	15	39.5
			F	48	27	56.3
			M + F	86	42	48.8

[a] Drinking water alone.

the present results, regulatory measures and preventive actions must be undertaken to prevent the carcinogenic risk of VAM, mainly among exposed workers and among consumers of the goods containing the monomer.

Of particular concern is the current use of VAM-based polymers as a component in contact with food and beverages and in the production of chewing gum, since the vinyl acetate monomer has been found to migrate from plastic materials into, for example, wine[18] and water,[19] (and therefore presumably into saliva and other biological fluids).

SUMMARY

Vinyl acetate monomer (VAM) was administered in drinking water at doses of 5,000, 1,000, and 0 ppm (v/v), to Swiss mice, 17 weeks old (breeders) or 12-day embryos (offspring) at the start of the experiment. The treatment lasted 78 weeks, and the animals were kept under control until spontaneous death. VAM has been shown to cause an increase in: (1) total malignant tumors; (2) carcinomas of the Zymbal glands, oral cavity, tongue, esophagus, and forestomach; (3) stomach tumors; (4) lung tumors; and (5) uterine tumors. A slight increase of hepatomas has been observed among male mice offspring treated with the higher dose. On the basis of these data VAM must be considered a multipotential carcinogen.

REFERENCES

1. International Agency for Research on Cancer. 1979. Monographs on the evaluation of the carcinogenic risk of chemicals to humans, Vol. 19. Some monomers, plastics and synthetic elastomers, and acrolein. IARC. Lyon.
2. International Agency for Research on Cancer. 1986. Monographs on the evaluation of the carcinogenic risk of chemicals to humans, Vol. 39. Some chemicals used in plastics and elastomers. IARC. Lyon.
3. International Agency for Research on Cancer. 1995. Monographs on the evaluation of the carcinogenic risk of chemicals to humans, Vol. 63. Dry cleaning, some chlorinated solvents and other industrial chemicals. IARC. Lyon.
4. United States Food and Drug Administration. 1984. U.S. Code Fed. Regul., *Title 21,* Parts 175.105, 175.300, 175.350, 176.170, 176.180, 177.1010, 177.1200, 177.1350, 177.1360, 177.1670, 177.2260, 177.2260, 177.2800, 178.3910: 133, 145, 160, 180, 189, 199, 211, 225, 255, 271, 289, 348.
5. Hazleton Laboratories Europe. 1979. Vinyl acetate. Unpublished reports Nos. 1910-51/8, 2511-51/11-14, 1835-51/3, 1884-51/3, 2286-51/5, 2303-51/5. Compilation of data. *In* Gesundheitsschädliche Arbeitsstoffe, Toxikologischarbeitsmedizische Begründungen von MAK-Werten. D. Henschler, Ed. Verlag Chemie. Weinheim, Germany.
6. Simon, P., V. G. Filser & H. M. Bolt. 1985. Metabolism and pharmacokinetics of vinyl acetate. Arch. Toxicol. **57:** 19–23.
7. Filov, V. A. 1959. The fate of complex esters of vinyl alcohol and fatty acid in the body. Gig. Tr. Prof. Zabol. **3:** 42–46.
8. International Agency for Research on Cancer. 1985. Monographs on the evaluation of the carcinogenic risk of chemicals to humans, Vol. 36. Allyl compounds, aldehydes, epoxides and peroxides. IARC. Lyon.
9. Soffritti, M., F. Belpoggi, A. Ciliberti *et al.* 1994. Long-term carcinogenicity bioassays of formaldehyde and acetaldehyde administered with drinking water: Results and implications. Presented at the International Conference on Drinking Waters, Other Beverages,

and Their Containers: A Present Problem of Public Health. Bologna, October 28, 1994. In press.
10. Maltoni, C. & G. Lefemine. 1974. Carcinogenicity bioassays of vinyl chloride. I. Research plan and early results. Environ. Res. **7:** 387-405.
11. Maltoni, C., G. Lefemine, P. Chieco *et al.* 1974. Vinyl chloride carcinogenesis: Current results and perspectives. Med. Lav. **65:** 421-444.
12. Maltoni, C. & G. Lefemine. 1975. Carcinogenicity bioassays of vinyl chloride: Current results. Ann. N.Y. Acad. Sci. **246:** 195-218.
13. Lijinsky, W. & M. D. Reuber. 1983. Chronic toxicity studies of vinyl acetate in Fischer rats. Toxicol. Appl. Pharmacol. **68:** 43-53.
14. Bogdanffy, M. S., H. C. Dreef-van der Meulen, R. B. Beems *et al.* 1994. Chronic toxicity and oncogenicity inhalation study with vinyl acetate in the rat and mouse. Fundam. Appl. Toxicol. **23:** 215-229.
15. Bogdanffy, M. S., T. R. Tyler, M. B. Vinegar *et al.* 1994. Chronic toxicity and oncogenicity study with vinyl acetate in the rat: In utero exposure in drinking water. Fundam. Appl. Toxicol. **23:** 206-214.
16. Waxweiler, R. J., A. H. Smith, H. Falk *et al.* 1981. Excess lung cancer risk in a synthetic chemical plant. Environ. Health Perspect. **41:** 159-165.
17. Ott, M. G., M. J. Teta & H. L. Greenberg. 1989. Lymphatic and hematopoietic tissue cancer in a chemical manufacturing environment. Am. J. Ind. Med. **16:** 631-643.
18. Noble, A. C., R. A. Flath & R. R. Forrey. 1980. Wine headspace analysis. Reproducibility and application to varietal classification. J. Agric. Food Chem. **28:** 346-353.
19. Montiel, A. & S. Rauzy. 1983. Dosage des monomères et solvants légers dans les matériaux plastiques en contact avec l'eau et dans l'eau en contact avec ces matériaux. Rev. Fr. Sci. Eau **2:** 255-266.

Mercurial Uncertainties in Environmental Health

PHILIPPE GRANDJEAN [a]

Institute of Community Health
Odense University
5000 Odense
Denmark
and
Departments of Neurology and Environmental Health
Boston University Schools of Medicine and Public Health
Boston, Massachusetts 02118

INTRODUCTION

A small percentage of environmental pollutants has been adequately characterized so far with regard to adverse health effects. While safety assessments are proceeding far too slowly to catch up in the near future, useful guidelines deserve to be extracted from the experiences with chemicals already studied in reasonable detail.[1]

Mercury has been known as a toxic metal for millenia. As learned from several outbreaks of methylmercury poisoning due to contaminated food, the most important environmental health risks are associated with the methylmercury species.[2] On the basis of available evidence, the International Programme of Chemical Safety determined that a risk to the fetus may occur at exposures associated with a maternal hair-mercury concentration of 10–20 μg/g.[2] Since large population groups depend on seafood, which may be contaminated with methylmercury, the validity of this limit is of considerable concern. Also, given that serious poisoning episodes have occurred, the usefulness of the information gathered deserves to be scrutinized.

POPULATIONS AT RISK

In the 1950s a new disease occurred in the town of Minamata, Japan.[3,4] The community includes a large chemical factory and a fishing harbor. The new disease especially hit fishermen's families, but the causation for a long time seemed mysterious. It was finally revealed that methylmercury was the cause and that it was released from the chemical factory to the Minamata Bay, where the fish became contaminated.

As confirmed later from other outbreaks,[5,6] major symptoms in adults included paresthesias, ataxia, dysphasia, decrease in visual fields, and deafness. Children were found to be more susceptible than adults with congenital methylmercury poisoning

[a] Address for correspondence: Philippe Grandjean, M.D., Institute of Community Health, Winslowparken 17, 5000 Odense C, Denmark. Phone: +45-6557.3769; fax: +45-6591.1458; e-mail: p.grandjean@winsloew.ou.dk

TABLE 1. Indicators of Early Exposure to Methylmercury and Their Association with the Cord–Blood Mercury Concentration (Spearman's Correlation Coefficient) in a Cohort of Faroese Children[a]

Mercury Concentration in	Number	Correlation
Umbilical cord	50	0.85
Maternal hair	891	0.75
Infant hair (12 months)	515	0.50
Hair at age 7 years	880	0.30

[a] From Dalgård *et al.*[8] and Grandjean *et al.*[15]

resulting in a cerebral palsy syndrome, even though the mother remained healthy or suffered only minor mercury-related symptoms. An important conclusion was therefore that risk assessment should be based on prenatal exposure.

EXPOSURE ASSESSMENT

Because the causation of Minamata disease remained unknown during the peak of the epidemic, data on individual mercury exposures were not obtained. However, according to local tradition, dried umbilical cords were sometimes saved, and cord tissue samples from patients and controls could therefore be analyzed for methylmercury. These analyses documented much higher mercury concentrations in Minamata patients compared to control groups,[7] but the distributions overlapped considerably, perhaps because of diagnostic misclassification and loss of mercury during storage. The data nonetheless support the notion that Minamata disease was due to methylmercury poisoning, but they are difficult to translate into useful dose-response relationships.

Any detailed evaluation of cord-mercury concentrations is also hampered by the fact that the toxicokinetic aspects of methylmercury retention in cord tissue are unknown. The most frequently used measures of methylmercury exposures are mercury concentrations in hair and in the blood. No such data were available from the Minamata incident. We therefore conducted parallel analyses of umbilical cords and other samples at the Faroe Islands (TABLE 1). These results document that, in a population with chronic exposure to methylmercury, mercury concentrations in cord, cord blood, and maternal hair correlate quite well. Further, a regression coefficient was derived so that the data from Minamata could be translated into more useful hair-mercury concentrations.[8] The variation in cord-mercury concentrations is substantial, and some low values are clearly not representative of Minamata disease. Nonetheless, it is surprising that the estimated median maternal hair concentration of 23 μg/g is only slightly above the preliminary threshold of 10–20 μg/g.

In the poisoning episode in Iraq, only maternal hair samples were obtained for analysis. Because of the temporal variations in exposure, the peak level measured in 1-cm hair segments was taken to indicate the causative exposure.[9] Adverse effects in infants were not recorded if the maternal hair-mercury concentrations did not exceed 10–20 μg/g. Each segment represented approximately a one-month period during pregnancy, and it was assumed that a peak level at any time would then indicate the magnitude of the causative exposure. Average mercury concentrations could be used as well, but then the assumption would be that peak levels would not exacerbate the effects.

Subsequent studies have also utilized maternal hair-mercury concentrations during pregnancy as a convenient indicator of fetal exposures.[10–13] Although the mercury concentration may be affected by external contamination, hair color, hair treatment, and growth rate,[14] the ease of hair sampling and storage has made this parameter useful for field studies. The distance of the hair sample from the root will determine the time period reflected by the analysis. Limited experience is available with infant hair, but it seems to retain lower mercury concentrations than adult hair.[15] Given the limited biological half-life of methylmercury in the body, the mercury concentration in the child's hair is unlikely to reflect prenatal exposures. Accordingly, correlations with cord-blood concentrations decrease with time (TABLE 1).

The cord-blood concentration directly reflects the exposure of the fetus and should therefore be preferred as the best indicator of fetal exposure. With a biological half-life of methylmercury in blood of up to two months,[2] this parameter reflects mainly exposures during the last trimester of gestation. Because cord blood is more difficult to obtain, this parameter has been less extensively used.[16]

SUSCEPTIBILITY FACTORS

The greatest susceptibility to methylmercury toxicity undoubtedly occurs during the gestational period, and a distinction has been made between congenital and infantile poisoning.[3,4] However, given the biological half-life of methylmercury of up to two months[2] and the long-term contamination of the fish in Minamata Bay,[3,4] most of the cases recorded were probably exposed both prenatally and postnatally. Exposure to methylmercury from human milk was apparently associated with the development of toxicity,[17] although the exact contribution by prenatal versus postnatal exposures could not be determined. In Iraq,[18] mercury from human milk gave rise to excessive blood-mercury concentrations above 1000 μg/L in five infants, although none of them showed immediate signs of poisoning.

Human milk contains essential nutrients that could possibly counteract the toxic effects of mercury. A surprising finding was made in a prospective study of Faroese infants.[19] Those who reached developmental milestone criteria early had significantly *higher* mercury concentrations in the hair at 12 months of age. However, these infants also had been nursed longer, and milestone development was not associated with indicators of prenatal methylmercury exposure in this cohort. The developmental milestone attainment therefore seemed to be primarily associated with breast-feeding, and methylmercury toxicity was not detected. These findings suggest that susceptibility to methylmercury decreases after birth, and that breast-feeding provides some protection against toxic effects in infants.

OUTCOME PARAMETERS

Methylmercury poisoning is unlikely to constitute a clinical entity that either appears in full scale or not at all. At lower exposure levels, less severe symptoms

TABLE 2. Tests Used to Reveal Dysfunction in Vigilance Associated with Prenatal Methylmercury Exposure (Cord-Blood Mercury Concentration) in a Cohort of Faroese Children[a]

	Number Examined	Number of Different Responses	*p* for Association with Mercury[b]
Catching a ball	864	3	0.71
Digit span score	867	10	0.06
Reaction time	878	312	0.003

[a] From Dahl *et al.*[13] and White *et al.*[16]

[b] Spearman's correlation coefficient, not adjusted for covariates.

would be expected, and the clinical picture may then become nonspecific and difficult to distinguish from variations within the normal range. Data from Minamata are in accordance with this notion. Of 72 children born in the area during 1953/1954 and 1959 (i.e., just before and just after the highest pollution period), 21 (29%) had an IQ below 70.[4] School children born in the Minamata area during 1955-1959 showed high prevalences of mental retardation, sensory disturbance, mild dysarthria, and adiodochokinesia.[4] Unfortunately, the epidemiological designs do not appear ideal, but this evidence suggests that delayed mental development may be an effect of early methylmercury exposure.

Neuropathological findings in Minamata disease[20] indicate that prenatal methylmercury exposure can cause diffuse brain damage, while lesions in adults are more focal. These results and the experience with, for example, early lead exposure in children, would suggest that several brain functions might be affected by prenatal exposure. To assess the effects clinically, a routine neurological examination[10] is unlikely to reveal subtle dysfunctions. IQ testing appears to offer some sensitivity to methylmercury toxicity at age six years,[11] although other omnibus tests used at younger ages[12] revealed only equivocal associations. Since the neuroanatomical basis is known, specific tests that reflect cognitive processing abilities would have important advantages and might be more sensitive.[21]

In a recently completed study at the Faroe Islands, we used both clinical and neuropsychological tests to determine the effects at age seven years of prenatal exposure to methylmercury.[13,16,21] Vigilance is one of the brain functions that might be affected by prenatal methylmercury exposure. A clinical test reflecting vigilance involved catching a ball with a diameter of 15 cm thrown from a distance of 3 m. The performance was rated as automatic, questionable, or poor. A simple neuropsychological test that also involves vigilance is the Digit Spans subtest of the Wechsler Intelligence Scale for Children–Revised. In this test, digit spans of increasing length were presented until the child failed both trials in a series of the same length. Score was total number of correct trials for the forward condition. As a third approach, we used a computerassisted assessment of reaction time on the Continuous Performance Test of the Neurobehavioral Evaluation System–2. The score was the average reaction time during a 3-minute period. As shown in TABLE 2, the three tests offered different degrees of quantitation of the response, with the computerassisted test providing the best separation. Also, since only eight children (1%) failed to catch the ball, this task may be too easy to reveal slight neurotoxic damages at this age. All associations with mercury exposure levels were in the direction expected, but the (two-sided) *p*-value was statistically significant only for the computerassisted test (TABLE 2).

TEMPORAL RELATIONSHIP

Effects incurred prenatally may not become apparent until the nervous system has matured sufficiently to express the dysfunctions.[22,23] Simple milestone data and early developmental tests may be too crude to reveal the neurotoxic effects, and their predictive validity is limited with regard to subsequent cognitive development.[23] Also in connection with exposures to lead during early life, available evidence suggests that the neurotoxicity is lasting and that its expression depends on age.[24,25] Dysfunctions associated with prenatal exposure to polychlorinated biphenyls also appear to depend on the age of assessment.[26,27] These studies are of particular interest, because the children examined may also have been exposed to methylmercury.[28]

As the mental sequelae cannot be reliably assessed at the time of the neurotoxic exposure, the developmental stage, both at the time of the exposure and at the time of examination, must be taken into regard. A detailed neurobehavioral examination may not be possible before a child has reached school age. Accordingly, attention must be paid to other factors that may affect neurological development during the interval between toxic exposure and the diagnostic testing.

PERSPECTIVES

The nervous system is particularly susceptible to toxic effects due to environmental exposures. For example, in an extensive review of human poisoning cases, the nervous system was the organ system most often involved in the clinical symptoms and signs.[29] As demonstrated by experiences with methylmercury and lead,[30] the brain appears to be most susceptible to adverse effects of chemicals during gestation and early postnatal life. Although some information is available on PCBs,[26,27] very little is known about other environmental chemicals that may affect brain development in humans. The paucity of evidence is perhaps surprising, and it is certainly unfortunate.

Even though methylmercury is one of the few substances documented as a developmental neurotoxicant, the evidence on this agent is uncertain. With regard to the Minamata outbreak, the circumstances did not allow detailed epidemiological studies with proper exposure assessment. The most useful dose-response data on congenital methylmercury poisoning was obtained in Iraq where delayed milestone development was used as an indication of neurotoxic effect.[5,9] Unfortunately, milestone attainment is a very crude parameter, and it is probably affected by breast-feeding.[19] Detailed information on breast-feeding was not available from the outbreak in Iraq. Although these data may therefore underestimate the toxic potential of prenatal methylmercury exposure, they have been applied as the main basis for the current preliminary exposure limit.[2]

In risk assessment, uncertainty factors may be used to take into account statistical variation and differences in susceptibility, among other factors. In the case of methylmercury, extensive epidemiological evidence is available, and there would appear to be little need for a large uncertainty factor. Nonetheless, considerable uncertainty is present because exposure assessments were imprecise, the outcome measures were crude, and the full extent of neurotoxic damage as expressed in the mature brain has not been determined. Unfortunately, the magnitude of this uncertainty is not yet known. Evidence in this area is badly needed to assess uncertainties that relate to neurotoxicants in general. Although decisions on safety must necessarily involve transscientific aspects,[31] a major goal of research is to provide the best possible documentation, including an estimate of the uncertainties.

REFERENCES

1. GRANDJEAN, P. 1994. Uncertainties in environmental health: Implications for research and policy-making. *In* The Identification and Control of Environmental and Occupational Diseases, A Tribute to Professor Irving J. Selikoff (1915-1992). M. A. Mehlman & A. Upton, Eds. Adv. Mod. Environ. Toxicol. **23:** 539-548.
2. INTERNATIONAL PROGRAMME ON CHEMICAL SAFETY. 1990. Methylmercury (Environmental Health Criteria 101). World Health Organization. Geneva.
3. KURLAND, L. T., S. N. FARO & H. SIEDLER. 1959. Minamata disease: The outbreak of a neurologic disorder in Minamata, Japan, and its relationship to the ingestion of seafood contaminated by mercuric compounds. World Neurol. **1:** 370-395.
4. HARADA, M. 1995. Minamata disease: Methylmercury poisoning in Japan caused by environmental pollution. Crit. Rev. Toxicol. **25:** 1-24.
5. MARSH, D. O., G. J. MYERS, T. W. CLARKSON, L. AMIN-ZAKI, S. TIKRITI & M. MAJEED. 1980. Fetal methylmercury poisoning: Clinical and pathological features. Ann. Neurol. **7:** 348-353.
6. DAVIS, L. E., M. KORNFELD, H. S. MOONEY *et al.* 1994. Methylmercury poisoning: Long-term clinical, radiological, toxicological, and pathological studies of an affected family. Ann. Neurol. **35:** 680-688.
7. NISHIGAKI, S. & M. HARADA. 1975. Methylmercury and selenium in umbilical cords of inhabitants of the Minamata area. Nature (Lond.) **258:** 324-325.
8. DALGÅRD, C., P. GRANDJEAN, P. J. JØRGENSEN & P. WEIHE. 1994. Mercury in the umbilical cord: Implications for risk assessment for Minamata disease. Environ. Health Perspect. **102:** 548-550.
9. COX, C., T. W. CLARKSON, D. O. MARSH, L. AMIN-ZAKI, S. TIKRITI & G. G. MYERS. 1989. Dose-response analysis of infants prenatally exposed to methylmercury: An application of a single compartment model to single-strand hair analysis. Environ. Res. **49:** 318-332.
10. EYSSEN, G. E. M., J. RUEDY & A. NEIMS. 1983. Methylmercury exposure in northern Quebec II. Neurologic findings in children. Am. J. Epidemiol. **118:** 470-479.
11. KJELLSTRÖM, T., P. KENNEDY & S. WALLIS. 1989. Physical and mental development of children with prenatal exposure to mercury from fish. Stage 2, Interviews and psychological tests at age 6. (Report 3642) National Swedish Environmental Protection Board. Stockholm.
12. DAVIDSON, P. W., G. MYERS, C. COX *et al.* 1995. Longitudinal neurodevelopmental study of Seychellois children following in utero exposure to methylmercury from a maternal fish ingestion: Outcomes at 19 and 29 months. Neurotoxicology **16:** 677-688.
13. DAHL, R., R. F. WHITE, P. WEIHE *et al.* 1996. Feasibility and validity of three computer-assisted neurobehavioral tests in 7-year old children. Neurotoxicol. Teratol. **18:** 413-419.
14. SUZUKI, T. 1988. Hair and nails: Advantages and pitfalls when used in biological monitoring. *In* Biological Monitoring of Toxic Metals, T. W. Clarkson, L. Friberg, G. F. Nordberg & P. R. Sager, Eds.: 623-640. Plenum. New York.

15. Grandjean, P., P. J. Jørgensen & P. Weihe. 1994. Human milk as a source of methylmercury exposure in infants. Environ. Health Perspect. **102:** 74-77.
16. White, R. F., P. A. Grandjean & P. Weihe. 1995. An overview of human studies on CNS effects of methylmercury. Proc. Nat. Forum on Mercury in Fish: 109-112. U.S. Environmental Protection Agency. Washington, D.C.
17. Kojima, K. & M. Fujita. 1973. Summary of recent studies in Japan on methyl mercury poisoning. Toxicology **1:** 43-62.
18. Amin-Zaki, L., S. El-Hassani, M. A. Majeed, T. W. Clarkson, R. A. Doherty & K. R. Greenwood. 1974. Studies of infants postnatally exposed to methylmercury. J. Pediatr. **85:** 81-84.
19. Grandjean, P., P. Weihe & R. F. White. 1995. Milestone development in infants exposed to methylmercury from human milk. Neurotoxicology **16:** 27-33.
20. Choi, B. H. 1989. The effects of methylmercury on the developing brain. Prog. Neurobiol. **32:** 447-470.
21. White, R. F., F. Debes, R. Dahl & P. Grandjean. 1994. Development and field testing of a neuropsychological test battery to assess the effects of methylmercury exposure in the Faroe Islands. Proc. Int. Symp. on Assessment of Environmental Pollution and Health Effects of Methylmercury. 127-140. Univ. of Kumamoto. Kumamoto.
22. Cravioto, J. & R. Arrieta. 1984. Malnutrition in childhood. *In* Developmental Neuropsychiatry, M. Rutter, Ed.: 32-51 Churchill Livingstone. Edinburgh.
23. Morgane, P. J., R. J. Austin-LaFrance, J. D. Bronzino & J. R. Galler. 1992. Malnutrition and the developing nervous system. *In* The Vulnerable Brain and Environmental Risks, Vol. 1, R. L. Isaacson and K. F. Jensen, Eds.: 3-44. Plenum Press. New York.
24. Damm, D., P. Grandjean, T. Lyngbye, A. Trillingsgaard & O. N. Hansen. 1993. Early lead exposure and neonatal jaundice: Relation to neurobehavioral performance at 15 years of age. Neurotoxicol. Teratol. **15:** 173-181.
25. White, R. F., R. Diamond, S. P. Proctor, C. Morey & H. Hu. 1993. Residual cognitive deficits 50 years after lead poisoning during childhood. Br. J. Ind. Med. **50:** 613-622.
26. Gladen, B. C., W. J. Rogan, P. Hardy, J. Thullen, J. Tingelstad & M. Tully. 1988. Development after exposure to polychlorinated biphenyls and dichlorophenyl dichloroethene transplacentally and through human milk. J. Pediatr. **113:** 991-995.
27. Jacobson, J. L., S. W. Jacobson & H. E. B. Humphrey. 1990. Effects of in utero exposure to polychlorinated biphenyls and related contaminants on cognitive functioning in young children. J. Pediatr. **116:** 38-45.
28. Humphrey, H. E. B. & M. L. Budd. 1996. Mercury exposure in the Michigan cohorts. Toxicol. Ind. Health **12:** 499-505.
29. Grandjean, P., S. H. Sandoe & R. D. Kimbrough. 1991. Nonspecificity of clinical signs and symptoms caused by environmental chemicals. Hum. Exp. Toxicol. **10:** 167-173.
30. Dietrich, K. N. & D. Bellinger. 1994. The assessment of neurobehavioral development in studies of the effects of prenatal exposure to toxicants. *In* Prenatal Exposure to Toxicants: Developmental Consequences, H. L. Needleman and D. Bellinger, Eds.: 57-85. Johns Hopkins Univ. Press. Baltimore.
31. Selikoff, I. J. 1984. Lessons for living in a chemical world. Bull. Environ. Contam. Toxicol. **33:** 682-695.

Long-term Health Effects of the Occupational Exposure to DDT

A Preliminary Report[a]

PIERLUIGI COCCO,[b,e] AARON BLAIR,[c]
PATRIZIA CONGIA,[b] GIOVANNA SABA,[b]
ANNA R. ECCA,[d] AND COSTANTINO PALMAS[d]

[b]*Istituto di Medicina del Lavoro*
Università di Cagliari
Cagliari, Italy

[c]*Occupational Studies Section*
Environmental Epidemiology Branch
National Cancer Institute
Bethesda, Maryland 20892

[d]*Istituto di Parassitologia*
Università di Cagliari
Cagliari, Italy

INTRODUCTION

Since World War II, the insecticide dichlorodiphenyltrichloroethane (DDT) has been used extensively worldwide for mosquito control in the prevention of malaria, typhus, yellow fever, and sleeping sickness, and as an agricultural insecticide, mostly for cotton, peanuts, and soybean crops.[1] Agricultural uses of DDT were restricted in the late 1960s to minimize residues in food and in animal feed, to reduce environmental contamination, and because of the increasing resistance of pests. DDT is still used for public health purposes, and to a lesser extent agricultural purposes, in some developing countries.[1] Because DDT and its metabolites break down slowly, they have a long persistence in sediments and soils. Plants and animals take up these chemicals from the environment and bioconcentrate them in the food chain.[1]

The DDT accumulation in the food chain has raised concern about human health effects, including cancer. The International Agency for Research on Cancer (IARC) considered the evidence of carcinogenicity of DDT as being sufficient in experimental animals.[1] Epidemiologic data on cancer risk associated with exposure to DDT are suggestive, but limitations in the exposure assessment and the finding of small and

[a] The work of one of the authors (P.C.) at the National Cancer Institute was supported with funding from the International Union Against Cancer (Geneva, Switzerland) and the NCI/EORTC Exchange Program (Brussels, Belgium).

[e] Address for correspondence and reprint requests: Pierluigi Cocco, M.D., Institute of Occupational Medicine, University of Cagliari, via San Giorgio 12, 09126 Cagliari, Italy. Phone: + 39 70 602-8278; fax: + 39 70 654350; e-mail: coccop@pacs.unica.it

inconsistent excesses of cancers of the lymphatic and hemopoietic system, lung, and pancreas complicate the evaluation.[1–8] More recently, interest has focused on a possible role of DDT and its metabolites in the etiology of breast cancer.[9–11]

The availability of records on individuals who took part in an antimalarial campaign in Sardinia, Italy, from 1946 to 1950 involving DDT provided the opportunity to evaluate the pattern of mortality associated with exposure to this pesticide. Here we report the results of a proportional mortality analysis conducted on 1043 deaths among these subjects.

METHODS

The Antimalarial Campaign in Sardinia

Immediately following World War II, the Rockefeller Foundation promoted and supported a DDT campaign to eradicate malaria in Sardinia, Italy, where mortality from this disease was 5–6 times higher than in the rest of Italy.[12] A special company was created named Regional Institution for the Anti-*Anopheles* Fight in Sardinia (ERLAAS). Its operations covered the period between November 1946 and September 1950, and were divided in two phases: the residual spraying and an antilarval campaign.

Residual Spraying

The interiors of all man-made structures underwent a complete DDT treatment to destroy the maximum number of overwintering *Anopheles labranchiae,* the vector for *Plasmodium falciparum,* the parasite responsible for malaria. Sardinia was divided into 5229 sectors (average area = 4.61 km^2), and each applicator was charged with the task of treating the structures in one sector. Applicators were organized in squads made up of five men and a group leader. Several squads in an area worked from a central warehouse, located in the main village of the area, where a storekeeper was responsible for checking the supplies of insecticides and equipment. Shoulder pumps were used to apply DDT at a concentration of 1.6–2.0 gm^2 of wall surface. In 1948, a small amount of chlordane was also applied indoors for fly control as an alternative to DDT at a concentration of 0.8 g/m^2 of wall surface.[12]

Antilarval Campaign

An effective larviciding required a DDT treatment for every water deposit on the surface of the island, which are potential shelters of mosquito larvae. The antilarval campaign was performed mostly in the summer, with the exception of 1948, when it covered the period from the middle of February through early December. Each of the 5229 sectors was divided into six approximately equal subsectors. Every water deposit in a subsector had to be treated once a week during the campaign. A 2.5–5% DDT solution in a light distillate or diesel fuel was applied by hand pumps or shoulder pumps at a concentration of 10–20 mg DDT/m^2.

Because of objections to the presence of oil in the drinking water following the DDT treatment, Paris green (lead arsenate) was also utilized in two localities in 1948, and for the treatment of wells in 1950. Small envelopes were issued containing 0.02 g Paris green mixed with talc to treat one square meter of water surface. The number of envelopes depended on the size of the well. Overall, more than 26,000 were used,[12] but the map of these treatments is not currently available.

Cohort Identification

A list of 2908 employees who applied DDT and made inspections after the applications as part of the antimalarial campaign was retrieved from the Archive of defunct Governmental Institutions of the State General Accounting in Rome. Information abstracted on each employee included: full name, date and place of birth, gender, residence, specific jobs, and dates the jobs were held. When company records were incomplete, the periods of work at ERLAAS were derived from certificates released by the National Institute of Social Security (INPS). Complete sets of data were also available for another 2285 employees hired for the campaign as supervisors, drivers, and laboratory, administrative and directive staff, who were considered unexposed to DDT. Apparently, an ERLAAS roster never existed. We are currently searching and assembling the list of all ERLAAS workers involved in the operations with the help of the local government agencies for pest control and survivors identified from the currently available list. Based on the total working population reported by Logan,[12] we estimate a total number of about 5715 exposed workers, 91% of whom were DDT applicators. We have so far identified 51% of these subjects (2908). Another 2807 have yet to be identified. The 2285 occupationally unexposed subjects are estimated to correspond to the total number of subjects hired on a permanent basis.

Vital status of the 5193 subjects identified to date was sought at the National Institute for Social Security and registers of the communes of residence, and death certificates are being requested for each deceased worker. As of February 15, 1995, 2086 subjects have been identified as deceased before December 31, 1992, and death certificates have been obtained thus far for 1107 subjects (53%). Only 13 of these were female, and they were excluded from this preliminary report. Another 9 male subjects were excluded because of missing date of death. Forty-two deaths between 1947 and 1955 were also excluded to allow a minimum 8-year latency period after initial employment in the antimalarial campaign. Thus, this preliminary proportional mortality analysis is based on 1043 deaths among men who worked in the antimalarial campaign and who died between January 1, 1956 and December 31, 1992.

The underlying causes of death have been coded according to the International Classification of Diseases (ICD) 9th Revision.[13] The expected number of events for each cause of interest was derived from the 5-year age group and 5-year calendar period-specific proportional mortality rates among the Italian male population, for the total study population (n = 1043), for exposed workers (n = 590; 57%), for unexposed workers (n = 453; 43%), and for categories of duration of employment in exposed jobs defined as the tertiles of the distribution of the number of days worked (<75, 75–149, ≥150 days). Variations in coding of specific causes of death were accounted for by calculating expected deaths for the broader group, which included all the different codes of a given cause of death in the subsequent ICD editions. For instance, liver cancer deaths were accounted for by joining codes for liver cancer and biliary tract cancer (ICD9 codes 155-156). Proportional mortality ratios (PMRs) for each cause of interest are expressed as 100 times the ratio of observed versus expected events. Ninety-five percent confidence intervals of PMRs were calculated according to Liddell.[14]

RESULTS

The mean age at the start of work was 37.4 years (sd = 10.4; median = 37). Twenty-five percent of the study population started work at age 30 or younger, and 12% was aged 51 or more. Mean age at death was 68.3 years (SD = 11.7; median = 69), and ranged from 30 to 99 years. Twenty-three percent of the study population died at age 59 or younger, and 15% died at age 80 or older.

Mortality from Nonmalignant Diseases

PMRs for selected causes of death are shown in TABLE 1, separately for the unexposed and exposed groups. Among the unexposed group, deaths from nonmalignant respiratory diseases showed a significant excess. However, the excess was smaller and not statistically significant among workers exposed to DDT. Significant deficits in proportional mortality were observed for cardiovascular diseases and liver cirrhosis in both groups. Accidental deaths showed a nonsignificant 16% elevation among exposed workers.

Cancer Mortality

The risk for all cancers was about as expected among unexposed and exposed employees. A few cancer sites, that is, stomach, colon, pancreas, larynx, and non-Hodgkin's lymphoma, were fewer than expected in both groups. Kidney cancer showed a significant 3-fold excess (PMR = 303) among the unexposed, but not among the exposed (PMR = 151). A significant increase in the PMR for liver and biliary tract cancer was observed in both groups (exposed: PMR = 228; unexposed: PMR = 210). Exposed workers showed a considerably larger PMR for multiple myeloma (PMR = 341) than did unexposed workers. Myeloid leukemia risk was elevated among the exposed (PMR = 184) and unexposed (PMR = 170), but neither number was statistically significant. Esophageal cancer was slightly elevated among exposed workers (PMR = 153), while there was a deficit among nonexposed (PMR = 65).

In 1948, small amounts of chlordane and lead arsenate started to be used in addition to DDT. To see whether risks for liver and biliary tract cancer, multiple myeloma, and myeloid leukemia varied depending on the possible exposure to other pesticides, we calculated PMRs according to whether subjects worked only before 1948 or only from 1948 onward. No changes were observed (data not shown in the tables).

TABLE 1. Proportional Mortality Ratios Among Unexposed Employees and Among Workers Exposed to DDT in the 1946–1950 Antimalarial Campaign in Sardinia, Italy

	Unexposed Subjects			Exposed Subjects		
Cause of Death	Obs	PMR	(95% C.I.)	Obs	PMR	(95% C.I.)
Infectious diseases	8	106	(45–208)	9	101	(46–191)
Pulmonary tuberculosis	4	78	(21–201)	5	86	(28–201)
All cancers	134	110	(92–130)	158	99	(84–115)
Oral cavity and pharynx	2	51	(6–182)	6	121	(44–263)
Cancer of the digestive system	39	88	(63–121)	57	99	(75–128)
Esophageal cancer	2	65	(7–233)	6	153	(56–332)
Stomach cancer	8	46	(20–91)	14	63	(35–106)
Colon cancer	6	93	(30–203)	2	23	(3–84)
Rectal cancer	4	101	(27–260)	2	38	(4–137)
Liver and biliary tract cancer	15	210	(117–346)	22	228	(143–345)
Pancreatic cancer	1	24	(0–135)	3	55	(11–160)
Cancer of the respiratory system	52	131	(98–171)	41	78	(56–106)
Laryngeal cancer	4	90	(24–230)	1	18	(0–99)
Lung cancer	44	127	(92–170)	40	87	(62–119)
Pleural cancer	1	180	(2–999)	0	—	—
Prostate cancer	9	126	(57–238)	7	68	(27–140)
Bladder cancer	6	107	(39–234)	8	103	(44–203)
Kidney cancer	6	303	(111–659)	4	151	(41–387)
Brain and CNS cancer	3	139	(28–406)	2	73	(8–263)
Hemolymphatic system cancer	6	80	(29–174)	12	123	(63–215)
Non-Hodgkin lymphomas	1	53	(1–295)	2	81	(9–294)
Multiple myeloma	1	94	(1–522)	5	341	(110–795)
All leukemias	4	111	(30–285)	5	107	(34–249)
Myeloid leukemia	2	170	(19–614)	3	189	(38–552)
Diabetes	12	137	(71–240)	6	50	(18–108)
Diseases of the nervous system	7	128	(51–264)	5	67	(22–157)
Cardiovascular diseases	143	80	(68–94)	179	74	(64–86)
Respiratory diseases	52	141	(105–185)	53	108	(81–142)
Digestive diseases	28	79	(52–114)	39	88	(63–120)
Liver cirrhosis	13	59	(31–101)	16	59	(34–96)
Genitourinary diseases	8	102	(44–201)	9	89	(41–169)
Accidental deaths	22	91	(57–137)	35	119	(83–165)

The archive of the regional agency that continued pest control operations after the end of the antimalarial campaign were searched to identify individuals who continued working in this agency and may have experienced further exposure to DDT and to other pesticides. Forty-nine deaths (9%) among exposed workers occurred among those who continued working in the regional pest control agency. The proportional mortality analysis restricted to these subjects is limited by the small sample size, but the observed versus expected ratios were similar to those observed for the rest of the exposed workers for all cancers, lung cancers, and liver and biliary tract cancer (data not shown).

In this analysis, we used the number of days of work in exposed jobs as a surrogate for the cumulative exposure to DDT. PMRs for specific causes were calculated for unexposed subjects and by categories of duration of employment defined by the tertiles of the distribution of the number of days of work among exposed subjects (TABLE 2). Liver cancer mortality showed an inconsistent pattern. It increased from 2.3-fold among exposed subjects employed for less than 75 days, to 2.8-fold among subjects employed for 75-149 days, and then decreased to 1.9-fold among exposed subjects employed for 150 days or more. Multiple myeloma showed the largest PMR among exposed subjects with the shortest duration of employment. Myeloid leukemia risk increased by number of days in exposed jobs, although deaths were very few and an increase in the PMR was also observed for unexposed subjects.

Risk for liver and biliary tract cancer increased by age at first exposure from 2.2-fold at age ≤ 30 to 3.3-fold at age 41-50, but no death from the cause occurred among subjects who were first exposed to DDT at age 51 or older. Deaths from multiple myeloma and myeloid leukemia were not concentrated in specific age groups at first exposure (data not shown in the tables).

Among the 37 deaths from cancer of the liver and biliary tract observed in the present study, 22 (59%) were due to primary liver cancer, which is more than the 16.9 expected deaths from liver cancer and cancer of the biliary tract combined, 13 deaths (35%) were due to cancer of the liver not specified whether primary or secondary, one to a malignant neoplasm of the gall bladder, and one to a neoplasia of the Vater's ampulla.

DISCUSSION

Although most industrialized countries have restricted or prohibited production and use of DDT for almost three decades, investigating long-term health effects of the human exposure to DDT is relevant to public and occupational health because it is still used in some developing countries.[1] Residues also continue to be found in various foodstuffs,[15] although surveys of the content of DDT and its most persistent metabolite dichlorodiphenyldichloroethylene (DDE) in the adipose tissue and serum of general-population samples have shown a worldwide decline from the 1970s onwards.[16–19] An elevated correlation of the body burden of organochlorine compounds and fish[20–22] and fatty food consumption[23] has been observed, and an association of DDE level in the serum and cancer of the breast and other sites has been recently reported.[2,9–11,24–26]

Our results show a significant excess for liver cancer and multiple myeloma among DDT-exposed workers. Liver cancer was significantly elevated also among unexposed workers, and it did not show a trend with duration of exposure. Myeloid leukemia was also elevated in both groups, although not significantly so, and increased up to 4.5-fold among subjects who spent ≥150 days in exposed jobs, although the figure was based on two deaths only and the trend was not statistically significant.

TABLE 2. Proportional Mortality Ratios for Selected Cancer Sites Among Subjects Exposed to DDT in the 1946–1950 Antimalarial Campaign in Sardinia, Italy, by Tertiles of Duration of Employment in Exposed Jobs

	Exposed < 75 Days (No. Deaths = 186)			Exposed 75-149 Days (No. Deaths = 204)			Exposed ≥ 150 Days (No. Deaths = 172)		
Cause of Death	Obs	PMR	(95% C.I.)	Obs	PMR	(95% C.I.)	Obs	PMR	(95% C.I.)
All cancers	51	102	(76-134)	52	91	(68-119)	50	109	(81-144)
Cancer of the digestive system	17	94	(55-151)	17	83	(48-133)	21	127	(78-194)
Liver and biliary tract cancer	7	234	(94-481)	10	281	(134-516)	5	188	(61-439)
Lung cancer	10	70	(33-129)	13	78	(42-134)	16	124	(71-201)
Kidney cancer	1	122	(2-677)	2	207	(23-748)	0	—	—
Cancer of the lymphohemopoietic system	4	136	(36-347)	4	109	(29-279)	4	146	(39-375)
Multiple myeloma	3	642	(129-1875)	1	191	(2-1064)	1	240	(3-1333)
Myeloid leukemia	0	—	—	1	173	(2-961)	2	446	(50-1609)

Multiple myeloma was significantly elevated only among exposed workers, but the highest risk was observed among workers with the shortest duration of employment. The lack of an increase in the PMRs for liver and biliary tract cancer and myeloid leukemia by number of days of exposure, and the finding of excesses among subjects whose job title did not imply direct contact with the pesticide, may indicate that DDT is not involved. On the other hand, the environmental exposure to DDT was presumably high for the total Sardinian population, and the number of days of work in exposed jobs may not be a good surrogate for dose in this study.

This preliminary report was designed as a proportional mortality analysis due to the incompleteness of the listing of temporary ERLAAS workers who applied DDT and those who inspected the results of these applications. Selection bias could have affected the results if the subjects identified for this report had a mortality figures that differed from the other ERLAAS workers. Although we cannot completely rule it out, we have no reason to suspect such an occurrence. Retrieval was complete for ERLAAS permanent staff, who did not have direct contact with the pesticide. All missing subjects were among workers temporarily hired to apply DDT or inspect the efficacy of the treatments. The group of exposed subjects in the present study population is a large sample of these workers, although not a randomized one, and we know of no reason why the records would have preferentially been available or selected by cause of death.

We used deaths among the Italian male population in 1956–1992 as the reference, since regional mortality figures by age groups and gender have been available only since 1970. Standardized mortality rates from all cancers, lung cancer, stomach cancer, and kidney cancer are, respectively, 16%, 12%, 41%, and 33% lower among the Sardinian male population than the total Italian male population, while liver cancer and leukemia mortality are, respectively, 14% and 11% higher among the Sardinian male population.[27] No figures have been published to date comparing multiple myeloma and single leukemia types. The PMRs for liver and biliary tract cancer and myeloid leukemia may be slightly elevated due to geographic factors, while PMRs for stomach cancer and kidney cancer may be underestimated.

Experimental administration of DDT and the DDT metabolites *p,p′*-DDE and dichlorodiphenyldichloroethane (TDE) in various rodent species have consistently shown dose-related increases of liver tumors, while inconsistent results have been obtained for lung cancer, malignant lymphomas, and thyroid tumors.[1] Despite the occurrence of liver cancer in laboratory animals, no evidence of hepatic disease has been described in the literature among DDT workers,[1] and temporal trends in liver cancer mortality in the United States were not correlated with amounts of this pesticide used.[28]

Numerous cases of multiple myeloma have been reported among farmers using DDT.[29] Elevated risks of non-Hodgkin's lymphoma have also been noted,[8,30] although we observed a deficit in this study. Reports of increased risk of lymphatic tissue cancer, multiple myeloma, kidney cancer, and testicular cancer among agricultural workers and pesticide users have also been published with mention of the possible role of exposure to DDT in generating the observed excess risks.[31–35]

A case-control study of pancreatic cancer found a strong association with exposure to DDT among manufacturers, unaccounted for by dietary, lifestyle, and social variables,[6] and mortality studies of organochlorine pesticides manufacturers[4,7] and users[2] have shown a slight excess risk of lung cancer. We observed a deficit of pancreatic cancer and no evidence of an increase in lung cancer risk.

Compared to previous epidemiologic studies on DDT-exposed workers, this preliminary report offers the advantage of a long duration of follow-up. A unique aspect that differs from most occupational studies conducted so far among pesticide users is that the exposure was limited to DDT for most of the study population. Exposure to chlordane and lead arsenate also occurred to a lesser extent from 1948, but these exposures do not appear to account for the observed excesses in this preliminary report. We observed interesting excesses of liver cancer, multiple myeloma, and myeloid leukemia. The occurrence of excesses among those workers thought to have less exposure and inconsistent risks for liver cancer and multiple myeloma by duration of employment complicate interpretation. Extension of the study, completing enrollment of exposed workers to increase the number of deaths for analysis, and a better characterization of individual levels of exposure will hopefully allow a better test of the findings herein reported and help clarify the observed inconsistencies.

SUMMARY

We conducted a proportional mortality study of 1043 deaths among men who took part in an antimalarial campaign in Sardinia, Italy from 1946 to 1950. DDT comprised 94% of the insecticide used during the campaign, and was sprayed over the soil of the entire region at an average concentration of 10 mg/m^2, as well as in all dwellings and animal shelters. Expected deaths were derived from the proportional mortality rates of the general Italian male population, specific by cause, 5-year age groups, and 5-year calendar periods in the period from 1956 to 1992. The proportional mortality ratio (PMR) for cardiovascular diseases was significantly decreased, while nonmalignant respiratory diseases showed a 22% increase in risk of borderline statistical significance. Significant increases in risk among workers exposed to DDT in application or inspection jobs were observed for liver and biliary tract cancer (PMR = 228; 95% C.I. = 143-345) and multiple myeloma (PMR = 341; 95% C.I. = 110-795). The PMR for myeloid leukemia was also increased (PMR = 189; 95% C.I. = 38-552), although it was not statistically significant. PMRs for liver and biliary tract cancer and myeloid leukemia were also elevated among workers who did not have direct occupational contact with DDT (liver and biliary cancer: PMR = 210; 95% C.I. = 117-346; myeloid leukemia: PMR = 170; 95% C.I. = 19-614). No trends occurred according to length of employment in exposed jobs. These preliminary results are somewhat in agreement with experimental studies in rodents and previous epidemiologic findings. Expansion of the cohort to include all applicators, and collection of information to improve exposure assessment is needed to clarify these findings.

REFERENCES

1. International Agency for Research on Cancer. 1991. IARC Monographs for the Evaluation of Carcinogenic Risk of Chemicals to Humans, Vol. 53, Occupational Exposures in Insecticide Application, and Some Pesticides: 179-249. IARC. Lyon.
2. Austin, H., I. E. Keil & P. Cole. 1989. A prospective follow-up study of cancer mortality in relation to serum DDT. Am. J. Public Health **79:** 43-46.

3. Brown, L. M., A. Blair, R. Gibson, et al. 1990. Pesticide exposure and other agricultural risk factors for leukemia among men in Iowa and Minnesota. Cancer **50:** 1685-1691.
4. Ditraglia, D., D. P. Brown, T. Namekata & N. Iverson. 1981. Mortality study of workers employed at organochlorine pesticide manufacturing plants. Scand. J. Work Environ. Health **7**(Suppl. 4): 140-146.
5. Flodin, U., M. Fredriksson, B. Persson & O. Axelson. 1988. Chronic lymphatic leukaemia and engine exhausts, fresh wood, and DDT: A case-referent study. Br. J. Ind. Med. **45:** 33-38.
6. Garabrant, D. H., J. Held, B. Langholz, J. M. Peters & T. M. Mack. 1992. DDT and related compounds and risk of pancreatic cancer. J. Natl. Cancer Inst. **84:** 764-771.
7. Wong, O., W. Brocker, H. V. Davis & G. S. Nagle. 1984. Mortality of workers potentially exposed to organic and inorganic brominated chemicals, DBCP, Tris, PBB and DDT. Br. J. Ind. Med. **41:** 15-24.
8. Woods, J. S., L. Polissar, R. K. Severson, L. S. Heuser & B. G. Kulander. 1987. Soft tissue sarcoma and non-Hodgkin's lymphoma in relation to phenoxyherbicide and chlorinated phenol exposure in Western Washington. J. Natl. Cancer Inst. **78:** 899-910.
9. Wolff, M. S., P. G. Toniolo, E. W. Lee, M. Rivera & N. Dubin. 1993. Blood levels of organochlorine residues and risk of breast cancer. J. Natl. Cancer Inst. **85:** 648-652.
10. Falck, F., Jr., A. Ricci, Jr., M. S. Wolff, J. Godbold & P. Deckers. 1992. Pesticides and polychlorinated biphenyl residues in human breast lipids and their relation to breast cancer. Arch. Environ. Health **47:** 143-146.
11. Krieger, N., M. S. Wolff, R. A. Hiatt, M. Rivera, J. Vogelman & N. Orentreich. 1994. Breast cancer and serum organochlorines: A prospective study among white, black, and Asian women. J. Natl. Cancer Inst. **86:** 589-599.
12. Logan, J. A. 1953. The Sardinian Project: An Experiment in the Eradication of an Indigenous Malarious Vector. The Johns Hopkins Press. Baltimore, MD.
13. International Classification of Diseases. 1977. 1975 revision, World Health Organization. Geneva.
14. Liddell, F. D. K. 1984. Simple exact analysis of the Standardized Mortality Ratio. J. Epidemiol. Community Health **38:** 85-88.
15. FAO/WHO. 1985. Pesticide residues in food—1984. Report of the Joint Meeting on Pesticide Residues, FAO Plant Production and Protection, Rome.
16. Mes, J., D. J. Davies & D. Turton. 1982. Polychlorinated biphenyl and other chlorinated hydrocarbon residues in adipose tissue of Canadians. Bull. Environ. Contam. Toxicol. **28:** 97-104.
17. Jani, J. P., I. S. Patel, M. P. Shah, et al. 1988. Levels of dichloro-diphenyl-trichloroethane and hexachlorocyclohexane in human adipose tissue of the Indian population. Scand. J. Work Environ. Health **14:** 201-204.
18. Mes, J., L. Marchand & D. J. Davies. 1990. Organochlorine residues in adipose tissue of Canadians. Bull. Environ. Contam. Toxicol. **45:** 681-688.
19. Burgaz, S., L. Afkham & A. E. Karakaya. 1994. Organochlorine pesticide contaminants in human adipose tissue collected in Ankara (Turkey) 1991-92. Bull. Environ. Contam. Toxicol. **53:** 50-58.
20. Kreiss, K., M. M. Zack, R. D. Kimbrough, L. L. Needham, A. L. Smrek & B. T. Jones. 1981. Cross-sectional study of a community with exceptional exposure to DDT. JAMA **245:** 1926-1930.
21. Hovinga, M. E., M. Sowers & H. E. B. Humphrey. 1993. Environmental exposure and lifestyle predictors of lead, cadmium, PCB, and DDT levels in Great Lakes fish eaters. Arch. Environ. Health **48:** 98-104.
22. Asplund, L., B.-G. Svensson, A. Nilsson, et al. 1994. Polychlorinated biphenyls, 1,1,1-trichloro-2,2-bis(p-chlorophenyl)ethane (p,p′-DDT) and 1,1-dichloro-2,2-bis(p-chlorophenyl)-ethylene (p,p′-DDE) in human plasma related to fish consumption. Arch. Environ. Health **49:** 477-486.

23. Kashyan, R., L. R. Iyer & M. M. Singh. 1994. Evaluation of daily dietary intake of dichloro-diphenyl-trichloroethane (DDT) and benzene hexachloride (BHC) in India. Arch. Environ. Health **49:** 63-66.
24. Wassermann, M., D. P. Nogueira, L. Tomatis, *et al.* 1976. Organochlorine compounds in neoplastic and adjacent apparently normal breast tissue. Bull. Environ. Contam. Toxicol. **15:** 478-484.
25. Unger, M. & J. Olsen. 1980. Organochlorine compounds in the adipose tissue of deceased people with and without cancer. Environ. Res. **23:** 257-263.
26. Saxena, S. P., C. Khare, A. Farooq, K. Murugesan, K. Buckshee & J. Chandra. 1987. DDT and its metabolites in leiomyomatous and normal human uterine tissue. Arch. Toxicol. **59:** 453-455.
27. Capocaccia, R., G. Farchi, S. Mariotti, *et al.* 1989. La mortalita' in Italia nell'anno 1985. Istituto Superiore di Sanita. Roma. (ISTISAN 89/6).
28. Deichmann, W. B. & W. E. MacDonald. 1977. Organochlorine pesticides and liver cancer deaths in the United States, 1930-1972. Ecotoxicol. Environ. Saf. **1:** 89-110.
29. Brown, L. M., L. F. Burmeister, G. D. Everett & A. Blair. 1993. Pesticide exposures and multiple myeloma in Iowa men. Cancer Causes Control **4:** 153-156.
30. Cantor, K. P., A. Blair, G. Everett, *et al.* 1992. Pesticides and other agricultural risk factors for non-Hodgkin's lymphoma among men in Iowa and Minnesota. Cancer Res. **52:** 2447-2455.
31. Pearce, N. E., A. H. Smith & D. O. Fisher. 1985. Malignant lymphoma and multiple myeloma linked with agricultural occupations in a New Zealand Cancer Registry-based study. Am. J. Epidemiol. **121:** 225-237.
32. Corrao, G., M. Calleri, F. Carle, R. Russo, S. Bosia & P. Piccioni. 1989. Cancer risk in a cohort of licensed pesticide users. Scand. J. Work Environ. Health **15:** 203-209.
33. Wiklund, K., J. Dich, L.-E. Holm & G. Eklund. 1989. Risk of cancer in pesticide applicators in Swedish agriculture. Br. J. Ind. Med. **46:** 809-814.
34. Stottrup Hansen, E., H. Hasle & F. Lander. 1992. A cohort study on cancer incidence among Danish gardeners. Am. J. Ind. Med. **21:** 651-660.
35. Faustini, A., F. Forastiere, L. Di Betta, E. M. Magliola & C. A. Perucci. 1994. Cohort study of mortality among farmers and agricultural workers. Med. Lav. **84:** 31-41.

Surveillance of Occupational, Accidental, and Incidental Exposure to Organophosphate Pesticides Using Urine Alkyl Phosphate and Phenolic Metabolite Measurements

JOHN E. DAVIES[a] AND JAMES C. PETERSON[b,c]

[a]*University of Miami*
School of Medicine
90555 N. 115 Terrace
Miami, Florida 33176

[b]*Pacific Toxicology Laboratories*
1545 Pontius Avenue
Los Angeles, California 90025

INTRODUCTION

Since continued pesticide usage is essential for modern agricultural technology, occupational health is vitally concerned with the protection of the exposed workers and with the development of a variety of strategies that are designed to minimize this exposure. Cholinesterase surveillance, the mainstay of present pesticide occupational surveillance, has many limitations and at times is inadequate, nonspecific, and unpredictable. Over the last two decades increased interest has been shown in surveillance by the urinary metabolites.[1-6] The potential of these metabolites as a surveillance instrument has been further stimulated by the significant developments in analytical methodologies.

The two types of metabolites that are identified following exposure to the organophosphate insecticides are the alkyl phosphate and phenolic metabolites. The six primary alkyl phosphate metabolites include dimethyl phosphate (DMP), diethyl phosphate (DEP), dimethyl thio phosphate (DMTP), diethyl thio phosphate (DETP), dimethyl dithio phosphate (DMDTP), and diethyl dithio phosphate (DEDTP). Nutley and Cocker[6] estimate that almost 80% of the organophosphorus pesticides approved for use in the United Kingdom should yield one or more alkyl phosphate metabolites. The metabolism of ethyl parathion illustrated in FIGURE 1 is characteristic of organophosphate pesticides. In this case, the urinary diethyl phosphate is a metabolite of the oxon of the intact pesticide. The oxons are toxic and inhibit the cholinesterase more than the thio organophosphate pesticides. The phenolic metabolites reflect the nitro and chlorophenol moieties of the insecticides. Being rapidly excreted, both types of metabolites have proven to be usable indices of recent exposure.

[c]Corresponding author. Phone: 310/479-4911; fax: 310/479-2894; e-mail: jcptrsn@aol.com

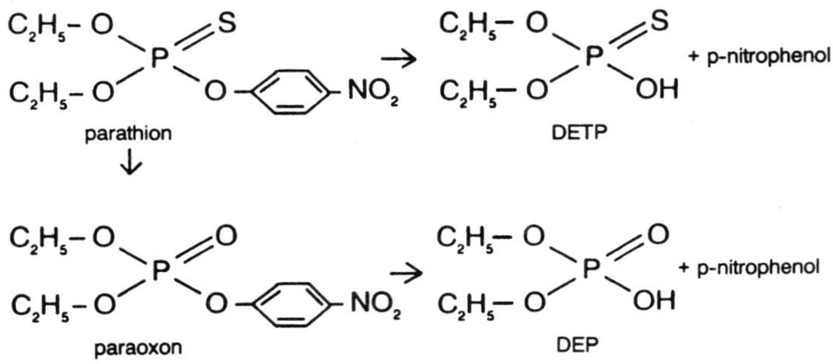

FIGURE 1. Metabolism of ethyl parathion in humans.

Today, man is vulnerable to three types of pesticide exposures; acute, chronic, and incidental. Acute exposure is an overexposure in which the illness develops shortly after exposure and is reflective of the toxicity of the offending pesticide. Chronic exposure is the exposure acquired by working day after day either in the manufacturing, formulation, mixing, handling, or application of pesticides. The population at risk is the occupationally exposed. Incidental exposure is the ubiquitous exposure of the general population to trace amounts of residues found in air, water, and food.

The urinary metabolites have been used to measure human exposures in acute poisonings, in the occupationally exposed, and in the general population in order to test (1) the diagnostic potential of the pesticide metabolites in acute poisoning, (2) the surveillance potential of the metabolites where surveillance has been equated with the assessment of the predictive potential for cholinesterase depression or illness, and (3) the epidemiologic evaluatory potential of the metabolites in exposures to the organophosphate group rather than to a single pesticide.

MATERIALS AND METHODS

Specimen Collection

Acute Poisoning Cases

Arrangements were made with physicians and nurses in the emergency rooms and Intensive care units of three Miami area hospitals to call us as soon as a pesticide poisoning case was admitted to the hospital. A program was instituted whereby all urines voided during the first two or three days were collected in hexane washed jars, labeled, and frozen for later urinary metabolite determinations. Ten milliters of blood were collected in a heparinized tube and 10 mL of clotted blood were also collected; the former for red blood cell and plasma cholinesterase determinations, and the latter for intact pesticides. Subsequent hospital and field visits were made by project personnel to review and document the clinical findings and to determine the mechanism of the poisoning and the most probable route of absorption.

Sequential urines were obtained from eleven cases of systemic poisonings due to organophosphate pesticides. Seven of these poisonings were due to ethyl parathion and all were the result of dermal exposures. Three cases of mevinphos (Phosdrin) poisoning were similarly investigated. Two cases of chlorpyrifos (Dursban) poisoning were due to ingestion of the insecticide. All patients were hospitalized shortly after becoming sick so that the initial urine voided almost certainly represented the first voided specimen after developing overt illness.

Occupational Exposure and General Population Studies

Workers agreed to provide all voided urine specimens over a continuous work period of between 4 and 5 days. These specimens were collected in hexane-washed jars, and the date and time of voiding noted. The volume of the urine voided was measured and the specimen frozen to be analyzed at a later date for alkyl phosphate and phenolic metabolites. General population studies—grab samples of urine were collected in hexane-washed jars, each specimen was labeled with the name, age, race, sex, and occupation of the participant.

Foliar Residue Exposure Studies

Twenty-seven agricultural laborers picking cotton in El Salvador were asked to participate in a protective clothing project where each would be provided with new sets of long-sleeved shirts, denim pants, cotton socks and heavy leather shoes purchased in a local market. Fourteen workers were given clothing that had been pretreated by spraying with a fluorocarbon solution provided by the 3M Company. Earlier laboratory studies had shown that penetration was reduced when a cloth was treated with a fluorocarbon solution and then sprayed with a 10% xylene dye extract. Thirteen workers were given new but untreated clothing. During the six-day study period, urines were collected consecutively at 12-h intervals in hexane-washed bottles. Temperatures during the six days ranged from 63°F at night to 80°F during the day. The fields had been sprayed from the air with mixtures of ethyl and methyl parathion five days before the study began.

Analytical Methods

Cholinesterase activity was measured by the Michel electrochemical method.[7] The phenolic metabolites were analyzed by an electron capture gas chromatographic method described by Shafik *et al.*[8] Urine osmolality determinations were made using the Fiske osmometer, and urinary metabolite concentrations were corrected to a standard osmolality of 800 mL/Osm/L.

Urinary Alkyl Phosphate Method Development

The measurement of urinary alkyl phosphates using an amberlite resin[9] was modified for these studies to enable the analysis to be performed rapidly, efficiently, and accurately. Urine is diluted with acetone and collected on an Amerlite CG400 resin. This resin is placed in a culture tube containing 0.05 mL 6N HCl and 1 mL acetone. After 30 min, 3 mL of diazopentane is added and the derivatization is complete in 1 h. The diazopentane derivatives are extracted with hexane and are concentrated to 1 mL for injection into the gas chromatograph equipped with an FPD detector. Recoveries of alkyl phosphates spiked in urine at 0.5, 0.1, and 0.05 mg/mL ranged from 63% to 91%.

Unfortunately, urinary inorganic phosphates are also derivatized by diazopentane, and while they do not interfere with alkyl phosphate peaks, they do slow down the analysis by showing up as very large and very late peaks. Attempts to precipitate the inorganic phosphate resulted in a large decrease of inorganic phosphates, but the results varied with different urines, probably because of the amount of phosphate present in the urine due to dietary habits. Also, a problem arose concerning interfering peaks originating from the reagent, diazopentane, or more specifically, the nitrosoguanidine.

Subsequent to the performance of these studies we decided to use another derivative and make the following modifications to improve the method.[10] After freeze-drying the 1-mL urine sample overnight, the dried alkylphosphate residues are dissolved in 1 mL acetone and derivatized with a triazine reagent (10% 3-benzyl-*l*-*p*-tolyltriazine, TCI America, Portland, OR) at 70°C for 2 h. Benzyl derivatives amenable to normal GC conditions are produced while inorganic phosphate is not derivatized. After acidification to stop the reaction, 10 mL saturated NaCl solution is added to the extract and the benzylated alkylphosphates are extracted into 1 mL cyclohexane, and the undesired amine derivatization by-product (*p*-toluidine) remains in the aqueous phase. Flame photometric gas chromatographic analysis has been improved by using a megabore fused-silica GC column (30 M, 0.53 mm i.d. DB-210, J&W Scientific, Folsom, CA). The analysis is unaffected by the presence of inorganic phosphate, and the chromatograms are free from interference. Good recoveries ranging from 90% to 100% are obtained for all six alkyl phosphate metabolites, including DMP and DEP. Precision of the method ranges from 4.7% to 14.5% (average: 11.1%), depending on the metabolite at spike level.

RESULTS AND DISCUSSION

Acute Pesticide-poisoning Studies

The objective of the acute-poisoning studies was to determine the diagnostic potential of the urinary alkyl phosphates. The major types of urinary metabolites detected in the urine of poisoning cases will vary with the chemical composition of the pesticide. Thus, with ethyl parathion, the DEP and the DETP and paranitrophenol (PNP) are the major alkyl phosphate and phenolic metabolites identified. With chlorpyrifos (Dursban) the diethyl alkyl phosphates, DEP, DETP, and the phenol, 3,5,6-trichloropyridinol (3,5,6-TCPyr), are the major metabolites excreted; and with mevinphos (Phosdrin), the DMP is the major metabolite observed.

TABLE 1. Levels of Metabolites in First Urine Samples and Cholinesterase Activities in Seven Cases of Ethyl Parathion Poisoning

Name	DEP (mg/L)	DETP (mg/L)	PNP (mg/L)	RBC ChE (dpH/h)	Plasma ChE (dpH/h)
Frank R.	0.46	0.28	0.44	0.21	0.49
Maynard W.	0.44	0.16	0.70	0.37	0.33
Chris W.	7.84	0.09	QNS[a]	0.30[b]	0.08
Jimmy J.	1.47	0.31	2.26	0.55[b]	0.20
Matthew P.	2.21	1.48	2.26	0.55[b]	0.18
Tony B.	0.88	0.30	2.14	0.55[b]	0.55
James D.	0.99	0.10	2.14	0.15	0.10

[a] QNS: Quantity not sufficient.
[b] Post-PAM blood.

TABLE 2. Urinary DEP:DETP Ratios from Patients with Parathion Poisoning Compared to Asymptomatic Occupationally Exposed Workers

	DEP:DETP Ratio					
Name	Number of Urines	Mean	Standard Deviation	Standard Error	Min	Max
Poisonings						
TB	6	3.95	3.24	1.32	1.40	9.75
JD	7	7.12	2.58	0.97	4.59	10.33
MP	7	1.79	0.69	0.26	0.90	2.58
Combined	20	4.14	3.21	0.70	0.90	10.83
Exposed workers						
WG #1	13	0.60	0.24	0.07	0.32	1.16
WG #2	11	0.17	0.21	0.06	0	0.69
FB	19	0.60	0.40	0.09	0	1.73
GJ	16	1.73	1.04	0.08	0	4.42
DA	12	1.17	0.29	0.26	0.64	1.76
Combined	71	0.88[a]	0.78	0.09	0	4.42

[a] *t*-Test—percent of significance of differences at <0.01.

Poisoning by Diethyl Organophosphate Insecticides

In order to show the correlations of the blood and urine laboratory confirmation tests, admission concentrations of diethyl alkyl phosphate metabolites (osmolar adjusted), paranitrophenol levels, and red blood cell and plasma cholinesterase were measured in seven cases hospitalized for parathion poisoning. These are shown in TABLE 1. DEP, reflective of paraoxon, was higher than DETP in all seven cases. The significance of the ratio of DEP to DETP was tested in three poisoning cases and compared with the same ratio in five asymptomatic but ethyl-parathion-exposed workers, as shown in TABLE 2. As can be seen from this comparison of symptomatic

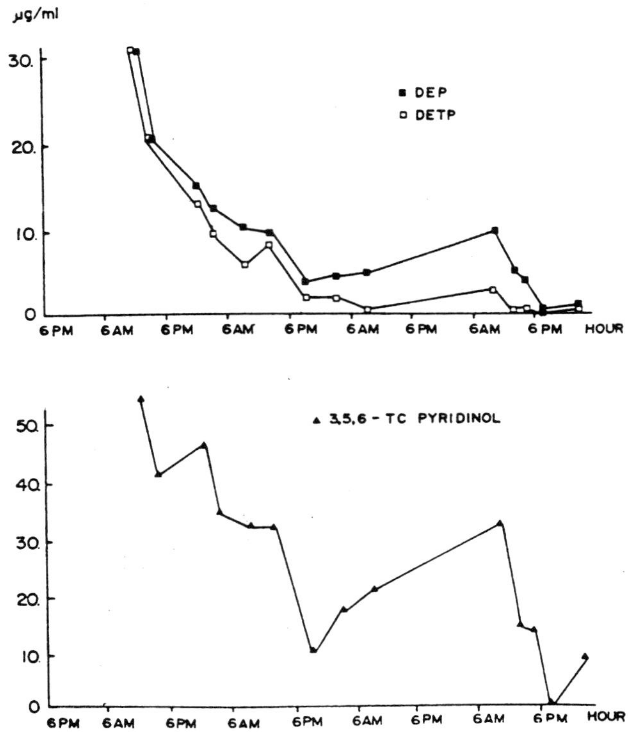

FIGURE 2. Sequential excretion of alkyl phosphate and phenolic metabolites following accidental oral ingestion of chlorpyrifos (Dursban) in a 3-year-old child.

cases versus the asymptomatic cases, the ratio of DEP to DETP was significantly higher in the poisoned cases, with symptoms having a mean of 4.14 mg/L compared to a mean of 0.88 mg/L in the exposed workers. This data suggested that alkyl phosphates, like paranitrophenol determinations, can predict poisoning and provide information as to when a worker should be taken off a job.

FIGURE 2 illustrates the excretion of DEP, DETP, and 3,5,6-TCPyr in a child who was poisoned as a result of ingestion of an unknown amount of chlorpyrifos. The presence of 3,5,6-TCPyr confirms the identity of the pesticide, and all three metabolites show a similar pattern of excretion. Again, in this case, DEP concentrations exceeded the DETP concentrations. The initial urinary DEP concentration of 30 mg/L was an order of magnitude greater than seen in cholinergic illness due to ethyl parathion; emphasizing the importance of the dose and the LD_{50} of the organophosphate from which the alkyl phosphate was metabolized rather than the absolute level of the DEP itself.

The significance of the physical-chemical properties of the pesticide causing the poisoning on the duration of metabolite excretion was illustrated by a dichlofenthion

TABLE 3. Selected Organophosphate Pesticides, Their Toxicities and the Major Metabolites Identified

Pesticides	Metabolites	Oral LD_{50} (mg/kg)	Dermal LD_{50} (mg/kg)
Diethyl organophosphates	*Alkyl Phosphates*		
Ethyl parathion	DEP, DETP	3-33	21
Chlorpyrifos	DEP, DETP	135	2000
Dichlofenthion	DEP, DETP	270	6000
Diazinon	DEP, DETP	100-150	900
Dimethyl organophosphates	*Alkyl Phosphates*		
Mevinphos	DMP	7	5-33
Methyl parathion	DMP, DMTP	9-25	67
Dichlorvos (DDVP)	DMP	56-80	75-107
Dimethoate	DMP, DMTP, DMDTP	215	
Naled (Dibrom)	DMP	430	1100
Organophosphates	*Phenols*		
Ethyl, methyl parathion	PNP		
Chlorpyrifos	3,5,6-TCPyr		
Dichlofenthion	2,4-DCP		

poisoning case. This organophosphate is highly soluble in adipose tissue, producing a slow release of the pesticide from the fat into the circulation. The initial concentrations of the urinary alkyl phosphates were greater than 10 mg/L and were still detectable in the urine for as long as 80 days after exposure. The cholinesterase activities remained depressed throughout the period of metabolite excretion.

These several poisoning case studies clearly demonstrate the diagnostic potential of the urinary metabolites if the exposure has been to a single pesticide. If additional phenolic metabolite data are available, more specific identification information is obtained. If the pesticide does not produce a phenolic metabolite, the identification of the organophosphate group is facilitated, but not the individual pesticide. Also, from a quantitative point of view there are no absolute concentrations of urinary alkyl phosphates that can be considered uniformly diagnostic of all organophosphate pesticides because common alkyl phosphates are derived from different pesticides with varying toxicities. The toxicity differences of several organophosphorus pesticides that yield the same alkyl phosphate metabolites are compared in TABLE 3. The phenolic metabolites are also listed in TABLE 3, with their respective organophosphate pesticides.

Ethyl parathion and mevinphos merit further discussion because these two pesticides are among the most toxic organophosphates used by agriculture, and in the past were the pesticides most often associated with poisoning and/or severe cholinesterase inhibition. In seven cases of parathion poisoning studied, the lowest concentration of DEP observed in the initial urine was 0.9 mg/L, with initial concentrations in all these cases ranging from 0.9 mg/L to 8.1 mg/L. These concentrations should be contrasted with DEP concentrations observed in 99 urines from 8 workers exposed primarily to these pesticides and found not to have depressed cholinesterase activities. The average DEP concentration was 0.14 mg/L, and only on one occasion was a DEP concentration greater than 0.4 mg/L identified. Two mevinphos poisoning cases were investigated and the initial urine concentration of DMP was 5 mg/L in both cases; these findings were very similar to those reported by Holmes *et al.*,[11] who found that initial urine concentrations of DMP were 4.7 and 4.0 mg/L respectively, in the two cases that they reported.

Occupational Exposure Studies

Surveillance of the worker exposed to organophosphate pesticides is designed to detect and prevent serious cholinesterase inhibition and cholinergic illness. These are two human health end points of special concern. In South Florida, past experience has suggested that these effects are most likely to occur with workers working with the more toxic pesticides such as parathion or mevinphos.[12] Sequential urinary metabolite studies[13] showed that applicators working with relatively nontoxic organophosphates such as chlorpyrifos, although exhibiting significant urinary excretions of the alkyl phosphates of this pesticide, did not demonstrate simultaneous cholinesterase depression. Thus, the surveillance potential of these metabolites to prevent cholinergic illness is of primary importance in situations where the worker is working with the more highly toxic organophosphates. We have also found that prediction is impossible when the worker is exposed to a mixture of pesticides, particularly when the mixture includes both highly toxic and relatively nontoxic organophosphate pesticides.[14]

Since today almost all agricultural practices call for the use of a variety of organophosphates, one must conclude that although the urinary alkyl phosphate metabolites are highly sensitive indicators of exposure to the organophosphates, they are not reliable nonspecific predictors of cholinesterase depression in mixed exposure situations where the pesticides involved differ greatly with regard to inherent toxicities. This broad generalization of the potential of the urinary alkyl phosphates as a surveillance instrument should be tempered by one clarification. If, in the future, occupational programs based on metabolite excretions are pursued, then standards might be set that would have to be based on the worst theoretically possible situations, namely exposures to ethyl parathion and mevinphos. DMP and DEP concentrations greater than the threshold of adverse health effect levels found in cases of exposure to the most toxic pesticides would justify temporary withdrawal of the worker from exposure.

Evaluation of Protective Clothing Effectiveness

The objective of these studies was to test the evaluatory potential of the urinary metabolites, imposing an intervention procedure designed to produce subtle differences in exposure to foliar residues in two groups of workers and to determine whether the urinary metabolites were sensitive enough to detect these differences. Mean differences in urinary alkyl phosphates between workers wearing fluorocarbon-

TABLE 4. Mean Differences in Urinary Alkyl Phosphate Levels between Agricultural Workers Wearing Untreated and Treated Fluorocarbon Clothing over a Six-day Period

	DMP (mg/L)	DEP (mg/L)	DMTP (mg/L)	DETP (mg/L)
Mean concentration (over 6 days)[a]				
Untreated clothing	0.20	0.22	0.14	0.11
Treated clothing	0.14	0.17	0.08	0.07
Mean difference (over 12-h time periods)[a]	0.06	0.05	0.06	0.04
Standard error	0.016	0.009	0.006	0.012
p	<0.01	<0.01	<0.01	<0.01

[a] The number of subjects each day varied from 10 to 13 workers.

treated clothing and workers wearing untreated clothing are shown in TABLE 4. The differences are the mean values of the untreated minus the treated for twenty-four 12-h urines collected over a 6-day study period. For all four metabolites these differences were significant at the $p < 0.01$ level. These showed that the workers wearing treated clothing excreted significantly lower levels of urinary alkyl phosphates than workers wearing untreated clothing. FIGURE 3, which graphically presents the

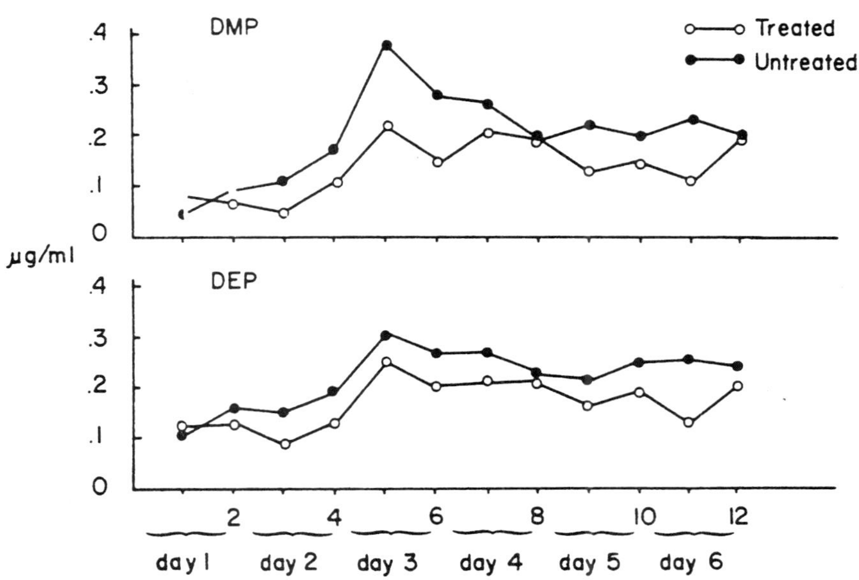

FIGURE 3. Comparison of mean urinary alkyl phosphates in workers wearing fluorocarbon-treated and untreated clothing.

TABLE 5. Mean, Ranges, and Detection Frequencies of Alkyl Phosphate and Selected Phenolic Urinary Metabolites in the General Population of Dade County, Florida

Metabolite	Number of Subjects	Mean (mg/L)[a]	Range (mg/L)[a]	% Detected
Alkyl phosphates				
DMP	36	0.008	N.D.[b]-0.053	56
DEP	36	0.012	N.D.-0.11	58
DMTP	33	0.027	N.D.-0.22	45
DETP	33	0.021	N.D.-0.3	36
Phenols				
3,5,6-TCPyr	37	0.003	N.D.-0.032	27
2,4,5-TCP	37	0.004	N.D.-0.10	14

[a] Detection limits (mg/L): DMP: 0.003; DEP: 0.005; DMTP: 0.010; DETP: 0.010; 3,5,6-TCPyr: 0.002; 2,4,5-TCP: 0.002.
[b] N.D.: Not detected (assumed to be 0 for mean calculation).

individual DMP and DEP excretion data summarized in TABLE 4, exhibits striking temporal parallelism between excretion values of the two groups, further emphasizing the unique sensitivity of these indices.

Urinary Organophosphate Pesticide Metabolite Levels in the General Population

The objective of this study was to measure the profiles of incidental exposure of a small sample of the general population of Dade County, Florida, to organophosphate pesticides. The mean, ranges, and detection frequency of the urinary alkyl phosphate and phenolic metabolites in TABLE 5 shows that there were minimal incidental exposures of the general population in this area to trace amounts of organophosphates in 1975. Based on a small sample size of 37 individuals, between 36% and 56% of the population had trace amounts of organophosphates in their urine. Since 11 (27%) of these had trace amounts of 3,5,6-TCPyr, this would suggest that chlorpryifos was one major source of this incidental organophosphate exposure.

Hill *et al.*[15] recently observed that 82% of the U.S. population had measurable concentrations of 3,5,6-TCPyr. These results differ significantly from the results of the second National Health and Nutrition Examination Survey (NHANES II)[16] collected between 1976 and 1980. In NHANES II, 5.8% of the 6990 people studied had concentrations of 3,5,6-TCPyr greater than its detection limit of 0.005 mg/L. Because Hill's method of detection limit was 0.001 mg/L for 3,5,6-TCPyr, part of the increase in the frequency of detection was due to the sensitivity of the method. Nevertheless, 31% of the population had concentrations of 0.005 mg/L or greater. This is a fivefold increase over concentrations observed in NHANES II. These results are likely due to the increased use of chlorpyrifos in the United States, particularly as a replacement for the termiticide chlordane.

CONCLUSIONS

The initial concentrations of the urinary pesticide metabolites in poisoning were related to (1) the chemical configuration of the pesticide, (2) its metabolism and toxicity (LD_{50}), and (3) the dose and route of absorption. Of the several variables influencing initial urinary concentrations of metabolites, it was found that the dose and toxicity were the most important. The dialkyl phosphates reflective of the oxon appeared to be more specifically related to cholinergic illness than did the dithio urinary derivatives. For example, in 32 of 40 urines from seven poisonings cases due to ethyl parathion, DEP concentrations were higher than DETP.

The urinary alkyl phosphates, while being highly sensitive indicators of organophosphate exposures, lacked specificity for individual organophosphate pesticides, making it impossible to uniformly predict cholinesterase-inhibition illness on the basis of a single urinary alkyl phosphate concentration after exposure to an unknown pesticide. Only in occupational exposures to a single pesticide, particularly to those that are highly toxic, can these urinary metabolites be used as a surveillance instrument. Under the circumstances, standards for safe and unsafe levels of urinary alkyl phosphates could be set that would be based on the metabolite concentrations observed with known exposures to parathion and mevinphos.

In contrast to specificity, however, the sensitivity of these indices was remarkable, often facilitating the identification of minute exposures from the environment or from contaminated clothing, which was not recognized by the worker himself or herself. It was concluded that the urinary metabolites were very reliable epidemiologic instruments of organophosphate exposures, capable of identifying subtle differences in groups of workers and able to measure small incidental exposure of the general population to these pesticides in the environment.

REFERENCES

1. Knaak, J. B., T. Jackson, A. S. Fredrickson, L. Rivera, K. T. Maddy & N. B. Akesson. 1980. Safety effectiveness of closed-transfer, mixing-loading, and application equipment in preventing exposure to pesticides. Arch. Environ. Contam. Toxicol. **9:** 231-245.
2. Hayes, A. L., R. A. Wise & F. W. Weir. 1980. Assessment of occupational exposure to organophosphates in pest control operators. Am. Ind. Hyg. Assoc. J. **41:** 568-575.
3. Franklin, C. A., N. I. Muir & R. P. Moody. 1986. The use of biological monitoring in the estimation of exposure during the application of pesticides. Tox. Lett. **33:** 127-136.
4. Coye, M. J., J. A. Lowe & K. T. Maddy. 1986. Biological monitoring of agricultural workers exposed to pesticides II. Monitoring of intact pesticides and their metabolites. J. Occup. Med. **28:** 628-636.
5. Krieger, R. I. & T. Thongsinthusak. 1993. Metabolism and excretion of dimethoate following ingestion of overtolerance peas and a bolus dose. Food Chem. Toxic. **31:** 177-182.
6. Nutley, B. P. & J. Cocker. 1993. Biological monitoring of workers occupationally exposed to organophosphate pesticides. Pestic. Sci. **38:** 315-322.
7. Michel, H. 1949. An electrometric method for the determination of red blood cell and plasma cholinesterase activity. J. Lab. Clin. Med. **34:** 1564.
8. Shafik, T. M., H. C. Sullivan & H. F. Enos. 1973. A multiresidue procedure for halo and nitrophenols—Measurement of exposure to biodegradable pesticides yielding these compounds as metabolites. J. Agric. Food Chem. **21:** 295-298.

9. SHAFIK, T. M., D. BRADWAY, H. ENOS & A. YOBS. 1973. Human exposure to organophosphorus pesticides: A modified procedure for gas liquid chromatographic analysis of alkyl phosphate metabolites in urine. J. Agric. Food Chem. **21:** 625-629.
10. PETERSON, J. C. 1993. Monitoring human exposure to organophosphate pesticides by measuring metabolites in urine. The 107th American Association of Official Analytical Chemists Annual Meeting, Washington, DC, July.
11. HOLMES, J. H., H. G. STARR JR., R. C. HANISCH & K. N. VON KAULIA. 1974. Short-term toxicity of mevinphos in man. Arch. Environ. Health **29:** 84-89.
12. REICH, G. A., J. H. DAVIS & J. E. DAVIES. 1968. Pesticide poisoning in South Florida: An analysis of mortality and morbidity and a comparison of sources of incidence data. Arch. Environ. Health **17:** 768.
13. DAVIES, J. E. 1974. Pesticides Epidemiological Field Studies. Environmental Health Effects Research Series. EPA-650/1-74-009. Office of Research and Development, U.S. Environmental Protection Agency, Washington, DC.
14. DAVIES, J. E. 1977. Occupational and Environmental Pesticide Study in South Florida. Environmental Health Effects Research Series. EPA-600/1-77-019. Office of Research and Development, U.S. Environmental Protection Agency, Research Triangle Park, NC.
15. HILL, R. H., S. L. HEAD, S. BAKER, M. GREGG, D. B. SHEALY, S. L. BAILEY, C. C. WILLIAMS, E. J. SAMPSON & L. L. NEEDHAM. 1995. Pesticide residues in urine of adults living in the United States: Reference range concentrations. Environ. Res. **71:** 1-10.
16. KUTZ, F. W., B. T. COOK, O. D. CARTER-POKRAS, D. BRODY & R. S. MURPHY. 1992. Selected pesticide residues and metabolites in urine from a survey of the U.S. general population. J. Toxicol. Environ. Health **37:** 277-291.

Agricultural Sustainability, Pesticide Exposures, and Health Risks: Israel, the Palestinian National Authority, and Jordan[a]

ELIHU D. RICHTER,[b] STEPHEN GASTEYER,[c]
SAMIR EL HAJ,[d] M. JAQHABIR,[e] AND J. SAFI[f]

[b]*Hebrew University School of Public Health
and Community Medicine
Jerusalem, Israel*

[c]*Iowa State University
Ames, Iowa*

[d]*Bir Zeit University Center for Occupational
and Environmental Medicine
Bir Zeit, Palestine National Authority*

[e]*University of Applied Sciences
Amman, Jordan*

[f]*Environmental Protection and Research Institute of Gaza
Gaza, Palestine National Authority*

INTRODUCTION: DR. SELIKOFF'S LAST CONVERSATION WITH ONE OF THE AUTHORS (E.D.R.)

To this day, I can still recall Dr. Selikoff's last words with me. He was on his deathbed in Ridgewood, New Jersey in 1992. He looked me straight in the eye and then gazed upward. "I could have saved the lives of a lot of those boys had I called for getting rid of asbestos in the 1960s . . . what I knew then was already more than enough . . . I should have spoken out earlier. . . ." Dr. Selikoff, attacked by many for his warnings that asbestos exposure was dangerous at levels once considered safe, himself felt, as he lay dying, that he had not spoken out soon enough and forcefully enough.

At the time, scientists in Israel, the West Bank-Gaza (now the Palestinian National Authority, PNA)[b] and Jordan had been working separately, with no contact with each other, on assessment of the risks from exposures to organochlorines, organophosphates, and heat stress in field workers; and, in Israeli, together with colleagues from

[a]We thank Econet and the Conanima Foundation for support.

[b]For simplicity's sake we are using the term Palestinian National Authority to represent the area of West Bank and Gaza. However, approximately 70 percent of West Bank and 30 percent of Gaza remain under the direct and full control of Israeli occupation forces, and are the subject of ongoing negotiations.

WHO-Europe, completing the final drafts of the Multinational Study on the Health Effects of Exposures to Organophosphate Pesticides.[1–5] All were moving towards the opinion that monitoring of air or dermal exposures—what today are called biomarkers of exposure—all too often is an inadequate substitute for the definitive solution: getting rid of the exposure to the hazard in the first place by stopping its use, in the classic tradition of Sir Thomas Legge's axioms on solutions external to the worker.[6]

In that last meeting, I remember saying to Dr. Selikoff that repetitive monitoring routines sometimes serve as fig leaves for permitting work conditions and exposures that should not have been tolerated to begin with. This point of view is often criticized as utopian and not fitting current fashions in cost-benefit analysis. But experiences in the control of health risks from pesticide use now suggest that that utopian hypothesis may sometimes generate more sustainable solutions than risk management strategies embedded in the inertia of the status quo, and that in the long run these solutions may be more cost-effective as well.

There has been a gradually growing awareness of the primacy of substitution, solutions external to the worker, and right-to-know and the obligation to inform. These principles are central to occupational medicine and were often quoted by Dr. Selikoff. Geoffrey Rose's axioms about the superiority of control based on prevention of sickness in populations compared to case finding of sick individuals restate these principles in more formal epidemiologic terms and present the theoretical reasons for their effectiveness and greater cost effectiveness relative to screening, monitoring, and case finding.[7]

In agriculture, the question, of course, is whether substantial reduction in pesticide use, and therefore exposure and risk, is compatible with sustaining crop yield and providing fresh wheat, rice, fruits, and vegetables in abundance—one of the cornerstones of a policy for global health promotion—for ever-growing populations.

AGRICULTURE IN ISRAEL AND THE PALESTINIAN NATIONAL AUTHORITY

Hazards and risks for many remain in agriculture in Israel and the Palestinian National Authority. This paper recalls the progress in the last two decades in applying the principle of reduction of pesticide use, but also calls attention to the unfinished agenda of control of hazards based on Legge's principles in a complex and brittle political, social, and ecological setting. Israel and the Palestinian National Authority are two separate political societies, but one ecosystem that now supports a total population of seven million (some 50-fold or more than the Judean hills in Josephus's time, when families fed themselves from crops grown on terraced plots of land of 60×60 m^2).[1,8]

Yet, most of Israel's agricultural landmass has been used not for growing food but for growing cotton; for the PNA, most of the land is for orchards and dry land crops. In Israel, cotton crops are the major consumer of water and pesticides; cotton is grown using mechanized plowing, fertilizers, irrigation, and pesticide spray technology and is dependent on extremely small numbers of field workers—itself an effective method of exposure restriction. Cotton's requirement for large amounts of water and land–both in scarce supply as ground water sources are contaminated and land prices are soaring–implies disappearance of land for cultivation in coming years. By contrast, orchard and vegetable growth involves larger numbers of people intensively working small plots of land in family moshavim, kibbutzim, greenhouses, and glass houses in Israel and in large and small family-based orchards in the PNA.

Less than 3% of Israel's population of some 5,800,000 and some 25–30% of the PNA population of some 2,200,000 persons are employed in agriculture. Large amounts of produce grown in the West Bank and Gaza are now marketed in Israel, and much of the produce consumed in the West Bank comes from Israel. Both export to Common Market countries, and there has been much back and forth movement of produce between the West Bank and Jordan. In Israel, there has been an upheaval in the employment picture, as migrant foreign workers, mainly from the Far East have been brought in to do field work formerly done by workers from the West Bank and Gaza. The hazards and risks to migrant laborers have been a regulatory wasteland.

Pesticide use has been part of the package associated with large-scale advances in agricultural productivity in earlier years, and was central to vector control programs against disease-bearing mosquitoes–notably malaria in the 1940s and 1950s.

In the 1960s and early 1970s, organochlorines, (OCl's), notably DDT, Lindane, and benzene hexachloride (BHC), as well as Hepatachor, Dieldrin, Endosulfan, and Endrin, were the most commonly used agents. By now, in Israel as in most Western countries, these agents have either been banned or withdrawn, but they remain in use for selected vector control activities. Endosulfan is still used for aerial spraying of cotton, but otherwise there has been massive restriction of organochlorines. By the mid-1970s, concentration of BHC in breast milk may have averaged as much as 2,500 parts per billion or some 800 times the 3-ppb level in U.S.A. samples; but now levels are not higher than those seen in Western countries.[9,10]

The earlier extremely high levels may have been implicated in the rise of breast cancer mortality in the 1960s and early 1970s in Israel; the subsequent fall in mortality has been attributed to the abrupt cessation of their use and drops in levels in milk to levels no higher than in other Western countries in which use was terminated.[9] We are now monitoring what is a possible trend in the leveling off in incidence of breast cancer in Israeli women (Israel Cancer Registry Data, 1993) after previous rises, but it is premature to draw any conclusions given uncertainties concerning changes in the population mix from massive recent immigration and reporting practices. If risks are shown not to be lower in immigrants and if current (relative) underreporting has been ruled out, then, it is possible that the drop in incidence may be attributable, at least in part, to the past termination of population-wide exposure to organochlorines, since cessation in rise in incidence cannot be explained by improved survival from more effective treatment.

In Gaza and the West Bank, however, the use of organochlorines remains widespread, although data on amounts applied on a crop-by-crop basis are not readily available.[4] Data also are not readily available on OCl levels in breast milk of Palestinian women. Preliminary hospital-based data from the Gaza Strip suggest a marked rise in the incidence of breast cancer relative to other cancers in women (J. Safi, 1997).

PHASE II. ORGANOPHOSPHATES AND MIXED EXPOSURES IN ISRAEL

In Israel, the massive reduction in the use of organochlorine pesticides was followed by their replacement by organophosphates in the 1970s, during which there was a big rise in their use.

In past years, there has been substantial documentation of the short-term health effects from pesticide exposures in workers in kibbutzim, moshavim, and factories, and in residents exposed to pesticide drift from aerial spraying and pesticide residues in foods and fruits.[11,13] In the 1980s, cotton field workers and residents complained frequently of illness episodes from exposure to spray drift, and these complaints were shown to be associated with high levels of metabolites of organophosphates in urine.[14]

There has been work on the possible etiologic role in Parkinson's disease of residential pesticide exposure in agricultural settings,[15] and work is now under way on the possible role of exposures to organophosphates in increasing risks for spontaneous abortion and birth defects (J. Goldsmith, personal communication). One study is also under way on hematolymphatic risks and occupational pesticide exposure (O. Paltiel, personal communication).

TRENDS IN USE, EXPOSURE, AND RISK: MORE COTTON YIELD AND LESS PESTICIDE USE

In Israel, in the past decade there has been a decline in spontaneous reports of mass outbreaks of illness in cotton field workers and residents.[8,14] There is evidence to indicate that reduction of risk resulted from reduced use of, and therefore reduced exposures to, organophosphates and other anticholinesterases, the dominant type of pesticide applied. This trend occurred during a period when cotton cultivation was reduced because of a severe water shortage and declining world prices of cotton.

During this period, cotton yield per hectare increased by 21% from 1.4 to 1.7 tons. The increased yield occurred despite, or perhaps because of, reduced pesticide use. Between 1979 and 1989, there was a massive reduction in both the total tonnage of pesticides in use and the amount of organophosphates in use per hectare cultivated (Fig. 1). Furthermore, there was a shift from the use of more to less toxic agents within the organophosphate family, notably as a result of reduced use of parathion (LD50: 3 mg/kg body weight, BW). This meant that the drop in use of organophosphates was even greater than indicated by data on tonnage (Fig. 2). There were massive reductions in nation-wide use of organophosphates from 1241 tons in 1979 to 350 tons in 1989—a drop of 72% in absolute tonnage (but 41% when corrected for reduction in cotton yield resulting from reduced cultivation). While factors such as better cultivation and selective use of more fertile land may have been involved, the fact still remains that reduced pesticide use, at the least, did not serve as an obstacle to increased crop yield per hectare cultivated. These trends have been seen on a far more massive scale in Egypt (B Otefa, personal communication; 1994 Meeting of Regional Collaborative Program on Pesticide Hazards, Cairo). They support the case for action for work on maintaining crop yield with integrated pest management and other reduction strategies.

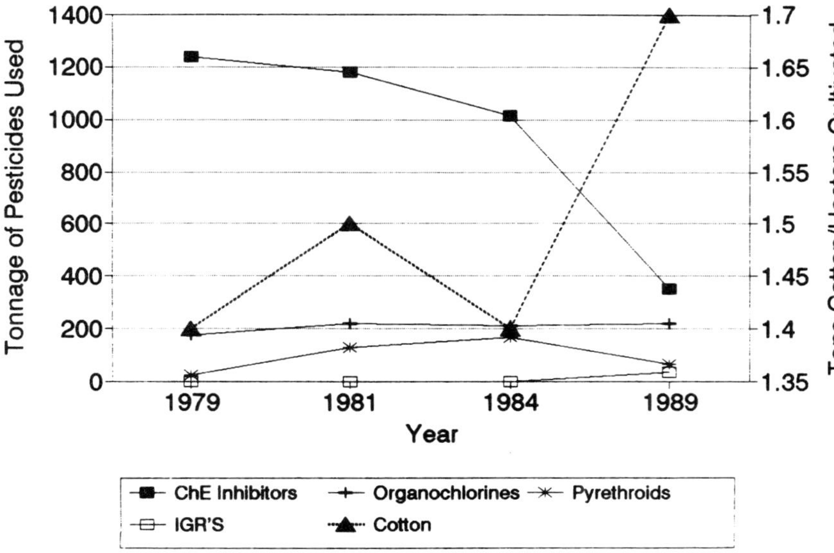

FIGURE 1. Cotton yield vs. pesticide use in Israel.

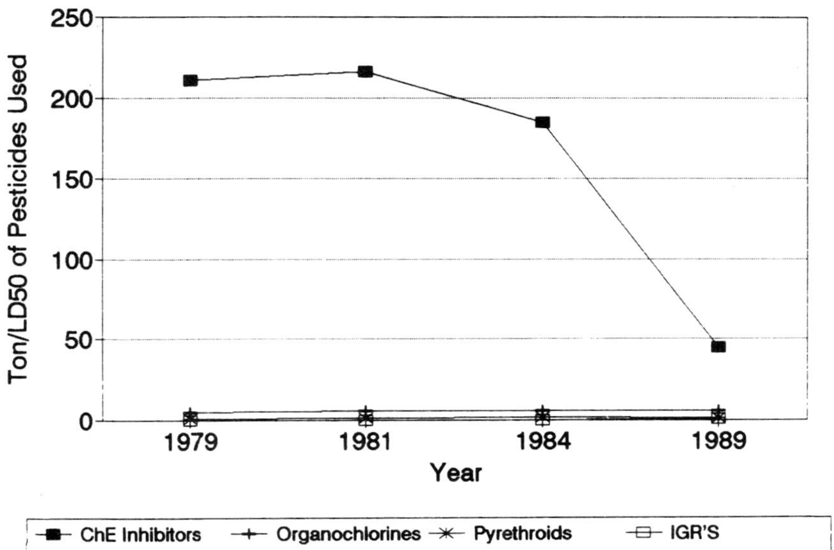

FIGURE 2. Insecticides used against cotton pests in Israel.

FIELD WORKER HEALTH RISKS IN AN ERA OF DECLINING PESTICIDE USE

Data from a field survey (1991) on work practices, symptoms, and cholinesterase and alkyl phosphate levels in a group of kibbutz cotton field workers ($n = 12$) and orchard workers ($n = 7$) suggest that health risks from reduced pesticide use (TABLE 1) are now submaximal.[16] This situation contrasts with evidence of much higher exposures in previous years, when application levels, though beginning to drop from peak amounts, were substantially higher. Interviews and walk-through surveys indicated that these workers had received little formal training in hazard prevention, they worked almost daily in irrigation and crop care, they wore short pants and sleeveless shirts in field work, they did not change their clothes daily, they acknowledged odors of pesticide in their field work, and they entered fields on the day of spraying. Yet our 1991 field survey indicated they were almost totally asymptomatic, and the degree of risk, as measured by erythrocyte and plasma cholinesterase (Elman Modified Test-Mate Method) (TABLES 2 and 3) and alkyl phosphate metabolites (TABLES 4 and 5), were far below levels considered to be acutely hazardous. While these observations should not be considered an endorsement for hazardous work practices and the nonuse of protective covering for feet, legs, hands, and arms, they suggest the hypothesis that much of the protection came from simple reduction of the amounts of pesticide applied.

By contrast, a group of moshav farmers, whose work involved intensive use and contact with pesticides in backyard greenhouses and orchards, were at greater risk, because use patterns had not been reduced over the years. Their exposures were to Cotnion, Divipan, Monocron, Marshall, and Supracide, and their work practices (TABLE 6) were far from adequate. TABLE 7 shows that for this group the situation was considerably different from that of kibbutz farmers working in open fields. Kibbutz urinary metabolites of organophosphates were more frequently detected, and at higher levels. Other data showed that headache, fatigue, nausea, and stomache aches, diarrhea, breathing difficulty and cough, running nose, muscle fatigue, and skin problems were frequent. A field survey showed that women who picked and cut flowers in glass houses were more likely to be ill than men, who sprayed and were more apt to use protective clothing. Other data showed that urine metabolites varied with the frequency of reported pesticide applications, but not with the reported frequency of use of protective clothing or gloves.[16]

The findings on exposure and symptoms in kibbutz workers working in open fields, compared with data from previous years showed the benefits of reducing risks from reduced pesticide use and substitution of less-toxic for more-toxic agents. But in the moshav, the enclosed greenhouse work conditions led to subacute and chronic illness in many men and women, which was not prevented, it appeared, even when they wore what they called protective clothing. These latter findings call for preventive measures in greenhouses based on a strategy similar to what was achieved in cotton—an integrated approach to risk prevention by reducing pesticide use, but at the same time maintaining crop yield.

TABLE 1. Potential Exposure: Agent, Toxicity, and Days of Use in Kibbutz Zora, March 16-September 15, 1991

Planting (Season)	Name	LD50[a] (mg/kg)	Category	Estimated Days of Use	Toxic Exposure Index[b]
Orchard (March-July)	Di-Syston	7.55	OP[c]	8	105.9
	Divipan	56	OP	8	14.28
	Novathion	490	OP	8	1.6
					Total: 121.78
Cotton (July-September)	Pirimore	147	carbamate	3	2.04
	Marshall	209	carbamate	2	0.47
	Lannate	17	carbamate	6	35.29
	Supracide	25	OP	8	32
	Novathion	490	OP	7	1.4
	Parathion	3	OP	6	200
					Total: 271.2

[a] Rcference 29.
[b] Toxic exposure index = days/LD50 × 100.
[c] OP = organophosphate.

TABLE 2. Erythrocyte Cholinesterase (AChE) Activities Adjusted by Hemoglobin (Hb) Concentrations in Students, Factory Workers, Fruit Growers, and Cotton Growers during Exposure Period for Field Workers

		Hb-Adjusted AChE (IU/g of Hb)			
		Baseline Estimated Measurement	In-Exposure Measurement	Intraindividual Variation (Decline)	
	No.	X1 (SD)	X2 (SD)	X (SD)[a]	% (Range)[b]
Students	11	32.7 (2.05)	31.7 (1.87)[c]	1.0 (2.13)	2.9% (−8.8–12.5%)
Factory workers	10	30.2 (3.71)	28.2 (3.49)[c]	2.1 (5.73)	5.3% (−8.9–46.0%)
Fruit growers	7	27.6 (2.31)	29.9 (2.79)[c]	−2.3 (1.75)	−8.6% (−19.1–1.6%)
Cotton growers	12	31.1 (3.07)	27.5 (3.45)[d]	3.6 (4.83)[e]	10.7% (−4.2–47.7%)

[a] Value of intraindividual variation = value of baseline estimated measurement (X1) − value of in-exposure measurement (X2).

[b] Percent of intraindividual variation = {value of baseline estimated measurement (X1) − value of in-exposure measurement (X2)} / value of baseline estimated measurement (X1).

[c] Paired sample *t*-test for difference between baseline estimated and in-exposure measurements: $p > 0.05$.

[d] Paired sample *t*-test for difference between baseline estimated and in-exposure measurements: $p < 0.05$.

[e] One-way analysis of variance for difference between baseline estimated intraindividual variations of group: $p > 0.05$.

TABLE 3. Plasma Cholinesterase (PChE) Activities in Students, Factory Workers, Fruit Growers, and Cotton Growers during Exposure Period for Field Workers

		PchE (IU/ml)			
		Baseline Estimated Measurement	In-Exposure Measurement	Intraindividual Variation (Decline)	
	No.	X1 (SD)	X2 (SD)	X (SD)[a]	% (Range)[b]
Students	11	3.143 (0.56)	3.067 (0.44)[c]	0.076 (0.28)	1.6% (−9.7–15.6%)
Factory workers	10	3.481 (0.48)	3.368 (0.50)[c]	0.113 (0.32)	3.0% (−17.5–20.3%)
Fruit growers	7	3.060 (0.58)	2.943 (0.35)[c]	0.117 (0.44)	2.4% (−10.9–24.1%)
Cotton growers	12	3.128 (0.63)	2.572 (0.82)[d]	0.556 (0.71)[e]	17.3% (−5.9–83.7%)

[a] Value of intraindividual variation = value of baseline estimated measurement (X1) – value of in-exposure measurement (X2).

[b] Percent of intraindividual variation = {value of baseline estimated measurement (X1) – value of in-exposure measurement (X2)} / value of baseline estimated measurement (X1).

[c] Paired sample *t*-test for difference between baseline estimated and in-exposure measurements: $p > 0.05$.

[d] Paired sample *t*-test for difference between baseline estimated and in-exposure measurements: $p < 0.05$.

[e] One-way analysis of variance for difference between baseline estimated intraindividual variations of group: $p > 0.05$.

TABLE 4. Urine Alkyl Phosphate Metabolites in Kibbutz (ppb) Field Workers and Comparison Groups

	DEP	DEDTP	DETP	DMTP	DMDTP
Cotton workers (n = 123)					
Baseline					
Mean	0	0	1.3	4.8	0
Range	0	0	0–16.8	0–28	0
No. positive	0	0	8%	12%	0
Exposure period					
Mean	7.9	0	3.6	11.6	2
Range	0–94.9	0	12	0–53.2	0–8.5
No. positive	2	0	4	10	5
Orchard workers (n = 2)					
Baseline					
Mean	0	0	0	0	0
Range	—	—	—	—	—
No. positive	0	0	0	0	0
Exposure period					
Mean	5.9	0	0	6.8	0
Range	0	0	0–7.54	0–48.7	0
No. positive	0	0	0	2	0
Factory workers (n = 10)					
Baseline					
Mean	0	0	0	0	0
Range	0	0	0	0	0
No. positive	0	0	0	0	0
Exposure period					
Mean	0	0	0.64	4.35	0
Range	0	0	0–6.4	0–21.0	0
No. positive	0	0	1	3	0
Student volunteers (n = 11)					
Baseline					
Mean	9.9	0	0	1.0	1
Range	0–90	0	0	0–10	0
No. positive	1	0	0	1	0

TABLE 5. Alkyl Phosphate Metabolites and ChE Depression in Kibbutz Groups

One or More Metabolite	Factory Workers		Orchard Workers		Cotton Workers	
	PChE	RChE	PChE	RChE	PChE	RChE
Yes						
n	3		3		10	
ChE depression						
Mean	3.2%	−1.3%	−7.8%	−8.03%	17.6%	10.3%
Range	(1.0->5.0%)	(−8.9->7.2%)	(−11.0->4.5%)	(−19->3.5%)	(−3.5->83.7%)	(−4.0->47%)
No						
n	7		4		2	
ChE depression						
Mean	2.8%	8.2%	9.9%	−8.9%	15.8%	9.1%
Range	(−17.5->8.5%)	(−8.2->46%)	(4.0->24.1%)	(−13.5->4.8%)	(14->17%)	(7.7->10.6%)

NOTES: χ_2 for linear trend: $p < 0.05$. Minus sign means that exposure value is higher than baseline.

TABLE 6. Work Practices and Habits among Moshav Farmers[a]

Safety	Male (n = 56)						Female (n = 22)					
	Never		Always		Unknown		Never		Always		Unknown	
Measure	n	%	n	%	n	%	n	%	n	%	n	%
Change clothes	18	32.1%	32	57.1%	6	10.7%	3	13.6%	1	4.5%	18	81.8%
Wash/shower	12	21.4%	39	69.6%	5	8.9%	4	18.2%	2	9.1%	16	72.7%
Protective suit	24	42.9%	26	46.4%	6	10.7%	2	9.1%	0	0.0%	20	90.9%
Mask	15	26.8%	34	60.7%	7	12.5%	1	4.5%	1	4.5%	20	90.9%
Gloves	40	71.4%	8	14.3%	8	14.3%	2	9.1%	1	4.5%	19	86.4%
Not eating	0	0.0%	49	87.5%	7	12.5%	0	0.0%	4	18.2%	18	81.8%
Not drinking	1	1.8%	48	85.7%	7	12.5%	0	0.0%	4	18.2%	18	81.8%
Not smoking	2	3.6%	48	85.7%	6	10.7%	0	0.0%	4	18.2%	18	81.8%

[a] Results of questionnaire distributed to farmers, including persons who did not give blood for ChE exposures to alkyl phosphates.

TABLE 7. DMTP in Urine of Kibbutz and Moshav Workers

	Kibbutz Workers	Moshav Workers[a]
Total (no. of urine samples)	58	65
Not detected	25 (43.2%)	30 (464%)
Detected	33 (56.8%)	35 (53.8%)
Distribution (ppb)		
Peak value	53	213
Top 10%	28	108
Top 20%	24	53.2
Top 50%	8	20.2
Mean (all positive)	13.6	39.2
Mean (all)	7.7	21.1

[a] Includes duplicates from some collection times, repeats at a later time, and several individuals not included in studies on symptoms and ChE who donated samples.

PESTICIDES USE AND EXPOSURES IN THE PNA (WEST BANK, GAZA) AND JORDAN

In the West Bank and Gaza, there was massive increase in use of organophosphates in the mid-1970s, slightly lagging behind trends in Israel. This coincided with a major change in the work economy of agriculture from a traditional, self-sufficient, and more or less integrated crop system of cereals, legumes, fruits, grapes and livestock to a commercial system dominated by fruit trees and vineyards, requiring less manpower. One major reason for this switchover was the migration of Palestinian laborers into Israel. This left fewer workers for everyday work in agriculture and created greater dependence on pesticides and other technologies to replace traditional labor-intensive manual crop tending.

Saleh *et al.* have reviewed the situation in the West Bank, where pesticides are widely used first in agriculture, followed by vector control, animal pest control, and household pest control.[17]

Some 400–500 tons of pesticides are used annually in the West Bank,[17,18] and some 100 tons in Gaza.[4] In the West Bank, some 40% of usage is of methyl bromide, for soil fumigation in irrigated agriculture against pests and diseases. Seventy-two percent of pesticide use is greatest in irrigated areas, which constitute 5% of cultivated land. Fifty-three percent of agents other than methyl bromide goes into irrigated agriculture. Usage rates per dunam were 4.4 kg in plastic houses, 2.1 kg in open irrigated areas, and 0.6 kg for fruit trees. FIGURE 3 presents data on crop area treated by crop type, and FIGURE 4 presents data on average pesticide consumption by crop pattern.

Of 123 agents in use, 14 are internationally suspended, canceled or banned, including 7 (Aldicarb, Chlordane, DDT, Lindane, Paraquat, Parathion, and Pentachlorophenol) that are members of the "dirty dozen." Other than methyl bromide, there are 122 other pesticides, including 17 organochlorine and 6 organophosphates (all with LD50 ratings less than 500 mg/kgBW), 5 carbamate agents, and 4 dithiocarbamates. Abu-Quare has reported similar findings.[19]

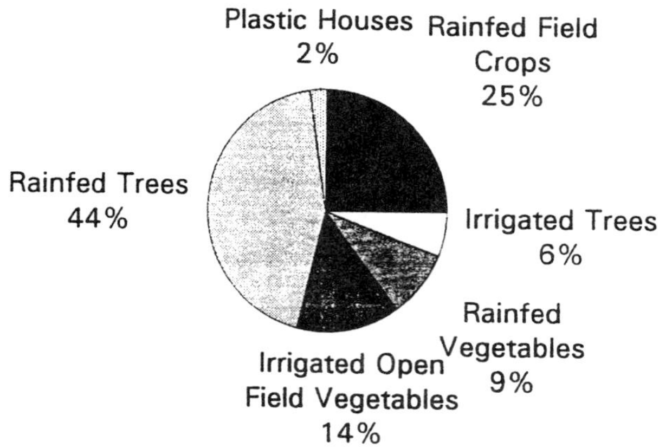

FIGURE 3. Pesticide use in the West Bank: average percent of 383,453 dunams devoted to various crops. (According to Salah *et al.*[17])

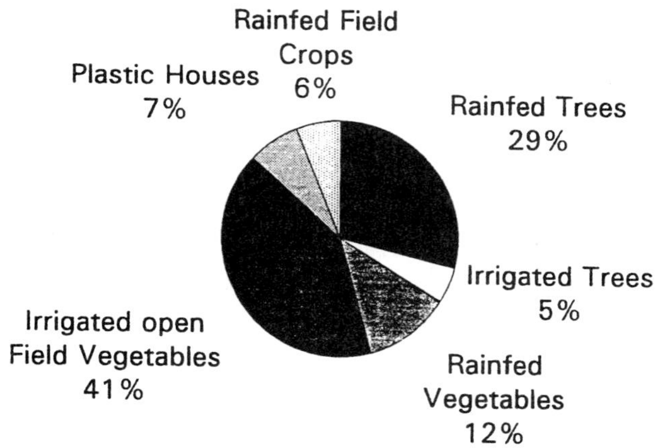

FIGURE 4. Pesticide use in the West Bank: average percent of 289,819 tons of pesticide devoted to treatment of various crops. (According to Salah *et al.*[17])

Data on pesticide use, field observations and interview data, and sporadic episodes of acute intoxication suggest that for field workers and others with adjacent exposures, the hazards and risks from pesticide use are more severe in the Palestinian National Authority than in Israel, if only because agriculture is a major sector its economy. But there are other problems as well. Salah et *et al.*'s report, based on a survey of 128 farmers in the West Bank, enumerates the following problems: absence of quality control on chemicals shipped from or through Israel, poor labeling, possible adulteration, faulty application equipment, laundering of pesticide-contaminated work clothes with regular household laundry, work and indirect exposures of children and pregnant women.

TABLE 8, from Salah, summarizes information on pesticide knowledge, uses, and practices among this group. Twenty-six percent of interviewees reported illness episodes involving themselves or their families, half of which were attributed to skin absorption and the remaining half to inhalation and ingestion equally. The large majority were aware in a general way of the potential for pesticide's environmental hazards and were interested in receiving training in IPM (Integrated Pest Management) were it available.

A study, reported by El Haj *et al.* from the Bir Zeit Center for Occupational and Environmental Health Sciences, disclosed substantial risks for potential dermal exposures, based on skin pad studies, in sprayers applying methamidophos (1/2 kg/ 500 L) in the Jordan Valley (Winter 1988, TABLE 9). Food residue analysis data, reported by the same team, indicated that 10 (24%) of 42 batches of fruits and vegetables contained concentrations above WHO tolerance levels for chlorpyrifos, diazinon, and methamidophos, and parathion (TABLE 10).

Al Shuraqi has shown that on the Jordanian Side of the Jordan Valley residues of organophosphates, dithiocarbamates, halogenated hydrocarbons, carbamates, and other agents detected in cucumbers, hot peppers, green beans, tomatoes, squash, green peppers, and eggplants grown under plastic exceeded German permitted residue levels in 3.6% to 28% of samples tested. Associations were seen between high residue levels and pesticide misuse.[20] Jaqhabir, using skin pad studies and cholinesterase, has demonstrated the dominant importance of skin absorption via the arms and legs in an open field situation. The implication of this work is that protecting the extremities alone was sufficient to prevent more than 85% of absorption in field workers exposed to organophosphates, for whom the skin has been shown to be the major absorption route in many field studies.[5,21]

NEGLECTED OR UNDERSTUDIED ISSUES

In both Israel and the PNA, data on the extent and distribution of pesticide contamination of groundwater supplies are not readily available, except for isolated sporadic probes showing massive contamination by pesticides in an agricultural area on the southern coastal area.[8,22,23]

In the PNA, severe problems in pesticide packaging and labeling and end-user lack of knowledge still produce episodes of acute poisoning from accidental ingestion in children. No information is available on sale of restricted pesticides from Israel to the PNA, and there are reports of buy-back by Israel of cut-rate pesticides sold to PNA distributors. The hazards and risks of foreign workers in Israel have so far fallen far beyond the scope of traditional surveillance. Information on imports of pesticides banned or restricted in first-world countries indicates the potential for many hazards. Child labor is a neglected issue, although it is suspected to be far more widespread in the PNA, given the much larger size of the agricultural sector and the large number of family orchards. Risks of cancer, spontaneous abortion, and birth defects have not been adequately explored, apart from the pilot studies alluded to above.

TABLE 8. Pesticide Knowledge, Uses, and Practices among 128 West Bank Farmers

Measure recommended dose	60%
Restrict dose to level recommended on label	70%
Reason for raising dose	
Pest resistance	51%
No reason	30%
Instructions not in Arabic	11%
Pesticide container damaged before disposal	73%
Pesticide storage in	
Special room	69%
Farm/barn	30%
House	1%
Disposal of pesticide waste	
Reuse it for spraying	
Same crop	34%
Adjacent crop	9%
Pour on soil	52%
No answer	5%
Disposal of container	
On farm	53%
Garbage	10%
Bury	10%
Burn	27%
Use of protective equipment	
Gloves	13%
Boots	51%
Mask	30%
Overalls	30%
Hat	48%
Glasses	8%
Reentry onto field	
Knowledge/belief: after 3 days	58%
Practice: prior to 3 days	98%
Availability of information on	
Use/concentration	>80%
Toxicity	53%
Reentry period	44%
Main source of information	
Agricultural extension worker	38%
Label	9%
Merchants	31%
Other farmers	22%
When spraying do not smoke, drink or eat	72%

TABLE 9. Concentration of Methamidophos (μg/cm2) on Skin Pads Collected from Two Groups of Male Farmers[a]

Pad No.	Source	Group I (n = 14)[b]		Group II (n = 10)[c]	
		Mean ± SE	Range	Mean ± SE	Range
1	left upper arm	0.70 ± 0.40	0–1.87	3.15 ± 1.41	0.20–13.86
2	left lower leg	26.62 ± 6.30	13.03–41.51	117.59 ± 34.21	10.26–303.60
3	left midthigh	10.78 ± 2.35	6.61–16.17	37.55 ± 16.98	2.91–174.68
4	chest over sternum	1.09 ± 0.43	0.21–2.26	1.67 ± 0.33	0.43–2.86
5	back between shoulder blades	0.34 ± 0.16	0–0.76	1.53 ± 0.57	0–5.08
6	forehead	1.19 ± 0.82	0–3.63	2.93 ± 1.22	0–12.51
7	belly under clothing	0	0	0.46 ± 0.20	0–1.37
Total		40.72 ± 1.74		164.88 ± 7.85	

[a] Methamidophos was used at Jiftlik in the Jordan Valley at a concentration of 1/2 kg/500 L. The study was conducted in winter 1988.
[b] Group I farmers had sprayed for 2 hours.
[c] Group II farmers had sprayed for 4 hours.

TABLE 10. Food Residue Analysis[a]

Serial No.	Product	Source	Chemicals Found	Concentration (ppm)
1.	Tomato	R. Eshkol	–	–
2.	Tomato	Surdah	–	–
3.	L. G. bean	Gaza	Chloropyrifos	2.50*
4.	Zucchini	Beirzeit	Chloropyrifos + Parathion	trace
5.	Grape	Beirzeit	Parathion	0.15
6.	Eggplant	Gaza	Parathion	trace
7.	Cauliflower	Jericho	Diazinon	0.38*
			Methamidophos	trace
8.	B. pepper	JRS	Chloropyrifos	0.30*
9.	Zucchini	Jericho	Methamidophos	trace
10.	Cauliflower	Ramallah	Parathion	0.16
			unknown	trace
11.	Tomato	JRS	Chloropyrifos	0.20
12.	Eggplant	Ramallah	–	–
13.	Spinach	Ramallah	–	–
14.	B. pepper	Ramallah	Chloropyrifos	0.36*
15.	Cucumber	Gaza	–	–
16.	Tomato	Gaza	–	–
17.	Grape	Hebron	Parathion	0.65*
18.	Cauliflower	Hebron	–	–
19.	Cucumber	Birzeit	Parathion	0.27
20.	Zucchini	Birzeit	Parathion	0.10
21.	Tomato	Golan Heights	Chloropyrifos	1.20*
22.	Cauliflower	–	2 unknown	–
23.	Zucchini	unknown	Parathion	0.19
24.	Grape	Israel P.	Chloropyrifos	0.12
25.	Cucumber	Jericho	Parathion	0.25
26.	Tomato	Jericho	Parathion	trace
27.	Strawberry	Gaza	unknown	–
28.	F. bean	Jericho	unknown	–
29.	Tomato	Israel	Diazinon	0.73*
30.	Tomato	Ramallah	–	–
31.	B. pepper	Ramallah	–	–
32.	H. pepper	Ramallah	unknown	–
33.	Zucchini	Ramallah	–	–
34.	Tomato	Ramallah	unknown	–
35.	Okra	JRS	Diazinon deomposition product	–
36.	Okra	Ramallah	Paraoxon	–
37.	B. pepper	JRS	–	–
38.	Grape	Ramallah	Parathion	0.40*
39.	Zucchini	Ramallah	–	–
40.	Tomato	Ramallah	–	–
41.	Grape	JRS	Chloropyrifos	0.23*
42.	Tomato	Bethlehem	Diazinon	0.78*

[a] Analysis conducted in April 1992 by the Center for Environmental and Occupational Health Sciences, Birzeit University. Tests are of single items based on random sampling from supermarkets. Method of analysis: gas chromatography using N-P detector.

* = concentration above WHO tolerance.

PHASE III. CUTTING DOWN ON PESTICIDE USE: THE NEED FOR POLICIES AND STRATEGIES

The scenario of ecological abuse and health risk from excessive pesticide use, as well as overuse of chemical fertilizers, has been seen worldwide.[24] There have been case studies of crops having become ''hooked''—increased pesticide use leading to increased pest resistance leading to still more use, with adverse human health effects and devastating ecosystem impact. At the same time, it has been suggested that ''Were farmers unable to use pesticides, their crop yields per acre would decline and more scarce land would be used to produce the same amount of food (or the costs of using alternative methods of pest control would increase). Either way, farmers would be forced to charge higher prices for their products. . . .''[25] The assumptions behind this statement have been challenged by Pimentel, who reports that a 50% increase in pesticide use between 1948 and 1992 was associated by a doubling in pest-related loss, from 17% to 34%.[26] The World Resources Institute has reported that in Indonesia, in the 1980s, an integrated pest management program that cut pesticide use by 60% produced a 15% rise in rice production. In Bangladesh in the 1990s, a pilot program with a 75% decrease in pesticide expenditures showed a 13.5% increase in rice production.[24]

The story of cotton in Israel suggests that by 1990, substantial reduction in pesticide use was associated with producing more, not less, cotton. What happened with cotton is a possible model for achieving similar results with other crops in the region. In cotton, the pesticides were used to control insects; in fruits and vegetables, the problem is to control insects, fungi, and plant viral diseases, and so the issues may be more complex. Indeed, there are some successful, sustained projects in the Beit Shean area in the Jordan Valley directed to the control of fruit and vegetable crops other than cotton, and similar new activities are under way in the Jericho area. But, as we see, in both Israel and the Palestinian National Authority, the situation with regard to growth of fruits and vegetables remains far from ideal, with exposure risks for workers and consumers from residues, and for local and migrant workers and possibly their families from exposures during application.

USE, EXPOSURE, AND RISK

Risk assessment, management, and control of the ecologic and health effects of pesticides should be based on a simple principle: risk is determined by exposure, but the best predictor of exposure is use. Therefore, reduction in use should lead to reduction of exposure and risk. Sometimes, however, such reductions are a consequence not of direct policy, but of trends having to do with conversion of agricultural land to other uses. Apart from cotton, in Israel, reductions in pesticide use have come from constriction of the agricultural sector and ''off-loading'' of crop growth to the PNA and surrounding regions—a trend with unforeseen social, political, and ecological implications.

The fact that the agricultural economies of Israel and the PNA are closely linked, with possible future linkages to Jordan as well, states the case for regional programs based on the establishment of a single uniform standard for protection of field workers and consumers, whatever the political climate. The fact that the entire region seeks markets in the European Community serves as a potential lever for achieving such standards over a period of years. On the other hand, Smith and Beckman reported that in 1990 the United States exported to Israel (includes exports to Gaza and the West Bank) 1,171,799 tons, to Jordan 89,773 tons, to Egypt 964,793 tons, and to Iraq 322,843 tons of pesticides, many banned, unregistered, or restricted for use in the United States.[27]

Alternatives to pesticide use and abuse have been understudied, despite rapidly growing awareness. The elements of a comprehensive program aimed at reducing risk from exposure and use include: banning use of agents outlawed elsewhere (the so-called dirty dozen); introduction of integrated pest management; effective, low-cost real-time surveillance and monitoring; delivery of information to end users; and using education, right-to-know and right-to-act in introducing such programs. Individuals, agricultural communities, farm workers, nongovernmental organizations, and, of course, academic and governmental agencies would do well if they were to adopt the action program of Pesticide Action Network, the group that has made these recommendations.[28]

WHAT NEXT? THE NEED FOR ACTION

It would be a mistake to focus attention on pesticides alone in relation to crop yield. Pesticide use is only part of the revolution in modern agriculture, which is based on use of fertilizers, intensive cultivation, monocropping, irrigation, and mechanization.

Can the lessons from the story of more cotton yield per dunam cultivated be replicated? Can crop yields and profits be sustained while reducing pesticide use through integrated pest management or rediscovery of organic farming-type practices? In Israel and the PNA projects are needed that are based on the following elements:

(1) A uniform regional standard for health protection of workers and consumers.
(2) Joint assessments of health risk and crop yield in relation to pesticide risk.
(3) Training joint health-agricultural teams to introduce and evaluate crop growth and management based on reduced pesticide use.
(4) Tracing and stopping trade in banned or restricted pesticides.
(5) Restricting child labor.
(6) Promoting information delivery and worker-community right to know and right to act.
(7) Extending first-world bans and restrictions on pesticides to other countries.

In conclusion, work on introducing safe and sustainable alternatives to pesticide use, as well as reducing excessive dependence on chemical fertilizers, is long overdue. It should be based on two questions: Can agricultural productivity be sustained and increased as pesticide use, exposure, and risk are reduced? What new organizational frameworks at the local, national, and regional levels need to be created to deliver programs aimed at reducing pesticide-associated risks? Such work would be a fitting memorial to Dr. Selikoff.

REFERENCES

1. Richter, E. D. 1994. Sustainable agriculture and pesticides: Problems, perspectives and programs. *In* Our Shared Environment. R. Twite & J. Isaak, Eds.: 182–196. Israel/Palestine Center for Research and Information. Jerusalem.
2. Sansur, R. M., S. Kuttab & S. Abu-El-Haj. 1990. Extent of Exposure of Farm Workers to Organophosphate Pesticides in Jordan Valley in Impact of Pesticide Use on Health in Developing Countries: Symposium: 1313–1400. Bir Zeit University.
3. Abu-El-Haj, S. 1994. The pesticide dilemma: Complete reliance or total abandonment in our shared environment. R. Twite & J. Isaak, Eds.: 197–213. Israel/Palestine Center for Research and Information. Jerusalem.
4. Safi, J. M., Y. Z. Ed-Hahhal, S. A. Soliman & A. H. El-Sebae. 1993. Mutagenic and carcinogenic pesticides used in the agricultural environment of Gaza Strip. Sci. Total Environ. **132:** 371–380.
5. WHO-Europe. 1993. Organophosphorus pesticides: A multinational epidemiological study. E. D. Richter, Ed. WHO. Copenhagen.
6. Hunter, D. 1971. The Diseases of Occupations. 4th edit. English Universities Press.
7. Rose, G. 1985. Sick individuals and sick populations. Int. J. Epidemiol. **14**(1): 32–38.
8. Richter, E. D. & J. Safi. 1997. Pesticide use, exposure and risk: A joint Israeli-Palestinian perspective. Env. Res. **73:** 211–218.
9. Westin, J. B. & E. D. Richter. 1990. The Israeli breast cancer anomaly. Ann. N.Y. Acad. Sci. **609:** 269–279.
10. Westin, J. B. 1993. Carcinogens in Israeli milk: A study in regulatory failure. Int. J. Health Serv. **23:** 279–297.
11. Cohen, B., E. Richter & M. Luria. 1979. Sources of parathion exposures for Israeli aerial spray workers. Pestic. Monit. J. **13**(3): 81–86.
12. Richter, E. D., Z. Rosenvald, L. Kaspi, S. Levy & N. Gruener. 1986. Sequential cholinesterase tests and symptoms for monitoring organophosphate absorption in field workers and in persons exposed to pesticide spray drift. Toxicol. Lett. **33:** 25–35.
13. Ratner, D., P. Bar-Sella, A. Schneeyour, A. Karodontchik & E. Eshel. 1989. Seasonal variation in blood cholinestererase activity. Isr. J. Med. Sci. **5:** 247–250.
14. Richter, E. D., P. Chuwers, Y. Levy, N. Gruener, *et al.* 1992. Health effects from exposure to organophosphate pesticides in workers and residents in Israel. Isr. J. Med. Sci. **28**(8–9): 584–597.
15. Goldsmith, J. R., Y. Herishanu, J. M. Abarbanel & Z. Weinbaum. 1990. Clustering of Parkinson's disease points to environmental etiology. Arch. Environ. Health **45:** 88–89.
16. Meng, Z., F. Grauer, E. Ben-Michael & E. D. Richter. 1996. Alkyl phosphates and cholinesterase in workers exposed to organophosphate pesticides. *In* Proceedings of the 6th International Conference of the Israeli Society for Ecological and Environmental Quality Sciences VIA: 283–287.
17. Saleh, A., F. Neiroukh, O. Ayash & S. Gasteyer. 1995. Pesticide Usage in the West Bank. Applied Research Institute. Jerusalem.
18. Ziller, K. 1995. Pesticide Related Problems in the Palestinian Territories. UNDP/PAPP Contract No. 95/02/022. Monograph, UNDP. Jerusalem.
19. Abu-Quare, A. W. 1994. List of banned or restricted pesticides in many countries and still in use in West Bank and Gaza. Bir Zeit University Unit for Pesticide Chemistry.
20. Al Shuraiqi, Y. T. 1987. Evaluation of Residue Situation of the Most Frequently Used Pesticides on and in the Economically Important Fruits and Vegetables in Jordan. Ph.D. thesis, Rhine Friedrich-Wilhelms University, Bonn.
21. Jaqhabir, M. 1993. Skin residues of organophosphates in field workers. Bull. Environ. Contam. Toxicol.
22. Muszkat, L., E. Rosenthal, D. Roenen & M. Magaritz. 1989. Organic contaminants in the Israeli coastal aquifer. *In* Proceedings of the 4th International Conference of the Israeli Society for Ecological and Environmental Quality Sciences, IV: 471–479.

23. MUSZKAT, L., L. RAUCHER, M. BIR, M. MAGARITZ & D. RONEN. 1992. Liability of groundwater and depth of soil to contamination by pesticides and other organic xenobiotics: Two case histories. *In* Proceedings of the 5th International Conference of the Israeli Society for Ecological and Environmental Quality Sciences: 360-367.
24. WORLD RESOURCES INSTITUTE. 1994-1995. People and the Environment: Resource Consumption, Population Growth, Women: 116-117. Oxford University Press. New York.
25. GRAHAM, J. 1995. Risk in perspective: How should pesticides be regulated? Harvard Center for Risk Analysis **3:** 1-2.
26. PIMENTEL, D., M. ACQUAY, M. BILTONEN, P. RICE, M. SILVA, J. NELSON, V. LIPNER, S. GIORDANO, A. HOROWITZ & M. D'AMORE. 1992. Assessment of Environmental and Economic Impacts of Pesticide Use in The Pesticide Question: Environment, Economics, and Ethics. D. Pimentel & H. Lehman, Eds.: 47-83. Chapman Hall. New York.
27. SMITH, C. & S. L. BECKMANN. 1991. Export of Pesticides from U.S. Ports in 1990: Focus on Restricted Pesticide Exports. Report to the U.S. Senate Committee on Agriculture, Nutrition, and Forestry, September 20, 1991.
28. PESTICIDE ACTION NETWORK. 1993. The Demise of the Dirty Dozen. Pesticide Action Network. San Francisco.
29. THOMPSON, W. T. 1985-1986. Agricultural Chemicals, Book I: Insecticides. Thomson Publications. Fresno, CA.

Occupational Exposure to Pentachlorophenol: The Portuguese Situation[a]

ANTÓNIO JORGE FERREIRA,[b,c] DUARTE N. VIEIRA,[d]
ESTELA P. MARQUES,[e] AND ISABEL S. PEDRO[f]

[b]*Respiratory Diseases Department*
Coimbra University Hospital
Coimbra, Portugal

[d]*Institute of Forensic Medicine*
Coimbra, Portugal

[e]*Toxicology Laboratory*
Institute of Forensic Medicine
Coimbra, Portugal

[f]*C. S. Montemor e Velho*
Figueira da Foz, Portugal

Pentachlorophenol (PCP) is a widely used, very versatile, pesticide, having excellent characteristics for use as a fungicide, insecticide, herbicide, and for slime control. Its low price, good chemical stability, and water insolubility have given this toxic substance a wide variety of applications and a wide presence in almost all ecosystems.[1–4]

This product was first synthesized in the last century; however, it began to be used only in the 1930s. Its main use occurs in the industrial environment, as a general microbiocide in wood, canvas, cotton, rope, twine, and burlap preservation, and as an antifungal agent in the textile industry.[4] In Portugal, it is used mainly for the preservation of wood and wood products.

Portugal has important forest resources, and wood production and export are very important economically.[5,6] In recent years (1994), our country exported 1,635,000 tonnes of wood and wood products, of which approximately 600,000 tonnes were cut wood (''palettes'', boxes, construction materials, among others). The value of these exports has been rising, with an increase of 27% from 1993 to 1994. These facts lead to the conclusion that, in general, wood preservation and related matters are very important for our export income.

In Portugal, PCP was used for several years by the general population, because it was an ingredient in a number of special-purpose commercial products (used especially in hobbies involving wood materials). However, recent European Union

[a] This work was supported by Grant/Project No. 24/95 from Comissão de Fomento da Investigação em Cuidados de Saúde.

[c] Address for correspondence: Rua Miguel Torga, 64-8B, 3030 Coimbra, Portugal.

directives confined the use of PCP to wood preservation, chemical synthesis, *in situ* treatment of historical buildings, and the textile industry; so commercial products with PCP stopped being sold to the general population in recent years; but PCP is still by far the microbiocide most used in the preservation of wood products.[5,6]

Nevertheless, around 200 tonnes/year of PCP are currently being imported by one Portuguese company, and probably more has been imported from oriental sources, with significant contamination with dibenzodioxins and dibenzofurans. (This data is uncertain, with no official confirmation.)

PCP does not degrade and decompose completely. These processes are greatly influenced by several ambient conditions (pH, temperature, soil humidity, and oxygenation).[4] In a country with our patterns of PCP use, it is to be expected that this substance might be present in most of the unexposed population, and in higher levels in the exposed workers in the wood industry.

Indeed, some Portuguese authors refer to cases of occupational exposure, some with severe results. In 1980, Lima *et al.*[7] mentioned six fatal cases in the wood transformation industry, and Vieira *et al.*[8] also cited six acute cases of toxic exposure (two resulting in death) in the same line of work. Suicide with PCP is rare; Vieira *et al.*[9] allude to a case of intentional death following the ingestion of a PCP solution. The international literature cites a large number of toxic exposure cases, mainly related to occupational exposure.[1]

The toxicokinetic profile of PCP is characterized by quick absorption through inhalation, dermal, and oral exposure, with extensive plasma protein binding, possibly with limited forms of metabolism.[3,4]

In chronic exposure situations, some distinct clinical findings have been made. Dermatological findings include urticaria, *pemphigus vulgaris,* and chloracne.[10–13] Renal effects such as decrease in the renal clearance of creatinine and phosphorus absorption anomalies have been found, and respiratory tract irritation has been described.[14,15] Hematological findings include anemia, hematocrit reduction, severe pancytopenia, and bone marrow aplasia.[16–18] Some authors refer to statistically significant differences in some parameters of exposed populations (alkaline phosphatase, cholinesterase, gamma globulin, basophil count, and serum calcium).[17]

Although PCP is considered a known animal carcinogenic, in the human species data is not always in agreement. There may be some relation between PCP (and other chlorophenols) exposure and the development of soft-tissue sarcomas, Hodgkin's disease, non-Hodgkin's lymphoma, and leukemia. However, these studies could be of only limited value when analyzing the occupational risk associated only with known exposure to PCP.[4,19,20]

EXPERIMENTAL STUDY: METHODS

Population

We have studied two different populations, one occupationally exposed at a wood transformation unit in the central region of Portugal, the other formed by 10 individuals

TABLE 1. Workers Exposed to PCP

Workers	Age	Years of Exposure	Days/Week	Hours/Day
1	42	2	5	7
2	26	2	5	7
3	24	5	5	7
4	31	0.5	5	7
5	32	3	5	7
6	29	8	5	7
7	38	13	5	7
8	53	20	5	7
9	39	4	5	7
10	39	8	5	7
11	38	2	5	7
Mean	35.54	6.13		
SD	8.26	5.87		

TABLE 2. Chromatography Systems

	GC/ECD	GC/MS
Chromatograph	Pye Unicam, model 204	Hewlett-Packard, model 5890, series II
Column	filling (5 ft × 4 mm) with 6% QFI + 4% SE 30 in Gas Chrom Q, 80/100 mesh	Silica capilar (12.5 m × 0.2 mm methylsilicone)
Detector	ECD, Ni^{63}	MSD, model 5970 B
Ionization mode	—	electronic impact
Operation mode	—	selective ion monitoring (SIM)
Temperature (°C)		
Injector	250	250
Column	210	150 during 1 minute
Detector	250	
MSD transfer zone	—	280

NOTE: MSD = mass spectrometry detector

from the same region with no known exposure to this product (occupational or ambient).

TABLE 1 shows the constitution of the exposed population.

Analysis of Blood and Urine

Urine samples from the exposed population were obtained during a 24-hour period and were homogenized. Urine samples were collected from the unexposed population

TABLE 3. Levels of PCP in Exposed Population

Workers	Age	Years of Exposure	Urine (A) (μg/ml)	Urine (B) (μg/ml)	Blood (μg/ml)
1	42	2	5.566	4.723	6.884
2	26	2	0.312	0.333	1.388
3	24	50	0.753	0.760	1.748
4	31	0.5	0.139	0.148	1.393
5	32	3	0.834	0.925	0.244
6	29	8	0.953	0.920	3.647
7	38	13	0.070	0.083	0.133
8	53	20	1.350	1.269	3.958
9	39	4	1.182	1.167	2.064
10	39	8	1.785	1.729	3.101
11	38	2	0.222	0.365	0.459
Mean ± SD	35.54 ± 8.26	6.13 ± 5.87	1.197 ± 1.548	1.129 ± 1.1296	2.273 ± 2.015

TABLE 4. Levels of PCP in General Population

Sample	Age	Urine (A) (μg/ml)	Urine (B) (μg/ml)	Blood (μg/ml)
1	65	0.004	0.004	0.007
2	51	0.009	0.008	0.0011
3	56	0.005	0.004	0.094
4	66	0.004	0.003	0.006
5	16	0.031	0.032	0.017
6	81	0.003	0.002	0.005
7	86	0.002	0.002	0.003
8	82	0.002	0.002	0.003
9	66	0.001	0.002	0.003
10	70	0.003	0.002	0.006
Mean ± SD		0.0064 ± 0.0089	0.006 ± 0.0093	0.0153 ± 0.028

in the morning. Blood was drawn from a peripheral vein into a vacutainer tube. All samples were kept frozen until analysis.

The analytical procedures applied to these samples included gas chromatography/mass spectrometry with selective ion monitoring (GC/MS-SIM) and, for the samples with PCP values lower than 0.008 μg/ml, gas chromatography with electron capture detection (GC/ECD).

For blood analysis aliquots were extracted with *n*-hexane after acidification with sulphuric acid, adapting the method suggested by Rick *et al.*[21] First, 2,4,6-tribromophenol (TBF) was added as internal standard.

Two methods were used for urine sample extraction: (1) The sample was acidified with sulphuric acid and kept at room temperature for one hour before extraction with *n*-hexane. (2) Aliquots were treated in an adaptation of the hydrolysis method suggested by Butte.[22] Acidification was carried out with concentrated hydrochloric acid; after this procedure, the samples were heated for one hour at 95°C.

Derivatization was undertaken following an acetylation method (using acetic anhydride), with prior extraction using potassium carbonate. The final *n*-hexane extracts obtained were injected in the chromatography systems shown in TABLE 2. Two ions were measured: 266 and 308 for PCP; 332 and 374 for TBF.

RESULTS

The levels of PCP found in the two populations are shown in TABLE 3. The results of the general population are shown in TABLE 4

DISCUSSION

The techniques used for determination of PCP in urine and blood samples seem to be accurate, having low detection levels (around 1 - 2 ppb). The variation coefficients were found to be between 3 and 12%, slightly superior in the GC/MS system. PCP levels found in the two populations studied were roughly similar to those cited in international literature, as shown in TABLE 5. The values determined in the current investigation seem to show some correlation between blood and urine levels, with no relevant differences between the two urine analysis methods. The levels found in the two populations seem not to show marked differences when compared with similar populations in other countries.

TABLE 5. Urine and Serum PCP Levels as Reported in the Literature

n	Urine Value	Serum Value	Reference
Unexposed population			
248	3.21 ± 5.32 μg/g creatinine	–	Angerer *et al.*, 1992[23]
117	40 ± ?	–	Bevenue *et al.*, 1967[1]
30	< 0.25 mg/L	–	Chou & Bailey, 1986[24]
37	4.7 μg/L	8.9 μg/L	Colosio *et al.*, 1993[25]
5	< 1 μg/g creatinine	< 1 μg/L	Colosio *et al.*, 1993[26]
61	35 ± 53 ppb	–	Gilbert *et al.*, 1990[27]
50	25 ± 3.9 ng/ml	–	Gómez-Catalán *et al.*, 1987[28]
100	–	21.9 ± 1.9 ng/mL	Gómez-Catalán *et al.*, 1987[28]
197	14 ppb	–	Hill, Jr. *et al.*, 1989[29]
16	–	22 ± 16 ppb	Jorens *et al.* 1991[30]
32	0.03 ± 0.18 ppm	0.32 ± 1.259 ppm	Klemmer *et al.*, 1980 [17]
Exposed workers			
18 (last day of work exposure before vacation)	1.31 ± 1.08 ppm	5.14 ± 3.23 ppm	Begley *et al.*, 1977 [14]
18 (twentieth day of vacation	0.59 ± 0.6 ppm	2.19 ± 1.39 ppm	Begley *et al.*, 1977[14]
11 (vat dipping)	2.6 ppm	–	Casarett *et al.*, 1969[31]
11 (tank)	1.6 ppm	–	Caserett *et al.*, 1969[31]
32	142 μg/L	207.7 μg/L	Colosio *et al.*, 1993[25]
11 (at 8.00 hours)	175 μg/g creatinine	742 μg/L	Colosio *et al.*, 1993[26]
11 (at 17.00 hours)	106 μg/g creatinine	703 μg/L	Colosio *et al.*, 1993[26]
3 (airbone)	45 ± 15 ppb	–	Embree *et al.*, 1984[15]
3 (dermal)	105 ± 18 ppb	–	Embree *et al.*, 1984[15]
5 (airborne)	–	241 ± 232 ppb	Embree *et al.*, 1984[15]
5 (dermal)	–	714 ± 383 ppb	Embree *et al.*, 1984[15]
88	174 ± 342 ppb	–	Gilbert *et al.*, 1990[27]

TABLE 5. Urine and Serum PCP Levels as Reported in the Literature (*Continued*)

n	Urine Value	Serum Value	Reference
26 exposed formulators	39.6 ± ?mmol/mmol creatinine	—	Jones *et al.*, 1986[32]
29 exposed formulators	—	1.3 ± ?mmol/L	Jones *et al.*, 1986[32]
112 exposed sprayers	274 ± ?mmol/mmol creatinine	—	Jones *et al.*, 1986[32]
108 exposed sprayers	—	6 ± ?mmol/L	Jones *et al.*, 1986[32]
22 open vat wood treaters	—	3.78 ± 3.998 ppm	Klemmer *et al.*, 1980[17]
18 open vat wood treaters	0.95 ± 1.93 ppm	—	Klemmer *et al.*, 1980[12]
230	0.9–7.8 μmol/L	—	Lindroos *et al.*, 1987[33]
20	—	23–775μg/L	Ziemsen *et al.*, 1987[34]

REFERENCES

1. BEVENUE, A. & H. BECKMAN. 1967. Pentachlorophenol: A discussion of its properties and its occurrence as a residue in human and animal tissues. Residue Rev. **19:** 83-134.
2. CROSBY, D. G., K. I. BEYNON, P. A. GREVE, F. KORTE, G. G. STILL & J. W. VONK. 1981. Environmental chemistry of pentachlorophenol. Pure Appl. Chem. **53:** 1051-1080.
3. U. S. DEPARTMENT OF HEALTH AND HUMAN SERVICES. PUBLIC HEALTH SERVICE. 1992. Draft. Toxicological profile for pentachlorophenol.
4. WHO. 1987. Environmental Health Criteria, 71: Pentachlorophenol. International Programme on Chemical Safety, World Health Organization. Geneva.
5. PEIXOTO, F. R., M. M. A. PEDROSO, L. NUNES & J. A. SANTOS. 1990: Ensaio de eficácia de produtos de tratamento contra o azulamento do pinho bravo: 1-33. Associação Portuguesa de Comércio e Indústria de Madeiras. Lisbon.
6. PEIXOTO, F. R., M. M. A. PEDROSO, L. NUNES & J. A. SANTOS. 1988. Ensaio de eficiência de produtos de tratamento contra o azulamento do pinho bravo (produtos alternativos ao pentaclorofenol). Associação Portuguesa de Comércio e Indústria de Madeiras.
7. LIMA, A. P., M. T. AVILA, R. P. COSTA, E. P. MARQUES & E. V. PINTO. 1980. Intoxicação pelo Xilofene e Basilit PN. Coimbra Med. Serie IV: 175.
8. VIEIRA, D. N., E. P. MARQUES, M. T. AVILA & M. F. MARTINS. 1988. Intoxicações pelo PCP. XXIII Jornadas de Medicina do Trabalho da Figueira da Foz. Figueira da Foz, Portugal.
9. VIEIRA, D. N., E. P. MARQUES, R. AZEVEDO-BERNARDA & J. PINHEIRO. 1991. Suicídio por PCP: Estudio toxicologico e anatomopatologico de un caso. IX Jornadas toxicológicas Espanolas. Santiago de Compostela, Spain.
10. CARPENTER, A. V., M. O'MALLEY, M. SWEENEY, M. A. FINGERHUT & D. A. MARLOW. 1991. Further study of chloracne and pentachlorophenol operations Am. J. Ind. Med. **20:** 817.
11. KENTOR, P. M. 1996. Urticaria from contact with pentachlorophenate. JAMA **256:** 3350.
12. LAMBERT, J., P. SCHEPHENS, J. JANSSENS & P. DOCKX. 1986. Skin lesions as a sign of subacute pentachlorophenol intoxication. Acta Dermato-Venereol. **66:** 170-172.
13. LEET, T. L. & J. J. COLLINS. 1991. Chloracne and pentachlorophenol operations. Am. J. Ind. Med. **20:** 815-816.
14. BEGLEY, J., E. L. REICHERT, M. N. RASHAD, H. D. KLEMMER & A. W. SIEMSEN. 1977. Association between renal function tests and pentachlorophenol exposure. Clin. Toxicol. **11:** 97-106.
15. EMBREE, V., D. A. ENARSON, M. CHAN-YEUNG, A. DYBUNCIO, R. DENNIS & J. LEACH. 1984. Occupational exposure to chlorophenates: Toxicology and respiratory effects. Clin. Toxicol. **22:** 317-329.
16. HAY, A. & C. R. J. SINGER. 1991. Wood preservatives, solvents, and thrombocytopenic purpura. Lancet **338:** 766.
17. KLEMMER, H. W., L. WONG, M. M. SATO, E. L. REICHERT, R. J. KORSAK & M. N. RASHAD. 1980. Clinical findings in workers exposed to pentachlorophenol. Arch. Environ. Contam. Toxicol. **9:** 715-725.
18. ROBERTS, H. J. 1981. Aplastic anemia due to pentachlorophenol. N. Engl. J. Med. **305:** 1650-1651.
19. ERIKSSON, M., L. HARDELL & H. ADAMI. 1990. Exposure to dioxins as a risk factor for soft tissue sarcoma: A population based case-control study. J. Natl. Cancer Inst. **82:** 486-490.
20. ROBINSON, C. F., R. J. WAXWEILER & D. P. FOWLER. 1986. Mortality among production workers in pulp and paper mills. Scand. J. Work Environ. Health **12:** 552-560.
21. RICK, D. L., C. F. LICHT & L. P. MCCARTHY. 1982. Determination of phenol and pentachlorophenol in plasma and urine samples by liquid gas chromatography. J. Anal. Toxicol. **6:** 297-300.
22. BUTTE, W. 1984. Determination of free and total pentachlorophenol in urine. Fresenius Z. Anal. Chem. **59:** 562-569.

23. Angerer, J., B. Heinzow, D. O. Reimann, W. Knorz & G. Lehnert. 1992. Internal exposure to organic substances in a municipal waste incinerator. Int. Arch. Occup. Environ. Health **64:** 265-273.
24. Chou, P. P. & J. L. Bailey. 1986. Liquid-chromatographic determination of urinary pentachlorophenol. Clin. Chem. **32:** 1026-1028.
25. Colosio, C., M. Maroni, W. Barcellini, P. Meroni & D. Alcini. 1993. Toxicological and immune findings in workers exposed to pentachlorophenol (PCP). Arch. Environ. Health **48:** 81-88.
26. Colosio, C., F. Barbieri, M. Bersani, H. Schlitt & M. Maroni. 1991. Markers of occupational exposure to pentachlorophenol. Bull. Environ. Contam. Toxicol. **51:** 820-826.
27. Gilbert, Jr. F. I., C. E. Minn, R. C. Duncan & J. Wilkinson. 1990. Effects of pentachlorophenol and other chemical preservatives on the health of wood-treating workers in Hawaii. Arch. Environ. Contam. Toxicol. **19:** 603-609.
28. Gomez-Catalán, J., J. To-Figueras, J. Planas, M. Rodamilans & J. Corbella. 1987. Pentachlorophenol and hexachlorobenzene in serum and urine of the population of Barcelona. Hum. Toxicol. **6:** 397-400.
29. Hill, Jr. R. H., T. To, J. S. Holler, D. M. Fast, S. J. Smith, L. L. Needham & S. Binder. 1989. Residues of chlorinated phenols and phenoxi acid herbicides in the urine of Arkansas children. Arch. Environ. Contam. Toxicol. **18:** 469-474.
30. Jorens, P. G., J. J. Janssens, I. Wouter, van Tichelen, W. van Paesschen, P. P. De Deyn & P. J. C. Schepens. 1991. Pentachlorophenol concentrations in human cerebrospinal fluid. Neurotoxicology. **12:** 1-8.
31. Casarett, L. J., A. Bevenue, W. L. Yauger, Jr. & S. A. Whalen. 1969. Observations on pentachlorophenol in human blood and urine. Am. Ind. Hyg. Assoc. J. **30:** 360-366.
32. Jones, R. D., D. P. Winter & A. J. Cooper. 1986. Absorption study of pentachlorophenol in persons working with wood preservatives. Hum. Toxicol. **5:** 189-194.
33. Lindroos, L., H. Koskinen, P. Mutanen & J. Jarvisalo. 1987. Urinary chlorophenols in sawmill workers. Int. Arch. Occup. Environ. Health **59:** 463-467.
34. Ziemsen, B., J. Angerer & G. Lehnert. 1987. Sister chromatid exchange and chromosomal breakage in pentachlorophenol (PCP) exposed workers. Int. Arch. Occup. Environ. Health **59:** 413-417.

Dibromochloropropane: Epidemiological Findings and Current Questions

JOHN R. GOLDSMITH [a]

Department of Epidemiology
Faculty of Health Sciences
Ben Gurion University of the Negev
P.O.B. 653
Beer Sheva 84105, Israel

INTRODUCTION

Communication between scientific specialists seems to stand in the way of effective use of our knowledge for prevention of health damage from the increasing use of chemical agents. Prevention seems to be treated as a matter of ideology, rather than as a principle to which our knowledge commits us. Experience with the agent dibromochloropropane (DBCP) illustrates our inadequacies, if not our incompetence. Bernardino Ramazzini, that incomparable seventeenth-century clinician, founder of the specialty of occupational medicine, might well cringe with shame could he hear this tale of the triumph of selfishness and irresponsibility over the humane use of medical knowledge.

We can still be true to the spirit of Ramazzini if, in reviewing the story and learning from the errors it documents, we vow to avoid these pitfalls in the future.

Part of the problem can be said to be the failure of communication between toxicologists, epidemiologists, endocrinologists and other clinicians.

I recall a conversation with the late Dr. Charles Hine from the University of California at San Francisco about 1960 at a party, when he said, "If anyone wants to use a male birth control drug, I think we have identified one, but it is not very pleasant to use." Dr. Hine at that time was doing toxicological work for Shell Development. DBCP was the drug. The results to which he was referring were published by Torkelson *et al.* in 1961.[1]

In 1976, production workers recognized that they had become infertile and sought medical help. The quantitative basis for this was reported by Whorton *et al.* in 1977 for California production workers[2] and by Potashnik *et al.* for Israeli production workers in 1978.[3]

Both sets of studies showed the progressive loss of spermatogenesis with increased duration of exposure. Pathological changes in spermatogenic cells and Sertoli cells were found on biopsy. This was accompanied with compensatory increases in follicle stimulating hormone (FSH) and luteinizing hormone (LH). Progressive drop in sperm count was felt to be a suitable indicator for the extent of gonadotoxicity.

[a] Phone: 972-7/640-0876; fax: 972-7/6277342; e-mail: gjohn@bgumail.bgu.ac.il

The number of production workers was small compared to the several thousands of agricultural workers *in California alone* who were exposed during the application of over 450,000 kg of DBCP to more that 20,000 hectares.

CALIFORNIA APPLICATORS STUDY 1977

A team from the California Department of Health, the United States Centers for Disease Control, the Environmental Protection Agency, and the California Department of Food and Agriculture set out to study pesticide applicators in five counties in California, each of which had reported heavy use of DBCP during 1976-1977.[4] Twenty-two firms employed the men, and, of these, twenty agreed to cooperate in the study. Originally the study was to have included 50 applicators who used DBCP in the previous 8-12 months and 50 other applicators with no recorded use of the agent, but of the same age group and employed in the same area. It turned out that a number of the presumably nonexposed workers really *were* exposed, so the design was altered to compare groups of workers according to the number of days of DBCP exposure in the current year, as determined from current work histories. Among the 96 men who came for examination and provided a semen specimen, results were the same for the whole cohort as for 31 age- and location-matched pairs.

Of the ten men with clinical infertility, two had sperm counts of less than one million, and one of them had a long-standing (prior to first exposure to DBCP) azospermia. Two of the remaining seven had no history of DBCP exposure. Four additional men had sperm counts below a million, but did not complain of infertility; of these, three had substantial DBCP exposures and the fourth only brief exposure.

Extensive DBCP exposure in the current year was significantly correlated with sperm count depression ($p < 0.01$). When the men were divided in four classes by exposure time, those with more than 2 months' exposure had significantly depressed counts; 11 irrigators who also worked in grapes and orchards were responsible for most of the occupationally significant exposures.

Ten specimens showed morphological abnormalities, but these were not correlated with sperm count depression or exposure. When data were classified according to 0, 1-29, and 30+ days of exposure FSH increased significantly with days of exposure, and LH also increased, but not significantly. There was no significant association of sperm count with number of years of exposure in the past when current year's exposure is included in the analysis.

The authors concluded that infertility was not a problem in this group. Concerning the lack of much effect of exposures in previous years, the authors wrote: "If the toxicity of DBCP were irreversible, we would have expected applicators with several years of experience to be more severely affected than applicators with only recent contact. This was not observed, which suggests that the sperm count in these men will return to normal. Repeat semen analyses on men with severely depressed sperm counts are needed to verify this conclusion."[4]

BANANA PLANTATION WORKERS STUDY, ISRAEL 1978

Following the reports of Wharton *et al.*[2] and Potashnik *et al.*,[3] the Israel Ministry of Labor in 1977 banned the production and use of DBCP. Because of the damage from the nematode *Heliocotylenchus multicintus* to banana plantations, an exception was made for application from May to July for that one crop alone. Protective clothing was required, and closed systems were used, with the material applied with irrigation water.

Cooperation was obtained from the banana-growing kibbutzim in the Jordan Valley, and 102 married banana workers from 14 kibbutzim were identified.[5] A total of 62 of the men were available for interview as to their exposure histories and the reproductive histories of their wives. Data on reproductive outcomes were also obtained from the regional hospital. Of a total of 76 pregnancies prior to the husbands' DBCP exposure, spontaneous abortion occurred among 5 (6.6%) in women of mean age of 25.6 years. But of 121 pregnancies after the men first had exposure to DBCP, there were 24 spontaneous abortions (19.8%), a highly significant increase. The mean age of postexposure mothers was 28.3, but this increase in abortions was far greater than could be accounted for by the normal increase of spontaneous abortion with maternal age. For a subset of couples, n = 16, with pregnancies both prior to and after first exposure, thus likely to have no other risk factor difference, 2 spontaneous abortions in 34 pregnancies (5.9%) occurred preexposure, and 11 spontaneous abortions among 40 pregnancies (27.5%) occurred after first exposure of the husband to DBCP, also a significant difference. No differences were found for interconception intervals before and after first exposure. Three men reported that at one time or another they had had a fertility problem; in one couple this preceded the exposure to DBCP. The men reported laboratory tests to be normal. In each case the first pregnancy ended with spontaneous abortion, and one of the two exposed men subsequently fathered a healthy child. No differences were found for postexposure and preexposure live births in sex, birth weight, type of delivery, congenital anomalies, diseases at birth, prematurity, or infant mortality.

These workers were exposed for relatively brief periods of the year, and if recovery from the toxic effects could occur as suggested by Glass *et al.*,[5] during much of the year they may have had no toxic effects. Resources were not available for sperm counts.

EFFECTS FOUND AMONG ISRAELI PRODUCTION WORKERS

Potashnik *et al.*[6] initially found that the more continuous exposures of production workers were closely associated with a drop in sperm count and, if sufficiently protracted, to oligospermia (sperm count 10 million or less), azospermia, and sterility. Among the pregnancies that did occur among these workers, increased spontaneous abortion was not found. After the cessation of exposures to DBCP, 30 workers were followed for *five years;* for some of them with azospermia or oligospermia, spermatogenesis recovered and they fathered children. While the babies born after initiation of exposure were otherwise healthy, 11 out of 13 were females, a highly significant shift in sex ratio.[7,8] Assuming the probability of boys and girls to be equal, $p = 0.011$.

Fifteen men with azospermia ($n = 8$) or oligospermia ($n = 7$) followed *eight years* after exposure were all found to be in good physical condition.[9] Three initially azospermic men recovered and fathered 10 children. The recovered men had exposure times of 114, 120, and 390 hours, and mean FSH levels in 1977 of 9.3 ± 2.9 mIU/ml, while the five who did not recover had exposure times of 100, 120, 618, 901, and 1504 hours and mean FSH levels in 1977 of 20.8 ± 5.3. Five of the seven oligospermic men recovered and fathered 12 children; all of the five had exposures of less than 100 hours, while the two who did not recover were exposed for 220 and 310 hours. No difference in FSH levels were found for the recovered and persistently oligospermic men. Reported recovery times were from 14 to 45 months. Of 19 live births completed during recovery (there were two therapeutic abortions and one uncomplicated ongoing pregnancy), 4 were male and 15 female. Assuming the probability of boys and girls to be equal, $p = 0.010$. The children born during recovery were all in good health.

In a 17-year follow-up of nine formerly azospermic and 6 formerly oligospermic men from this cohort, Potashnik and Porath[10] did not find recovery of spermatogenesis for additional men. The 3 recovered azospermic men fathered 5, 5, and 8 additional children (the latter with a second wife), thus contributing during recovery 9, 8, and 11 children overall. One of the originally oligospermic men fathered 8 additional children, bringing his total to 13. Of a total of 48 recorded pregnancies for the 7 recovered men, there were 6 spontaneous abortions, 1 fetal death, and 17 out of 41 male babies, for a male sex ratio of 41.4%. This suggests some recovery in whatever mechanism was responsible for alteration in the sex ratio.

DISCUSSION

Such changes in the sex ratio of a small population exposed to a toxin should be evaluated in the context of the overall population sex ratio. In virtually every population studied, there is a slight excess of newborn males. Medawar[11] cites as the sex ratio the number of live born boys per 1000 live born girls. The ratio was 1038 in Britain during 1911–1915 and rose to 1051 in the next 5-year period. Part of this wartime increase in boy babies may have been related to the higher ratio, 1074 for mothers under 20, compared to 1026 for mothers between 40 and 44. These "physiological" changes in sex ratio are really quite small compared to the changes produced by DBCP.

Recently, observations on the sex ratio of families with pesticide exposures have shown that those with greater exposures tend to have a longer interpregnancy interval (evidence of hypofecundicity) and more girls than they do boys.[12,13] Such observations may be a very sensitive way of studying sex ratio, but covariates such as age of parents should still be checked.

Thus a single agent to which working men have been exposed has numerous different outcomes, all of which are related to the known testicular toxicity. Decreased sperm count was found in both production workers and applicators, along with secondary increases in FSH and LH. Recovery of testicular function and fertility is less likely if FSH levels are high. Sterility has resulted among production workers, but in the two applicator studies reported here it was not observed. Spontaneous abortion was found to be more frequent in one set of applicators, but not in the smaller population of production workers. Spontaneous abortion was not enquired about in the initial study of applicators. Finally, in one set of recovering production workers, a high proportion of live births resulted in female children. The proportion seemed to be related to the duration of exposures. As recovery proceeded, there seemed to be less effect on sex ratio. The numbers of years of exposure seemed less important in the study of decreased sperm count in applicators, presumably because they had sufficient time with no exposure to allow for some recovery.

Experimental studies of effects related to spontaneous abortion and sex ratio changes from DBCP have not been reported. Thus, originally the toxicological studies were not taken seriously; the result was extensive use, followed by epidemiological evidence of gonadal toxicity. Aspects of that toxicity seem not to have attracted the experimental attention that would have been expected.

DBCP is an animal carcinogen. Fortunately, until now large numbers of humans have not been exposed with a long enough latency period so that excess human cancer could be demonstrated. Olsen *et al.*[14] have reported on the mortality of 548 potentially exposed chemical plant employees. No overall increase in mortality or cancer occurred, but of the 81 with direct exposure, 3 developed lung cancer compared to 0.9 expected. Two of these men were known to be long-term cigarette smokers; for the third there was no smoking history. Wesseling *et al.*[15] are studying a large population of banana workers in Costa Rica–29,565 men and 4,822 women. Cancer among men is less than expected and among women more than expected based on the National Cancer Registry. Nonsignificant increases were found for men for melanoma and penile cancer; and for women for leukemia and cervical cancer. Follow-up of the cohort is continuing.

DBCP is also a potent mutagen. The prompt onset of reduced sperm counts after exposure provides a warning, and avoidance of such effects should make an important contribution to prevention of DBCP-related cancer. This principle of using unfavorable reproductive outcomes (UROs) as sentinel events for protection against cancer is being used for other suspected carcinogens. Similarly, the increase in female births is being observed among workers exposed to other and unspecified pesticides in association with orchard spraying in Holland and South Africa. Reversal of such effects presumably is preventive with respect to cancer.

QUESTIONS RAISED BY THESE FINDINGS

1. Is the sex ratio change due to a specific toxic effect, or is it primarily a reflection of low sperm count?
2. Given that there is evidence that some effects of DBCP are reversible, is this repair capacity universal, and are there likely to be long-term consequences of repeated exposures?
3. Does DBCP have a toxic effect on oocytes?
4. How can one best study analogues of spontaneous abortion in experimental animals?
5. Are the spermatogenic effects of DBCP a sufficient sentinel for cancer risk?
6. What legal and administrative procedures are needed in order to prevent further damage from this agent?
7. What other agents have similar patterns of effects, and how can what we have learned be best used for protection?

8. What sort of evidence of predominance of female births is needed to guide a preventive program?

The importance of cancer prevention makes it all the more appalling to learn that the experiences in Israel and the United States (and other Western countries) are being ignored in subtropical countries such as Honduras, Costa Rica, the Ivory Coast, and the Philippines. Thousands of banana field workers have not only been exposed to this carcinogen, but have been rendered sterile as a result of this exposure. Since sterility was not found for the applicators in either California or Israel, it must follow that the exposures in this new wave are more persistent or larger than they were in California or Israel. One can only see this as retrogression in occupational health and take the most vigorous steps to assure that this selfish policy becomes too costly for those who are engaged in it. Anything less is professionally irresponsible.

SUMMARY

Dibromochloropropane, DBCP, has had a seminal role in our current understanding of how to prevent chemical risks to health. Early toxicological studies showed its special impact on the testes, and detection of its mutagenic potency was soon followed by demonstration of its carcinogenicity to animals. Its commercial use as a useful nematocide ignored, at first, these warnings from the laboratory. When production workers, first in California and then in Israel, found they were sterile as a result of their exposure, this was convincing evidence that prevention had failed. The evidence, azospermia, oligospermia, and gonadotrophin response to testicular damage, were found first in production workers. In agricultural applicators in California who used the material, decreased sperm count and increased gonadotrophin levels were found. While production in California, Texas, and Israel was halted, studies continued and so, it seems, did use. Our first Israeli study was of workers on banana crops, and we found convincing evidence of increased spontaneous abortion in their family histories. Follow-up studies among production workers in Israel showed that some recovered testicular function, but among their offspring, otherwise in good health, there was a predominance of females. Those who did not recover from azospermia were those with high levels of follicle stimulating hormone. However data for production workers did not show increased spontaneous abortion. Nor have any studies so far shown increased birth defects or increased infant mortality. Unfavorable reproductive outcomes can be due to other agents, as shown by sprayers in Dutch orchards having hypofecundity (increased interpregnancy period) and sex ratio changes; but the agents responsible have not yet been identified.

These experiences have lead to the general acceptance of some implications: (1) Paternal exposures can lead to a variety of unfavorable effects on reproductive outcome, including infertility, spontaneous abortion, and altered sex ratio. (2) Patterns of effects of potent agents in production workers and in applicators or users of chemicals may differ. (3) Although human carcinogenesis has not yet been confirmed, unfavorable reproductive outcomes are a reasonable early indicator of such risk. (4) Shifts in sex ratios of populations may be a subtle sign of more serious risks. (5) Continued use of an agent such as this under circumstances in which these UROs cannot be prevented is unconscionable.

REFERENCES

1. TORKELSON T. R., S. E. SADEK, V. K. ROWE, J. K. KODAMA, H. H. ANDERSON, G. S. LOZUVAM & C. H. HINE. 1961. Toxicologic investigations of 1,2 dibromochloropropane. J. Toxicol. Appl. Pharmacol. **3:** 549-559.
2. WHORTON, D., R. M. KRAUSS, S. MARSHALL & T. H. MILBY. 1977. Infertility in male pesticide workers. Lancet. **ii:** 1259.
3. POTASHNIK, G., N. BEN-ADERET, R. ISRAELI, I. YANAI-INBAR & I. SOBER. 1978. Suppressive effect of 1,2 dibromo-3-chloropropane on human spermatogenesis. Fertil. Steril. **30:** 444-447.
4. GLASS, R. I., R. N. LYNESS, D. C. MENGLE, K. E. POWELL & E. KAHN. 1979. Sperm count depression in pesticide applicators exposed to dibromochloropropane. Am. J. Epidemiol. **109:** 346-351.
5. KHARRAZI, M., G. POTASHNIK & J. R. GOLDSMITH. 1980. Reproductive effects of dibromochloropropane. Isr. J. Med. Sci. **16:** 403-406.
6. POTASHNIK, G. 1983. A four-year reassessment of workers with dibromochloropropane-induced testicular dysfunction. Andrologia **15:** 164-170.
7. POTASHNIK, G., J. GOLDSMITH & V. INSLER. 1984. Dibromochloropropane-induced reduction of the sex-ratio in man. Andrologia **16:** 213-218.
8. GOLDSMITH, J. R., G. POTASHNIK & R. ISRAELI. 1984. Reproductive outcomes in families of DBCP exposed men. Arch. Environ. Health **39:** 85-89.
9. POTASHNIK, G. & H. YANAI-INBAR. 1987. Dibromochloropropane (DBCP): An eight year reevaluation of testicular function and reproductive performance. Fertil. Steril. **47:** 317-322.
10. G. POTASHNIK & A. PORATH. 1995. Dibromochloropropane (DBCP): A 17-year reassessment of testicular function and reproductive performance. J. Occup. Environ. Med. **37:** 1287-1292.
11. MEDAWAR, P. 1960. The Future of Man. Basic Books. New York.
12. DE COCK, J., K. WESTVEER, E. TE VELDE & R. VAN KOOIJ. 1994. Time to pregnancy and occupational exposures to pesticides in fruit growers in The Netherlands. Occup. Environ. Med. **51:** 693-699.
13. DE COCK, J., D. HEEDERIK, E. TIELEMANS, E. VELDE & R. VAN KOOIJ. 1995. Offspring sex ratio as an indicator of reproductive hazards associated with pesticides (Abstr.). Epidemiology **6:** S110.
14. OLSEN, G. W., K. M. BODNER, B. A. STAFFORD, J. B. CARTMILL & M. R. GONDEK. 1995. Update of the mortality experience of employees with occupational exposure to dibromochloropropane (DBCP). Am. J. Ind. Med. **28:** 399-410.
15. WESSELING, C., A. AHLBOM, D. ANTICH, A. C. RODRIGUEZ & R. CASTRO. 1996. Cancer in Banana Plantation workers in Costa Rica. Int. J. Epidemiol. **25:** 1125-1131.

Liver and Kidney Function Tests as a Tool for Periodic Health Evaluation of Laboratory Workers

A. PINES,[a,e] D. ALKASLASSY,[a,c] M. KLEBANOV,[a]
C. LEMESCH,[a,b] J. RIBAK,[d] AND Y. LERMAN[d]

[a]*General Health Insurance Fund*
Occupational Medicine Clinic
Jerusalem, Israel 91440

[b]*Ministry of Labour and Social Affairs*
Jerusalem, Israel 91008

[c]*Ministry of Health*
Ha-Dov Street
Jerusalem, Israel 96952

[d]*Department of Epidemiology and Preventive Medicine*
Sackler School of Medicine
101 Arlozorov Street
Tel-Aviv, Israel 62092

INTRODUCTION

A laboratory can be somewhat loosely defined as "a building or part of a building equipped to conduct scientific experiments, tests, investigations, etc., or to manufacture chemicals, medicines, or the like."[1] All those employed at such premises are considered for the purposes of this paper as laboratory workers.

During the last decades laboratory workers have become a subject of concern for occupational health services due to their probable, but rather poorly documented, association with the excessive development of various malignancies[2–4] and adverse reproductive outcomes.[5–7] Media interest in alleged clusters of such events in specific institutions contributed significantly to the wide public interest in the subject.

While studies on the mortality of laboratory workers and related occupational groups are scarce and not always consistent, investigations of the health status of these populations are almost nonexistent. As a matter of fact, up to now no answer exists as to whether laboratory work affects the health conditions of those engaged in it. This great gray area in occupational health reflects the real-life situations, whereas any epidemiological study of the probable relationships between laboratory work and its potential health effects has to deal with a number of common methodological obstacles, intrinsic to the virtuality of laboratory work. Among these obstacles are:

[e]Address for correspondence: A. Pines, M.D., General Health Insurance Fund, Occupational Medicine Clinic, P.O. Box 44016, Jerusalem, Israel 91440. Phone: 972-2/571-3694; fax: 972-2/571-3906; e-mail: tola@inter.net.il

- The diversity of laboratories by type, size, functional objectives, and methods of investigation interferes with the basic requirements of epidemiological study, such as the homogeneity of any subject population of sufficient size.
- Whereas chemical hazards are predominant, a large variety of chemicals being used simultaneously or in succession should be considered. The toxic properties of most or even all of these chemicals may be well known, but the type of possible health effects resulting from their interactions in the human body remains obscure.
- The common pattern of laboratory work is characterized by short-term, relatively intense exposures to specific chemical(s), followed by long periods of nearly zero exposure to this (those) chemical(s). The time-weighted average of laboratory exposures are presumed and proved[8] to be low or very low, sometimes below the detectability level. The toxicological consequences of such intermittent exposure are poorly understood in most cases. Whereas multiple exposures are considered, composite pictures of highs and lows are unknown.

From the previous considerations it follows that neither environmental measurements nor the results of biological monitoring can be used to assess the potential health risks associated with laboratory work.

It can be assumed from the preceding discussion that quantitative hazard evaluation of the laboratory environment, in particular where research laboratories are concerned, appears to be a virtually unattainable goal. At the same time, assessment of the health risks associated with laboratory employment remains not only a long-term objective but a daily requirement of the occupational health services. Detection of early nonspecific changes in the various organs and bodily functions of laboratory workers and the evaluation of their causal relationships with chronic occupational exposure, as well as their significance to the workers' health, appears to be the only available method for risk assessment in this occupational group.

The purpose of this paper is to assess, from the preceding point of view, how useful routine laboratory liver and kidney function tests are for health screening and long-term health surveillance of laboratory workers.

MATERIALS AND METHODS

Study Population

The study included 783 persons employed at scientific research, industrial research, and applied medicobiological laboratories in the Jerusalem region in Israel who had undergone periodic medical examination in the Jerusalem Occupational Health Clinic *at least* once during the years 1980 to 1996. In all these laboratories the main type of exposure was a chemical one, with organic solvents, in particular aromatic hydrocarbons, being the most common. Among these two-thirds of the subjects were strictly laboratory workers, whereas one-third were clerical and managerial staff at the same laboratories. It was originally hypothesized that the latter composed a control group, rather than a study population, but analysis[8] showed just the opposite: only two out of 29 hematological and biochemical variables compared differed significantly between these subgroups, while 27 variables were similar (sign test: $p < 0.001$). Therefore these two study subpopulations were considered to be identical.

In order to judge on normal values of the concerned variables common for Jerusalem population and to assess the influence on them of potential confounders, e.g., age and sex, a control group comprising 1393 persons (47% of them clerical workers and 43% skilled and unskilled laborers) was examined. No known hazardous occupational exposure was reported, for examinees included in the control group.

Age distribution in both groups was almost identical (FIG. 1), but sex distribution was not: males comprised about two-thirds of the control group, but only half of the laboratory workers.

Approximately half of the examined laboratory workers were employed at the current laboratory for not more than two years, while those employed for more than 10 years constituted one-fifth of the total group. With regard to seniority (longevity) it should be noted that:

- duration of laboratory employment was considered to be the best available quantitative exposure estimate;
- from the point of view of exposure assessment, the term *seniority* has no meaning with respect to the control group;
- no data were available concerning the length of laboratory employment of laboratory workers, so duration of current employment, being the only available measure, may be a source of assessment error.

Three hundred and forty-four laboratory workers underwent additional medical examinations during the study period, as a routine of periodic medical examinations of workers exposed to hazardous factors in their working environment. Frequency distribution of these exams is presented in FIGURE 2.

Methods

The epidemiological design of the study was conceived as a bipartite one with two major components:

- a cross-sectional, baseline examination of laboratory workers and control group;
- a historical cohort study of laboratory workers for a period of one to fifteen years.

The findings analyzed in this paper include the results of routine liver [activity of the serum glutamic oxalocetic transaminase (SGOT), alkaline phosphatase (AP), lactate dehydrogenase (LDH), gamma-glutamyl transpeptidase (GGTP)] and kidney (blood serum levels of urea and creatinine) function tests usually applied in medical screening and periodic surveillance of chemically exposed workers, such as laboratory workers. These results were subjected to comprehensive statistical scrutiny in order to obtain valid conclusions. The differences between the groups were considered statistically significant when the probability of the first type of error was lower than 5% ($p < 0.05$). Time trends were evaluated in the follow-up examinations by applying a simple linear regression model. Age, seniority, and span were used as alternate

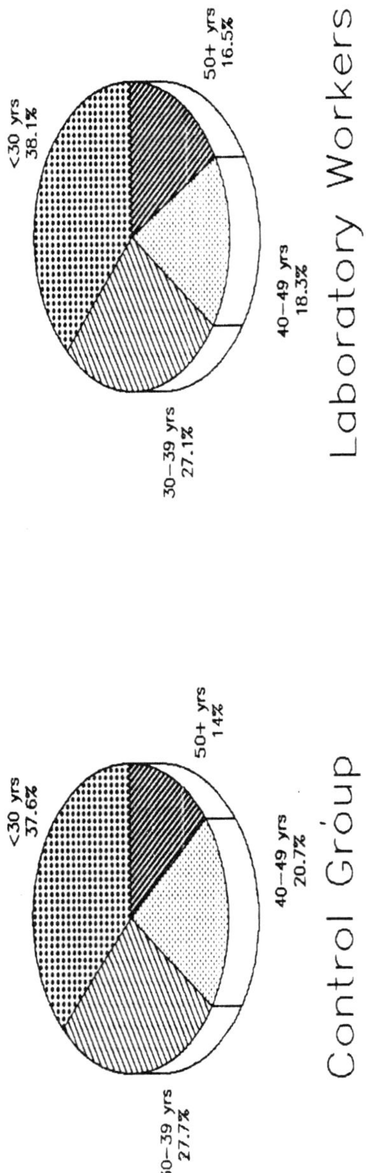

FIGURE 1. Distribution of the examined population by age.

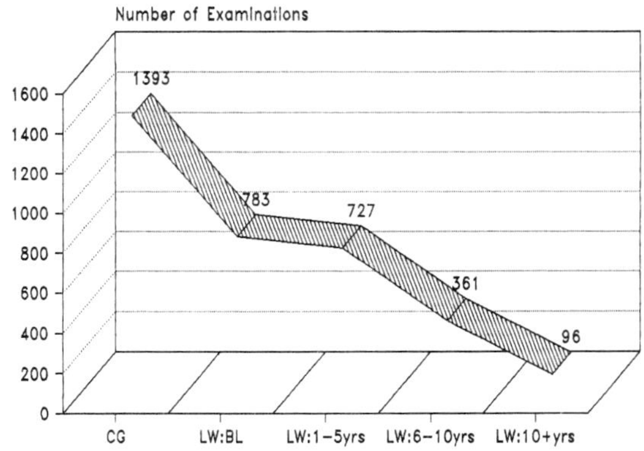

FIGURE 2. Number of examinations by exposure and duration of follow-up. CG = control group; LW = laboratory workers; BL = baseline; 1-5, 6-10, 10+ yrs = duration of follow-up.

independent (time) variables in this model. The term "span" was introduced to denote the time lapsed between *i*-examination and the first one. Age and seniority were determined for each examinee by subtracting the year of birth or the year of onset of current employment, respectively, from the year of inclusion in the study group, that is, from the year of the first examination. Age and seniority with respect to specific examination were calculated similarly, but instead of the year of the first examination, the year of the *i*-examination was used.

All statistical processing was performed with the help of SPSS (Statistical Package for Social Sciences, Chicago) release 6.0 for Windows.

RESULTS

It may be seen from the TABLE 1 that mean levels of activity of all four liver enzymes at a baseline examination were the same or somewhat lower than in the control group. During the follow-up period they changed in a very similar pattern: almost no change within first five years, moderate changes in the five-ten year period, and a manifest rise in activity (compared both to control group or to baseline levels) during the period of ten or more years. It should be noted that even in this latter group, mean enzyme activity levels in blood did not exceed the normal range.

While individual enzyme activity levels were considered, the number of values in excess of the upper normal limit followed a similar pattern of change. (FIG. 3).

Changes in kidney function tests (TABLE 2) appeared to be inconsistent: while urea tended to decrease in the follow-up examinations, creatinine, on the contrary, exhibited a slight upward trend. No characteristic pattern in individual urea- and creatinine-level changes was observed during the follow-up.

Time trends were investigated with respect to the potential influence of gender on the dependent variables. Therefore regression coefficients were calculated for each of the genders separately and for both together. For the sake of brevity, TABLE 3 presents only the slopes and their standard errors for the combined population data.

TABLE 1. Summary of Liver Function Tests

		Laboratory Workers										
	Control Group	Baseline		1-5 Years Follow-up			6-10 Years Follow-up			10+ Years Follow-up		
Tests	Mean (SE)	Mean (SE)	p vs. CG	Mean (SE)	p vs. CG	p vs. BL	Mean (SE)	p vs. CG	p vs. BL	Mean (SE)	p vs. CG	p vs. BL
GGTP	17.0 (0.34)	14.8 (0.51)	↓↓↓	15.5 (0.61)	NS	NS	16.4 (0.57)	NS	↑	19.5 (1.28)	NS	↑↑
SGOT	15.7 (0.18)	15.7 (0.31)	NS	15.6 (0.24)	NS	NS	16.0 (0.40)	NS	NS	20.0 (0.88)	↑↑↑	↑↑↑
AP	61.2 (0.53)	51.3 (0.66)	↓↓↓	52.3 (0.78)	↓↓↓	NS	58.1 (1.01)	↓↓	↑↑↑	74.2 (3.87)	↑↑↑	↑↑↑
LDH	198.5 (1.41)	192.1 (1.76)	↓↓↓	200.4 (1.76)	NS	↑↑	212.2 (4.07)	↑↑	↑↑↑	288.5 (7.46)	↑↑↑	↑↑↑

NOTES:
Test results are expressed in IU.
CG = control group; BL = baseline examination of laboratory workers.

Statistical significance testing of follow-up findings:

	$p > 0.05$	$p < 0.05$	$p < 0.01$	$p < 0.001$
Higher than CG or BL:	NS	↑	↑↑	↑↑↑
Lower than CG or BL:	NS	↓	↓↓	↓↓↓

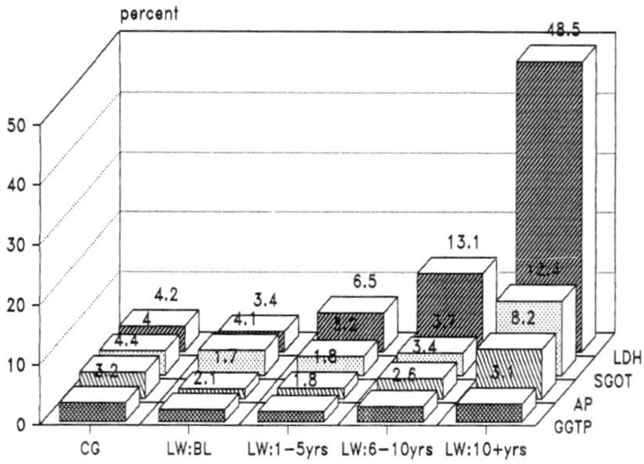

FIGURE 3. Frequency of abnormal enzyme values (in excess for the upper normal limit; mean + 2 SD for the control group). CG = control group; LW = laboratory workers; BL = baseline; 1–5, 6–10, 10+ yrs = duration of follow-up.

b-coefficients were somewhat higher, though not statistically significant, in females as compared with males, with the exception of SGOT in laboratory workers.

Age did not appear to be a satisfactory predictor of changes in enzyme activity levels, with the exception of GGTP in the control group, and LDH and AP in laboratory workers. The latter enzymes were as satisfactory predicted by seniority and even better by span (FIG. 4). The strength of all these effects should not be overestimated: the determination coefficient (R^2) was as low as 0.069–0.081 (i.e., the time trend accounted for 7 to 8% of the total variation of these variables). Time-associated effects in the variability of SGOT and GGTP were considerably lower ($R^2 = 0.007$–0.017).

Age appeared to be a statistically significant, though slight predictor of changes in urea and creatinine blood serum levels in the control group. In laboratory workers this was true for urea, and not only for age but for seniority as well (TABLE 3).

The strength of the associations between the levels of enzyme activity in the blood was in general low, though statistically significant, because of the large number of examinations in each (sub)group. It should be pointed out that in the control group the only essential correlation was observed between AP and SGOT ($r = 0.59$), while in the laboratory workers it was low. A small but essential correlation emerged instead between LDH and SGOT ($r = 0.32$), which repeated in all follow-up subgroups: $r = 0.22$ in baseline and 1–5 yr subgroups, with twofold increases in 5–10 and 10 yr and more span subgroups ($r = 0.45$).

DISCUSSION

The main findings of this study may be briefly summarized as follows.

In the baseline examination, statistically significant lower values as compared with the control group were observed in the blood serum levels of three (GGTP, AP,

TABLE 2. Summary of Kidney Function Tests

		Laboratory Workers										
	Control Group	Baseline		1–5 Years Follow-up			6–10 Years Follow-up			10+ Years Follow-up		
Tests	Mean (SE)	Mean (SE)	p vs. CG	Mean (SE)	p vs. CG	p vs. BL	Mean (SE)	p vs. CG	p vs. BL	Mean (SE)	p vs. CG	p vs. BL
Urea	31.3 (0.23)	31.7 (0.37)	NS	30.1 (0.43)	↓↓	↓↓	31.9 (0.47)	NS	NS	30.0 (0.66)	NS	↓
Creatinine	0.94 (0.011)	0.93 (0.012)	NS	0.96 (0.014)	NS	NS	0.96 (0.009)	NS	↑	1.01 (0.015)	↑↑↑	↑↑↑

NOTES:
Test results are expressed in mg/dL.
CG = control group; BL = baseline examination of laboratory workers.

Statistical significance testing of follow-up findings.

	$p > 0.05$	$p < 0.05$	$p < 0.01$	$p < 0.001$
Higher than CG or BL:	NS	↑	↑↑	↑↑↑
Lower than CG or BL:	NS	↓	↓↓	↓↓↓

TABLE 3. Regression Coefficients ($b \pm se_b$) for Various Time-trend Models for Liver and Kidney Function Tests

Dependent Variables	Control Group	Laboratory Workers		
	Age	Age	Seniority	Span
GGTP	0.37 ± 0.124***	0.12 ± 0.082	0.08 ± 0.043	0.05 ± 0.197
SGOT	0.06 ± 0.070	0.05 ± 0.017	0.04 ± 0.026	0.16 ± 0.049**
AP	0.07 ± 0.102	0.37 ± 0.046***	0.43 ± 0.067***	1.35 ± 0.126***
LDH	0.21 ± 0.137	1.49 ± 0.139***	1.48 ± 0.212***	4.83 ± 0.384***
Urea	0.23 ± 0.019***	0.22 ± 0.021***	0.26 ± 0.030***	–0.06 ± 0.055
Creatinine	0.005 ± 0.0006***	–0.003 ± 0.0035	–0.001 ± 0.005	–0.007 ± 0.009

NOTE: Statistical significance testing of *b*-coefficient's (slope's) statistical significance: $^{**}p < 0.01$; $^{***}p < 0.001$.

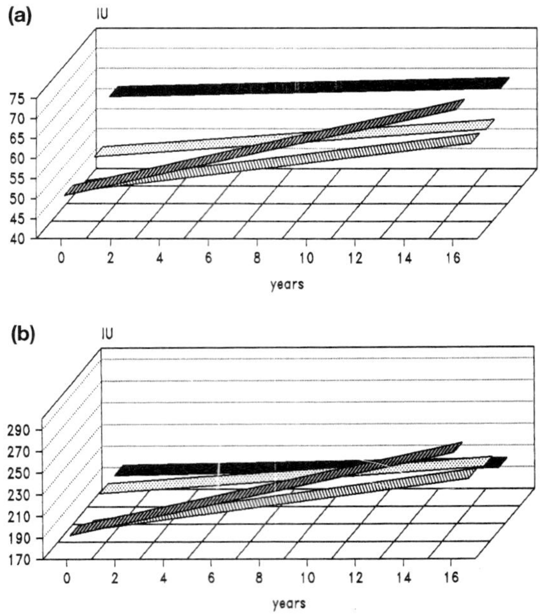

FIGURE 4. Time trends of changes in alkaline phosphatase (**a**) and lactate dehydrogenase (**b**) activity by various independent variables. For (**a**) and (**b**): ▨ by span in LW; ▩ by seniority in LW; ▧ by age in LW; ■ by age in CG; age = 20 + 2× (years); LW—laboratory workers; CG—control group.

and LDH) out of the four enzymes studied. These findings may be cautiouosly interpreted as a manifestation of a healthy worker effect in laboratory workers due to preemployment selection. The slightly higher incidence of higher social classes among laboratory workers as compared with the control group should be considered as well.[9–11] The mortality rates of professional[12] and research[13] chemists, which may be considered as being very similar if not the same occupational groups as laboratory workers, support this hypothesis.

Conversely, an elevation in enzyme activity levels was evident during long-term tracking of laboratory workers, particularly in the group followed up for more than 10 years. Though mean enzyme activity levels remained well within the normal limits, they were statistically significantly higher than both baseline and control group levels. Changes in individual enzyme values appeared more pronounced, in particular when LDH was concerned—almost half of its measurements were higher than the normal upper limit (the normal limits were obtained from the control group in the framework of this study as mean ± 2 SD). The existence of a few to a moderate number of abnormalities in SGOT and AP was also statistically significantly higher than in the control group or at baseline examination. In the 6- to 10-yr follow-up category the observed changes in liver function tests were similar but less pronounced.

Such a pattern of changes observed during 15 years of surveillance is very likely to be of a dose-related nature. Therefore it may be cautiously suggested that, as a result of long-term occupational exposure, at some moment adverse health changes began to supress the healthy-worker effect, characteristic of the baseline examination.

Serum creatinine levels changed in a similar, though less manifest pattern, which may indicate a low degree of kidney involvement in the health responses to laboratory exposures. It should be recognized that the changes in the urea blood content were just the opposite, for which we have no plausible explanation.

Qualitative identification of the occupational exposures in laboratory settings, as was explained in the introduction, may encounter a lot of obstacles and is not always attainable. In very basic terms, laboratory exposure in most of the institutions included in the study can be approximated by exposure to aromatic solvents, such as toluene and xylene.

Data in the literature were expected to be useful in explaining the changes observed in this study as a result of exposure to aromatic solvents. A few studies, including some of the case-control type, reported that both liver[14–16] and kidney[17–19] may be implicated to a certain degree as target organs in organic solvents exposure. However, these communications should be treated cautiously because of certain flaws inherent in their epidemiological design, inadequate information on the type of solvents under consideration (usually mixtures or unidentified compounds), the use of occupational groups with a higher level of exposure than in laboratory workers, etc. We conclude that the specific cause of the observed changes in our study remain obscure and require additional examination, as well as assessment of their clinical significance.

Two main conclusions can be drawn from this study.

- Laboratory workers with relatively low seniority appear to be healthier than the control population, in particular with respect to certain liver functions, according to serum enzyme levels. Frequent health screening of these workers, especially during the early stages of their laboratory employment (first 5 to 10 years) appear to be of low, if any, diagnostic significance.
- As the length of laboratory employment increased, these functions began to deteriorate. Long-term (as a matter of fact, more than 10 years) health surveillance can detect clinically asymptomatic adverse health effects of laboratory employment.

REFERENCES

1. WEBSTER'S ENCYCLOPEDIC UNABRIDGED DICTIONARY OF THE ENGLISH LANGUAGE. 1989. Portland House. New York.
2. CORDIER, S., *et al.* 1995. Cancer risk among workers in biomedical research. Scand. J. Work Environ. Health **21:** 450–459.
3. BELLI, S. 1992. Mortality study of workers employed by the Italian Institute of Health, 1960–1989. Scand. J. Work Environ. Health **18:** 64–67.
4. CARPENTER, L., *et al.* 1991. Cancer in laboratory workers. Lancet **8774:** 1080–1081.
5. TASKINEN, H. *et al.* 1994. Laboratory work and pregnancy outcome. J. Occup. Med. **36:** 311–319.
6. MEIRIK, O., *et al.* 1979. Major malformations in infants born to women who worked in laboratories while pregnant. Lancet **8133:** 91.
7. LEMESCH, C. & P. MAGNUS. 1996. Occupational health in laboratories: Cancer, effects on reproduction, and Israeli legislation. Israel J. Occup. Health **1:** 119–121.

8. PINES, A. *et al.* Environmental monitoring and health screening of laboratory workers: A useful or wasteful practice. Submitted for publication.
9. ARRIGHI, H. M. & I. HERTZ-PICCIOTTO. 1994. The evolving concept of the healthy worker survivor effect. Epidemiology **5:** 189-196.
10. ARAKI, S., *et al.* 1986. Mortality of medical practitioners in Japan: Social class and the healthy worker effect. Am. J. Ind. Med. **10:** 91-99.
11. DAHL, E. 1993. High mortality in lower salaried Norwegian men: The healthy worker effect? J. Epidemiol. Community Health **47:** 192-194.
12. HUNTER, W. J., *et al.* 1993. Mortality of professional chemists in England and Wales, 1965-1989. Am. J. Ind. Med. **23:** 615-627.
13. MAHER, K. V. & L. R. DEFONSO. 1986. A historical cohort study of mortality among chemical researchers. Arch. Environ. Health **41:** 109-116.
14. NASTERLACK, M. 1994. Hepatotoxic effects of solvent exposure around permissible limits and alcohol consumption in printers over a 4-year period. Int. Arch. Occup. Environ. Health **66:** 161-165.
15. TAGESSON, C. 1985. Liver damage and laboratory diagnostics. Scand. J. Work Environ. Health **11** (Suppl. 1): 101-103.
16. CHEN, J. D., *et al.* 1991. Exposure to mixtures of solvents among paint workers and biochemical alterations of liver function. Br. J. Ind. Med. **48:** 696-701.
17. MEYER, B. R., *et al.* 1984. Increased urinary enzyme excretion in workers exposed to nephrotoxic chemicals. Am. J. Med. **76:** 989-998.
18. STENGEL, B. 1995. Organic solvent exposure may increase the risk of glomerular nephropathies with chronic renal failure. Int. J. Epidemiol. **24:** 427-434.
19. SESSO, R., *et al.* 1990. Exposure to hydrocarbons and rapidly progressive glomerulonephritis. Braz. J. Med. Biol. Res. **23:** 225-233.

Two NIOSH Resources for Implementing Workplace Safety and Health Surveillance

LEELA I. MURTHY

National Institute for Occupational Safety and Health
4676 Columbia Parkway
Cincinnati, Ohio 45226

INTRODUCTION

Health practitioners and researchers alike are concerned with high rates of disease that occur in smaller populations. Some of these diseases may be of occupational origin. The frequency of occupational illnesses and diseases varies depending upon the individual work conditions; yet, their occurrence is sufficient to warrant active surveillance of such workers. Two resources from the National Institute for Occupational Safety and Health (NIOSH) are described herein for the implementation of workplace safety and health surveillance: (1) the Occupational Sentinel Health Events (SHEO) list,[1,2] which provides the involved occupations, industries, and agent(s) for a specific occupational disease or condition; and (2) a table of medical screening and biological monitoring tests that are currently available in the literature for monitoring workers potentially exposed to OSHA-regulated substances.[3]

PROVISION OF OCCUPATIONAL MEDICAL SERVICES

The provision of some aspects of medical care to workers in manufacturing and nonmanufacturing facilities seems to have changed during the 1980s from that noted in the 1970s, according to two observational surveys conducted by NIOSH (TABLE 1).[4] The first NIOSH survey, the National Occupational Hazard Survey (NOHS), was conducted between 1972 and 1974. Because of the continuing need for information on nationwide patterns of occupational exposure to health hazards, NIOSH conducted a second survey, the National Occupational Exposure Survey (NOES), during 1981-1983. The surveyed facilities in both NOHS and NOES were designed to be representative of virtually all the nonagricultural, nonmining, and nongovernmental businesses covered under the Occupational Safety and Health Act of 1970.

TABLE 1 shows that the proportion of the workforce with access to physician services in off-site clinics was 19.6% in the survey conducted between 1972 and 1974. In the second survey (1981-1983), the proportion of the workforce with access to physician services in off-site clinics rose to 57.8%, almost threefold from that used a decade earlier. On-site physician services (employed or contract) remained stable during both surveys—i.e., approximately 20%.[4] Information was not collected on the training of the physicians providing these services.

TABLE 1. Proportion of Workforce With Access to Physician Services from Two Surveys Conducted by the National Institute For Occupational Safety and Health (NIOSH)[a]

Off-Site Physician Services		On-Site Physician Services	
1972-1974	1981-1983	1972-1974	1981-1983
19.6%	57.8%	20.8%	19.1%

[a] Adapted from Ref. 4.

Even though the NIOSH survey data is over 10 years old, it does show that occupational health activities were being conducted by off-site and/or contractual physicians, many of whom may not have been adequately trained in occupational medicine. From the data available to NIOSH, comparative analyses of the data between on-site and off-site practice of medicine showed that use of off-site medical practice apparently resulted in diminished provision of screening tests and medical examinations of workers; this tendency may have been due to the recent decline of the presence of on-site physicians and the subsequent rapid growth of off-site medical practice.[5]

An Occupational Safety and Health Administration (OSHA) survey conducted in 1990-1991 estimated that only 6.3% of United States industries currently had a medical surveillance program at the individual establishment.[6,7]

An increased interest in academic training for occupational medicine has also been shown in the United States. Although there has been a growth in the number of accredited occupational medicine residencies from 10 in 1976 to 39 in 1993 (NIOSH, unpublished), the number of residents now being trained in occupational health is probably still too few to handle the problems of the numerous workers exposed to occupational hazards.

Some problems have been noted in the provision of occupational medical services:[3,5–8]

(1) The off-site, nonoccupational physicians often may have very little formal training in occupational medicine.
(2) Since they are practicing away from their on-site industrial hygienist and occupational nurse colleagues, these physicians may or may not be familiar with the type of work being conducted or the existing work conditions.
(3) They may have very little information on the various hazards that workers are exposed to and may not be aware of the toxicity of all hazards of each exposed worker.
(4) There are so many medical tests recommended in the literature for the various substances that they may not be able to decide which tests are to be performed on a worker at that specific worksite.
(5) Very few industries have an ongoing medical surveillance program.

Occupational Illnesses and Injuries

What is the magnitude of occupational illnesses, injuries, and deaths occurring in the United States?

According to estimates obtained by the National Traumatic Occupational Fatality (NTOF) surveillance system administered by NIOSH, 63,589 workers died from injuries sustained while working (1980-1989); 62,289 (98%) were workers in the civilian labor force. The average annual occupational fatality rate for the United States workforce was 7.0 per 100,000 workers.[9]

In 1992, the Bureau of Labor Statistics (BLS) implemented a new plan to conduct a systematic, verifiable count of all fatal occupational injuries and to obtain descriptive data on the circumstances surrounding these events.[10] Statistics reported to the National Safety Council (NSC)[10,11] for occupational injuries, illnesses, and deaths for the years 1992 through 1995 are presented in TABLE 2. From 1992 to 1993, the number of occupational illnesses seems to have increased almost 5% (from 457,000 to 482,000).[10] The data for 1994 show 514,700 illnesses, an increase of over 1 percent from 1993.[11] The occupationally related illnesses for 1995, however, decreased to 494,800 illnesses.

The number of disabling injuries has steadily risen from 3.2 million in 1993 to 3.6 million in 1995. There is an upward trend in the total number of occupationally related deaths (including suicides and homicides) from 6,217 in 1992 to 6,588 in 1994;[10,11] however, for 1995, the estimated number of all deaths including homicide and suicide was 5,300.[11]

TABLE 2. Number of Occupationally Related Illnesses and Deaths from the Bureau of Labor Statistics, 1992-1995[a]

	1992	1993	1994	1995
Illnesses	457,000	482,000	514,700	494,800[b]
Disabling injuries	3.3 million	3.2 million	3.5 million	3.6 million
Deaths (total)	6,217	6,271	6,588	5,300
Homicides, suicides	1,252	1,297	1,281	1,239[b]

[a] Adapted from Refs. 10 and 11.
[b] Not yet published.

CONTROL OF OCCUPATIONAL DISEASE

The successful control of occupational disease depends upon two factors: the recognition and diagnosis of cases by physicians and the implementation of epidemiologic surveillance, prevention, and control programs. Unfortunately, these factors have historically received inadequate attention.

Recognition and Diagnosis of Occupational Diseases

An instructive example of how occupationally related illnesses can be underdiagnosed can be found in a letter written to the editor of the New England Journal of

Medicine in 1980.[12] Sixty-seven physicians, more than half of whom were board-certified pathologists, were interested enough to take a one-week postgraduate course on pathology of the lung. A microscopic section was shown to demonstrate a straightforward example of asbestosis. Fewer than 10 percent (6 of 67) of the physicians suspected and diagnosed asbestosis. On the other hand, 75–80 percent of them diagnosed successfully "mystery" cases of non-occupationally related disease.[12]

Further documentation of the isolation of occupational disease was published in an editorial in the *Annals of Internal Medicine* by L. Rosenstock.[13] The systematic estimates of the magnitude of occupationally related illnesses and injuries available during the 1970s and 1980s are believed by many to be gross underestimates of the extent of the occupational health problems in the United States, due, perhaps, to various factors: (1) failure to identify diseases as occupational; (2) if an occupational cause is suspected, failure to report it; (3) the link between work and ill-health is often obscured by the long lag time from exposure to a subsequent illness; (4) the multiple and often poorly characterized hazardous exposures in the workplace; and (5) the multifactorial causation of many illnesses.[13]

Prevention and Control of Occupational Disease

The control of occupational disease has its genesis in methodologies used in the health-care field that were found to be successful. As an example, the approach of identifying and counting the number of preventable tragedies in the health-care field was successfully used in the 1930s, when every maternal death occurring in New York City was vigorously pursued; pertinent facts were collected and later evaluated by a group of obstetricians. The evolution and implementation of this process was followed by a rapid drop in maternal mortality in New York City.[14]

The above principles were applied to infant deaths in 1967 and 1968 in Massachusetts. Such evaluations demonstrated that about one-third of infant deaths in the state of Massachusetts were preventable by medical means.[15]

Based on the experience with the identification and prevention of maternal and infant mortality, the late Dr. Rutstein coined the term *Sentinel Health Event* for diseases and disabilities that were preventable. Thus, "The occurrence of an unnecessary disease, disability, or untimely death is a *Sentinel Health Event* (SHE) that justifies carefully controlled scientific research for remediable underlying causes."[16]

The occurrence of a SHE serves as a warning signal that the quality of preventive and/or therapeutic medical care may need to be improved. Thus, according to Rutstein, the SHEs serve as negative indexes of the quality of medical care where unnecessary disease or untimely death occurs. For example, a case of polio is a SHE. The occurrence of this preventable disease signals a breakdown in immunization programs.[16]

Occupational Sentinel Health Event

The Sentinel Health Event (SHE) approach was subsequently modified and successfully applied to the field of occupational disease.[1] Thus, an occupational sentinel health event (SHEO) is a preventable disease, a preventable disability, or a preventable untimely death that is occupationally related.

The occurrence of a SHEO indicates that (1) epidemiologic studies or industrial hygiene studies should be conducted; (2) control technology should be implemented to prevent that disease, disability, or death; and (3) appropriate medical care should be provided.[1]

Two broad categories of SHEOs have been recognized. The first group includes diseases or conditions that, by their inherent nature, are occupationally related. Such conditions include the pneumoconioses; it is unlikely that these diseases would occur in the absence of an occupational exposure to the inciting agent. The second set of conditions include such diseases as lung cancer, leukemia, peripheral neuropathy, leptospirosis, and ornithosis, which may or may not be occupationally related. For the latter set of conditions, further information on the industry and occupation is required to establish a causal link between disease condition and occupation.[1,2]

The occupational health literature was surveyed, and a list of SHEOs was assembled, each of which met three criteria of scientific proof: documentation of associated agent or agents, of involved industries, and of involved occupations. In addition, the disease or condition must be codable within the framework of the Ninth Revision of the International Classification of Diseases Adapted for Use in the United States, 1975–i.e., ICD-9.[1,2]

The first list of 50 work-related conditions was published in 1983.[1] Most of the reports included in the list were epidemiologic studies; few of them were case reports. An updated list of SHEOs was published in 1991.[2] (This is included below as APPENDIX 1.) For the updated SHEO list, additional criteria were used, since many studies were found to be equivocal.

First, the report had to be a sound epidemiologic study with appropriate controls, end point, and specifics concerning occupation, industry, and agent.[2] Second, in the case of lung cancer, the study must have been controlled for smoking history. A few epidemiologic studies were noted in which lung cancer was the end point but there was no mention of smoking characteristics as a confounding factor; such studies were not included in the SHEO list. Third, for death certificate studies, confirmatory studies must have been done using more rigorous methodologies–e.g., case control study or a retrospective mortality study, etc.[2]

The updated SHEO list contained 64 diseases or conditions and over 140 agents. Of the 14 new conditions included in the list, 7 belonged to the infectious disease group. These were "Fish fancier's finger," "Herpetic whitlow," "HIV infection," "Rocky Mountain spotted fever," "Leptospirosis," "Histoplasmosis," and "Sporotrichosis." None of these conditions was solely related to occupation. Details of the occupations/industries dealing with the new infectious disease conditions are presented in TABLE 3.[2]

METHODS OF SURVEILLANCE OF OCCUPATIONAL DISEASES

Two approaches are useful in the surveillance of occupational disease conditions: medical screening and biological monitoring. Medical screening is the search for early signs or symptoms of disease *before* the patient is symptomatic. Biological

TABLE 3. Occupations, Industries, and Agents Noted for Seven New Infectious Diseases in the Occupational Sentinel Health Event (SHEO) Update[a]

ICD-9	Condition	Industry/Process/Occupation	Agent
031.1	Fish-fancier's finger	Aquarium worker/cleaner, owner/breeder	*Mycobacterium marinum*
		Longshoreman	*Mycobacterium marinum*
054.6	Herpetic whitlow	Surgical resident, student nurse, nurse, dental assistant, physician, orthopedic scrub nurse, psychiatric nurse	Herpes simplex virus
042	Human immunodeficiency virus	Health care worker	Human immunodeficiency virus
082.0	Rocky Mountain spotted fever	Laboratory technician, tick breeder, virologist, microbiologist, physician	*Rickettsia rickettsii*
100.8	Leptospirosis	Farmer/laborer	*Leptospira*
115	Histoplasmosis	Bridge maintenance worker	*Histoplasma capsulatam*
117.1	Sporotrichosis	Nurseryman, forester, florist, equipment operator	*Sporothrix schenkii*

[a] Adapted from Ref. 2.

monitoring is the testing of a specimen from the patient for the presence of a hazardous intoxicant or its metabolite.[3]

A simple guide containing specific medical tests for medical screening and biological monitoring of specific substances would be helpful to both the occupational health professional and the general practitioner. Hence, to provide the practicing physician with a roadmap to the literature of the available recommendations for medical screening and biological monitoring, a literature search was conducted to obtain information on medical tests that were available for these substances. The medical tests recommended by the federal government (NIOSH/OSHA) and other researchers for substances regulated by OSHA in 1989 and revised in 1993 were summarized, in tabular format. There are so many agents being used in the workplace, and a start had to be made somewhere; hence, for this report, medical tests available for screening workers exposed to the substances regulated by OSHA were chosen.[3]

The criteria for an effective screening test are: safety, reliability, validity, positive results in presymptomatic period, and positive predictive value.[17]

The medical tests recommended for substances regulated by OSHA (and for which permissible exposure limits had been specified) were tabulated.[3] (This is included below as APPENDIX 2.) Included in the table were the name of the substance, the Chemical Abstracts Service Registry (CAS) number, and recommendations for specific medical tests made by NIOSH/OSHA[18,19] and by other data sources.[20–28] A glossary was also provided in the table to define the terms or abbreviations used in the table. The intent of this table was not to provide an evaluation of the recommendations or a validation of the medical tests for use in surveillance, but to provide a source for the medical tests described in the literature for the specific regulated agent. The efficacy of these tests for screening workers exposed to the specific substances was not evaluated.[3] This table is now available from NIOSH as a poster.

When a worker is exposed to a specific substance–e.g., trichloroethylene–the occupational health professional needs to know the specific medical test or tests to detect this agent or its effects on the worker. Most often, only the agent under question gets screened for, in this case, trichloroethylene. There are agents whose metabolites are also toxic. In such cases the worker should be screened not only for the specific agent but also for its metabolites. In the case of trichloroethylene, the metabolites are trichloroacetic acid and trichloroethanol, both of which are toxic. Hence, the worker should be screened for trichloroethylene as well as the two metabolites that are also toxic. The media that are to be used are urine, blood, and exhaled air.[3]

Medical tests recommended by NIOSH/OSHA and other researchers for acetone, benzene, and carbon tetrachloride are presented in TABLE 4.

Regarding medical tests for acetone, for example, though there is a NIOSH recommended exposure level and an OSHA permissible exposure level for acetone, this chemical was not yet included in the *Occupational Health Guidelines for Chemical Hazards* (1981-1989);[18,18a] however, in the *Occupational Diseases* book published by NIOSH, preplacement examinations were recommended for acetone to evaluate the worker's skin and respiratory conditions.[19]

In addition to NIOSH's recommendations, four other sources have recommended sampling for acetone in whole blood;[20,21] in expired air;[21,22] by urinalysis (in general);[20] by urinalysis at the end of work shift;[21] and by urinalysis during exposure.[23]

TABLE 4. Medical Tests Recommended for Acetone, Benzene, and Carbon Tetrachloride by NIOSH/OSHA and Other Researchers[a]

Name of Substance	CAS Number	Recommendations by NIOSH/OSHA	Recommendations by Other Researchers
Acetone	00067-64-1	Pulmonary function tests	Whole blood, expired air, urinalysis at end of exposure, urinalysis during exposure
Benzene	00071-43-2	Complete blood count, pulmonary function tests	Urinalysis, urinalysis at end of shift, expired air, expired air prior to next shift, whole blood
Carbon tetrachloride	00056-23-5	Liver function tests, urinalysis	Liver function tests, kidney function tests, urinalysis, urinalysis (24 h), whole blood, expired air

[a] Adapted from Ref. 3.

Taking another example, benzene exposure has been associated with leukemia. Thus, preplacement and periodic examinations should include the effects of benzene on the blood and bone marrow and a history of exposure to other myelotoxic agents or drugs or of other diseases of the blood.[18] According to the *Occupational Diseases* book, preplacement laboratory examinations should include (1) a complete blood count–i.e., hematocrit, hemoglobin, mean corpuscular volume, white blood count, differential count, and platelet estimation; (2) reticulocyte count; (3) serum bilirubin; and (4) urinary phenol.[19]

Eight other data sources have recommended sampling by using one or more of the following media for benzene exposure: urinalysis;[20–22,24–26] urinalysis at end of shift;[27] expired air;[20–22,26] expired air prior to next shift–i.e., pre- and postshift;[27] and whole blood.[20,21,23,26]

A discussion is presented herewith regarding recommendations for urinalysis. If the substance under question or its metabolite has a half-life of less than five hours, the term "end of shift" is used. That means sampling can be done during the last two hours of exposure of that day's shift. For the term "end of workweek," the sampling should be done after four to five consecutive days of exposure since the half-life of the substance is greater than five hours. If "end of shift at end of workweek" is specifically mentioned, the sampling should be done during the last hour of the fifth day; in other words, the exposure of the fifth day also needs to be taken into consideration before sampling is done.

Taking the medical tests for carbon tetrachloride as another example, the *NIOSH/OSHA Occupational Health Guidelines* recommended that the examination of liver and kidneys should be stressed.[18] For preplacement examination, liver function tests and urinalysis should be conducted, and these tests should be repeated on an annual basis.[18]

Other than NIOSH/OSHA, one data source recommended liver function tests, kidney function tests, and urinalysis for the monitoring of carbon tetrachloride.[28] Another data source recommended 24-hour urinalysis,[23] two sources recommended whole blood sampling,[21,23] and three sources recommended the sampling of carbon tetrachloride in expired air.[21–23]

CONCLUSIONS

The occurrence of occupational illnesses and diseases warrants the implementation of active safety and health surveillance in the workplace. To assist the occupational health provider in this effort, two NIOSH resources, (1) a list of SHEOs from the published literature, and (2) recommended medical screening and biological monitoring methods for OSHA regulated substances, have been described in this report.

It is advisable that a list of SHEOs be developed in each workplace by occupation, process, or work unit. When the process is changed, the agents used may also change, and hence, a new list of SHEOs will have to be developed.

Also, specific medical tests should be performed by the occupational health professional on each worker depending upon the particular agent and the extent of exposure of the worker to that agent. To effectively and appropriately utilize these techniques, the occupational health professional delivering occupational medical services must:

(1) understand the role of medical screening and biological monitoring in the full spectrum of approaches to occupational disease prevention;
(2) be knowledgeable of the chemical, physical, and biological hazards (including toxicity) to which the workers are exposed; and
(3) have access to scientific and regulatory literature.

The occupational health program should not be cast in stone for a particular industry or occupational group. With newer processes and agents entering the industrial environment, there will be a continual change in the nature of work, and occupational diseases will also change. For example, if another agent, say X, is substituted for carbon tetrachloride, the required medical screening and biological monitoring would be different if X does not cause liver or kidney dysfunction. Thus, the toxicity of the new agent X is to be first determined, and appropriate medical tests should be performed. Preventive measures should be taken to control the worker's exposure to agent X in order to prevent occupational diseases due to exposure of the worker to agent X.

Thus, from the perspective of a health care provider, appropriate questions regarding work history should be asked. To cite an example, Ramazzini (1713) would ask the worker what kind of work he performed. Specifically, the question asked was, "What trade are you of?"[29] Hence, the specific industry (4-digit Standard Industrial Classification [SIC] code), the specific occupation (3-digit occupation code), the various agents used, the duration of exposure, whether part-time or full-time exposure to the agent, etc. are all important parameters that a health provider should ascertain before a diagnosis of the illness is made.

SUMMARY

To improve safety and health in the workplace, appropriate occupational health programs should be implemented utilizing expertise from multiple disciplines. In other words, the occupational health program should be a *team effort.* Expertise from all aspects of occupational health should be utilized, from the industrial hygienist, to the safety officer, to the occupational health nurse, and the practicing physician—all should be involved in the program to maintain a safe and healthy workplace.

Two NIOSH resources have been described to assist the occupational health professional in the improvement of safety and health in the workplace. First, the SHEO approach, where a separate SHEO list is to be developed for each workplace. This may be a problem when the physician is an outside contractor, but with the help of the team approach, a list of SHEOs can be developed. Second, medical screening and biological monitoring is often required. While we realize that medical screening and biological monitoring is part of the complete occupational health program, the table of medical tests that we have prepared[3] may give some leads into the type(s) of medical tests to be conducted on the individual worker at a particular worksite.

REFERENCES

1. RUTSTEIN, D. D., R. J. MULLAN, T. M. FRAZIER *et al.* 1983. Sentinel Health Events (Occupational): A basis for physician recognition and public health surveillance. Am. J. Public Health **73:** 1054-1062.
2. MULLAN, R. J. & L. I. MURTHY. 1991. Occupational Sentinel Health Events: An up-dated list for physician recognition and public health surveillance. Am. J. Ind. Med. **19:** 775-799.
3. MURTHY, L. I. & W. E. HALPERIN. 1995. Medical screening and biological monitoring—A guide to the literature for physicians. J. Occup. Environ. Med. **37:** 170-184.
4. PEDERSEN, D. H. & K. W. SIEBER. 1989. Some trends in worker access to health care in the United States (1974-1983). Am. J. Ind. Med. **15:** 151-165.
5. PEDERSEN, D. H., H. L. VENABLE & K. W. SIEBER. 1990. An examination of occupational medical practices. J. Occup. Med. **32:** 1037-1041.
6. CONWAY, H., J. SIMMONS & T. TALBERT. 1993. The Occupational Safety and Health Administration's 1990-1991 survey of occupational medical surveillance prevalence and type of current practices. J. Occup. Med. **35:** 659-669.
7. HATHAWAY, J. A. 1993. Medical surveillance: Extent and effectiveness? J. Occup. Med. **35:** 698-700.
8. LEVY, B. A. 1980. The teaching of occupational health in American medical schools. J. Med. Educ. **55:** 18-22.
9. FATAL INJURIES TO WORKERS IN THE U.S. 1980-1989: A Decade of Surveillance. US DHHS PHS CDC NIOSH, DHHS (NIOSH) Number 93-108S, August 1993.
10. NATIONAL SAFETY COUNCIL. 1994. Accident Facts. National Safety Council. Itasca, IL.
11. NATIONAL SAFETY COUNCIL. 1996. Accident Facts. National Safety Council. Itasca, IL.
12. ABRAHAM, J. L. 1980. Underdiagnosis of pulmonary asbestosis (Letter to the Editor). N. Engl. J. Med. **302:** 464.
13. ROSENSTOCK, L. 1981. Occupational medicine: Too long neglected. Ann. Intern. Med. **95:** 774-776.
14. NEW YORK ACADEMY OF MEDICINE, COMMITTEE ON PUBLIC HEALTH RELATIONS. 1933. Maternal Mortality in New York City: A Study of All Puerperal Deaths 1930-1932. The Commonwealth Fund. New York.
15. MASSACHUSETTS MEDICAL SOCIETY, PERINATAL WELFARE COMMITTEE. 1971. Report on Perinatal and Infant Mortality in Massachusetts, 1967 and 1968. Massachusetts Medical Society. Boston.
16. RUTSTEIN, D. D., W. BERENBERG, T. C. CHAMBERS *et al.* 1976. Measuring the quality of medical care: A clinical method. N. Engl. J. Med. **294:** 582-588.
17. SILVERSTEIN, M. A. 1990. Medical screening, surveillance, and the prevention of occupational disease. J. Occup. Med. **32:** 1032-1036.
18. U.S. DEPARTMENT OF HEALTH AND HUMAN SERVICES, PUBLIC HEALTH SERVICE, CENTERS FOR DISEASE CONTROL, NATIONAL INSTITUTE FOR OCCUPATIONAL SAFETY AND HEALTH, AND U.S. DEPARTMENT OF LABOR, OCCUPATIONAL SAFETY AND HEALTH ADMINISTRATION. 1981, 1988, 1989, 1992, 1995. NIOSH/OSHA Occupational Health Guidelines for Chemical Hazards (1981, 1988, 1989, 1992, 1995). F. W. Mackison, R. S. Stricoff, L. J. Partridge, Jr. & A. D. Little, Inc., Eds. DHHS (NIOSH) Publication Nos. 81-123 and Supplement I-IV U.S. Department of Health and Human Services. Washington, DC.

18a. U.S. DEPARTMENT OF LABOR, OCCUPATIONAL SAFETY AND HEALTH ADMINISTRATION. 1996. Code of Federal Regulations. 29 CFR 1910 (1910.1000 to end). Air Contaminants. Revised as of July 1, 1996. U.S. Government Printing Office. Washington, DC.

19. U.S. DEPARTMENT OF HEALTH, EDUCATION, AND WELFARE, PUBLIC HEALTH SERVICE, CENTERS FOR DISEASE CONTROL, NATIONAL INSTITUTE FOR OCCUPATIONAL SAFETY AND HEALTH. 1977. Occupational Diseases: A Guide to Their Recognition. Marcus Key *et al.,* Eds. DHEW (NIOSH) Publication No. 77-181. U.S. Government Printing Office. Washington, DC.

20. Lauwerys, R. R. & P. Hoet. 1993. Industrial Chemical Exposure. Guidelines for Biological Monitoring. 2d edit. R. R. Lauwerys & P. Hoet, Eds. Lewis Publishers. CRC Press. Boca Raton, FL.
21. Baselt, R. C. 1988. Biological Monitoring Methods for Industrial Chemicals. 2d edit. Year Book Medical Publishers. Littleton, MA.
22. Linch, A. L. 1974. Biological Monitoring for Industrial Chemical Exposure Control. CRC Press. Cleveland, OH.
23. LaDou, J. 1990. Occupational Medicine. J. LaDou, Ed. A Lange Medical Book. Appleton & Lange. East Norwalk, CT.
24. Kneip, T. J. & J. V. Crable. 1988. Methods for Biological Monitoring—A Manual for Assessing Human Exposure to Hazardous Substances. T. J. Kneip & J. V. Crable, Eds. American Public Health Association. Washington, DC.
25. Ho, M. H. & H. K. Dillon. 1987. Biological Monitoring of Exposure to Chemicals. Organic Compounds. M. H. Ho & H. K. Dillon, Eds. John Wiley & Sons. New York.
26. Atio, A., V. Riihimaki & H. Vainio. 1984. Biological Monitoring and Surveillance of Workers Exposed to Chemicals. A. Atio, V. Riihimaki & H. Vainio, Eds. Hemisphere Publishing Corporation. New York.
27. ACGIH. 1996. 1996 Threshold Limit Values for Chemical Substances and Physical Agents and Biological Exposure Indices. American Conference of Governmental Industrial Hygienists Worldwide. Technical Affairs Office. Cincinnati, OH.
28. Proctor, N. H. & J. P. Hughes. 1978. Chemical Hazards of the Workplace. N. H. Proctor & J. P. Hughes, Eds. JB Lippincott Company. Philadelphia.
29. Ramazzini, B. [1713] 1933. Diseases of Tradesmen. Translated by Herman Goodman. Medical Lay Press. New York.

APPENDIX 1

Occupationally Related Unnecessary Disease, Disability, and Untimely Death[a,b]

ICD-9	Condition[c]	Industry/Process/Occupation	Agent
011	Pulmonary tuberculosis (O)	Physician, medical personnel, medical laboratory worker	*Mycobacterium tuberculosis*
011, 502	Silicotuberculosis	Quarryman, sandblaster, silica processor, mining, metal foundry, ceramic industry	Silica + *Mycobacterium tuberculosis*
020	Plague (O)	Shepherd, farmer, rancher, hunter, field geologist	*Yersinia pestis*
021	Tularemia (O)	Hunter, fur handler, sheep industry worker, cook, veterinarian, rancher, veterinarian pathologist, laboratory worker, soldier	*Francisella tularensis, Pasteurella tularensis*
022	Anthrax (O)	Shepherd, farmer, butcher, handler of imported hides or fibers, veterinarian, veterinarian pathologist, weaver	*Bacillus anthracis*
023	Brucellosis (O)	Farmer, shepherd, veterinarian, laboratory worker, slaughterhouse worker, field officer	*Brucella abortus, suis*
031.1[d]	Fish-fancier's finger (O)	Aquarium worker/cleaner, breeder/owner, longshoreman	*Mycobacterium marinum*
037	Tetanus (O)	Farmer, rancher	*Clostridium tetani*
042[e]	Human immunodeficiency virus (O)	Health care worker	Human immunodeficiency virus
054.6	Herpetic whitlow (O)	Surgical resident, student nurse, nurse, dental assistant, physician, orthopedic scrub nurse, psychiatric nurse	Herpes simplex virus
056	Rubella (O)	Medical personnel, intensive care personnel	Rubella virus
070.0 .1	Hepatitis A (O)	Day care center staff, orphanage staff, mental retardation institution staff, medical personnel	Hepatitis A virus
070.2 .3	Hepatitis B (O)	Nurse and nurses' aide, anesthesiologist, orphanage and mental institution staff, medical laboratory personnel, general dentist, oral surgeon, physician	Hepatitis B virus

***Occupationally Related Unnecessary Disease, Disability, and Untimely Death*[a,b] (*Continued*)**

ICD-9	Condition[c]	Industry/Process/Occupation	Agent
070. 4	Non-A, non-B Hepatitis (O)	As above for hepatitis A and B	Unknown
071	Rabies (O)	Veterinarian, animal and game warden, laboratory researcher, farmer, rancher, trapper	Rabies virus
073	Ornithosis (O)	Psittacine bird breeder, pet shop staff, poultry producer, veterinarian, zoo employee, duck processing and rearing	*Chlamydia psittaci*
082.0	Rocky Mountain spotted fever (O)	Laboratory technician, tick breeder, virologist, microbiologist, physician	*Rickettsia rickettsii*
100.8	Leptospirosis (O)	Farmer/laborer	*Leptospira*
115	Histoplasmosis (O)	Bridge maintenance worker	*Histoplasma capsulatam*
117.1	Sporotrichosis (O)	Nurseryman, forester, florist, equipment operator	*Sporothrix schenkii*
147	Malignant neoplasm of nasopharynx (O)	Carpenter, cabinet maker, sawmill worker, lumberjack, electrician, fitter	Chlorophenols
155M[f,g]	Hemangiosarcoma of the liver	Vinyl chloride polymerization industry	Vinyl chloride monomer
		Vintner	Arsenical pesticides
158, 163	Mesothelioma (MN of peritoneum and pleura)	Asbestos industries and utilizers	Asbestos
160.0	Malignant neoplasm of nasal cavities (O)	Woodworker, cabinet and furniture maker	Hardwood dusts
		Boot and shoe industry	Unknown
		Radium chemist and processor, dial painter	Radium
		Chromium producer, processor, user	Chromates
		Nickel smelting and refining	Nickel
		Sawmill worker, carpenter	Chlorophenols
161	Malignant neoplasm of larynx (O)	Asbestos industries and utilizers	Asbestos
162	Malignant neoplasm of trachea, bronchus, and lung (O)	Asbestos industry and utilizers	Asbestos
		Topside coke oven workers	Coke oven emissions
		Uranium and fluorspar miner	Radon daughters

		Chromium producer, processor, user	Chromates
		Nickel smelter, processor, user	Nickel
		Smelter	Arsenic, arsenic trioxide
		Mustard gas formulator	Mustard gas
		Ion exchange resin maker, chemist	Bis(chloromethyl)ether, chloromethyl methyl ether
		Iron ore (underground) miner	Radon daugthers
		Plant protection worker/agronomist	Pesticides, herbicides, fungicides, insecticides
		Welder	Unknown
		Copper smelter and roaster worker	Inorganic arsenic, sulfur dioxide, copper, lead, sulfuric acid, arsenic trioxide
		Welder, gas cutter	Asbestos, hexavalent chromium
		Foundry—floor molders and casters	Polyaromatic hydrocarbons
		Dichromate production—floor molder/caster	Unknown
		Chromate production	Chromium dust
		Chromate pigment production worker	Lead chromate, zinc chromate
		Pigment production	Zinc chromate dust
		Steel industry—furnace/foundry worker	Unknown
		Rubber reclaim operations	Unknown
170	Malignant neoplasm of bone (O)	Radium chemist and processor, dial painter	Radium
187.7	Malignant neoplasm of scrotum	Automatic lathe operator, metalworker	Mineral/cutting oils
		Coke oven worker, petroleum refiner, tar distiller	Soots/tar/tar distillates
		Tool setter, fitter, cotton spinner, chimney sweep, machine operator	Mineral oil, pitch, tar
188	Malignant neoplasm of bladder (O)	Rubber and dye worker	Benzidine, alpha- and beta-naphthylamine, magenta, auramine, 4-aminobiphenyl, 4-nitrophenyl
189	Malignant neoplasm of kidney, other, and unspecified urinary organs (O)	Coke oven worker	Coke oven emissions

Occupationally Related Unnecessary Disease, Disability, and Untimely Death*[a,b] *(Continued)

ICD-9	Condition[c]	Industry/Process/Occupation	Agent
204.0	Lymphoid leukemia, acute (O)	Rubber industry	Unknown
		Radiologist	Ionizing radiation
205.0	Myeloid leukemia, acute (O)	Occupations with exposure to benzene	Benzene
		Radiologist	Ionizing radiation
207.0	Erythroleukemia (O)	Occupations with exposure to benzene	Benzene
283.1	Hemolytic anemia, nonautoimmune (O)	Whitewashing and leather industry	Copper sulfate
		Electrolytic processes, arsenical ore smelting	Arsine
		Plastics industry	Trimellitic anhydride
		Dye, celluloid, resin industries	Naphthalene
284.8	Aplastic anemia (O)	Explosives manufacture	Trinitrotoluene
		Occupations with exposure to benzene	Benzene
		Radiologist, radium chemist, dial painter	Ionizing radiation
288.0	Agranulocytosis or neutropenia (O)	Occupations with exposure to benzene	Benzene
		Explosives and pesticide industries	Phosphorus
		Pesticides, pigments, pharmaceuticals	Inorganic arsenic
289.7	Methemoglobinemia (O)	Explosives and dye industries	Aromatic amino and nitro compounds. (e.g., aniline, trinitrotoluene, nitroglycerin)
		Rubber worker	Aniline, o-toluidine, nitrobenzene
323.7	Toxic encephalitis (O)	Battery, smelter, and foundry workers	Lead
		Electrolytic chlorine production, battery maker, fungicide formulator	Inorganic and organic mercury
332.1	Parkinson's disease (secondary) (O)	Manganese processing, battery maker, welder	Manganese
		Internal combustion engine industries	Carbon monoxide
334.3	Cerebellar ataxia (O)	Chemical industry using toluene	Toluene
		Electrolytic chlorine production, battery maker, fungicide formulator	Organic mercury

354M[h]	Carpal tunnel syndrome (O)	Meat packer, deboner	Cumulative trauma
354.0	Mononeuritis of upper limb and mononeuritis multiplex (O)	Dental technician	Methyl methacrylate monomer
.2		Poultry processing—turkey	Cumulative trauma
.3		Meat packer, deboner	Cumulative trauma
357.7	Inflammatory and toxic neuropathy (O)	Pesticide industry, pigments, pharmaceuticals formulator	Arsenic/arsenic compounds
		Furniture refinisher, degreasing operations	Hexane
		Plastic-coated fabric worker	Methyl n-butyl ketone
		Explosives industry	Trinitrotoluene
		Rayon manufacturing	Carbon disulfide
		Plastics, hydraulics, coke industries	Tri-o-cresyl phosphate
		Battery, smelter, and foundry workers	Inorganic lead
		Dentist, chloralkali workers	Inorganic mercury
		Chloralkali plants, fungicide maker, battery maker	Organic mercury
		Plastics industry, paper manufacturing	Acrylamide
		Ethylene oxide sterilizer operator	Ethylene oxide
366.4	Cataract (O)	Microwave and radar technicians	Microwaves
		Explosives industries, trinitrotoluene worker	Trinitrotoluene
		Radiologist	Ionizing radiation
		Blacksmith, glass blower, baker	Infrared radiation
		Moth repellant formulator, fumigator	Naphthalene
		Explosives, dye, herbicide, and pesticide industries	Dinitrophenol, dinitro-o-cresol
		Ethylene oxide sterilizer operator, microbiology supervisory, inspector	Ethylene oxide
388.1	Noise effects on inner ear (O)	Occupations with exposure to excessive noise	Excessive noise
443.0	Raynaud's phenomenon (secondary) (O)	Lumberjack, chain sawyer, grinder, chipper, rock driller, stone cutter, jackhammer operator, riveter	Whole body or segmental vibration
		Vinyl chloride polymerization industry	Vinyl chloride
493.0, 507.8	Extrinsic asthma (O)	Jewelry, alloy, and catalyst makers	Platinum
		Polyurethane, adhesive, paint workers	Isocyanates

Occupationally Related Unnecessary Disease, Disability, and Untimely Death[a,b] (Continued)

ICD-9	Condition[c]	Industry/Process/Occupation	Agent
		Alloy, catalyst, refinery workers	Chromium, cobalt
		Solderer	Aluminum soldering flux
		Plastic, dye, insecticide makers	Phthalic anhydride
		Foam worker, latex maker, biologist	Formaldehyde
		Printing industry	Gum arabic
		Nickel plater	Nickel sulfate
		Baker	Flour
		Plastics industry, organic chemicals manufacture	Trimellitic anhydride
		Woodworker, furniture maker	Red cedar (plicatic acid) and other wood dusts
		Detergent formulator	*Bacillus*-derived exoenzymes
		Crab processing worker	Unknown
		Hospital and geriatric department nurses	Psyllium dust
		Laxative manufacture and packing	Psyllium dust
		Prawn processing worker	Unknown
		Snow crab processing worker	Unknown
495.4	Maltworker's lung	Maltworker	*Aspergillus clavatus*
495.5	Mushroom worker's lung	Mushroom farm/spawning shed, farmer	Pasteurized compost
495.8	Grainhandler's lung	Grain handler	*Erwinia herbicola (Enterobacter agglomerans)*
	Sequoiosis	Red cedar mill worker, woodworker, sawmill, joinery	Redwood sawdust, *Thuja plicata*
495.9	Unspecified allergic alveolitis	Cinnamon processing worker	Cinnamon dust, cinnamaldehyde
		Distillery, vegetable compost plant worker	*Aspergillus fumigatus*
		Sawmill worker	Unknown
		Paper manufacture/wood room	*Alternaria,* wood dust

		Snow crab processing worker	Unknown
500	Coalworker's pneumoconiosis	Coal miner	Coal dust
501	Asbestosis	Asbestos industries and utilizers	Asbestos
502M[i]	Silicosis	Quarryman, sandblaster, silica processor, mining, metal, and ceramic industries	Silica
		Cryolite refining	Cryolite (Na_3AlF_6), quartz dust
	Talcosis	Talc processor, soapstone mining/milling, polishing, cosmetics industry	Talc
503M[j]	Chronic beryllium disease of the lung	Beryllium alloy worker, ceramic and cathode ray tube makers, nuclear reactor worker	Beryllium
504	Byssinosis	Cotton industry worker	Cotton, flax, hemp, and cotton-synthetic dusts
506.0, 506.1	Acute bronchitis, pneumonitis, and pulmonary edema due to fumes and vapors (O)	Refrigeration, fertilizer, oil refining industries	Ammonia
		Alkali and bleach industries	Chlorine
		Silo filler, arc welder, nitric acid industry	Nitrogen oxides
		Paper and refrigeration industries, oil refining	Sulfur dioxide
		Cadmium smelters, processors	Cadmium
		Plastics industry	Trimellitic anhydride
		Boilermaker	Vanadium pentoxide
		Organic chemicals manufacture	Trimellitic anhydride
570, 573.3	Toxic hepatitis (O)	Solvent utilizer, dry cleaner, plastics industry	Carbon tetrachloride, chloroform, tetrachloroethane, trichloroethylene, tetrachloroethylene
		Explosives and dye industries	Phosphorus, trinitrotoluene
		Fire and waterproofing additive formulator	Chloronaphthalenes
		Plastics formulator	Methylenedianiline
		Fumigator, gasoline and fire extinguisher formulators	Methyl bromide
			Ethylene dibromide
		Disinfectant, fumigant, synthetic resin formulators	Cresol
584, 585	Acute or chronic renal failure (O)	Battery maker, plumber, solderer	Inorganic lead
		Electrolytic processes, arsenical ore smelting	Arsine

***Occupationally Related Unnecessary Disease, Disability, and Untimely Death*[a,b] (*Continued*)**

ICD-9	Condition[c]	Industry/Process/Occupation	Agent
		Battery maker, jeweler, dentist	Inorganic mercury
		Fluorocarbon formulator, fire extinguisher maker	Carbon tetrachloride
		Antifreeze manufacture	Ethylene glycol
		Chromate pigment production worker	Inorganic lead
606	Infertility, male (O)	Kepone formulator	Kepone
		DBCP producer, formulator, and applicator	Dibromochloropropane
692	Contact and allergic dermatitis (O)	Leather tanning, poultry dressing plants, fish packing, adhesives and sealants industry, boat building and repair	Irritants (e.g., cutting oils, phenol, solvents, acids, alkalis, detergents); allergens (e.g., nickel, chromates, formaldehyde, dyes, rubber products)
733.9M[k]	Skeletal fluorosis (O)	Cryolite worker (grinding room), cryolite refining worker	Cryolite (Na_3AlF_6)

[a] Modified from TABLE I of R. J. Mullan & L. I. Murthy, 1991, Occupational Sentinel Health Events: An Up-Dated List for Physician Recognition and Public Health Surveillance, Am. J. Ind. Med. **19:** 775–799.
[b] External causes of injury and poisoning (occupational), including accidents, are classified in the ICD-9 Manual under the E codes.
[c] (O) indicates that condition is specifically occupation related.
[d] Original ICD rubric = Cutaneous Diseases Due to Other Mycobacteria.
[e] From the International Classification of Diseases, 9th Revision, Clinical Modification (ICD-9-CM).
[f] M = Modified ICD rubric.
[g] Original ICD rubric = Malignant Neoplasm of Liver and Intrahepatic Bile Ducts.
[h] Original ICD rubric = Mononeuritis of Upper Limb and Mononeuritis Multiplex.
[i] Original ICD rubric = Pneumoconiosis Due to Other Silica or Silicates.
[j] Original ICD rubric = Pneumoconiosis Due to Other Inorganic Dust.
[k] Original ICD rubric = Other Disorders of Bone and Cartilage.

APPENDIX 2

Specific Medical Tests Published in the Literature for OSHA-Regulated Substances[a]

NOTES TO APPENDIX 2:

- Efficacy of medical tests has not been evaluated.
- NIOSH references include diagnostic, screening, and other tests.
- OSHA-mandated medical tests are shown in **BOLD**, underlined, and are listed separately.
- Only OSHA-regulated substances with published medical tests are included.
- Abbreviations and references are at end of APPENDIX 2.

Name of Substance	CAS Number	Specific Medical Tests (References in Superscript)
Acetaldehyde	00075-07-0	BL[3] ExA[3,4] U[3]
Acetone	00067-64-1	BL[3,5] BL(DE)[15] ExA[3,4] ExA(DE)[15] PFT[2] U[5] U(DE)[15] U(EOS)[3,18]
Acetonitrile	00075-05-8	BLC[2,3,16] BLP[2,3] ExA[4] U[3] Ua[2]
Acetylaminofluorene, 2-	00053-96-3	**RIC**[1] U[2]
Acetylene tetrabromide	00079-27-6	ExA[4] LFT[2,7]
Acrolein	00107-02-8	CXr[2,7] ExA[4] PFT[2,7]
Acrylamide	00079-06-1	NCS[15]
Acrylonitrile	00107-13-1	**CXr**[1] **FOB**[1] BLC[3] BLP[3] BLS[15] ExA[4] PFT[2] U[3,15]
Aldrin	00309-00-2	BLP[3] CBC[2] LFT[2] ReC[2] Ua[7]
Allyl chloride	00107-05-1	CBC[2] CXr[2,7] ExA[4] LFT[2] PFT[2,7] Ua[2]
Aluminum metal	07429-90-5	BLS[9] CXr[7] U[5,9,10,17]
Aminodiphenyl, 4-	00092-67-1	**RIC**[1] U[2]
Ammonia	07664-41-7	CXr[2,7] ExA[4] PFT[2,7]
Aniline	00062-53-3	BL[5,7] BL(COHb)[4] BL(DE)[11] BL(Hgb)[7] BL(MHgb)[2-5,8,11,15,16] BL(MHgb EOS)[15] CBC[2] ReC[2] U[3-6,12] U(EOS)[2,11,15,18] U(EWW)[18] Ua[2] Ua(Cyt Hmt)[2,16]
Anisidine (o-,p-isomers)	Varies	BL(Hgb)[7] BL(MHgb)[2,7,8,11] CBC[2] ReC[2] Ua[2]
Antimony and compounds	Varies	BL[9,17] BT[9] Cxr[7] PFT[2,7] U[3-5,9,13]
Arsenic, inorganic and compounds	Varies	**CXr**[1] **SpC**[1] BT[6] CXr[7] NCS[14] PFT[2,7] U[3-5,9,10,12-14] U(EWW)[11,15,16,18]

Specific Medical Tests Published in the Literature for OSHA-Regulated Substances (Continued)

Name of Substance	CAS Number	Specific Medical Tests (References in Superscript)
Arsine	07784-42-1	BL[7,13] BLP(Hgb)[16] LFT[7] PFT[2] ReC[16] U[9,10] U(EWW)[11] Ua[7] Ua(Hgb)[16] WBC[16]
Asbestos	Varies	**CXr**[1] **PFT**[1] CXr[2] PFT[2]
Azinphos-methyl (Guthion®)	00086-50-0	BF[2] BLS[9] CH[7] CH(BLS RBC)[2] CH(RBC)[11]
Barium and compounds	Varies	CXr[2] Ecg[2] PFT[2] U[9,17]
Benzene	00071-43-2	**CBC**[1] BL[3,5,12] BL(PNS)[15] ExA[3-5,12] ExA(EWW)[18] ExA(PNS)[11,15] ExA(PTS)[18] PFT[2] U[3-5,9,10,12] U(EOS)[11,15,18] U(PPS)[17] U(EWW)[18]
Benzidine	00092-87-5	**RIC**[1] PFT[2] U[2,3,17] Ua(Cyt[6M] Hmt[EM])[2] Ua(EM)[2]
Benzyl chloride	00100-44-7	CXr[2] ExA[4] PFT[2]
Beryllium and compounds	Varies	BT[9] CXr[2,7,16] PFT[2,7] U[3,4,10] WBC(LTT)[2]
Bis(chloromethyl) ether	00542-88-1	**RIC**[1] PFT[2] SpC[15]
Boron trifluoride	07637-07-2	CXr[2,7] PFT[2,7] U(PPS)[2]
Bromine	07726-95-6	CXr[2,7] PFT[2,7]
Butoxyethanol, 2-	00111-76-2	CBC[2,7] RBC(Frg)[2]
Butyl alcohol, n-	00071-36-3	BL[3] ExA[4]
Butyl chromate, tert-	00189-85-1	CXr[2] U[2]
Butyl glycidyl ether, n- (BGE)	02426-08-6	ExA[4] PFT[2]
Butyl mercaptan, n-	00109-79-5	ExA[4] PFT[2]
Butyltoluene, p-tert-	00098-51-1	CBC[2] Ecg[2] ExA[4]
Cadmium dust and fume	Varies	**U**[1] **BL**[1] BL[3-5,9,11,13,15,17,18] BT[9] CXr[2,4,7] LFT[2] PFT[2,7] U[3-5,7,9,11,13-15,18] Ua[7] Ua(Cyt)[2]
Camphor, synthetic	00076-22-2	BLP[3] U[3]
Carbaryl (Sevin®)	00063-25-2	BL(EOS)[15] BLS[9] CH[7] CH(PPS)[2,3] U[3-5,7] U(EOS)[15] Ua[2]
Carbon black	01333-86-4	PFT[2]
Carbon disulfide	00075-15-0	BL[3] Ecg[2,7] ExA[4] LFT[2,7] Oph[2,7] U[3-5] U(EOS)[3,11,15,18] U(EWW)[18] Ua[2,7]
Carbon monoxide	00630-08-0	BL[5] BL(COhb)[2-5,7,8,12] BL(COHb EOS)[11,18] BL(COHb EWW)[18] BL(EOS)[15] CBC[2] ExA[3-5] ExA(EOS)[11,18] ExA(EWW)[18]

Carbon tetrachloride	00056-23-5	BL[3,6] ExA[3,4] KFT[7] LFT[2,7] Ua[2,7]
Chlordane	00057-74-9	BL[3,15] BLS[9] BT[3] Ua[2,7]
Chlorinated diphenyl oxide	55720-99-5	LFT[2]
Chlorine	07782-50-5	CXr[2,7] ExA[8] PFT[2,7]
Chlorine dioxide	10049-04-4	CXr[2,7] PFT[2,7]
Chlorine trifluoride	07790-91-2	CXr[2,7] PFT[2,7]
Chlorobenzene	00108-90-7	U(EOS)[18] U(EWW)[18]
Chloroform (trichloromethane)	00067-66-3	ExA[3,4] LFT[2,7] Ua[2,7]
Chloromethyl methyl ether	00107-30-2	**RIC**[1] PFT[2] SpC[15]
Chloropicrin	00076-06-2	CXr[2,7] ExA[4] PFT[2,7]
Chloroprene, beta-	00126-99-8	CXr[2,7] PFT[2]
Chromic acid and chromates	Varies	BL[17] CBC[2] CXr[2,7] LFT[2] PFT[2,7] U[7] Ua[2]
Chromium, metal and compounds	Varies	BL[9,12] BT[9] CXr[2,7,9] PFT[2] U[4,5,9,11–13,17] U(EOS)[3,15,18] U(ESW)[11] U(EWW)[15,18]
Coal dust	68131-74-8	CXr[7] PFT[7]
Coal tar pitch volatiles	65996-93-2	CBC[2] CXr[2,7] PFT[2,7] PpT[2] SpC[2,7] Ua[2] Ua(Cyt Hmt)[2]
Cobalt metal, dust, and fume	07440-48-4	BL[9,13,17] BL(EOS)[18] BL(EWW)[18] BT[9] CXr[2,7] PFT[2,7] U[4,5,9,13] U(EOS)[3,18] U(EWW)[18]
Coke oven emissions	—	**CXr**[1] **PFT**[1] **SpC**[1] **Ua**[1] **Ua(Cyt Hmt)**[1]
Copper dust and mist	07440-50-8	BL[4,9,17] BLS[3] BT[9] U[9,17] U(24H)[3]
Cotton dust	—	**PFT**[1] CXr[2] PFT(PPS)[2]
Cresol, p-isomer	00106-44-5	LFT[2] PFT[2] U[3,9] U(PPS)[17]
Cumene	00098-82-8	U(L2H)[3,5]
Cyanide	00057-12-5	BL[3,5] BLC[16] BLP[3] CXr[2] PFT[2] U[3,5,15]
Cyclohexane	00110-82-7	BL[3,5] BL(DE)[15] ExA[3–5] ExA(DE)[15] U[5,10] U(EOS)[3] U(L4H)[15]
Cyclohexanone	00108-94-1	ExA[4] PFT[2] U[5]
Demeton (Systox®)	08065-48-3	CH[10] CH(BL BLP RBC)[5,16] CH(BLS RBC)[2] CH(RBC)[7,11]
Diacetone alcohol	00123-42-2	ExA[4] PFT[2]
Diazomethane	00334-88-3	CXr[2,7] PFT[2,7]
Diborane	19287-45-7	CXr[2,7] PFT[2,7]
Dibromo-3-chloropropane, 1,2- (DBCP)	00096-12-8	**BLS (FSH LH SCt TE)**[1] **GUT**[1] PFT[2]
Dibutyl phosphate	00107-66-4	Ecg[7] SpC[7] WBC[7]

***Specific Medical Tests Published in the Literature for OSHA-Regulated Substances** (**Continued**)*

Name of Substance	CAS Number	Specific Medical Tests (References in Superscript)
Dichlorodiphenyltrichloroethane (DDT)	00050-29-3	AdT[3] BL[12] BLS[3,9] BT[3] U[3,4]
Dichlorophenoxyacetic acid,2,4- (2,4-D)	00094-75-7	BLP[3] U[3,4] U(24H)[12]
Dichlorobenzene, p-	00106-46-7	BL(MHgb)[6] ExA[4] LFT[2,7] U[2-5]
Dichlorobenzidine, 3,3′-	00091-94-1	**RIC**[1] PFT[2]
Dichloro-5,5-dimethyl hydantoin, 1,3-	00118-52-5	Ecg[7] SpC[7] WBC[7]
Dichloroethyl ether	00111-44-4	CXr[2,7] ExA[4] PFT[2,7]
Dichlorvos (DDVP)	00062-73-7	BLS[9] CH[3,10] CH(BLP RBC)[16] CH(BLS RBC)[2] CH(RBC)[7,11] U[3]
Dieldrin	00060-57-1	BL[3,5,15] BLS[9] BT[3]
Diglycidyl ether (DGE)	02238-07-5	CBC[7] CXr[7] PFT[2,7]
Diisobutyl ketone	00108-83-8	PFT[2]
Dimethyl acetamide	00127-19-5	LFT[2,7] U(EOS)[18] U(EWW)[18]
Dimethyl sulfate	00077-78-1	CXr[2,7] LFT[2,7] PFT[2,7] Ua[2,7]
Dimethylaminoazobenzene, 4-	00060-11-7	**RIC**[1]
Dimethylaniline (N,N-dimethylaniline)	00121-69-7	BL(MHgb)[2,7,8,11,16] CBC[2,7] U(Cyt Hmt)[16]
Dimethyl-1,2-dibromo-2,2-dichloroethyl phosphate (Naled)	00300-76-5	BLS[9] CH(BLP RBC)[16] CH(BLS RBC)[2] CH(RBC)[7,11]
Dimethylformamide (DMF)	00068-12-2	BL[5] ExA[4,5] LFT[2,7] U[5,10,12] U(24H)[3] U(EOS)[11,15,18] U(EWW)[18]
Dimethylhydrazine, 1,1-	00057-14-7	CBC[7] LFT[7] PFT[2]
Dinitrobenzene, (all isomers)	Varies	BL(EOS)[15] BL(MHgb)[2,7,8,11,16] CBC[2,7] LFT[2,7] U(Cyt Hmt)[16]
Dinitro-o-cresol	00534-52-1	BLW[3,5]
Dinitrotoluene, 2,4-	00121-14-2	BL(MHgb)[2,7,8,11] CBC[2,7] LFT[2,7]
Dioxane (diethylene dioxide)	00123-91-1	BL(DE)[15] BLP[3] BUN[7] CXr[2] ExA[4] KFT[7] LFT[2,7] PFT[2] U(EOS)[3,15] Ua[2]
Endrin	00072-20-8	BL[5] BL(EOS)[15] BLP[3] BLS[9] U[3,5] U(EOS)[15]
Epichlorohydrin	00106-89-8	CXr[2,7] ExA[4] LFT[2] PFT[2,7] Ua[2]
EPN	02104-64-5	BLS[9] CH(BLS RBC)[2] CH(RBC)[7,11] U[10]
Ethyl alcohol (ethanol)	00064-17-5	BL[3,17] BLS[9] ExA[3,4] U(EOS)[3]

Ethyl benzene	00100-41-4	BL[5] ExA[4,5,11] ExA(EWW)[15] ExA(PNS)[15] U[5,9,10] U(EOS)[15,18] U(ESW)[11] U(EWW)[18] U(L2H)[3]
Ethyl ether (ether)	00060-29-7	BL[3] ExA[4]
Ethyl mercaptan	00075-08-1	ExA[4] PFT[2]
Ethylene chlorohydrin	00107-07-3	ExA[4] LFT[2,7] Ua[2,7]
Ethylene dibromide	00106-93-4	BUN[7] CXr[2] Ecg40[2] ExA[4] LFT[2,7] PFT[2]
Ethylene dichloride	00107-06-2	ExA[4] LFT[7] PFT[2]
Ethylene glycol dinitrate	00628-96-6	BL[3,12] BL(DE)[5,15] CBC[7] Ecg[7] ExA(DE)[5] U[3,12]
Ethylene oxide	00075-21-8	**<u>CBC</u>**[1] CBC[7] CXr[7] ExA[4] PFT[2]
Ethyleneimine	00151-56-4	**<u>RIC</u>**[1] CXr[7] ExA[4] PFT[2]
Ferrovanadium dust	12604-58-9	CXr[2] PFT[2]
Fluoride, inorganic	16984-48-8	BLP[3,12] CXr[2,7] PFT[2,7] PXr[2,7] U[2,4,5,9,10,12] U(EOS)[11,15,18] U(EWW)[15,18] U(PNS)[15] U(PPS)[7,17] U(PTS)[11] Ua[2]
Fluorine	07782-41-4	CXr[2,7] PFT[2,7]
Formalydehyde	00050-00-0	**<u>PFT</u>**[1] BL[3,9] CXr[7] PFT[7] PFT(PPS)[2] U[3,9]
Furfural	00098-01-1	U(EOS)[18]
Furfuryl alcohol	00098-00-0	ExA[4] PFT[2]
Graphite, natural	07782-42-5	CXr[2,7] PFT[2,7]
Hexachloronaphthalene (Halowax 1014)	01335-87-1	LFT[2,3,7]
Hexane, n-	00110-54-3	BL[3,5] ExA[3-5,11] ExA(DE)[15] U[3,5,10] U(EOS)[11,15,18] U(EWW)[18]
Hydrazine	00302-01-2	CXr[7] PFT[2,7]
Hydrogen chloride (hydrochloric acid)	07647-01-0	CXr[2,7] PFT[2,7]
Hydrogen cyanide (hydrocyanic acid)	00074-90-8	BL(COHb)[4] Ecg40[2] ExA[4]
Hydrogen fluoride (hydrofluoric acid)	07664-39-3	CXr[2,7] KFT[6] PFT[2,7] PXr[2,7] U[2,10] U(PPS)[7] Ua[2]
Hydrogen sulfide	07783-06-4	BL[3] BL(COHb)[4] BLP[3] CXr[2,7] PFT[2,7]
Hydroquinone	00123-31-9	Oph[7] PFT[2]
Iodine	07553-56-2	CXr[2,7] PFT[2,7]
Iron oxide fume	01309-37-1	BL[9,17] BT[9] CXr[2,7] PFT[2,7] U[9,17]
Isophorone	00078-59-1	CXr[2] PFT[2]
Isopropyl alcohol (isopropanol)	00067-63-0	BL[3] ExA[4] U[3]
Isopropyl glycidyl ether (IGE)	04016-14-2	PFT[2]
Ketene	00463-51-4	CXr[2,7] PFT[2,7]

Specific Medical Tests Published in the Literature for OSHA-Regulated Substances **(*Continued*)**

Name of Substance	CAS Number	Specific Medical Tests (References in Superscript)
Lead, inorganic	07439-92-1	**BLL**[1] **BUN**[1] **Hgb**[1] **SCr**[1] **U**[1] **ZPP**[1] BL[3,5,9,11–13,15–17] BLL[2,7,14,16,18] BT[9] CBC[2,7] RBC[2,5] RBC(ZPP)[2] U[3–5,9,11–17] U(EOS)[17] Ua[7] ZPP[2,13] ZPP(1M)[2,11,15,16]
Lindane	00058-89-9	BL[2,3,5,7,12] BLS[3,15] CBC[2,7] U[4]
Lithium hydride	07580-67-8	BL[2,9,17] BLS[3] BT[9] U[3]
Magnesium oxide fume	01309-48-4	BL[17]
Malathion	00121-75-5	BLS[9] CH[3,10] CH(BLS RBC)[2] CH(RBC)[7,11] CXr[2] LFT[2] PFT[2] U[3,4]
Manganese and compounds	Varies	BL[9,13,17] BT[9] CBC[2] CXr[2] Neur[6] PFT[2] U[2–4,9,13,17] Ua[2]
Mercury, inorganic and compounds	Varies	BL[3–5,12,14,16] BL(EOS)[18] BL(ESW)[11] BL(EWW)[18] BT[9] BUN[7] NCS[14,16] TFT[7] U[2–5,7,9,10,12–15] Ua[2,7] U(PTS)[11,18]
Mercury, organo alkyl compounds	Varies	BL[2,3,7,9] Emg[7] U[7,9] Ua[2,7]
Methyl alcohol (methanol)	00067-56-1	BL[16] BLP[16] ExA[4] LFT[2] U[3,5,7,10,16] U(EOS)[11,15,18] U(EWW)[15] U(PNS)[15] U(PWW)[11]
Methyl n-amyl ketone	00110-43-0	PFT[2]
Methyl bromide	00074-83-9	BL[15,16] BLS[3] BUN[7] CXr[2] ExA[4] PFT[2]
Methyl n-butyl ketone (MBK)	00591-78-6	BL[3] Emg[7] ExA[3] PFT[2] U(EWW)[5]
Methyl cellosolve	00109-86-4	CBC[2,7] U[4,9]
Methyl chloride	00074-87-3	BL[3] ExA[3,4]
Methyl chloroform	00071-55-6	BL[3,5,10,12] BL(EOS)[15,18] BL(ESW)[11] BL(EWW)[10,15,18] ExA[3,4,10,12] ExA(16H)[5] ExA(EWW)[10,15,18] ExA(PNS)[15] ExA(PTS)[18] ExA(PWW)[11] LFT[7] U[3,5,12] U(EOS)[15,18] U(ESW)[11] U(EWW)[5,11,15,18]
Methyl ethyl ketone (MEK)	00078-93-3	BL[3,9,10,17] ExA[3,4,10] PFT[2] U[3,5,10] U(EOS)[11,15,16,18]
Methyl hydrazine	00060-34-4	BL(MHgb)[16] PFT[2] U[16] U(Cyt Hmt)[16]
Methyl isobutyl ketone (MIBK)	00108-10-1	ExA[4] PFT[2] U[5] U(EOS)[11,18] U(EWW)[18]
Methyl isocyanate	00624-83-9	CXr[2,7] PFT[2,7]
Methyl mercaptan	00074-93-1	CXr[7] ExA[4] PFT[2,7]
Methyl propyl ketone	00107-87-9	CXr[2] PFT[2]
Methylene bisphenyl isocyanate (MDI)	00101-68-8	CXr[2,7] PFT[2,7]

Methylene chloride	00075-09-2	BL[3,5] BL(COHb)[2–5,16] BL(COHb EOS[15] BL(COHb PNS)[15] BL(EOS)[15] CBC[2,7] ExA[3–5,16] ExA(EOS)[15] LFT[2] U[4,16]
Methylene dianiline, 4,4′-	00101-77-9	**LFT**[1] **U**[1] U[16]
Mica	12001-26-2	CXr[2,7] PFT[2,7]
Molybdenum and compounds	Varies	BL[4,9,17] BT[9] U[4,9,17]
Monomethyl aniline	00100-61-8	BL[7] BL(MHgb)[2,7,8,11,16] CBC[2,7] U[7] U(Cyt Hmt)[16] Ua[7]
Naphthalene	00091-20-3	BL[7] BLP(Hgb)[7] CBC[2,7] LFT[7] RBC(Hem)[2] U[7] Ua[2] WBC[7]
Naphthylamine, alpha-	00134-32-7	**RIC**[1] Ua[7] Cys[7]
Naphthylamine, beta-	00091-59-8	**RIC**[1] Ua[7] Cys[7]
Nickel carbonyl	13463-39-3	BLP[3] CXr[2,7] ExA[3,9] PFT[2,7] SpC[2] U[3,7,12,16,17] Ua[2]
Nickel, metal and compounds	Varies	BLP[3,9,12] BLP(EOS)[15] BLS[13,16] BT[9] CXr[2,7] PFT[2] PPS[2,13] U[3,5,9,12,13,16,17] U(EOS)[15]
Nicotine	00054-11-5	BLP[3] BUN[7] U[3]
Nitric acid	07697-37-2	CXr[2,7] PFT[2,7]
Nitric oxide	10102-43-9	CXr[2,7] Ecg40[2] ExA[4] PFT[2,7]
Nitroaniline, p-	00100-01-6	BL[7] BL(MHgb)[2,7,8,11,16] CBC[2,7] LFT[2,7] U[16] U(Cyt Hmt)[16]
Nitrobenzene	00098-95-3	BL[7] BL(COHb)[4,11] BL(EOS)[15] BL(MHgb)[2,3,5,7,8,11,16] CBC[2,7] U[2,3,5,7] U(EOS)[15,18] U(ESW)[11] U(EWW)[12,18]
Nitrobiphenyl, 4-	00092-93-3	**RIC**[1] U[2]
Nitrochlorobenzene, p-	00100-00-5	BL(MHgb)[2,7,8,11,16] CBC[2,7] U[16] U(Cyt Hmt)[16]
Nitrogen dioxide	10102-44-0	CXr[2,7] Ecg40[2] ExA[4] PFT[2,7]
Nitrogen trifluoride	07783-54-2	BL[7] BL(MHgb)[2,7,8,11] CBC[2,7]
Nitropropane, 2-	00079-46-9	CXr[2] LFT[7] PFT[2] WBC[7]
Nitrosodimethylamine, N-	00062-75-9	**RIC**[1] LFT[7] PFT[2]
Nitrotoluene (all isomers)	Varies	BL[7] BL(MHgb)[2,7,8,11,16] CBC[2,7] U[7,16] U(Cyt Hmt)[16]
Octachloronaphthalene	02234-13-1	LFT[2,7]
Oxalic acid	00144-62-7	BUN[7] U[3]
Oxygen difluoride	07783-41-7	CXr[2,7] PFT[2,7]
Ozone	10028-15-6	BL(PMN)[16] CXr[2,7] PFT[2,7,16]
Paraquat	04685-14-7	CXr[2,7] LFT[2] PFT[2,7] U[3] Ua[2]
Parathion	00056-38-2	BLS[9] CH[3,7,10,15] CH(BLP)[16] CH(BLP RBC)[16] CH(BLS RBC)[2] CH(RBC)[7,11] U[3–5,10] U(EOS)[11,15,18] U(EWW)[18]
Pentachloronaphthalene	01321-64-8	LFT[2,7]

Specific Medical Tests Published in the Literature for OSHA-Regulated Substances (Continued)

Name of Substance	CAS Number	Specific Medical Tests (References in Superscript)
Pentachlorophenol	00087-86-5	BL[9,17] BLP[3,5] BLP(EOS)[11,18] BLS[9] U[2-5,7,9] U(EWW)[17,18] U(PTS)[18] U(PWW)[11]
Perchloroethylene (tetrachloroethylene)	00127-18-4	BL[3,12,16] BL(16H)[5] BL(EWW)[15,18] BL(PNS)[15] BL(PTS)[18] BL(PWW)[11] ExA[3,4,10,12,16] ExA(16H)[5] ExA(DE)[5] ExA(EOS)[6,15] ExA(EWW)[15,18] ExA(PNS)[15] ExA(PTS)[18] ExA(PWW)[11] LFT[2,7] U[2,16] U(16H)[5,11] U(EOS)[15,18] U(EWW)[5,11,18] Ua[2]
Perchloromethyl mercaptan	00594-42-3	CXr[2,7] LFT[2] PFT[2,7] Ua[2]
Perchloryl fluoride	07616-94-6	BL[7] BL(MHgb)[2,7,8,11,16] CBC[2,7] CXr[2,7] PFT[2,7] U[16] U(Cyt Hmt)[16]
Phenol	00108-95-2	LFT[2,7] U[2,5,7,9,12] U(L2H)[3,15] U(EOS)[11,15,18] U(PPS)[17] Ua[2,7]
Phenyl glycidyl ether (PGE)	00122-60-1	PFT[2]
Phenylhydrazine	00100-63-0	BL[7] BLP(Hgb)[7] CBC[7] LFT[7] PFT[2] U[7] Ua[7]
Phosdrin (Mevinphos®)	07786-34-7	BLS[9] CH[7] CH(BLS RBC)[2] CH(RBC)[11]
Phosgene (carbonyl chloride)	00075-44-5	BGa[16] CXr[2,7] Ecg[16] ExA[4] PFT[2,7] SpC[16] WBC[16]
Phosphine	07803-51-2	CXr[7] PFT[7]
Phosphorus (Yellow)	07723-14-0	CBC(Anm)[2] DXr[2,6,7] KFT[6] LFT[2,7]
Phosphorus pentachloride	10026-13-8	CXr[2,7] PFT[2,7]
Phosphorus pentasulfide	01314-80-3	CXr[2,7] PFT[2,7]
Phosphorus trichloride	07719-12-2	CXr[2,7] PFT[2,7]
Phthalic anhydride	00085-44-9	CXr[7] PFT[7] U[5]
Picric acid	00088-89-1	BUN[7] LFT[2,7] Ua[2]
Pindone (2-pivalyl-1,3-indandione)	00083-26-1	BL[7] BLP(PTT)[2,7] CBC[7] Ua(RBC)[7]
Platinum, metal, and compounds	Varies	BL[9,17] BT[9] U[9,17]
Polychlorobiphenyl (42% chlorine) (PCB)	53469-21-9	AdT[3] BL[3,15] BLP[3] BLS[9,17] LFT[2,7]
Polychlorodiphenyl (54% chlorine) (PCB)	11097-69-1	AdT[3] BL[3,15] BLP[3] BLS[9,17] LFT[2,7]
Portland cement	65997-15-1	CXr[2,7] PFT[2,7]
Propiolactone, beta-	00057-57-8	**RIC**[1] PFT[2]
Propyl nitrate, n-	00627-13-4	BL[7] BL(MHgb)[2,8,11,16] CBC[2,7] Ua[7] Ua(Cyt Hmt)[16]

Propyleneimine	00075-55-8	BL[7] CBC[7] CBC(GL)[2]
Pyridine	00110-86-1	ExA[4] LFT[2] Ua[2]
Quinone	00106-51-4	Oph[2,7]
Selenium compounds, except SeF_6	Varies	BH[3] BL[7,9,13] BLP[15] LFT[2] U[3,7,9,15] U(24H)[13] WBC[7]
Selenium hexafluoride (SeF_6)	07783-79-1	CXr[2,7] PFT[2,7]
Silica, amorphous, diatomaceous earth	61790-53-2	CXr[2,7] PFT[2,7] Rdg[7] SpC[7] TBS[7]
Silica, crystalline cristobalite	14464-46-1	CXr[2,7] PFT[2,7] Rdg[7] SpC[7] TBS[7]
Silicates—soapstone	—	CXr[2,7] PFT[2,7]
Silicates—talc (without asbestos)	14807-96-6	CXr[2,7] PFT[2,7] Rdg[7] SpC[7] TBS[7]
Silver, metal and compounds	Varies	BL[9,17] BT[9] Pgm[2] U[9,17]
Sodium fluoroacetate	00062-74-8	Ecg[2,7] Ua[2,7]
Sodium hydroxide	01310-73-2	CXr[2] PFT[2]
Stibine	07803-52-3	BL[7] BLP(Hgb)[7] CBC[7] LFT[2,7] RBC(Hem)[2] U[7] Ua[2,7] WBC[7]
Stoddard solvent	08052-41-3	CBC[2] ExA[4] LFT[2] Ua[2]
Strychnine	00057-24-9	BUN[7] Cnv[2,7,16]
Styrene	00100-42-5	BL(16H)[5] BL(EOS)[11,15,18] BL(EWW)[18] BL(PNS)[11,15] BL(PTS)[18] ExA[4,5,9,12] ExA(DE)[15] ExA(PNS)[15] Neur[7] U[3,5,7,9,10,12] U(EOS)[10,11,15,18] U(EWW)[18] U(PNS)[11] U(PTS)[18]
Sulfur dioxide	07446-09-5	CXr[2,7] ExA[4] PFT[2,7]
Sulfur monochloride	10025-67-9	CXr[2] PFT[2]
Sulfur pentafluoride	05714-22-7	CXr[2,7] PFT[2,7]
Sulfuric acid	07664-93-9	CXr[2,7] PFT[2,7]
Sulfotep (TEDP)	03689-24-5	BLS[9] CH[7] CH(BLS RBC)[2] CH(RBC)[11]
Tellurium hexafluoride	07783-80-4	CXr[7] PFT[7] U[6]
Tetraethyl pyrophosphate (TEPP)	00107-49-3	BLS[9] CH[7] CH(BLP RBC)[16] CH(BLS RBC)[2] CH(RBC)[7,11]
Tetrachloroethane, 1,1,2,2-	00079-34-5	BUN[7] LFT[2,7] Ua[2,7]
Tetrachloronaphthalene	01335-88-2	LFT[2,7]
Tetraethyl lead	00078-00-2	BL[3] BMU[2,7] U[3,7,16] U(EOS)[4] Ua[2,7]
Tetramethyl lead	00075-74-1	BMU[2,7] U[7] U(EOS)[4] Ua[2,7]
Tetranitromethane	00509-14-8	BL[7] BL(MHgb)[2,7,8,11] CBC[2,7] CXr[2,7] PFT[2,7]
Tetryl	00479-45-8	CBC[7] CBC(Anm)[2] LFT[7]
Thallium and compounds	Varies	BH[7] BL[3,9,17] BT[9] NCS[15] U[3,4,7,15,16] Ua[2,7]

Specific Medical Tests Published in the Literature for OSHA-Regulated Substances (*Continued*)

Name of Substance	CAS Number	Specific Medical Tests (References in Superscript)
Tin, inorganic compounds (exc oxide)	Varies	BL[13] CXr[15] U[3,9,17]
Tin, organic compounds	Varies	Ecg40[2,15] Glau[2] KFT[15] LFT[2,7,15] RBC(Hem)[2] U[2,3,15]
Toluene	00108-88-3	BL[3,5,9,10,15,17] BL(EOS)[11,15,18] BL(EWW)[18] ExA[3-5,9,11] ExA(DE)[9,15] U[2-5,7,9] U(EOS)[10,11,15,18] U(EOS 2D)[17] U(L2H)[15] Ua[2,7]
Toluene-2,4-diisocyanate (TDI)	00584-84-9	CXr[2,7] PFT[7] PFT(PPS)[2]
Toluidine, o-	00095-53-4	BL[7] BL(MHgb)[2,8,11,15] CBC[2] Ua[2]
Trichloroethane, 1,1,2-	00079-00-5	ExA[4]
Trichloroethylene	00079-01-6	BL[3,12] BL(EOS)[15,18] BL(ESW)[11] BL(EWW)[15,18] BLP[5] ExA[3-5,7,11,12] ExA(EWW)[15] ExA(PNS)[15] PFT[2] U[3-5,12] U(EOS)[15,18] U(ESW)[11] U(EWW)[11,15,18]
Trichloronaphthalene	01321-65-9	LFT[2,7]
Trinitrotoluene, 2,4,6- (TNT)	00118-96-7	BL[7] BL(MHgb)[15] CBC[7] CBC(ApA)[2] LFT[2,7] Ua[2]
Trichlorophenoxyacetic acid (2,4,5-T)	00093-76-5	BLP[3] U[3,4] U(24H)[12]
Trichloropropane, 1,2,3-	00096-18-4	ExA[4]
Uranium and compounds	07440-61-1	BL[7] CBC[2,7] CXr[2,7] U[2-4,7,9] Ua[2,7]
Vanadium fume (pentoxide)	01314-62-1	BL[17] CXr[2,7] PFT[2,7] U[5,7,13,15] U(EOS)[18] U(EWW)[18]
Vinyl chloride	00075-01-4	**APh**[1] **Br**[1] **GGT**[1] **SGOT**[1] **SGPT**[1] APh[9] Br[7] CXr[7] ExA[3,4] GGT[7] LDH[7] LFT[15] PFT[2,7] SGOT[7] SGPT[7] U[3,15] Ua[7] Usg[9]
Warfarin	00081-81-2	BL[7] BLP[3] BLP(Hyt)[2] BLP(PTT)[2,7,12] CBC[7] Ua(RBC)[2,7]
Xylene, all isomers	Varies	BL[3,7,12] BL(DE)[5] BL(EOS)[15] CBC[7] CBC(HeD)[2] ExA[3,4,10] LFT[2,7] U[3,5,9,10,12] U(EOS)[11,15,18] U(EOS 2D)[17] U(EWW)[18] U(L2H)[15] Ua[2,7]
Xylidine	01300-73-8	BL[7] BL(MHgb)[2,7,8,11] CBC[2,7]
Zinc chloride fume	07646-85-7	BL[9,17] BT[9] CXr[2,7] PFT[2,7] U[2,3,7,9,15]
Zinc oxide fume	01314-13-2	BL[9,17] BT[9] CXr[2] PFT[2] U[2,3,7,9,15] WBC[7]
Zirconium and compounds, except ZrCl4	Varies	BL[9,17] BT[9] (GraS)[2]

[a] This is an updated version of TABLE 2 of L. I. Murthy & W. E. Halperin, 1995, Medical Screening and Biological Monitoring: A Guide to the Literature for Physicians, J. Occup. Environ. Med. **37**(2): 170–184.

Abbreviations Used in Appendix 2

1M = After 1 month's exposure
2D = After 2 days' exposure
6M = Every 6 months
16H = 16 hours after end of exposure
24H = 24-hour collection
AdT = Adipose tissue
Anm = Anemia
ApA = Aplastic anemia
Aph = Alkaline phosphatase
BF = Body fluid (chemical/metabolite)
BGa = Blood gas analysis
BH/N = Body hair/nail
BL = Whole blood (chemical/metabolite)
BLC = Blood cyanide
BLL = Blood lead
BLM = Metabolite in blood
BLP = Blood plasma
BLS = Blood serum
BLW = Blood analyzed weekly
BMU = Biologic monitoring of urine every 3 months
Br = Bilirubin
BT = Biologic tissue/biopsy
BUN = Blood urea nitrogen
CBC = Complete blood count
CH = Blood cholinesterase
CXr = Chest X-ray
Cnv = Convulsions
COHb = Carboxyhemoglobin
Cyt = Cytology
DE = During exposure
DXr = Dental X-ray
Ecg = Electrocardiogram
Ecg40 = Electrocardiogram on workers over 40 years
EOS = End of shift
Emg = Electromyogram
ESW = End of shift at end of worksheet
EWW = End of workweek
ExA = Expired air
FOB = Fecal occult blood screening
Frg = Fragility
FSH = Follicle stimulating hormone
GGT = Gamma glutamyl transpeptidase
GL = Granulocytic leukemia
Glau = Glaucoma
GraS = Granuloma of the skin
GUT = Genito-urinary tract
Hem = RBC hemolysis
HeD = Hematopoietic depression
Hmt = Hematuria
Hyt = Hypoprothrombinemia
Hgb = Hemoglobin
KFT = Kidney function tests
L2H = Last 2 hours of 8-hour exposure
L4H = Last 4 hours of 8-hour exposure
LDH = Lactic dehydrogenase
LFT = Liver function tests

Abbreviations Used in Appendix 2 (Continued)

LH	= Luteinizing hormone	Rdg	= Radiography
LTT	= Lymphocyte transformation test	ReC	= Reticulocyte count
MHgb	= Methemoglobin	Ria	= Radioimmunoassay
NCS	= Nerve conduction studies	RIC	= Reduced immunologic competence
Neur	= Neurologic examination	SCr	= Serum creatinine
Oph	= Ophthalmic examination	SCt	= Sperm count
PFT	= Pulmonary function tests	SGOT	= Serum glutamic oxalacetic transaminase
Pgm	= Pigmentation evidence	SGPT	= Serum glutamic pyruvic transminase
PMN	= Polymorphonuclear leukocytes	SpC	= Sputum cytology
PNS	= Prior to next shift	TBS	= Tuberculin skin test
PPS	= Pre- and postshift	TE	= Total estrogen (females)
PpT	= Photopatch testing	TFT	= Thyroid function test
PTS	= Prior to shift	U	= Urine (chemical/metabolite)
PTT	= Prothrombin time	Ua	= Urinalysis (routine)
PWW	= Prior to last shift of workweek	Usg	= Ultrasonography of the liver
PXr	= Pelvic X-ray	WBC	= White blood cell count/differential
RBC	= Red blood cells	ZPP	= Zinc protoporphyrin

References in Appendix 2

1. U.S. Department of Labor, Occupational Safety and Health Administration. 1996. Code of Federal Regulations. 29 CFR Part 1910 (1910.1000 to end). Air Contaminants. Revised as of July 1, 1996. U.S. Government Printing Office. Washington, DC.
2. U.S. Department of Health and Human Services, Public Health Service, Centers for Disease Control, National Institute for Occupational Safety and Health, and U.S. Department of Labor, Occupational Safety and Health Administration. 1981, 1988, 1989, 1992, 1995. NIOSH/OSHA Occupational Health Guidelines for Chemical Hazards (1981, 1988, 1989, 1992, 1995). F. W. Mackison, R. S. Stricoff, L. J. Partridge, Jr. & A. D. Little Inc., Eds. DHHS (NIOSH) Publication Nos. 81-123 and Supplement I-IV. U.S. Department of Health and Human Services. Washington, DC.
3. Baselt, R. C. 1988. Biological Monitoring Methods for Industrial Chemicals. 2d edit. Year Book Medical Publishers. Littleton, MA.
4. Linch, A. L. 1974. Biological Monitoring for Industrial Chemical Exposure Control. CRC Press. Cleveland, OH.
5. Lauwerys, R. R. & P. Hoet. 1993. Industrial Chemical Exposure. Guidelines for Biological Monitoring. 2d edit. R. R. Lauwerys & P. Hoet, Eds. Lewis Publishers. CRC Press. Boca Raton, FL.
6. Brown, K. K., A. W. Teass, S. Simon & E. M. Ward. 1995. A biological monitoring method for o-toluidine and aniline in urine using high performance liquid chromatography with electrochemical detection. Appl. Occup. Environ. Hyg. **10**(6): 557-565.
7. Proctor, N. H. & J. P. Hughes. 1978. Chemical Hazards of the Workplace. N. H. Proctor & J. P. Hughes, Eds. JB Lippincott Company. Philadelphia.
8. Hathaway, G. J., N. H. Proctor, J. P. Hughes & M. L. Fischman. 1991. Chemical Hazards of the Workplace. 3d edit. G. J. Hathaway, N. H. Proctor, J. P. Hughes & M. L. Fischman, Eds. Van Nostrand Reinhold Publishers. New York.
9. Kneip, T. J. & J. V. Crable. 1988. Methods for Biological Monitoring—A Manual for Assessing Human Exposure to Hazardous Substances. T. J. Kneip & J. V. Crable, Eds. American Public Health Association. Washington, DC.
10. Ho, M. H. & H. K. Dillon. 1987. Biological Monitoring of Exposure to Chemicals. Organic Compounds. M. H. Ho & H. K. Dillon, Eds. John Wiley & Sons. New York.
11. ACGIH. 1996. 1996 Threshold Limit Values for Chemical Substances and Physical Agents and Biological Exposure Indices. American Conference of Governmental Industrial Hygienists Worldwide. Technical Affairs Office. Cincinnati, OH.
12. Atio A., V. Riihimaki & H. Vainio, Eds. 1984. Biological Monitoring and Surveillance of Workers Exposed to Chemicals. Hemisphere Publishing Corporation. New York.
13. Clarkson, T. W., L. Friberg, G. F. Nordberg & P. R. Sager. 1988. Biological Monitoring of Toxic Metals. Rochester Series on Environmental Toxicity. T. W. Clarkson, L. Friberg, G. F. Nordberg & P. R. Sager, Eds. Plenum Press. New York.
14. Dillon, H. K. & M. H. Ho. 1991. Biological Monitoring of Exposure to Chemicals. Metals. H. K. Dillon & M. H. Ho, Eds. John Wiley & Sons. Somerset, NJ.
15. LaDou, J., Ed. 1990. Occupational Medicine: 459-466. Appleton and Lange.

References in Appendix 2 (Continued)

16. 1996. Proctor and Hughes' Chemical Hazards of the Workplace. 4th edit. G. J. Hathaway, N. H. Proctor & J. P. Hughes, Eds. Van Nostrand Reinhold. New York.
17. U.S. Department of Health and Human Services, Public Health Service, Centers for Disease Control, National Institute for Occupational Safety and Health. NIOSH Manual of Analytic Methods. 4th edit. DHHS (NIOSH) Publication No. 94-113. U.S. Department of Health and Human Services. Washington, DC.
18. Fiserova-Bergerova, V. & J. Vlach. 1997. Timing of sample collection for biological monitoring of occupational exposure. Ann. Occup. Hyg. **41**(3): 345-353.

Molecular Epidemiology and Occupational Health

FREDERICA P. PERERA [a] AND
CHRISTOPHER DICKEY

Division of Environmental Health Sciences
School of Public Health
Columbia University
60 Haven Avenue, B-116
New York, New York 10032

For more than a decade, there has been wide agreement that most cancer results from industrial and environmental exposures (such as tobacco smoke; chemical pollutants in air, water, and food; drugs; radiation; dietary constituents; radon; and infectious agents) acting in concert with both genetic and acquired characteristics.[1–6] It has been estimated that without these environmental factors, cancer incidence would be dramatically reduced, by as much as 80–90%.[3,5] Cancer risk is strongly influenced by genetic composition, age, ethnicity, gender, immune function, preexisting disease, and nutritional levels, but each of these factors in isolation contributes little to overall cancer risk. Genetic predisposition, for example, in the absence of external environmental influence, probably explains no more than 5% of all cancers in the United States.[7] Thus, most cancer is by nature preventable.

Given the multifactorial nature of cancer, a practical approach to reducing the incidence of the disease combines active intervention on two fronts: modifying hazardous lifestyles, such as smoking and diets high in fat and low in protective antioxidants and fibers; and reducing or eliminating exposure to carcinogenic pollutants that pose substantial risks. Molecular epidemiology, a preventive approach that incorporates laboratory methods to analyze environmental and host factors (e.g., genetic polymorphisms), has the potential to give early warning by documenting the preclinical effects of exposure and increased susceptibility to cancer. Thus, molecular epidemiology can flag opportunities to avert cancer through timely intervention. Moreover, biomarker data on the distribution of procarcinogenic changes and susceptibility factors in the population can improve estimation of cancer risk from a given exposure.[8]

Significant exposure to carcinogens occurs for many in the workplace. Such exposures might include industrial or man-made chemicals, pesticides, metals, and fibers (for review, see references 9,10). Occupationally exposed persons are often faced with the choice between the immediate necessity to work and the long-term avoidance of a possible devastating chronic illness related to their job. Most workers given such a choice will continue to work despite the knowledge that they may be endangering their health. In addition, since most of the industrial chemicals produced

[a] Corresponding author. Phone: 212/304-7280; fax: 212/544-1943; e-mail: fpp1@columbia.edu

and released into the environment each year are untested, persons exposed occupationally to carcinogens may never even be aware of their increased risk.

Biologic markers can be incorporated into analytic epidemiologic studies of occupationally exposed individuals to help identify a causal relationship between exposure to a specific agent and increased risk of cancer. For example, urinary mandelic acid and 1-hydroxypyrene are considered reliable indicators of exposure and internal dose of styrene and benzo(a)pyrene (BaP), respectively. Styrene-DNA or BaP-DNA adducts provide further information on the biologically effective dose of these carcinogens. As such, both types of markers can serve to assign subjects to "exposed" and "unexposed" groups on a more meaningful basis than self-reported exposure, job history, or environmental monitoring, thereby reducing random exposure misclassification. In addition, biomarkers like the ones just listed can provide information on interindividual variation in response to carcinogen exposure, potentially eliminating the assumption of homogeneity.

Moreover, certain biologic markers of preclinical response (correlated with cancer and occurring prior to malignancy) have the potential to serve as intermediate markers, replacing clinical disease as an outcome. Possible candidates include specific alterations of oncogenes (e.g., ras) or tumor suppressor genes (e.g., P53). By providing an earlier and more commonly occurring outcome, such markers could mitigate the latency problem in cancer epidemiology, increase study power, and allow effective intervention.

Finally, biologic measures of molecular dose and effect coupled with biomarkers of susceptibility can be used to identify subgroups of workers at highest potential risk. Those workers can then be targeted for epidemiologic follow-up and intervention.

The class of polycyclic aromatic hydrocarbons (PAH) are common pollutants found in cigarette smoke, the workplace, air, drinking water, and diet. PAH are formed mainly as a result of pyrolytic processes, especially the incomplete combustion of organic materials; for example, fossil fuels in internal combustion engines, coke production, and power plants. The natural background PAH level may be near zero, but often ranges from 1-3 ng/m^3 in urban areas with exceptions in heavy coal-burning areas.[11] High concentrations on the order of 5 μg/m^3 can occur indoors when certain types of heating oils are used without chimneys or ventilation. Occupationally exposed coke oven and iron foundry workers can be exposed in the range of 4-40 μg/m^3.[12]

The best characterized PAH in terms of metabolism, detoxification, DNA binding, and cancer risk is BaP. BaP is metabolized by the cytochrome p450 monoxygenase system and epoxide hydrolase to a reactive molecule [7,8-dihydrodiol-9,10-epoxide, (BPDE)] that can ultimately react with DNA to form a covalently bound adduct.[13] The reactive epoxide may also undergo glutathione conjugation via glutathione *S*-transferase (GST) or detoxification by another phase II enzyme system.[14]

Cytochrome p450 1A1 (CYP1A1) is a membrane-bound phase I biotransformation enzyme that catalyzes the hydroxylation of BaP to its reactive metabolite. CYP1A1 contains two closely linked polymorphisms that have been associated with significantly increased risk of lung cancer in Japanese populations; one a restriction fragment-length polymorphism downstream from the coding region known as MspI; and the other a point mutation in exon 7 that results in the substitution of valine for isoleucine in the protein.[15] Several studies have shown an increase in CYP1A1 enzyme activity in lymphocytes or placental tissue that contain one or both of the polymorphisms.[16] Increased enzyme activity may lead to an increase in reactive metabolites of compounds like BaP, and a subsequent increase in covalently bound adducts to DNA. The pathway just described may partially explain the observation in some studies of a relatively high risk of cancer in persons with polymorphisms in CYP1A1.[15]

Similarly, deletions of GSTM1, a noninducible phase II cytosolic detoxification enzyme that catalyzes the conjugation of reactive electrophiles to reduced glutathione, have also been associated with increased risk of lung cancer.[17] Benzo(a)pyrene metabolites (e.g., BPDE) generated by activation of BaP in phase I, are covalently bound to glutathione in phase II by glutathione transferases. It is estimated that 30–60% of populations studied to date have the null (deleted) genotype.[18] The GSTM1 was reported to have a differential distribution across ethnic groups in the United States, with a 49% prevalence of the null genotype in Caucasians and a 35% prevalence among African Americans.[19] A positive association has been shown between the GSTM1 null genotype and PAH-DNA adducts in lung tissue.[20]

If unrepaired, DNA adducts can lead to gene mutation and neoplasia, possibly via activation of protooncogenes or inactivation of tumor suppressor genes. DNA adducts are considered a necessary (but not sufficient) event in carcinogenesis.[21] There are several methods available to measure DNA adducts. The most common of these methods are the enzyme-linked immunosorbent assay (ELISA) and ^{32}P-postlabeling (32P).

A 4-year study of Finnish iron foundry workers has recently been completed that evaluated a number of biomarkers, including carcinogen-DNA adducts in peripheral leukocytes, mutation at the HPRT locus and genetic polymorphisms in CYP1A1 and GSTM1. Iron foundry workers have long been known to be at increased risk for lung cancer,[22,23] and therefore constitute a model population for validating biologic markers.[24–29] The increased risk is primarily due to the high levels of PAH normally present in the foundry air.[30]

It is of interest that all of the exposures are much lower than those workers might have incurred in the past. The BP levels in the foundry are at least an order of magnitude lower than they were even a decade ago.[31] There are several reasons for this decline. First, the two processes used to cast iron in this foundry, the automatic and Zimmermann processes, which are normally in operation concurrently, have been staggered over the years so that the foundry could be operated with reduced manpower. This has substantially lowered the overall dust and particulate exposure at any given time. Second, in response to concern about the levels of PAH in foundry air resulting from combustion and release of organics, the composition of the mold has been steadily changing over the years, using fewer organic compounds in the binding material. Finally, improved industrial hygiene in the foundry has significantly reduced exposure to PAH each year.

A total of 100 persons were sampled in November/December of four successive years from 1990 to 1993. After adjusting for smoking, levels of PAH-DNA and aromatic-DNA adducts increased with exposure among the 100 workers sampled during the 4-year period ($p < 0.05$).[32,33] The difference in PAH-DNA adduct levels between workers with varying exposure to PAH has been consistent and demonstrable even at relatively low exposure levels.[28,31,32,34–36] In this study, significant correlations were seen between PAH-DNA adduct levels and both urinary 1-hydroxypyrene (a marker of internal dose of PAH) and HPRT mutation frequency in T-lymphocytes (a marker of preclinical biologic effect).[28,31] There was also a significant correlation ($p < 0.05$) between the adducts measured by immunoassay (PAH-DNA) and aromatic-DNA adducts measured by a ^{32}P-postlabeling procedure.[32]

In the initial year of sampling, PAH-DNA adducts in peripheral white blood cells increased with exposure to PAH in 38 iron foundry workers compared to controls.[29] The same relationship was seen in the enrollment sample from 85 workers exposed from 1990 to 1993. In addition, a dose-response relationship between levels of PAH-DNA adducts in peripheral white blood cells was detected, even though exposures to PAH in the same foundry were relatively low and varied from year to year. Independent variables other than BP exposure (smoking and dietary–charcoal-broiled food consumption, for example) were not significantly related to PAH-DNA adduct levels. The PAH-DNA adduct levels fluctuated in parallel with changes in workplace exposure. In the first year of the study, exposure to PAH, measured by personal and area monitoring, ranged from <2 ng/m^3 to 60 ng/m^3. The mean PAH-DNA adduct level for the entire cohort was 7.2 ± 6.2 adducts/10^8 nucleotides (n = 38). In the second year samples, when the foundry was operating at 60% of the schedule in year 1, the overall mean adduct level was 2.7 ± 2.9 adducts/10^8 nucleotides (n = 40). In the third year, when the foundry workers were again working on a 5-day schedule, albeit for only several weeks before the sample collection (possibly too soon to see a major effect of the exposure increase), the overall mean adduct level for the population was 2.9 ± 3.7 adducts/10^8 nucleotides (n = 57). Finally, in the last year, when the estimated comparable exposures were back to the levels measured in 1990, the overall mean PAH-DNA adduct level in peripheral white blood cells was 8.1 ± 11.3 adducts/10^8 nucleotides. Student's t-test analysis confirms that the mean PAH-DNA adduct levels in 1991 and 1992 are significantly different ($p <$ 0.01) than those in 1990 and 1993 (the high exposure years), but not from one another. Similarly, the mean adduct levels in 1990 and 1993 are not statistically different from one another. On a population scale, therefore, PAH-DNA adducts were a sensitive biomarker of the exposure changes experienced in this iron foundry.

In the first year, urinary 1-hydroxypyrene was associated with BP exposure (r = 0.27, p = 0.07).[29] Urinary 1-hydroxypyrene and aromatic-DNA adducts were strongly related to cigarette smoking exposure in the enrollment samples over the entire study and in the repeated measurements from the same workers. This relationship held true in multivariate analysis when controlling for other independent variables (estimated BP exposure and dietary charcoal-broiled food consumption). In terms of occupational exposure to PAH in the foundry, the level of DNA damage expressed as aromatic-DNA adducts was significantly lower in the low- versus high-exposure groups among the enrollment samples (n = 95). Moreover, aromatic-DNA adducts were significantly correlated with BP exposure as a continuous variable ($p < 0.05$). Urinary 1-hydroxy-pyrene was highly correlated with aromatic-DNA adducts in the enrollment samples, and this relationship held even in multivariate analysis when controlling for estimated BP exposure and cigarette smoking.[33]

In the first year HPRT Mf and PAH-DNA adducts were highly correlated (r = 0.67, $p < 0.01$).[29] In the second year of analysis, we did not see a significant relationship between DNA adducts and HPRT Mf, probably because a large number of individuals (approximately 40%) in the second year had nondetectable adduct levels, presumably due to the reduction in exposure in 1991. PAH-DNA adduct levels in total white blood cells decline more rapidly than HPRT mutant frequency in the longer-lived lymphocytes. It is therefore relevant that when detectable levels of adducts (>1 adduct/10^8) were plotted against HPRT mutant frequency for 67 individuals enrolled in years 1 and 2, there was a significant positive correlation ($r = 0.67$; $p < 0.01$) between these two endpoints.[36]

About 36% of the foundry workers revealed a deletion in GSTM1. Alone, the GSTM1 polymorphism appeared to have no effect on either PAH- or aromatic-DNA adduct levels. There was no difference at any time point or in the overall sample in adduct levels by GSTM1 genotype. This was true even when exposure to PAH either in the foundry air or from other exposures was controlled for. In contrast, PAH-DNA adduct levels were higher in the subset of workers who had one or both of the polymorphisms in CYP1A1 (13% of the cohort). This difference was most pronounced in the group with the lowest PAH exposure in the foundry. There was no difference in aromatic-DNA adduct levels related to polymorphisms in CYP1A1.[33]

The foundry worker study just discussed is an example of the potential contribution of molecular epidemiology to occupational health. Biomarkers of exposure to chemicals in the foundry air thought to significantly increase risk of lung cancer were validated in peripheral blood and urine from foundry workers. The molecular "footprint" on DNA left by metabolites of PAH was related to estimates of external exposure, even at the lowest exposures analyzed to date in the foundry. In year one, PAH-DNA adduct levels were significantly correlated with somatic cell mutation frequency in the HPRT gene, suggesting that the adducts were responsible for somatic mutations. Finally, many workers were identified who had one or more genetic susceptibility markers that have been linked to increased cancer risk in other studies. When the presence of one or both of the so-called "at risk" CYP1A1 genotypes was analyzed together with DNA adduct levels, the group of workers presumed to have the greatest risk of lung cancer due to genetic factors had the highest DNA adduct levels.[33]

The next steps in the cooperative effort between molecular epidemiology and occupational health are (1) the cancer risk to the most exposed/susceptible group of workers must be estimated; and (2) intervention efforts should be targeted to protect the high-risk persons more vigorously than to the rest of these workers as well as the rest of the population. Targeting of interventions and chemoprevention efforts is likely to be more effective and economical than blanket efforts to reduce risks in the overall population.

Molecular epidemiology has the potential to significantly contribute to the field of occupational health by providing early warning of the molecular and preclinical effects of exposure to carcinogens as well as increased susceptibility to cancer. Timely intervention in carcinogenesis will prevent disease in many workers. The distribution of procarcinogenic changes and susceptibility factors in the population can be used to ensure that those interventions will protect those most sensitive to carcinogen exposure, an effort that is both practical and fair.[1]

REFERENCES

1. PERERA, F. P. 1996. Molecular epidemiology: Insights into cancer susceptibility, risk assessment, and prevention. JNCI **88:** 496–509.

2. DOLL, R. & R. PETO. 1981. The Causes of Cancer: Quantitative Estimates of Avoidable Risk of Cancer in the United States Today. Oxford Univ. Press. New York, NY.
3. HIGGINSON, J. & C. S. MUIR. 1976. The role of epidemiology in elucidating the importance of environmental factors in human cancer. Cancer Detect. Prev. **1:** 79-105.
4. PERERA, F. P. & I. B. WEINSTEIN. 1982. Molecular epidemiology and carcinogen-DNA adduct detection: New approaches to studies of human cancer causation. J. Chron. Dis. **35:** 581-600.
5. WEINSTEIN, I. B., R. M. SANTELLA & F. P. PERERA. 1995. Molecular biology and epidemiology of cancer. *In* Cancer Prevention and Control, P. Greenwald, Ed.: 83-110. Marcel Dekker. New York, NY.
6. TOMATIS, L., A. AITIO, J. WILBOURN & L. SHUKAR. 1987. Human carcinogens so far identified. Jpn. J. Cancer Res. **78:** 887-898.
7. VENITT, S. 1994. Mechanisms of carcinogenesis and individual susceptibility to cancer. Clin. Chem. **40:** 1421-1425.
8. NATIONAL RESEARCH COUNCIL. 1994. Science and Judgement in Risk Assessment. National Academy Press. Washington, DC.
9. PERERA, F. P. & P. BOFFETTA. 1988. Perspectives on comparing risks of environmental carcinogens. JNCI **80:** 1282-1293.
10. LANDRIGAN, P. J. 1992. Commentary: Environmental disease—A preventable epidemic. Am. J. Public Health **82:** 941-943.
11. FAORO, R. 1990. EPA. Aerometric Information Retrieval System (AIRS), Data for 1985-1990. Environmental Protection Agency. Research Triangle Park, NC.
12. STERN, R. M. 1991. Assessing environmental carcinogens: Review of an approach adopted by the expert groups of the World Health Organization regional office for Europe. Ann. Ist. Super. Sanita **27**(4): 559-574.
13. GUENGERICH, F. P. 1993. Cytochrome p450 enzymes. Am. Sci. **81:** 440-447.
14. GUENGERICH, F. P. 1991. Interindividual variation in biotransformation of carcinogens: basis and relevance. *In* Molecular Dosimetry and Human Cancer. J. D. Groopman and P. L. Skipper, Eds. CRC Press. Boca Raton, FL.
15. HAYASHI, S., J. WATANABE & K. KAWAJIRI. 1992. High susceptibility to lung cancer analyzed in terms of combined genotype of P450IA1 and Mu-class glutathione S-transferase genes. Jpn. J. Cancer Res. **83:** 866-870.
16. COSMA, G., F. CROFTS, E. TAIOLI, P. TONIOLO & S. GARTE. 1993. Relationship between genotype and function of the human CYP1A1 gene. J. Toxicol. Environ. Health **40:** 309-316.
17. MCWILLIAMS, J. E., B. J. S. SANDERSON, E. L. HARRIS, K. E. RICHERT-BOE & W. D. HENNER. 1995. Glutathione S-transferase M1 (GSTM1) deficiency and lung cancer risk. Cancer Epi. Biomed. Prev. **4:** 589-594.
18. BELL, D. A., C. L. THOMPSON, J. TAYLOR, G. CLARK, C. R. MILLER, F. PERERA, L. HSIEH & G. W. LUCIER. 1992. Genetic monitoring of human polymorphic cancer susceptibility genes by polymerase chain reaction: Application to glutathione transferase. Environ. Health Perspect. **98:** 113-117.
19. BELL, D. A., J. A. TAYLOR, D. F. PAULSON, C. N. ROBERTSON, J. L. MOHLER. & G. W. LUCIER. 1993. Genetic risk and carcinogen exposure: A common inherited defect of the carcinogen-metabolism gene glutathione S-transferase M1 (GSTM1) that increases susceptibility to bladder cancer. JNCI **85:** 1159-1164.
20. SHIELDS, P. G., N. E. CAPORASO, R. T. FALK, H. SUGIMURA, G. E. TRIVERS, B. F. TRUMP, R. N. HOOVER, A. WESTON & C. C. HARRIS. 1993. Lung cancer, race, and a CYP1A1 genetic polymorphism. Cancer Epi. Biomed. Prev. **2:** 481-485.
21. PERERA, F. P. 1991. Emerging science of molecular epidemiology. Cancer Bull. **43:** 585-587.
22. INTERNATIONAL AGENCY FOR RESEARCH ON CANCER. 1984. Polynuclear Aromatic Compounds. Part 3. Industrial Exposures in Aluminium Production, Coal Gasification: 34.

IARC Monographs on the Evaluation of the Carcinogenic Risk of Chemicals to Humans. International Agency for Research on Cancer. Lyon, France.
23. SORAHAN, T. & M. A. COOKE. 1989. Cancer mortality in a cohort of United Kingdom steel foundry workers: 1946-85. Br. J. Ind. Med. **46:** 74-81.
24. PERERA, F. P., K. HEMMINKI, T. L. YOUNG, D. BRENNER, G. KELLY & R. M. SANTELLA. 1988. Detection of polycyclic aromatic hydrocarbon-DNA adducts in white blood cells of foundry workers. Cancer Res. **48:** 2288-2291.
25. SHERSON, D., P. SABRO, T. SIGSGAARD, F. JOHANSEN & H. AUTRUP. 1990. Biological monitoring of foundry workers exposed to polycyclic aromatic hydrocarbons. Br. J. Ind. Med. **47:** 448-453.
26. SHAMSUDDIN, A. K., N. T. SINOPOLI, K. HEMMINKI, R. R. BOESCH & C. C. HARRIS. 1985. Detection of benzo(a)pyrene DNA adducts in human white blood cells. Cancer Res. **45:** 66-68.
27. SAVELA, K., K. HEMMINKI, A. HEWER, D. H. PHILLIPS, K. L. PUTNAM & K. RANDERATH. 1989. Interlaboratory comparison of the 32P-postlabelling assay for aromatic DNA adducts in white blood cells of iron foundry workers. Mutation Res. **224:** 485-492.
28. SANTELLA, R., K. HEMMINKI, D. TANG, M. PAIK, R. OTTMAN, T. YOUNG, K. SAVELA, L. VODICKA, C. DICKEY, R. WHYATT, *et al.* 1993. PAH-DNA adducts in white blood cells and urinary 1-hydroxypyrene in foundry workers. Cancer Epi. Biomed. Prev. **2:** 59-62.
29. PERERA, F. P., D. TANG, P. O'NEILL, W. BIGBEE, R. ALBERTINI, R. SANTELLA, R. OTTMAN, W. Y. TSAI, C. DICKEY, L. MOONEY, *et al.* 1993. HPRT and glycophorin A mutations in foundry workers: Relationship to PAH exposure and to PAH-DNA adducts. Carcinogenesis **14:** 969-973.
30. KNECHT, U., H. U. ELLIEHAUSEN & H. J. WOITOWITZ. 1986. Gaseous and absorbed PAH in an iron foundry. Br. J. Ind. Med. **43:** 834-838.
31. PERERA, F. P. 1993. Molecular epidemiology in cancer prevention. *In* Cancer Epidemiology and Prevention, D. Schottenfeld and J. Fraumeni, Eds. Oxford Univ. Press. New York, NY.
32. DICKEY, C. P., D. A. BELL, K. HEMMINKI, R. SANTELLA, R. OTTMAN, W. Y. TSAI, K. SAVELA, G. LUCIER, & F. P. PERERA. 1995. GSTM1, CYP1A1 MspI and DNA adducts in workers exposed to PAH. Proc. Am. Assoc. Cancer Res. **36:** 120.
33. HEMMINKI, K., C. P. DICKEY, S. KARLSSON, D. BELL, Y. HSU, W. TSAI, L. A. MOONEY, K. SAVELA & F. P. PERERA. 1997. Aromatic-DNA adducts in foundry workers in relation to exposure, lifestyle and CYP1A1 and glutathione transferase M1 genotype. Carcinogenesis. **18:** 345-350.
34. PERERA, F. P. 1988. Biological markers in risk assessment. *In* Carcinogen Risk Assessment, C. C. Travis, Ed. Plenum Press. New York, NY.
35. HEMMINKI, K., K. RANDERATH, M. V. REDDY, K. L. PUTNAM, R. M. SANTELLA, F. P. PERERA, T. L. YOUNG, D. H. PHILLIPS, A. HEWER & K. SAVELA. 1990. Postlabeling and immunoassay analysis of polycyclic aromatic hydrocarbons—Adducts of deoxyribonucleic acid in white blood cells of foundry workers. Scand. J. Work Environ. Health **16:** 158-162.
36. PERERA, F. P., C. DICKEY, R. SANTELLA, J. P. O'NEILL, R. J. ALBERTINI, R. OTTMAN, W. Y. TSAI, L. A. MOONEY, K. SAVELA & K. HEMMINKI. 1994. Carcinogen-DNA adducts and gene mutation in foundry workers with low lever exposure to polycyclic aromatic hydrocarbons. Carcinogenesis **15:** 2905-2910.

The Historical Basis for Ecological Risk Assessment[a]

JOANNA BURGER

Ecology and Evolution Graduate Program
Rutgers University
Piscataway, New Jersey 08855-1059
and
Environmental and Occupational Health Sciences Institute
Piscataway, New Jersey 08855-1179

INTRODUCTION

Ecological risk assessment has emerged as a method for evaluating past and future damage to species, populations, communities, and ecosystems from a variety of stressors. Stressors can be natural, such as hurricanes, earthquakes, fire, or pests, or anthropocentric, such as agriculture and forestry, land development, or chemical contamination. In most cases, species and ecosystems are exposed to a combination of stressors, and risk assessment provides a methodology to compare relative risks, and serves as a tool for managers. In this paper, I examine the historical roots of ecological risk assessment.

THE ENVIRONMENTAL MOVEMENT

The growth of world population, the mass movement of peoples around the world, and the ascendancy of multinational corporations have increased the necessity for concern for protecting natural resources and the environment. Local people no longer have sole responsibility and jurisdiction over their local resources. Subsistence hunting and fishing gives way to a cash economy, followed by exportation of natural resources to distant lands. As Garrett Hardin suggested in his classic *Tragedy of the Commons,* with increased concentration of people in towns and cities comes decreased stewardship of natural resources, and those who monopolize "common" resources benefit at the expense of the human community.[1]

The environmental movement has moved forward by fits and starts over the last century. At least six major movements can be easily identified, although the progression of these movements in different countries and in different cultures varies. The general movements are: (1) species protection (i.e., the protection of migratory birds); (2) habitat protection (i.e., establishment of parks in the 1920s and the creation of

[a]This work was partially supported by the Consortium for Risk Evaluation with Stakeholder Participation (CRESP, AI DE-FC01-95EW 55084), which is funded by the Department of Energy, NIEHS Grants ES 05022 and ES 05955, the U.S. Environmental Protection Agency, and the Environmental and Occupational Health Sciences Institute.

habitat in the 1930s for ducks and other waterfowl following the dust bowl days); (3) soil conservation in the late 1930s; (4) forest conservation in the 1940s; (5) chemical protection (i.e., regulation and control of pesticides and other chemicals in the late 1960s and early 1970s); and (6) the recent concern that several anthropocentric activities threaten the health of the environment and the structure and function of both natural and man-altered ecosystems. This latter concern has prompted the need for a method to evaluate the importance of the different risks to these systems; leading directly to the need for ecological risk assessment.

In the late 1800s and early 1900s many species of birds were overexploited, and populations declined precipitously. The form of exploitation varied, but included hunting for food, sport, and plumes for the millinery trade. In the height of the fashion, whole terns and shorebirds were put on women's hats in America and Europe. Many species, particularly colonially nesting birds such as herons, egrets, and terns, were eliminated from some states. This led to a conservation movement to protect migratory birds and to limit hunting of all but game birds, that would be closely monitored and regulated so that hunting pressures did not destroy populations. The Migratory Bird Treaty, signed by Canada, Mexico, and the United States, provided for the protection of all birds that regularly migrated over the borders. It was not passed easily, however, and considerable effort was required by the National Audubon Society, the American Ornithologists' Union, and several other conservation organizations to persuade the United States to become a signatory.

The deliberate slaughter of animals for food or to collect parts that are valuable for aphrodisiacs, medicine, carvings, or adornments may be largely ended in the United States and Europe, but it continues elsewhere, notably in most of Africa and Asia.[2] In general, it is still the largest and scarcest animals that are most heavily exploited.[3]

With the immediate threat of avian extinction past in the United States, the emphasis of conservationists and scientists switched to habitat preservation, not only for birds but for all natural resources. National parks and national wildlife refuges were created by the federal government to protect geological beauty, aesthetics, and biological diversity, as well as to create nesting and breeding habitat for valuable game birds and mammals. In the 1930s when much of the West was in the grip of a dust bowl, waterfowl suffered dramatically because there were few prairie potholes where they could reproduce. Agriculture had eliminated most of the postglacial prairie marshes, and only small potholes remained.

In the late 1930s several national wildlife refuges were created by the federal government to protect duck-nesting habitat. Large tracts of land were purchased by the federal government, and diked and filled, by government work programs, with water to produce large prairie marshes. In most cases, this land was originally marshland that had been drained for farming in the late 1800s. Although initially created to protect duck populations, these habitats preserved the biodiversity of many other, nongame animals.

Up until this point, the anthropocentric threats to environmental health were largely from direct disturbance (killing of wildlife) or from habitat loss because of agricultural or suburban development. Farming practices included the use of inorganic compounds for insect control, such as arsenic, but use was low.

During World War II agents of chemical warfare were developed, and many proved to be potent insecticides. Initially chemists developed synthetic insecticides such as compounds of arsenic, copper, lead, manganese, and zinc; pyrethrum from chrysanthemums; and rotenone from leguminous plants from the East Indies. These chemicals had two functions, to enter the body to change reproductive and physiological processes, and to kill.

When the war ended it was an easy leap to use these chemicals for insect control for agricultural, industrial, and suburban uses. In 1947, only 259,000 pounds of synthetic pesticides were used in the United States; in 1960, this amount had risen 250-fold to 637,660,000 pounds. Two main types of pesticides were in use: chlorinated hydrocarbons such as DDT, chlordane, heptachlor, and dieldrin, and organic phosphorus insecticides such as malathion and parathion. The organophosphorus compounds are highly toxic to vertebrates as well as to insects, and even today are a cause of considerable human morbidity and occasional mortality. Their impact on vertebrate populations, however, is difficult to assess, since one must track the effects of reducing populations of insects on their predator populations.

The chlorinated hydrocarbons had the advantage of lower vertebrate toxicity (though far from innocuous), but even low-level exposures results in bioaccumulation through the food chains such that top predatory species could accumulate relatively high levels, particularly in their adipose tissue. Moreover, unlike the organophosphorus compounds, these insecticides biodegrade very slowly, so the accumulation in food chains can have far-reaching effects. The most severe effects are those on reproduction, which ultimately results in reduced population sizes.

As early as 1950 the Federal Food and Drug Administration recognized that it was ''extremely likely'' that the potential hazards from chemicals such as DDT were underestimated. The modern environmental era, however, can be traced to Rachel Carson's *Silent Spring,*[4] which clearly and eloquently forced us to face the consequences of the unthinking, unrestricted, and unregulated use of chemicals. Her interest was on the role of pesticides on bird and other wildlife populations. Her message was simple: unless we do something, we will one day wake up to a silent spring, for there will be no more birds to sing.

Even then, her emphasis was on direct toxicity of pesticides to birds, but by 1970, the effects of bioaccumulation of chlorinated hydrocarbons on the reproduction of birds that survived acute toxicity was recognized. Entire populations of eagles, peregrine falcons (*Falco peregrinus*), and pelicans (*Pelecanus occidentalis*) were eliminated.[5,6] Within a few years, the direct effects on populations decreased, but we began to see indirect effects from this same class of compound that function as endocrine disruptors. The consequences on populations and communities are as severe, but they are less obvious.[7]

Although many dismissed Carson's message as that of hysteria, gradually people began to notice that, indeed, there were fewer birds, frogs, insects, and butterflies. Within only a few years, stimulated by a wide coalition of organizations in addition to conservation ones, the country as a whole demanded environmental protection. It was not a matter of a few environmental or conservation groups, but middle America wanted to see protection of our air and water. Environmental protection became a national priority, not a partisan issue. Environmental protection was a broad mandate that included protection for human health, nature, and wildlife.

Many of the current issues that affect environmental management are fraught with a lack of basic information on the status and trends of the particular environment being considered.[8] This has led to calls for monitoring programs to assess changes in a variety of populations, communities, and chemicals.

LAWS GOVERNING ENVIRONMENTAL ASSESSMENT

With the groundswell of concern for the environment there was a national mandate, at least in the United States and many other Western countries, for laws and agencies that would develop legislation and regulations that would protect our environment. The concern was bipartisan and central to political thought, rather than being considered at one end of a continuum.

The first step was the creation of the U.S. Council on Environmental Quality in the late 1960s. Its function was to analyze and coordinate federal environmental policy. The problem with the council was that it had no authority and was only advisory, reporting directly to the president. The council, composed of 35–40 people, was placed in the Office of the President. Its main contribution was to write a "toxic substances" report that laid the groundwork for the Toxic Substances Control Act (TSCA). The report noted that the rate of use of toxic chemicals was increasing, that many posed a hazard, and that they were inadequately controlled.

This led directly to the formation of the Environmental Protection Agency in 1970, under President Richard M. Nixon. William Ruckelshaus was the first administrator, and he recognized that there was a public outcry for environmental protection. His initial assumptions were that (1) if the government set standards, polluters would comply; (2) we know who the bad polluters are; (3) we know the levels that cause adverse environmental and health effects, and (4) environmental protection can be accomplished at a reasonable cost, and in a reasonable time frame. It took him just three months in office to question these assumptions.

Ruckelshaus believed that he must establish the credibility of the agency, demonstrate a willingness of the federal government to act, and set out some achievable goals. He had a total work force of only about 1500 people, very small for a federal agency. Surprisingly, in these early days, much of the agenda of the environmental movement was embraced by the EPA, certainly very different from present-day reality when environmental groups are often at odds with EPA.

At about the same time, there were a number of laws passed that directly regulated different aspects of the environment (TABLE 1). From the perspective of ecological risk assessment, the most important of these was the National Environmental Policy Act (NEPA, 1969) which requires the analysis and disclosure of the effects of any human-induced (anthropogenic) factors, including chemicals; and requires the prediction of all consequences of an action or chemical. This led to the requirement for environmental impact assessments (EIS) that were to be performed uniformly in all states.

Environmental impact assessments were to be multidisciplinary approaches to understanding consequences and impacts of actions or chemicals. The intent was to provide information so that decision makers could balance effects against other factors such as economic development. This landmark legislation required that the consequences of human actions would be considered in environmental decisions.

TABLE 1. Major Legislation for Protection of the Environment[a]

Year	Legislation
1910	Federal Insecticide Act
1916	Migratory Bird Treaty
1947	Federal Insecticide, Fungicide and Rodenticide Act (FIFRA) (major changes and additions relevant to ecological risk were made in 1972 and 1978)
1965	Water Quality Act
1969	National Environmental Policy Act (NEPA)
1970	Clean Air Act
1972	Marine Protection, Research, and Sanctuaries Act
1973	Federal Water Pollution Control Act
1974	Safe Drinking Water Act
1976	Resource Conservation and Recovery Act (RCRA)
1976	Toxic Substances Control Act (TSCA)
1977	Wetlands Protection Executive Order
1977	Surface Mining Control and Reclamation Act
1980	Comprehensive Environmental Response, Compensation and Liability Act (CERCLA/Superfund Act)
1982	Nuclear Waste Policy Act
1983	Endangered Species Act
1986	Superfund Amendment Reauthorization Act (SARA)

[a] After Openchowski[45] and Cairns.[2]

There are several difficulties with the environmental impact assessment process, however, including an emphasis on cataloging species and on endangered species, no requirement for experts, no consistency among approaches or methods used, no consistency in end points, no requirement for consideration of uncertainties, and no requirement for evaluating the correctness of conclusions.[9,10] Also, monitoring after the action or exposure is conspicuously absent.[10] One never knew or had to know whether an EIS was correct. This means when making future decisions, it is impossible for the manager or regulator to know whether past mitigations or restorations were successful.[10]

In some ways, the role of science has been unclear in the EIS process, and it is possible for people with little biological training to conduct these, based largely on endangered and threatened plant and animal lists. Community- and ecosystem-level effects were completely ignored. Protection of the environment or evaluation of the effects of hazards has not been adequately served by this process.

The role of risk in EIS, has also been largely ignored.[11] Despite the large number of laws, regulations, programs, and agencies devoted to environmental protection, many national environmental goals have not been met, and many large-scale environmental problems remain.[12] This is partly the result of the fragmentary nature of environmental policy, laws, and tools. The emergence of ecological risk assessment provides another powerful tool to address the fragmentary and evaluative nature of environmental problems.

BISECTING FIELDS

Several fields have been involved with evaluating the effects of physical, biological, and chemical stressors on organisms, populations, communities, and ecosystems, including ecology, ecotoxicology, and wildlife and land management. Ecology mainly concentrated on understanding the structure and function of ecosystems and their component parts. Although ecologists primarily study natural systems, they also examine systems perturbed by man. Often understanding how organisms and ecosystems respond to natural disturbances such as fire and hurricanes can provide models for understanding at least the physical perturbations caused by man. Recently the subfield of restoration ecology has developed to help people understand how to restore damaged ecosystems to functioning systems that provide ecological services.[13–15] The emphasis on understanding changes in biodiversity is fundamental to examining the effects of humans on biological diversity.[16,17]

Ecotoxicology has been concentrating on understanding the effects of toxic chemicals on organisms, largely in laboratory settings.[18] Thus ecotoxicologists have been able to examine carefully the effect of dose and exposure on organisms, but frequently they work on only a few species of organisms that can be maintained in a laboratory setting. Moreover, they often concentrate only on establishing lethal doses or the no-observed-effect level (NOEL), without considering subtle behavioral and behavioral effects that may be significant in the wild.[19,20] The results of such laboratory studies can be extrapolated to the field; however, this assumption is seldom tested. More recently, ecotoxicologists have recognized the importance of developing predictive models that address ecosystem function and resiliency, particularly for hazardous-waste sites.[21,22]

Wildlife and land management are fields that deal with the practical aspects of managing resources, presumably to the benefit of both the exploited populations and for humans in general. To maintain suitable populations for exploitation, it is necessary to understand the factors that control these populations, and the effects that perturbations have on the system. A recent dialog between wildlife management biologists and toxicologists promised fruitful results in modeling effects of chemicals on populations.[23]

All three of these disciplines have been examining the effects of anthropogenic forces on organisms, populations, communities, and ecosystems; but they have done so largely in isolation.[10] Moreover, the levels of study have varied: ecologists have studied the whole continuum from organisms to ecosystems and the landscape; ecotoxicologists have largely concentrated on effects on the individual (similar to human health considerations); and wildlife and land managers have largely concentrated on exploitable lands and organisms.

At the same time that these three disciplines were examining the effects of physical, biological, and chemical stressors on ecological systems, human health risk assessors were developing paradigms and methodologies to assess the risk from various factors (usually chemicals) on various human health end points, particularly cancer.[24,25]

Recently, ecologists and environmentalists have been evaluating the possibility of using the human health risk assessment paradigm for ecological systems. The human health risk assessment paradigm, formalized by the National Research Council,[24,25] consists of four phases: hazard identification, dose-response analysis, exposure assessment, and risk characterization.

EMERGENCE OF ECOLOGICAL RISK ASSESSMENT

For a variety of reasons, there is a clear public mandate for the maintenance of environmental "health."[26–28] Although there is debate about the nature of ecological systems, and whether the health paradigm is useful, the public clearly is interested in examining the effects of physical, biological, and chemical hazards on ecosystems and their component parts (see references 29 and 30). Moreover, most people, both experts and the general public, can agree on what clearly constitutes an unhealthy ecosystem and one that is no longer providing ecological services.

Ecological risk assessment has emerged as a useful method for examining the effects of perturbations on ecosystems.[10,31–33] Perturbations can be natural and anthropogenic, or both. Ecological risk assessment can be used for single species or local natural communities, as well as for regional and landscape problems.[10,34] It can deal with chemical pollutants, biotechnology introductions, or proposed developments.

Over the last several years, the four phases of human risk assessment have been modified substantially for ecological risk assessment.[12,25,31,35–38] The primary modifications have included the addition of a more detailed initial problem-formulation phase, a recognition that dose-response data may not be available for most organisms and most ecosystem functions, and a formalization of the importance of a dialog between scientists and managers in all phases. Lack of dose-response data, however, does not mean a lack of hazard and response data. Two current models for ecological risk assessment are shown in FIGURES 1 and 2.

More recently, Burger and Handel[39] have suggested that restoration evaluation should be added as an important component of risk characterization. They added this component because there is a very real need to provide a science-based mechanism for evaluating the risks among sites. For example, one pressing problem facing Western countries today is how to deal with nuclear wastes.[40] Indeed, the international community and United Nations consider these substantive issues for worldwide cooperation and agreement.

The money required for the cleanup of all hazardous-waste sites to residential standards is exorbitant, and some relative ranking is required, both for the sites that will be cleaned up, and for the level of clean up. One way to do this is to evaluate the time, cost, and energy required to restore the degraded systems to functioning ecosystems that provide the ecological services desired for that site. Ecological risk assessment and restoration ecology provide tools for this task.

With the ending of the Cold War, the nearly 40 Department of Energy sites in the United States that manufactured nuclear weapons and thereby became repositories of chemical and nuclear wastes (as well as countless other federal and contractor facilities that were involved) are slated for cleanup. The task is daunting in terms of time, money, and energy, and critical management decisions are required regarding which sites to clean up, when and how to clean them up, and what the criteria are for a clean site.

The problem of evaluating degraded and contaminated sites is even more critical in some Eastern Block nations, because there were few environmental controls.

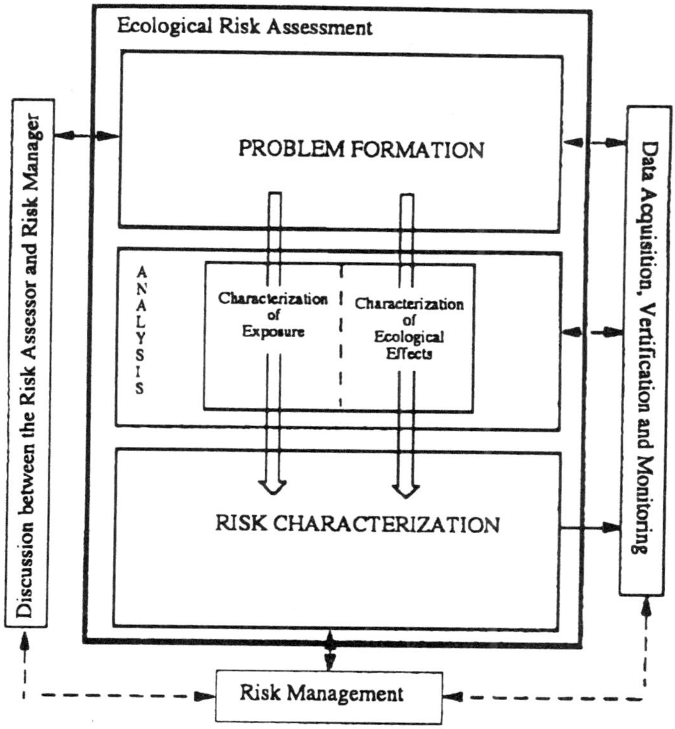

FIGURE 1. Ecological risk assessment paradigm as proposed by the EPA.[31]

Massive amounts of industrial, oil, and nuclear wastes currently render large tracts of land unusable. The international community, as well as national agencies, will have to determine which problems are the most acute and pose the greatest risk to ecosystems and humans.

Ecological risk assessment will also be useful for evaluating physical damage caused by natural events such as fires, hurricanes, and tornadoes, and by anthropogenic events such as clear-cutting, water diversion, development, and the introduction of exotic (or bioengineered) species.

CONCLUSIONS

Ecological risk assessment has a special role in the decisions required in the next century; with human populations increasing and resources decreasing, there is an even greater need to make choices about the risks of chemicals and other perturbations to our fragile environment. Some of these choices will result in mitigation or cleanup, some may dictate habitat management, while others may involve little or no interven-

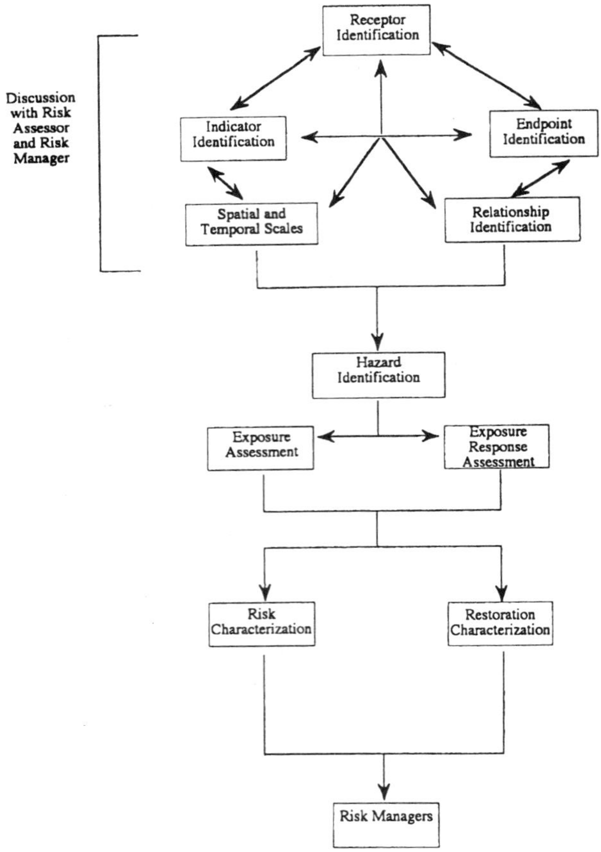

FIGURE 2. Ecological risk assessment paradigm as proposed by the NRC[25] and modified by Burger[10] and Burger and Handel.[39]

tion. These choices must have a sound scientific basis, and ecological risk assessment can provide this basis. Risk assessments for different degraded habitats can be used in the process of triaging which sites to clean up or mitigate.

Each of our current state and federal agencies, and our environmental laws, have responsibility for some fragment of environmental protection or management.[2] This often results in a great deal of regulation without improvement in overall environmental quality.[41] Ecological risk assessment has the potential of overcoming the fragmented nature of environmental assessment by examining all the factors that affect environmental "health," and by providing scientific data to make difficult management choices. Ecological risk assessment can be used in a landscape context to help make the best available decision when there are management options. It takes into account long-term changes that transcend the traditional 70-year lifetime.[42]

One key advantage of ecological risk assessment is that it provides a uniform methodology for evaluating the magnitude and probability of adverse effects of both natural and anthropogenic catastrophes, and of evaluating a range of diverse hazards such as chemicals, physical disruptions, and hunting and fishing (plus many, many others[43]). By using a common methodology, we can compare risks, leading to sound management decisions (i.e., lead[44]). Further, ecological risk assessment provides the opportunity for stakeholder participation in the initial scoping of the problem, and in the final risk characterization stage.

Although the ecological risk assessment process itself is science-based, a variety of stakeholders, including the government and the private sector, can influence both the types of risk assessments to be conducted, and the valuation of these assessments. Stakeholders can broaden or narrow the future land-use scenarios that risk assessors can incorporate. Risk assessment provides a way for expert knowledge to be used objectively to determine the risk of a hazard, while allowing for continuous stakeholder participation. Risk assessment is thus an iterative process, with risk assessors evaluating the hazards, while managers, regulators, and the general public can influence the selection of assessments and their ultimate valuation.

Ecological risk assessment is a fitting next step to the environmental movement of the twentieth century, because it provides a common method for evaluating the wide range of environmental problems that led directly to our environmental protection laws. The assessment process can be used for single stressors, or a combination, and for different types such as chemical, physical, and biological.

ACKNOWLEDGMENTS

I thank S. Bartell, L. Barnthouse, K. Cooper, B. D. Goldstein, M. Gochfeld, M. Greenberg, J. Ehrenfeld, M. Lee, J. Moore, S. Norton, D. Policansky, C. Powers, M. Robson, C. Safina, and D. Wartenberg for valuable discussions about ecological risk and the environmental movement.

REFERENCES

1. Hardin G. 1968. The tragedy of the commons. Science **162:** 1243-1248.
2. Cairns, J., Jr. 1994. The study of ecology and environmental management: Reflections on the implications of ecological history. Environ. Manage. Health **5**(4): 7-15.
3. Redford, K. H. 1992. The empty forest. BioScience **42**(6): 412-422.
4. Carson, R. 1962. Silent Spring. Fawcett. Greenwich, CT.
5. Hickey, J. J. 1969. The Peregrine Falcon Populations: Their Biology and Decline. Univ. of Wisconsin Press. Madison.
6. Lincer, J. L. 1975. DDE-induced eggshell thinning in the American Kestrel: A comparison of the field and the laboratory results. *J. Appl. Ecol.* **12**(3): 781-793.
7. Colburn, T. & C. Clement, Eds. 1992. Chemically-induced Alterations in Sexual and Functional Development: The Wildlife/Human Connection. Princeton Scientific. Princeton, NJ.
8. Eichibaum, W. M. & B. B. Bernstein. 1990. Current issues in environmental management: A case study of Southern California's marine monitoring system. Coastal Manage. **18**(3): 433-445.

9. SUTER, G. W. II. 1990. Endpoints for regional ecological risk assessment. Environ. Manage. **14**(1): 9–23.
10. BURGER, J. 1994. How should success be measured in ecological risk assessment? The importance of predictive accuracy. J. Toxicol. Environ. Health **42**(3): 367–376.
11. SUTER, G. W. II, L. W. BARNTHOUSE & R. V. O'NEILL. 1987. Treatment of risk in environmental impact statements. Environ. Manage. **11**(3): 295–303.
12. ENVIRONMENTAL PROTECTION AGENCY. 1990. Reducing risk: Setting priorities and strategies for environmental protection. U.S. EPA, SAB-EC 90-021, Washington, DC.
13. JORDAN, W. R. III, M. E. GILPIN & J. D. ABER, Eds. 1987. Restoration Ecology: A Synthetic Approach to Ecological Research. Cambridge Univ. Press. Cambridge.
14. ROBINSON, G. R. & S. N. HANDEL. 1993. Forest restoration on a closed landfill: Rapid addition of new species by bird dispersal. Conserv. Biol. **7**(2): 271–278.
15. HANDEL, S. N., G. R. ROBINSON & A. J. BEATTIE. 1994. Biodiversity resources for restoration ecology. Restor. Ecol. **2**(4): 230–241.
16. WILSON, E. O. 1986. Biodiversity. National Academy Press. Washington, DC.
17. RISSER, P. G. 1995. Biodiversity and ecosystem function. Conserv. Biol. **9**(4): 742–746.
18. BASCIETTO, J., D. HINCKLEY, J. PLAFKIN & M. SLIMAK. 1990. Ecotoxicity and ecological risk assessment: Regulatory applications at EPA. Environ. Sci. Technol. **24**(1): 10–14.
19. CAIRNS, J., JR. 1992. The threshold problem in ecotoxicology. Ecotoxicol. **1**(1): 3–16.
20. HOEKSTRA, J. A. & P. H. VANEWIJK. 1993. Alternatives for the no-observed-effect level. Environ. Toxicol. Chem. **12**(1): 187–194.
21. HOFFMAN, D. J., B. A. RATTNER & R. J. HALL. 1990. Wildlife toxicology. Environ. Sci. Technol. **24**(3): 276–283.
22. LINTHURST, R. A., P. BOURDEAU & R. G. TARDIFF, Eds. 1995. Methods to Assess the Effects of Chemicals on Ecosystems. SCOPE **53:** 1–416.
23. KENDALL, R. J. & T. E. LACHER, JR. 1991. Ecological modeling, population ecology, and wildlife toxicology: A team approach to environmental toxicology. Environ. Toxicol. Chem. **10**(3): 297–299.
24. NATIONAL RESEARCH COUNCIL. 1983. Risk Assessment in the Federal Government: Managing the Process. National Academy Press. Washington, DC.
25. NATIONAL RESEARCH COUNCIL. 1993. Issues in Risk Assessment. National Academy Press. Washington, DC.
26. RAPPORT, D. J. 1989. What constitutes ecosystem health? Perspect. Biol. Med. **33**(1): 120–132.
27. NATIONAL RESEARCH COUNCIL. 1986. Ecological Knowledge and Environmental Problem-solving. National Academy Press. Washington, DC.
28. NATIONAL RESEARCH COUNCIL. 1991. Animals as Sentinels of Environmental Health Hazards. National Academy Press. Washington, DC.
29. SUTER, G. W. 1993. A critique of ecosystem health concepts and indexes. Environ. Toxicol. Chem. **12**(9): 1533–1539.
30. SUTER, G. W. 1993. Ecological Risk Assessment. Lewis Press. Boca Raton, FL.
31. NORTON, S. B., D. R. RODIER, J. H. GENTILE, W. H. VAN DER SCHALIE, W. P. WOOD & M. W. SLIMAK. 1992. A framework for ecological risk assessment at the EPA. Environ. Toxicol. Chem. **11**(12): 1663–1672.
32. TRAVIS, C. C. & J. M. MORRIS. 1992. The emergence of ecological risk assessment. Risk Anal. **12:** 167–168.
33. LANDIS, W. G., J. S. HUGHES & M. A. LEWIS, Eds. 1993. Environmental Toxicology and Risk Assessment. ASTM STP 1179. American Society for Testing and Materials. Philadelphia.
34. GRAHAM, R. L., C. T. HUNSAKER, R. V. O'NEILL & B. L. JACKSON. 1991. Ecological risk assessment at the regional scale. Ecol. Applic. **1**(2): 196–206.
35. BURGER, J. & M. GOCHFELD. 1993. Temporal scales in ecological risk assessment. Arch. Environ. Contam. Toxicol. **23:** 484–488.

36. Burger, J. & M. Gochfeld. 1996. Ecological and human risk assessment: A comparison. In Interconnections Between Human and Ecosystem Health, R. T. DiGiulio and E. Monosson, Eds. Chapman & Hall. London.
37. Lipton, J., H. Galbraith, J. Burger & D. Wartenberg. 1993. A paradigm for ecological risk assessment. Environ. Manage. **17:** 1-5.
38. Karr, J. R. 1994. Risk assessment: We need more than an ecological veneer. Hum. Ecol. Risk Assess. **1:** 159-162.
39. Burger, J. & S. Handel. Using Restoration Ecology as A Tool for Risk Assessment. Risk Anal. CRESP. Unpublished Report 20.
40. Department of Energy. 1995. Risks and the Risk Debate: Searching for Common Ground. U.S. Dept. of Energy, Office of Environmental Management. Washington, DC.
41. Patrick, R., F. Douglas, D. M. Palavage & P. M. Stewart. 1992. Surface Water Quality: Have the Laws been Successful? Princeton Univ. Press. Princeton, NJ.
42. Gochfeld, M. & J. Burger. 1993. Evolutionary consequences for ecological risk assessment and management. Environ. Monit. Assess. **28:** 161-168.
43. Bartell, S. M. R. H. Gardner & R. V. O'Neill. 1992. Ecological Risk Estimation. Lewis Press. Boca Raton, FL.
44. Burger, J. 1995. A risk assessment for lead in birds. J. Toxicol. Environ. Health **45**(4): 369-396.
45. Openchowski, C. 1990. A Guide to Environmental Law in Washington, D.C. Environmental Law Institute. Washington, DC.

Paradigms for Ecological Risk Assessment[a]

JOANNA BURGER[b,c,e] AND MICHAEL GOCHFELD[c,d]

[b]*Ecology and Evolution Graduate Program*
Rutgers University
Piscataway, New Jersey 08855-1059

[c]*Environmental and Occupational Health Sciences Institute*
Piscataway, New Jersey 08855-1179

[d]*UMDNJ/Robert Wood Johnson Medical School*
Piscataway, New Jersey 08854

INTRODUCTION

Risk assessment examines the potential risk to target organisms or systems from chemical, physical, or other environmental hazards. In 1983 the National Research Council[1] formalized the human health risk assessment paradigm to include four parts: hazard identification, dose-response assessment, exposure assessment, and risk characterization. Although there have been considerable refinements in this process over the years,[2] the basic paradigm has remained the same, and has been extremely useful in providing consistency in methods (if not in assumptions) for identifying the risks to human health.

Several disciplines have studied or evaluated risks to nonhuman populations and the environment, including ecology, wildlife and land management, ecotoxicology, and more recently, restoration ecology and ecological engineering.[3–10] Yet these separate disciplines using different approaches and different languages have often failed to evaluate overall risks to the environment—both in terms of the levels and complexity of ecosystems and of the diverse and complex hazards.

Ecological risk assessment has emerged as an important discipline because it fulfills three needs: it can be used to assess the general health and well being of animal and plant populations, communities, and ecosystems; it can be used to evaluate competing risks, either past, present, or future; and it can inform decision makers about future use of contaminated land. In an age where time, money, and personnel resources are subject to competing demands, ecological risk assessment can provide a framework for evaluating and ranking sites. This is particularly critical for Department of Energy and other sites, where physical, chemical, and nuclear wastes may be intermixed.

[a]This work was partially supported by the Consortium for Risk Evaluation with Stakeholder Participation (CRESP, AI DE-FC01-95EW 55084), which is funded by the Department of Energy by NIEHS Grants ES 05022 and ES 05955, the U.S. Environmental Protection Agency, and the Environmental and Occupational Health Sciences Institute.

[e]Corresponding author.

In this paper we review briefly the differences between human and ecological risk assessment, examine the complexity of ecological risk assessment, describe the different ecological risk methods and models, and discuss advantages and disadvantages of these approaches to ecological risk assessment.

HUMAN RISK ASSESSMENT PARADIGM

The human health risk assessment paradigm was codified by the National Research Council[1] to provide consistency and comparability among assessments for the effects of different hazards on human health. Four steps are clearly recognized: hazard identification, dose-response assessment, exposure assessment, and risk characterization, although the role of risk managers and stakeholders in risk assessment is often debated.[2] Hazard identification involves specifying the hazards and the biological end points of concern. Dose-response assessment reviews the toxicologic and epidemiologic literature to establish the relationship between dose and the type and magnitude of effects. Exposure assessment examines contaminant levels in various media, bioavailability, and the pathways of exposure, and may even estimate dose-to-target tissues. Risk characterization estimates the probability of an adverse outcome or a threshold below which the probability of an adverse outcome is negligible.

COMPLEXITIES OF ECOLOGICAL SYSTEMS

Ecological risk assessment differs from human health risk assessment, primarily because it deals with ecosystems and their component species and populations, rather than only one species (humans). An ecosystem is a spatial entity comprising biotic components (bacteria, fungi, plants, animals) and abiotic components (air, water, soil), through which energy flows, nutrients move, and matter is cycled.[11] Ecosystems can range from a tiny puddle to the Great Lakes, or indeed to the earth or biosphere.

In most ecosystems, the flow of energy involves the fixation of solar energy through photosynthesis by plants, the consumption of plants by animals, the consumption of animals by other animals, and the ultimate decomposition of both plants and animals by microorganisms, which renders their chemical constituents available for recycling within the system. Ecosystems can contain hundreds or thousands of different organisms, one or more habitats (pond, marsh, field), and one or more communities (assemblages of organisms). Thus, evaluating the risks to ecosystems and their component parts is a monumental task, compared to only examining the risks to humans.

Ecosystems can be characterized by structure and function. Structure involves the species and populations. Function covers the magnitude and pathways of energy flow and the recycling dynamics of matter. One or both of these can be included among the end points.

Intrinsic to the definition of ecosystems are the homeostatic processes that stabilize ecosystems, the checks, balances, and feedback controls between production and consumption.[12–15] The functional relations among the biotic and abiotic components contribute to homeostasis, allowing ecosystems to recover from short-lived stresses such as hot or cold weather, dry or wet seasons, fire, hurricanes or volcanoes, chemical or physical perturbations, or even global climate changes. Since all organisms have evolved within a system that has been exposed to change, they have evolved mechanisms to cope with these changes. Most systems have some mechanisms for self-repair,[16] and it is this capacity that allows restoration of damaged ecosystems to functioning systems.

These repair mechanisms account for both the stability and resiliency of communities and ecosystems in the face of change, and should be an important part of any ecological risk assessment. Stability should not be interpreted as meaning fixed and immutable, since ecosystems undergo succession and dynamic changes with environmental conditions. Rather, stability includes the orderly or regular changes that occur through time that allow the ecosystem and its components to function and provide ecological services.

HUMAN AND ECOLOGICAL RISK ASSESSMENT DIFFERENCES

Human health risk assessment involves identifying hazardous agents (often chemicals), establishing the effects and the relationship between levels and effects, establishing how people are exposed, and identifying the target or at-risk human populations. All of these aspects apply equally to individual species in ecological risk assessment. However, even the simplest ecosystem has several species, and most have hundreds or even thousands of different species to consider.

Species must not only be considered in isolation, but the effects of a hazard on the relationships among species must also be evaluated. This includes examining the effect of hazards on competition, predation, mutualism, and a variety of other relationships between species pairs and groups. For example, the removal or decrease in population levels of one organism may result in its prey increasing (direct effects), its competitors increasing or decreasing in population levels (indirect effects), changes in the population levels of the competitors of its prey because of changes in the prey (second-order effects), or a combination of these. In other words, there are many pathways in ecological systems where feedback can effect several levels of the ecosystem.

Often it is the indirect effects that result in instability in the ecosystem, or the need for ecosystem repair or management. Thus, evaluating the effect of any hazard, chemical or otherwise, on an ecosystem and its component parts entails understanding the structure and function of that ecosystem. This may be easier in less complex systems such as the tundra, but is much more difficult in tropical ecosystems with high species diversity and complex interrelationships.[17]

Three factors differ dramatically between human and ecological risk assessment: species diversity and complexity, spatial considerations, and temporal considerations. As mentioned earlier, ecological risk assessment must take into consideration a variety of species in a matrix of structural and functional relationships. Human risk assessment takes people into account.

Spatial considerations are an important part of ecological risk assessment because the limits of the system examined must be defined. Since there are no clear boundaries, except in the case of the earth biosphere, the delineation of boundaries has inherent problems in the movement of organisms, matter, and energy into and out of the system. Ecological evaluations range from small systems such as a pond, to regional-scale assessments.[18–22]

Temporal considerations are an equally important part of ecological risk assessment because different species and ecosystems have different longevities and periodicities of processes.[23] For example, some organisms may live for only a period of minutes, while others may live for hundreds of years. Moreover, there are also differences in that for some species, there are unpredictable lengths of life-stages and different metamorphic stages, and others have indeterminate growth. When these differences are considered for multispecies assemblages, the impact on the food web will result in exposures of different magnitudes affecting different species.[23]

Similar differences in temporal scales exist for ecosystems. There are temporal differences in almost all functional aspects, from nutrient cycling, growth rates, decomposition time, growing season, recovery time, and succession time. For example, although tundra systems are less complex than tropical systems, the time required for decomposition or the return of nutrients to the system is much longer because of the cold climate.

Temporal considerations do not just apply to the lifespan of an individual, but also include evolutionary constraints.[24] For human risk assessment, the health and well-being of each individual is important; however, for ecological risk assessment the important unit is the population (except in the case of endangered species).

ECOLOGICAL RISK ASSESSMENT MODELS

In the early phases of ecological risk assessment, people concentrated on identifying or assessing the hazards of a given chemical or perturbation, and later moved to examining all phases of the ecological risk process, including risk characterization. Moreover, early assessments concentrated on single-species populations, and only later moved to systems-level testing (i.e., references 25–27).

Much of the literature on ecological risk assessment derives from regulatory mandates to protect the environment and human health, and has a toxicological or management approach.[22,28–31] Indeed, the United States Environmental Protection Agency and the National Research Council defined ecological risk assessment as a systematic means of developing a scientific basis for regulatory decision making. Thus, different agencies have proposed ecological risk assessment schemes to meet their particular regulatory needs. The National Research Council, academics, and others, however, have tried to formulate general ecological risk assessment paradigms that will have general applicability for chemical, biological, and physical hazards. In this section we will review the agency models, and then discuss the more general ecological risk assessment models.

The Department of Energy, recognizing the need to evaluate and deal with risks on their sites, has proposed a process that involves stakeholders up front in the initial scoping of the problem (FIG. 1). They have concentrated on the range of stakeholders to be involved,[32] more so perhaps, than any other agency. Partially this is a function of the truly national nature of both the risks at the sites, and the potential costs of remediation and restoration.

Their risk assessment process includes both human and ecological risk, as well as both cancer and noncancer. Their scoping phase identifies the potential human

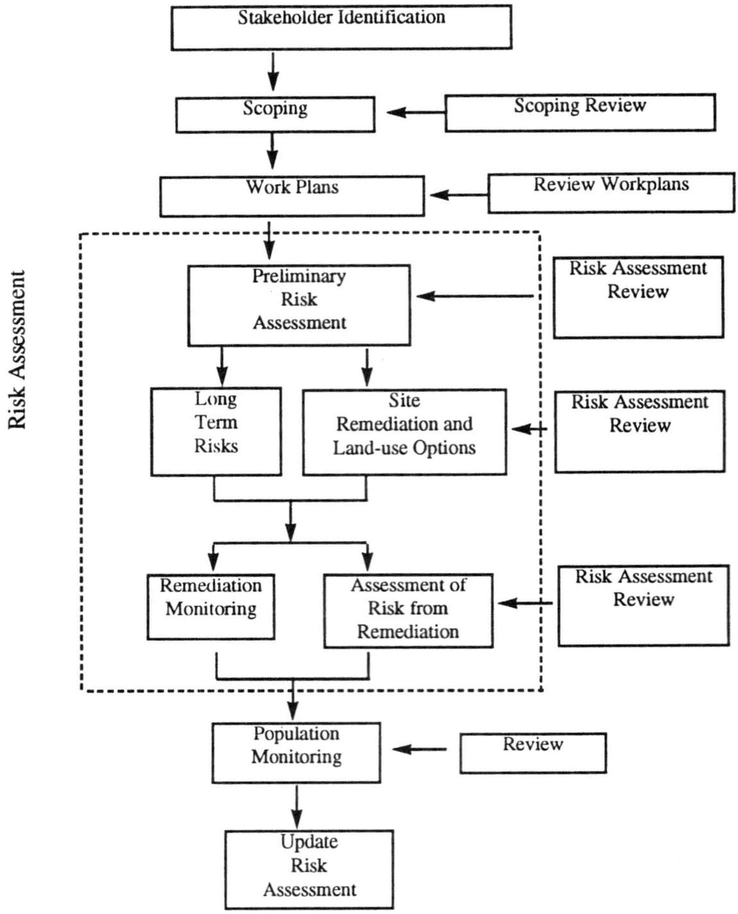

FIGURE 1. Department of energy ecological risk assessment model with stakeholder participation. (Abstracted from text, NRC 1993.)

and nonhuman targets of pollution and possible adverse consequences of exposure. Their risk assessments include an important role for public review at all stages, both at the local and national level. To some extent, the Department of Energy's view of risk assessment takes into account the iterative process necessary to make management decisions at their sites.[32]

Several offices, within the U.S. Environmental Protection Agency (EPA) have proposed ecological risk models to deal with their needs. The Office of Toxic Substances proposed an ecological risk assessment process to deal with their regulatory responsibilities under the Toxic Substances Control Act (TSCA). Their initial model (FIG. 2) deals mostly with chemical identification, hazard assessment, exposure assess-

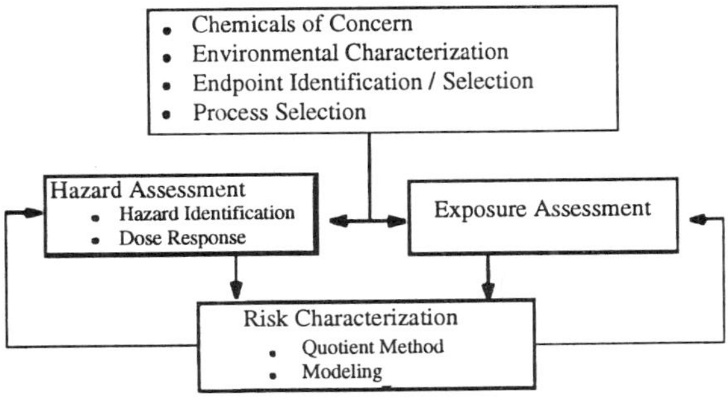

FIGURE 2. Toxic Substance Control Act (TSCA) view of ecological risk assessment. (Modified from Zeeman and Gilford.[33])

ment, and risk characterization; thus it is similar to the human health risk model.[33] This was amplified to illustrate the components of a risk assessment model (FIG. 3).[34]

The Federal Insecticide, Fungicide, and Rodenticide Act (FIFRA) is administered by EPA, and they are charged with protecting the environment from the unreasonable adverse effects of pesticides. They have dealt with developing ecological risk assessment methodologies for aquatic systems.[35] Their model is a simple one (FIG. 4), involving the use of toxicological and exposure data to estimate the hazards from pesticides. Their toxicological testing involves a tiered approach including acute tests, fish life-cycle tests, plant tests, sediment toxicity tests, microcosms, and mesocosms. They also mandate a scientific advisory panel to review the assessments.

Other countries, such as the United Kingdom, have also dealt with ecological risk issues concerning pesticides.[36] The European perspective concentrates on developing

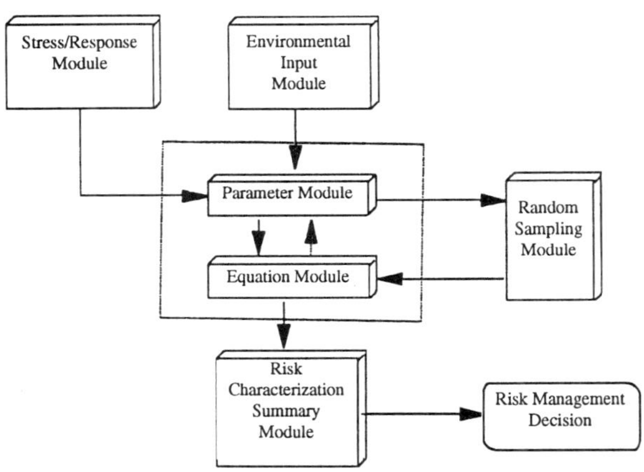

FIGURE 3. Expanded risk assessment model for TSCA. (Modified from Rodier and Mauriello[34].)

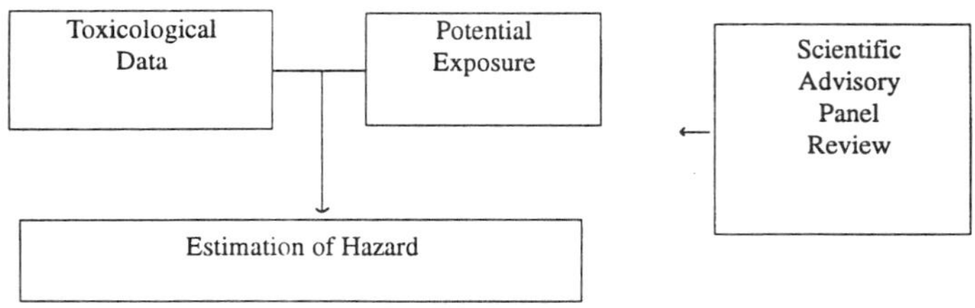

FIGURE 4. The Federal Insecticide, Fungicide and Rodenticide Act and ecological risk. (Modified from Resolve[35].)

consistent, yet flexible, decision-making procedures in which uncertainty is recognized and expert judgement is included. They identified a set of 10 issues that should be considered in the design of a risk assessment (FIG. 5). In our view, these are critical issues, but it provides less of a paradigm for practical ecological assessments.

The Environmental Protection Agency itself has worked for over a decade to formulate a generalized ecological risk paradigm that could be applied to all hazards: chemical, physical, and biological.[37] Their model (FIG.6) clearly separates risk assessment as a science-based process, with discussions between managers occurring at the beginning and end of the ecological risk assessment process. This has been an important dialogue involving hundreds of scientists, regulators, and managers over a long period, and their risk assessment model has general applicability.

The National Research Council convened a large committee to examine ecological risk,[2] and they modified the risk paradigm to include both ecological and human health (FIG. 7). The main modification was to add exposure-response assessment, acknowledging that for ecological systems, dose-response data are not always available. They also recognize the important role of research, validation, and monitoring. They further defined the role of laboratory and field observations of adverse effects on hazard identification, and of field measurements and the characterization of populations.[2]

Individual scientists have also proposed a series of modifications to the ecological risk models, often to address the complexity of ecological systems. Suter and Loar[38] emphasized the importance of feedback between the different stages (FIG. 8), rather than thinking of ecological risk assessment as a straight-line process (as most earlier models do). This is an important point, as most aspects of the assessment should be reevaluated with the completion of each succeeding phase.

We have proposed a more complex model for ecological risk assessment that takes into account the complexities of the system, feedback loops, evaluation of the process, and stakeholder participation.[39–41] We propose that at all phases, both the stakeholders and the managers should be involved, not in conducting or evaluating the science, but in fine-tuning the goals and objectives of the assessment.

Conceptual models have been augmented by mathematical models for ecological risk assessment.[42–44] For these to be useful, they must transcend the population and ecological models of the past; be broadly applicable to a variety of environmental problems on the local, regional, and global scale; and be applicable to the different

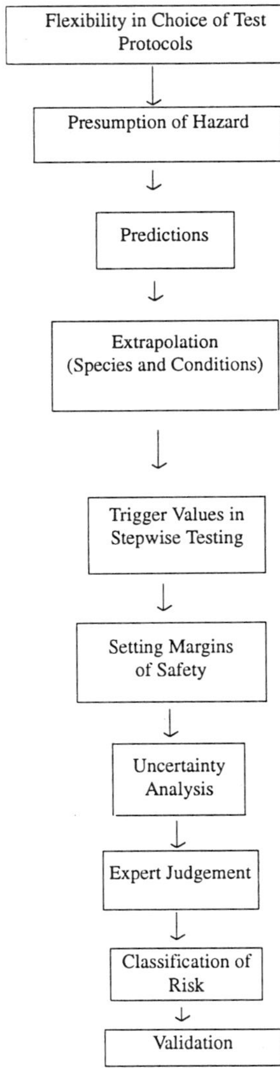

FIGURE 5. The European perspective on ecological risk assessment models for pesticides. (Modified from Grieg-Smith[36].)

components of the risk assessment process.[42] The use of models, however, introduces uncertainties in extrapolation, although they lead to probabilities of adverse outcomes.[45] Although extrapolation from laboratory data on single species to population effects on single species in the wild is sound, extrapolations from single-species laboratory data to ecosystem-level functions is fraught with difficulties.[46,47]

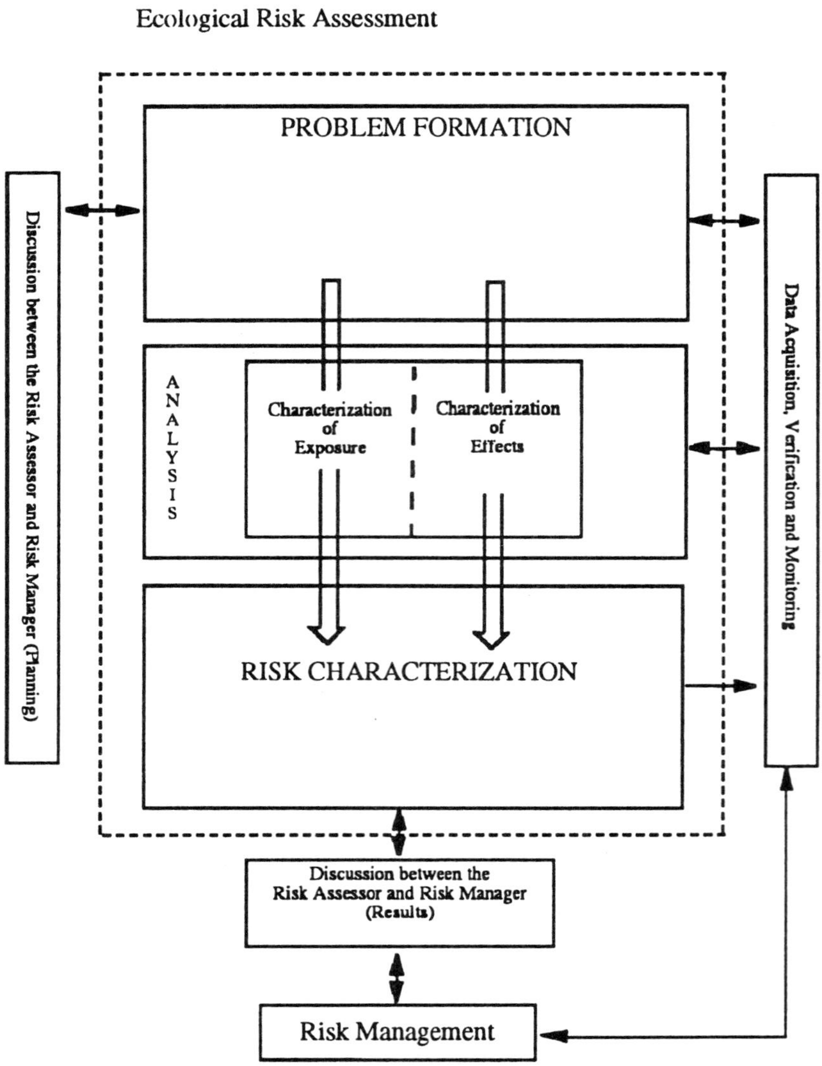

FIGURE 6. The Environmental Protection Agency's (EPA) ecological risk model. (Modified from Norton *et al.*[37].)

ADVANTAGES AND DISADVANTAGES OF ECOLOGICAL RISK APPROACHES

One of the primary criticisms of ecological risk assessment questions the concept of ecosystem health; proponents of this view claim that the "health" metaphor is

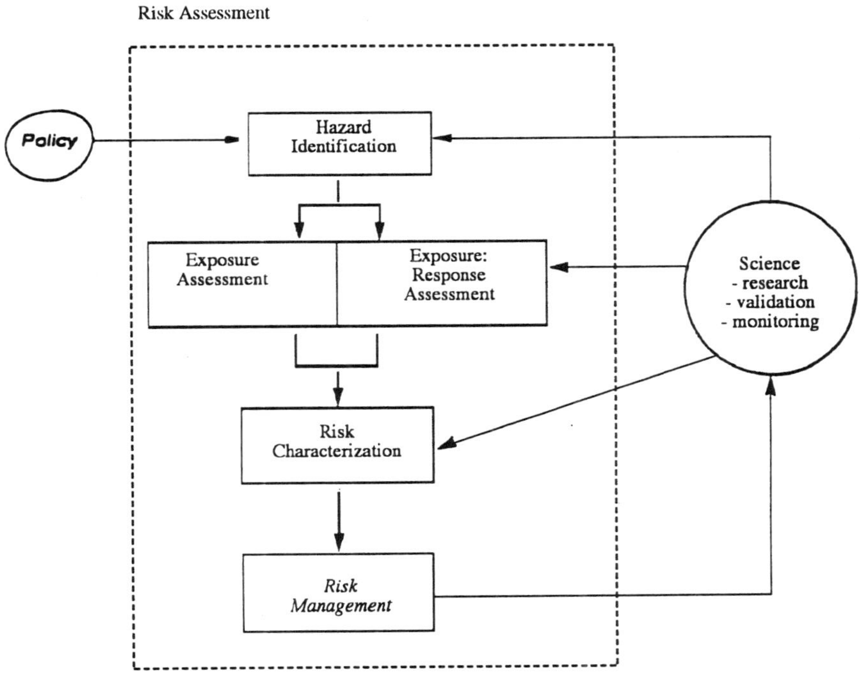

FIGURE 7. The National Research Council's modified model to include both human health and ecosystems. (After NRC[2].)

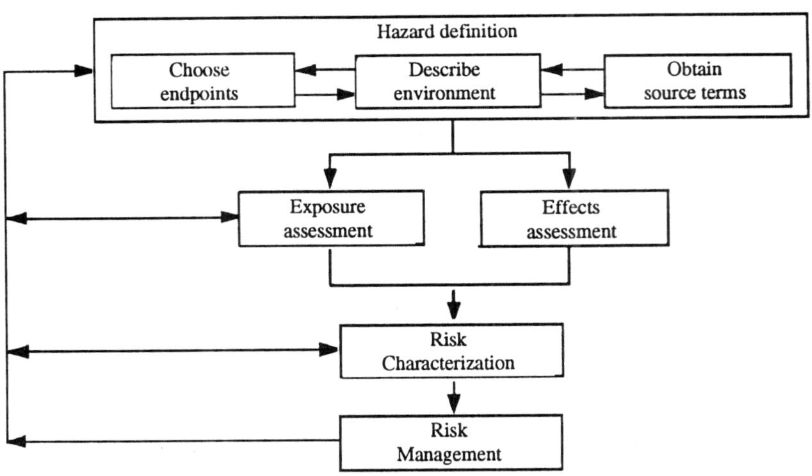

FIGURE 8. Ecological risk assessment as proposed by Suter and Loan.[38]

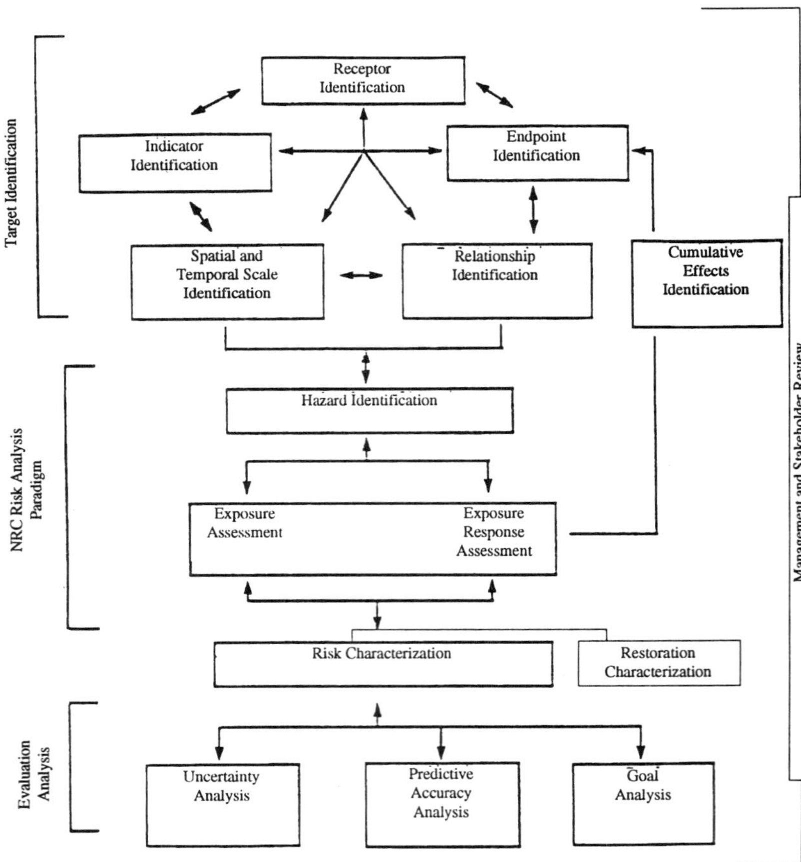

FIGURE 9. Ecological risk assessment model proposed by Burger and Gochfeld (this paper).

flawed. Suter[47] and others argue that ecosystems are not organisms, and that indices to measure their health are meaningless and have no diagnostic power. Others, however, argue that the metaphor is useful, and leads to productive examination of ecosystems.[48]

The health metaphor leads to examining signs and symptoms of ecosystem pathology, monitoring recovery after disturbance, and examining health status on the basis of potential threats from exposures to known stresses.[48] Since these three approaches are useful in examining the functioning of ecosystems, it seems unproductive to argue about whether the health metaphor is truly useful.

Another difficulty with ecological risk assessment is determining the level of ecosystem health or well being that is acceptable. Recently, it has become fashionable to talk about sustainable ecosystems and a sustainable biosphere.[49] Although this is a laudable goal, it simply removes the problem of defining ecosystem health to defining *sustainable* (and sustainable to what level, for whom, and for how long?).

These difficulties notwithstanding, it is clear that we must have some way of evaluating the risks posed by chemical, physical, and biological hazards, and of ranking these risks. Not only must we evaluate competing risks, but we must be able to determine risk when there are several hazards present at the same time. Ecological risk assessment allows for these two analyses, albeit with difficulty at the moment because the science base is not always present.

Ecological risk assessment provides a sound approach because it organizes scientific knowledge into a coherent framework for risk managers, regulators, and the public to make meaningful regulatory and cleanup decisions. This, it seems to us, is the primary advantage of ecological risk assessment. It is a uniform process whereby science can have a role in decisions concerning populations, communities, and ecosystems.

CONCLUSIONS

Ecological risk assessment provides a paradigm for evaluating the potential effects of chemical, physical, and biological hazards to organisms, populations, communities, and ecosystems. Because of the complexity in targets and end points, ecological risk assessment must involve some selection of indicators (both species and processes), and this requires a detailed knowledge of the structure and function of ecosystems. Nonetheless, ecological risk assessment is our best current method for evaluating competing hazards, and can be used to compare past, present, and future risks.

SUMMARY

Ecological risk assessment developed from the convergence of human health risk assessment, ecology, and ecotoxicology to provide data for environmental management and decision making. There has been an emphasis on using the health risk paradigm. However, ecological systems are much more complex than the single-species, single-lifetime approach used in human health risk assessment; hence several modifications are necessary, as ecological risk assessment evolves for particular uses. The advancement of ecological risk assessment is particularly timely, given competing considerations for cleanup of a variety of hazardous-waste sites, including the huge Department of Defense and Department of Energy sites, as well as the 1000+ Superfund sites. Sufficient resources are not available to clean up all sites completely, much less at the same time. Some sites pose no current identifiable risk to human receptors, but may be unusable for human habitation. Where human receptors are not the targets, ecological risk assessment can be used not only to evaluate the risks to ecosystems, but to help determine the degree of cleanup required to restore degraded environments to functioning ecosystems that provide valuable ecological services, and to rank sites for possible cleanup.

ACKNOWLEDGMENTS

We thank S. Bartell, L. Barnthouse, K. Cooper, B. D. Goldstein, M. Greenberg, J. Ehrenfeld, M. Lee, J. Moore, S. Norton, D. Policansky, C. Powers, M. Robson, C. Safina, and D. Wartenberg for valuable discussions about ecological risk and the environmental movement.

REFERENCES

1. National Research Council. 1983. Risk Assessment in the Federal Government. National Academy Press. Washington, DC.
2. National Research Council. 1993. Issues in Risk Assessment. National Academy Press. Washington, DC.
3. Paine, R. T. 1966. Food web complexity and species diversity. Am. Nat. **100**(1): 65-75.
4. National Research Council. 1986. Ecological Knowledge and Environmental Problem-solving. National Academy Press. Washington, DC.
5. Hoffman, D. J., B. A. Rattner & R. J. Hall. 1990. Wildlife toxicology. Environ. Sci. Technol. **24**(3): 276-283.
6. Baumann, P. C. 1992. The use of fish tumors in wild populations of fish to assess ecosystem health. J. Aquat. Ecosyst. Health **1**(1): 135-146.
7. Mitsch, W. 1993. Ecological engineering. Environ. Sci. Technol. **27**(3): 438-445.
8. Sheehan, P. J. 1984. Effects on community and ecosystem structure and dynamics. *In* Effects of Pollutants at the Ecosystem Level, P. J. Sheehan, D. R. Miller, G. C. Butler, and P. Bourdeau, Eds. Wiley. Chichester, England.
9. Cairns, J. 1991. Restoration ecology: A major opportunity for ecotoxicologists. Environ. Toxicol. Chem. **10**(4): 429-432.
10. Cairns, J. 1993. The balance of ecological destruction and repair. Environ. Health Perspect. **101**(3): 206.
11. Odum, E. T. 1957. Fundamentals of Ecology. Saunders. Philadelphia.
12. Beddington, J. R. 1984. *In* Exploitation of Marine Communities, R. M. May, Ed. Dahlem Konferenzen, Springer-Verlag, Berlin.
13. Sousa, W. P. 1984. The role of disturbance in natural communities. Annu. Rev. Ecol. **15:** 353-391.
14. Ojima, D. S., T. G. F. Kittel, T. Rosswall & B. H. Walker. 1991. Critical issues for understanding global change effects on terrestrial ecosystems. Ecol. Appl. **1**(3): 316-325.
15. Stiling, P. D. 1992. Introductory Ecology. Prentice Hall. Englewood Cliffs, NJ.
16. Pace, M. L. & E. Funlie. 1991. Regulation of planktonic microbial communities by nutrients and herbivores. Ecology. **72**(3): 904-914.
17. Wilson, E. O. 1986. Biodiversity. National Academy Press. Washington, DC.
18. Hunsaker, C. T., R. L. Graham, G. W. Suter II, R. V. O'Neill, L. W. Barnthouse & R. H. Gardner. 1990. Assessing ecological risk on a regional scale. Environ. Manage. **14**(3): 325-332.
19. Hunsaker, C., D. Carpenter & J. Messer. 1991. Ecological indicators for regional monitoring. Bull. Ecol. Soc. Am. **71**(3): 165-172.
20. Suter, G. W. II. 1990. Endpoints for regional ecological risk assessments. Environ. Manage. **14**(1): 9-23.
21. Graham, R. L., C. T. Hunsaker, R. V. O'Neill & B. L. Jackson. 1991. Ecological risk assessment at the regional scale. Ecol. Appl. **1**(2): 196-206.
22. Bartell, S. M., R. H. Gardner & R. V. O'Neill. 1992. Ecological Risk Estimation. Lewis Press. Boca Raton, FL.
23. Burger, J. & M. Gochfeld. 1992. Temporal scales in ecological risk assessment. Arch. Environ. Contam. Toxicol. **23**(4): 484-488.

24. Gochfeld, M. & J. Burger. 1993. Evolutionary consequences for ecological risk assessment and management. Environ. Monit. Assess. **28**(1): 161-168.
25. Heimbach, F., W. Pflueger & H. Ratte. 1992. Use of small artificial ponds for assessment of hazards to aquatic ecosystems. Environ. Toxicol. Chem. **11**(1): 27-34.
26. Weber, E. C., W. G. Deutsch, D. R. Bayne & W. C. Seesock. 1992. Ecosystem-level testing of a synthetic pyrethroid insecticide in aquatic mesocosms. Environ. Toxicol. Chem. **11:** 87-105.
27. Kendall, R. J. & J. Akerman. 1992. Terrestrial wildlife exposed to agrochemicals: An ecological risk assessment perspective. Environ. Toxicol. Chem. **11**(12): 1727-1749.
28. Environmental Protection Agency. 1982. Pesticide Assessment Guidelines. E: Hazard Evaluation: Wildlife and Aquatic Organisms. Office of Pesticide and Toxic Substance. Washington, DC.
29. Bascietto, J., D. Hinckley, J. Plafkin & M. Simak. 1990. Ecotoxicity and ecological risk assessment. Environ. Sci. Technol. **24**(1): 10-15.
30. Rifkin, E. & J. LaKind. 1991. Dioxin bioaccumulation: Key to sound risk assessment methodology. J. Toxicol. Environ. Health **33**(1): 103-111.
31. Bilyard, G. R., J. J. Bascietto & H. Beckert. 1993. Regulatory and institutional considerations in the application of ecological risk assessment at federal facilities. Fed. Fac. Environ. J. Autumn: 337-348.
32. National Research Council. 1994. Building Consensus Through Risk Assessment and Management of the Department of Energy's Environmental Remediation Program. National Academy Press. Washington, D.C.
33. Zeeman, M. & J. Gilford. 1993. Ecological hazard evaluation and risk assessment under EPA's Toxic Substances Control Act (TSCA): An introduction. Environ. Toxicol. Risk Assess. 7-21. (ASTM STP 1179, W. G. Landis, J. S. Hughes, and M. A. Lewis, Eds. Am. Soc. Testing Mater. Philadelphia.
34. Rodier, D. J. & D. A. Mauriello. 1993. The quotient method of ecological risk assessment and modeling under TSCA: A review. Environ. Toxicol. Risk Assess. 80-91. (ASTM STP 1179, W. G. Landis, J. S. Hughes & M. A. Lewis, Eds. Am. Soc. Testing Mater. Philadelphia.)
35. Resolve. 1992. Improving aquatic risk assessment under FIFRA. World Wildlife Fund. Washington, DC.
36. Grieg-Smith, P. W. 1992. A European perspective on ecological risk assessment, illustrated by pesticide registration procedures in the United Kingdom. Environ. Toxicol. Chem. **11**(12): 1673-1689.
37. Norton, S. B., D. J. Rodier, J. H. Gentile, W. H. van der Schalie, W. P. Wood & M. W. Slimak. 1992. A framework for ecological risk assessment at the EPA. Environ. Toxicol. Chem. **11**(12): 1663-1672.
38. Suter, G. W. II & J. M. Loar. 1992. Weighing the ecological risk of hazardous waste sites: The Oak Ridge Case. Environ. Sci. Technol. **26:** 432-438.
39. Burger, J. 1994. How should success be measured in ecological risk assessment? The importance of predictive accuracy. J. Toxicol. Environ. Health **42**(2): 367-376.
40. Burger, J. & M. Gochfeld. 1996. Ecological and human risk assessment: A comparison. *In* Interconnections Between Human and Ecosystem Health, R. T. DiGiulio and E. Monosson, Eds. Chapman & Hall. London.
41. Burger, J. & S. Handel. Using restoration ecology as a tool for risk assessment. CRESP. Unpublished Report 20.
42. Barnthouse, L. W. 1992. The role of models in ecological risk assessment: A 1990s perspective. Environ. Toxicol. Chem. **11**(12): 1751-1760.
43. Barnthouse, L. W., R. V. O'Neill, S. M. Bartell & G. W. Suter II. 1986. Population and ecosystem theory in ecological risk assessment. *In* Aquatic Toxicology and Environmental Fate, Vol. 9, T. M. Poston and R. Purdy, Eds.: 82-106. Am. Soc. Testing Mater. Philadelphia, PA.

44. Emlen, J. M. 1989. Terrestrial populations models for ecological risk assessment: A state-of-the-art review. Environ. Toxicol. Chem. **8:** 831-842.
45. O'Neill, R. V., R. H. Gardner, L. W. Barnthouse, G. W. Suter, S. G. Hildebrand & C. W. Giehrs. 1982. Ecosystem risk analysis: A new methodology. Environ. Toxicol. Chem. **1**(1): 167-177.
46. Cairns, J., Jr. 1992. The threshold problem in ecotoxicology. Ecotoxicology **1**(1): 30-16.
47. Suter, G. W. II. 1993. A critique of ecosystem health concepts and indexes. Environ. Chem. **12:** 1533-1539.
48. Rapport, D. J. 1989. What constitutes ecosystem health? Perspect. Biol. Med. **33**(1): 120-132.
49. Risser, P. G., J. Lubchenco & S. A. Levin. 1991. Biological research priorities—A sustainable biosphere. BioScience. **41**(9): 625-627.

Probabilistic Risk Assessment: Lessons from Four Case Studies[a]

LAURA C. GREEN[b] AND EDMUND A. C. CROUCH

Cambridge Environmental Inc.
58 Charles Street
Cambridge, Massachusetts 02141

INTRODUCTION AND SUMMARY

The past few years have seen legislative and other calls for "risk assessment reform." Congressional bills such as S.R. 343 and H.R. 1022, for example, sought, among other things, to make risk assessment more "realistic" and explicit. The belief is that current standard methods for risk assessments, typified by approaches taken by the U.S. EPA, are usually designed (1) deliberately to overestimate risks, and (2) to do so in such a way that the extent of overestimation in the risk estimates is impossible to discern. The former property, that of producing an overestimate, may often be desirable and/or mandatory, depending upon the context. But the latter property–obscuring the extent of overestimation–was thought to be neither desirable nor mandatory. Risk-assessment reformers typically seek both a greater emphasis on "best estimates" of risk and greater clarity in derivation of risk estimates.[c]

In particular, in standard-risk assessments, overestimates arise from a number of causes, principally:

- The selection of models (either statistical or physical) that are inherently conservative;
- The selection for those models of parameter estimates that are at the conservative end of their plausible ranges;
- The use of conservative values selected as a matter of policy for some parameters;
- The concatenation in the risk assessment of many parameters, many chosen to be conservative, without any account of the probability for all such parameters to be simultaneously at the high end of their range.

[a] This work was supported in part by the Commission on Risk Assessment and Risk Management. The opinions expressed herein are those of the authors, who accept responsibility for any errors or omissions.

[b] Corresponding author. Phone: 617/225-0810; fax: 617/225-0813; e-mail: green@cambridgeenvironmental.com

[c] In this discussion, we deliberately oversimplify by stereotyping risk-assessment reformers. Obviously, some who wish to reform current methods of risk assessment hold beliefs different from, even opposite to, those here ascribed to all reformers.

Without a mechanism to account for the implausibility of the concatenation of extreme values, or to moderate the conservatism of each parameter during such a concatenation, one cannot evaluate the extent of the overestimate. Many reformers believe that this obfuscation is inappropriate. Many believe further that illumination might be achieved by performing risk assessments in a probabilistic, rather than deterministic, fashion.

We undertook case studies designed to illustrate risk-assessment techniques that take account of the probabilities for extreme values in parameter estimates, and so can meet some of the requirements of the bills just alluded to (a full report of our work is presented in Crouch *et al.*[1]). The relevant requirements are to provide (1) more complete uncertainty analyses, and (2) more complete descriptions of the ranges of risk estimates, including–indeed, featuring–"best estimates" (as demanded in S.R. 343 and H.R. 1022), at least in some sense. In particular, the case studies undertaken describe and, when feasible, incorporate quantitatively by using probabilistic techniques the uncertainty or variability in each parameter used in estimating risks to human health. These parameters include those used to describe toxicity, to model fate and transport, and to estimate doses to exposed humans. The resulting estimates of risk include "best estimates," together with the surrounding uncertainty distributions.

We performed four case studies: three involving exposure to 1,1-dichloroethylene (11-DCE); the fourth involving exposure to vinyl chloride. Our principal findings were these:

- There is no single "best estimate." Indeed, risk-assessment reformers rarely define precisely what they mean by "best estimate." We examined the expectation values (means) and medians of the distributions obtained, since these are central tendency estimates for distributions that could be considered "best" for certain applications, but other interpretations are quite possible and may be desirable. Indeed, different legislative mandates are likely to require different definitions of "best" estimate, and without specification of such a mandate, the term is meaningless.

- Using *standard* assumptions, the mean estimate in our first case study is close to the 95th percentile, and the latter estimate may be preferable to the mean if a point estimate is required. In other situations, the mean estimate could be considerably larger or considerably smaller than the 95th percentile. In our case studies, however, the median (50th percentile) estimate is always substantially smaller in magnitude than either the mean or the 95th percentile.

- Using *nonstandard* assumptions (that could be equally defensible), the mean estimate of risk may be very much larger or very much smaller in magnitude than the 95th percentile upper confidence limit, and may indeed be of different sign (and so, from the point of view of decision making, infinitely different). Indeed, for the two case studies performed on 1,1-DCE in drinking water, a simple, quite defensible change in model for evaluation of the dose-response data yielded mean and median estimates of risk of opposite sign compared with the values estimated using the standard set of assumptions (that is to say, suggesting that 1,1-DCE likely *prevents* cancer, under the conditions specified). Nonetheless, the 95th percentile estimates of risk were *essentially identical* for both models.

- The point estimates obtained using standard assumptions can be extremely conservative. This is not to say that such a result will always obtain, but it did in the four case studies evaluated.

- To the uninitiated, the uncertainties inherent in the standard methodologies will appear to be surprisingly large, even with the (probably incorrect) assumption that all the incorporated models are correct.

- A precise definition of the measure(s) of risk to be evaluated is required. We evaluated just one measure of risk in the main case study—risks to a randomly chosen individual in an exposed population—but other measures may be what are wanted in particular cases.

- One cannot, in general, draw conclusions about particular measures of risk unless those measures have been evaluated specifically (although limited inferences may be possible in particular cases). For example, we cannot draw conclusions about population risks, since we evaluated risks only to a random individual. The distribution of risk estimates obtained is an uncertainty distribution for such an individual; and the uncertainty is due to a combination of a lack of knowledge about (among others):

  (i) The characteristics of that individual;
  (ii) The representatives of the particular outcome observed in the rodent bioassays;
  (iii) The interspecies extrapolation to apply to 1,1-DCE;
  (iv) Various parameters in the fate, transport, and exposure models.

The various statistics of the distribution thus apply only to the uncertainty about risks to the randomly chosen individual. The percentiles indicate that we are, for example, 50% sure (median) or 95% sure (95th percentile) that the risks are less than those indicated *for a randomly chosen individual* (and this statement is conditional on all the models being correct). The mean estimate of risk we obtain (expectation value of the distribution) strictly indicates a value that would be the best to use *if* we were interested in simultaneously summing up or averaging risks to many individuals, from many chemicals, using many rodent bioassays, and taking account of many other sets of measurements of various model parameters.

- Implementation of these methods reveals areas where the standard point estimate glosses over, or ignores entirely, important problems that ought to be addressed. One such problem, for example, is whether the uncertainty in interspecies extrapolation is correlated for different routes of exposure.

- Implementation of the methods apparently called for by many risk-assessment reformers is possible but fairly demanding. Readily available standard software is not adequate. There is a relatively large "up-front" burden in evaluating standard distributions (e.g., for carcinogenic potencies).

Our primary case study was one in which a population is exposed to 1,1-DCE through contaminated drinking water. The environmental data were abstracted from a real site, and used in a hypothetical and relatively simple exposure scenario in which the population has characteristics indistinguishable from the United States as

TABLE 1. Some Statistics of the Distributions of Risk Estimates from the Case Studies

Case	Median (50th Percentile)	Mean	95th Percentile	Point Estimate
1,1-DCE, standard	1.2×10^{-9}	1.6×10^{-6}	1.7×10^{-6}	1.3×10^{-4}
1,1-DCE, nonstandard	-2.0×10^{-9}	-9.5×10^{-6}	1.7×10^{-6}	—
Vinyl chloride (standard)	1.4×10^{-6}	8.8×10^{-5}	2.0×10^{-4}	4.1×10^{-4}
1,1-DCE workers	1.4×10^{-8}	3.6×10^{-3}	8.4×10^{-3}	2.7×10^{-2}

a whole. We evaluated a particular measure of risk—the lifetime excess carcinogenic risk to an individual chosen randomly from such a population. This measure was chosen to simplify our task, since all the variabilities in population characteristics are thus transformed to uncertainties for this individual measure of risk.

In addition to the case study using measurements of 1,1-DCE, we performed an additional case study in which the chemical contaminant was assumed to be vinyl chloride at the same concentrations as the measurements of 1,1-DCE, while all the other parameters of the assessment remained the same. This assessment was performed to evaluate the effect on the risk estimates of a substantial change in the uncertainty distribution for carcinogenic effects. For vinyl chloride, the rodent bioassay data upon which estimates of human risk are based unequivocally show carcinogenic effects (and it is, of course, an established human carcinogen). In contrast, the results for 1,1-DCE in laboratory rodent bioassays have generally been either null or equivocal, and there are certainly no compellingly positive epidemiologic studies.

Preliminary results indicated that the exposures to 1,1-DCE in the hypothetical situation considered, that is, by exposure to contaminated drinking water, would give negligible risks with near certainty, even though the standard point estimate[d] might indicate some need for regulatory action. We wondered what might happen in higher, but still plausible, exposure conditions—in part to determine whether a probabilistic methodology would generate risk estimates that merited a regulatory response when the situation warranted it. We thus also evaluated hypothetical exposures of workers to 1,1-DCE in workplace air. For this exercise, we chose plausible occupational levels of exposure based on OSHA standards for 1,1- DCE.

RESULTS AND DISCUSSION

Some of our specific numerical results are as shown below. In TABLE 1 we summarize the median, mean, 95th percentile, and point estimates of individual

[d] The "point" estimate is the value obtained using a selection of parameter values typical of those used in current, deterministic, regulatory approaches to risk assessment, such as those employed in evaluating Superfund sites.

carcinogenic risk from 1,1-DCE or vinyl chloride for the four case studies examined. For the primary case study–that involving a standard but probabilistic assessment of risk from 1,1-DCE in contaminated water at a Superfund site–the differences between the 95th percentile estimate of risk and the point estimate of the same may make all the difference in the world. The point estimate of risk, 1.3×10^{-4}, would be taken (and indeed was taken, in the actual case upon which our study was based) to be a clear, risk-based signal for groundwater remediation; and that remediation might well cost on the order of \$10,000,000-\$20,000,000. It would not matter that this point estimate is at the 99.8th percentile of the distribution of risk estimates–indeed, one would not even know its percentile rank using only point-estimate techniques. On the other hand, the 95th percentile estimate of risk, shown here to be only slightly more than one-in-one million, might be taken as risk-based grounds for *not* undertaking remediation; or at least for choosing a "remedy" that would be far less expensive and/or extensive.

This point requires some elaboration. Risk-management decisions, as they are called, change with time, across regions, and between decision makers. At some times and in some regions, individual, upper-bound risk estimates of greater than 10^{-6} suffice (or sufficed) for demanding remediation at Superfund sites; but for other situations, remediation is only required if risks exceed 10^{-5} (or higher, in specific cases). Several states now use the 10^{-5} risk level as their "bright line" for decision making; and some of those had preferred the 10^{-6} benchmark until it became clear how many sites/situations violated such a guideline, at which point their expectations relaxed.

The "standard" and "nonstandard" analyses of 1,1-DCE (which differ only in the model used to interpolate the dose-response data from the rodent bioassay) show substantial–indeed, diametric–differences in the median and mean estimates. These two "best estimates" of risk in the nonstandard analysis have a negative sign, indicating that exposure to 1,1-DCE at the low levels postulated might confer a net benefit! Clearly the definition of what statistic is the "best" estimator must be carefully made to match the desired end point, since different choices of statistic may lead to diametrically opposed choices for policy.

In either the standard or nonstandard analyses, the median estimates of risk (for carcinogenesis in the standard case, and for anticarcinogenesis in the nonstandard case) are extremely small, that is, quite close to zero. Moreover, the *upper end* of the uncertainty distribution is not substantially changed by the change in analysis method: indeed, at the 95th percentile of the distribution, the risk estimates for both the standard and the nonstandard approaches are identical for all practical purposes.

Such identical results for the high-end estimate might, at first blush, seem peculiar. After all, the standard approach assumes that all doses of 1,1-DCE, however small, may be carcinogenic. As it happens, there is no evidence of carcinogenesis between zero dose and the lowest dose level tested in the rodent bioassays; empirically, the slope of the dose-response line is slightly negative here (that is, indicating anticarcinogenesis), but the uncertainty is large (see FIG. 1). The nonstandard approach permits the dose-response line in this region to be as negative as allowed by the uncertainty. These different approaches do indeed give vastly different sorts of risk-estimate distributions at the low and midranges; but if one wishes to be 95% certain

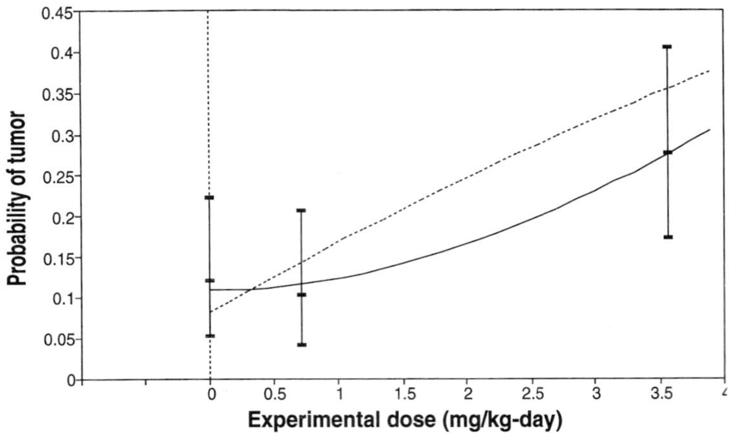

FIGURE 1. Dose-response data for 1,1-DCE ingestion (NCI/NTP).[3] *Key:* —■— Experimental; ——— maximum likelihood; ------ 95th percentile on $q1$.

that a random individual's risk is a certain value or lower, then that value turns out to be the same for both approaches.

This point is lost on many critics of EPA-style risk assessment. Many such critics, believing that standard, regulatory risk assessments are heavily biased toward overestimating the "real" risk, suppose that a full and honest incorporation of uncertainty and variability will vastly lower estimates of risk, even for those at the high end. Forgotten in this notion is that uncertainties and variabilities run in both directions: a compound may indeed be much less carcinogenic than the EPA-style point estimate of potency suggests, for example, but it may also be more carcinogenic than EPA's point estimate allows.

Comparison of the standard analyses of 1,1-DCE and vinyl chloride is also illuminating. The only differences between these two case studies are the carcinogenic potency estimates for the two substances—all other details are assumed to be the identical. The standard EPA point estimate of carcinogenic potency for vinyl chloride is approximately a factor of 3 higher than that for 1,1-DCE, and the unit risk estimate is only 60% higher. These differences account for the relatively small difference (a factor of 3) in the point estimates of risk.

Many will feel that the proximity of the point estimates for risks from equal exposures to 1,1-DCE and vinyl chloride signals the erroneous nature of the point estimate approach. Vinyl chloride is a clear and strong carcinogen in both rodents and people; 1,1-DCE is a marginal rodent carcinogen at best. Surely the risks from the two compounds should differ by more than a factor of 3.

The distributions provided by the Monte Carlo approach do indeed display a much greater disparity between 1,1-DCE and vinyl chloride, a disparity that reflects the very real differences in the weight of evidence for the carcinogenicity of 1,1-DCE compared with vinyl chloride. In addition, the 95th percentile risk estimate for vinyl chloride is only a factor of 2 lower than the point estimate, indicating that in the case of a clear carcinogen, the 95th percentile estimate may give results comparable with the current point estimates.

Working through the case studies, we developed certain opinions about the proposed risk-assessment reforms. We wondered about the emphasis on best estimate(s) of risk, as opposed to the old (and current) emphasis on an upper-bound estimate of risk. Best estimate, *per* the Congressional bills, means a "central estimate of risk," arrived at using the "most plausible and realistic assumptions ... given current scientific information." As noted earlier, we suppose that this emphasis, and the specific language, is an expression of the belief that current risk assessments inappropriately concatenate many upper-bound factors, so that the product is a highly implausible estimate of risk that applies to few or no real people exposed in the real world. We know of at least three groups who often share this view.

First are the regulated communities, whether private companies, municipalities, or others, that bear many of the costs of complying with certain regulations that may do little to reduce actual risk to the public health. The second is the research toxicology community, at least some members of which wonder why information they generate regarding mechanisms of carcinogenesis, for example, is largely ignored in favor of default assumptions such as that essentially all chemical carcinogens are likely to be equally potent at all nonzero levels of exposure.

The third group, perhaps less well known, are the local regulatory authorities: some of those responsible, for example, for writing or rewriting permits for facilities express frustration at U.S. EPA risk estimates for regulated chemicals. The agency explains that the risk estimates are upper-bound values; and that the true value is likely to be lower, and may even be zero. But the local permit writer may not wish to know what the risk "might be," or "might be less than"; he or she wants to know what the risk *is,* at least given current scientific evidence and expert judgment.

Some people therefore believe that a focus on a best estimate of risk would help. Perhaps those paying for compliance with regulations would feel (if not be) less burdened; perhaps results from the laboratory would be translated into more chemical-specific inputs for risk assessment; and perhaps permit writers would be better able to match permit conditions with actual, or at least expected, risk reduction.

But there are two distinct problems that are not acknowledged by such people or in the proposed legislation. First, there is no single estimator of risk that can be used in all situations, and the definition of the estimator is what is most important. Second, no matter what estimator of risk is chosen, the estimate has to be compared with some standard or another, and the choice of standard is what is most important.

It is plainly inadequate to perform a risk estimate such as that we have performed (for the risk to a randomly chosen individual), and then use a central-tendency estimator (e.g., the median estimate), if the legislative requirement is, for example, to set a standard that protects everybody with an adequate margin of safety. What is required in such a situation is to analyze the legislative requirement (protection of everybody with a margin of safety), and then to choose a suitable measure of risk, for example, an estimate of the risk to the most exposed member of the population might be a suitable choice. Given such a choice, one could demand that the estimator for this most exposed member of the population be the median for the uncertainty distribution of risk to that person (and then apply a safety factor of some sort—to afford the "adequate margin"). However, many of the parameters going into the evaluation of risk would certainly not be central-tendency values, since the most exposed person will be extreme in some ways. Similar considerations apply in every other situation.

The second problem is the selection of the standard against which to compare. Why perform a risk estimate if not to compare the result to some standard? The current standard is an upper-bound ''risk estimate'' of 10^{-4} to 10^{-7}, depending on the situation. If one simply demands that the current upper-bound estimate be replaced with a central-tendency value, what is to prevent the standard of comparison from changing to 10^{-8} or 10^{-11} or whatever? If one is going to change the rules of evaluation of risk estimates, one also has to take care to accurately define the standards against which those estimates will be compared.

More useful might be new rules of thumb based on both central-tendency and 95th percentile estimates of risk, or on other properties of the distribution of risk. Imagine two scenarios; air pollutant α poses a central-tendency risk estimate of 1 in 100,000,000 and a 95th percentile risk estimate of 1 in 1000, while air pollutant β poses a central-tendency risk of 1 in 10,000 and an upper-bound risk that is the same as for air pollutant α, 1 in 1000. The current practice in risk management would be to regard both air pollutants as equally risky, equally in need of reduction by regulation. Perhaps the new approach would make air pollutant β a much stronger candidate for regulation, because the ''real'' risk (*per* risk assessment focused on best estimates) is 10,000 times greater for β than for α, even though, at the upper bound, each could be equally risky.

More fundamentally, credible efforts at risk-assessment reform should recognize that the notion of an entirely scientifically objective risk assessment is a mirage. To the extent that risk-assessment reformers believe otherwise, we believe they have been misled.

Science is a method of observing the natural world and conducting tests of various hypotheses about how the world operates. Good science elicits a high degree of consensus among those who analyze it exactly because of its objectivity, reproducibility, and explanatory power.

Of course, science contributes heavily to risk assessment: it does so in such areas as identifying physical relationships that govern the transport of underground pollutants to the air, testing the ability of a chemical to cause cancer in laboratory animals, and measuring the volume of air inhaled in a day by persons of different ages. In each case, a scientific goal is clearly specified and can be reached by measurement of the quantities or processes of interest.

Unfortunately for those desiring certainty and consensus, risk-assessment problems are frequently unresolvable by purely scientific methods. Only scientific questions can be answered by scientific methods, and risk-assessment problems are often largely or entirely nonscientific. Thus, the solutions (or resolutions) to risk-assessment questions vary greatly in the degrees to which they are rooted in scientific observations and deduction. The critical factors determining whether a risk-assessment question can be satisfactorily answered using only scientific tools include: has careful science been done on this or similar problems in the past? If so, have scientists been able to observe this problem on a scale that is directly useful for public policy? Usually, the answers are "no."

A typical risk-assessment problem is one like that examined in the case studies presented here: what are the chances that exposure to a certain amount of a chemical will cause cancer in people? Were scientists assigned this problem, given no additional information about the particular concerns of the questioner, and forced to answer it as "scientifically" as possible, they would be limited in their work to one area of study: epidemiology. They would find people exposed to the chemical at the proper level and people with no exposure, monitor their health, and use statistics to evaluate the significance of any differences in cancer rates between the two groups. In other words, the scientists would look to actual instances of the problem of interest. Few inferences would be needed in applying the results of exposure to one group of people to another.

Alas, epidemiology is like a low-powered telescope–it does not allow one to see very far. The scientist's unarguable, objective conclusion might be that the exposure of interest may, at most, double one's rate of cancer, or may have no effect. This sound scientific answer[e] to the question posed may be useless for public policy, which might wish to discriminate very small increases in cancer risk.

In order to produce results that are useful for policy, scientists must turn away from the most relevant and objective information–that gained from deliberate or accidental human exposure–toward other branches of science, such as rodent toxicology. The study of carcinogenesis in laboratory animals is a science in its own right, but the demand that it be applied to the human situation *ipso facto* introduces unscientific elements into the analysis. The less like the situation of interest are the phenomena that science has been able to observe and test, the more inferences and assumptions must be made. Many inferences are chains of reasoning that have not been, or cannot be, adequately tested by scientific method.

Risk-assessment problems of concern to legislators and regulators are rife with such questions that science cannot answer. Whether a novel chemical that causes cancer in one strain of rat, but not in others or in mice, is able to cause cancer in humans is an issue science cannot answer at the present. It is conceivable, however, that this question could be answered in the future, either because accidental human exposure supplies the response, or because the biochemistry and molecular biology of rodents and humans is learned in such detail that the inferential gaps narrow to insignificance.

Importantly, other elements of risk-assessment problems will *never* be answerable by scientific methods. Such elements include future behaviors by persons, institutions, molecules, and the weather, none of which can be predicted in detail. Past experience guides scientists in making long-term predictions about average or typical behaviors, but is of less use in predicting outcomes for particular individuals at particular points in time; indeed, there is no guarantee even that past trends will continue.

[e] Of course, we are simplifying even here. The soundness of the epidemiologic study itself is subject to many things: how well the exposures can or have been quantified; how well exposures to other potentially harmful or helpful substances have been accounted for; how representative are the study subjects relative to "ordinary Americans," and so on.

Limits to the knowable are inescapable. As Ralph Gomory[2] has written:

> We are all taught what is known, but we rarely learn about what is not known, and we almost never learn about the unknowable. That bias can lead to misconceptions about the world around us. . . .
>
> [People do not] try to predict the automobile accidents they will be involved in. To know that we will be struck by a car next year, we would have to know, with impossible accuracy, the particulars of the life of the driver, his habits, his timing, his way of pressing the accelerator, and so forth. . . . It is clear that all these details are unknown, and we do not try very hard to learn about them because we instinctively realize they are also unknowable.
>
> In distinguishing the known or the unknown from the unknowable, the level of detail can be decisive. The level of detail is what separates the delusion of the gambler from the wealth of the casino owner. The gambler attempts to predict the individual and unpredictable spins of the roulette wheel; the owner concerns himself with the quite predictable average outcome.

Risk assessment almost always depends upon details that are inherently unknowable. Accordingly, how could anyone suppose there is one way to do it right?[f]

REFERENCES

1. Crouch, E. A. C., R. R. Lester, T. L. Lash, S. R. Armstrong & L. C. Green. 1995. Health risk assessments prepared *per* the risk assessment reforms under consideration in the U.S. Congress, Report to the Commission on Risk Assessment and Risk Management. Washington, DC.
2. Gomory, R. E. 1995. The known, the unknown and the unknowable. Sci. Am. **272:** 120.
3. National Cancer Institute/National Toxicology Program. 1982. NTP technical report on the carcinogenesis bioassay of vinylidene chloride in F344/N rats and B6C3F1 mice (Gavage study). Tech. Rep. No. 228. NTP No. 80-82. NIH Pub. No. 82-1784. NTP, Research Triangle Park, NC. U.S. Department of Health and Human Services, Public Health Service, National Institute of Health. Bethesda, MD.

[f] Of course, this does not mean that all ways are equally correct, nor that there are not parts of risk assessments where only one way is right.

Disconnect Brain and Repeat after Me: "Risk Assessment Is Too Conservative"[a]

ADAM M. FINKEL[b]

Director of Health Standards Programs
Occupational Safety and Health Administration
200 Constitution Avenue
Room N3718
Washington, DC 20210

My first task is to make some amends for the sarcastic title of this talk. I do intend to explore in a detailed manner the half-truths and untruths that form the foundation of the growing "conventional wisdom" about risk assessment–that it deliberately and invariably produces widely exaggerated or "conservative" estimates of harm. I do believe that many of the critics leading the charge against conservatism, having discovered that they can get away with making pronouncements based at best on anecdotes and more often on pure speculation, have in effect disconnected some of their faculties and are making exaggeration of risk into a mantra rather than a theorem. I do not mean to suggest, however, that anyone who inveighs against conservative aspects of risk assessment has abandoned critical thinking in favor of propaganda. To the contrary–the arguments do contain kernels of truth, and risk assessors and policy makers ignore them at their own peril. The title is also meant to be cautionary. Those of us who believe the facts support a different conclusion–that risk assessment often *underestimates* risk and that more stringent regulation would often be needed before costs were in danger of exceeding benefits–must guard against responding to half-baked arguments with reflexive and simplistic counters of our own. No matter how overwrought the criticism may be, "no it's not" is hardly an adequate response. My goal in this discussion is to trace the evolution of the attacks on the alleged conservatism of risk assessment (especially as practiced by federal environmental, health, and safety regulatory agencies); to suggest two unifying ideas that persons truly interested in improving the performance of regulatory risk assessment ought to keep in mind; and to dissect, as time permits, ten separate flaws in the summarial denunciation of risk assessment as a tool of exaggeration and overregulation.

THE STAKES ARE HIGH

The furor over whether current methods of risk assessment exaggerate risk is more than an arcane scientific debate; it has repercussions in virtually every aspect

[a]The opinions expressed here are those of the author and do not necessarily reflect the views of the United States Occupational Safety and Health Administration. This article is an edited version of remarks delivered at the Rammazzini Symposium.

[b]Phone: 202/219-7075; fax: 202/219-7125; e-mail: adam.finkel@osha-no.osha.gov

of environmental, health, and safety regulation. The crux of the matter really is our ability to protect human health and the environment; our ability to improve the basic science upon which regulations are promulgated; our ability to make more efficient and cost-effective the regulations that we promulgate; and our ability to provide some measure of environmental equity across various populations. All of these are increasingly being held hostage to the belief that overregulation is the problem and risk assessment is the solution, but only if risk assessment is remade in the image advocated now by the "reformers" in Congress and elsewhere.

This notion that regulation is out of control, and that the reason regulation is out of control is that the risk science that underlies regulation is out of control, is really beginning to dominate the landscape, both in terms of what politicians are doing and also to a large extent what both the general-interest media and the special-interest media are saying. The derisive characterization of a gullible public whose fears are inflamed by deliberate exaggeration of risk estimates has gone by many names over the years: "chemophobia," "toxic terror," "junk science," "mouse terrorism," etc. Generally, the critics posit a reinforcing relationship between a populace demanding a risk-free society and a cadre of regulatory scientists eager to concoct nonzero risks out of harmless exposures. As Peter Huber wrote in the 1980s, "It is very easy to overestimate risk, especially when the national mood is receptive to claims of new and lurid risks." Perhaps a more sober characterization comes from John Graham, who has written extensively about what he sees as the public's fixation on trivial risks rather than more significant ones (e.g., the risk of an unhealthy diet), which he has termed "a syndrome of paranoia and neglect."

THE POLITICAL LANDSCAPE

At the outset, I want to make three points about personal ideology. To begin with, risk assessment is something I'm trained in and believe in. I think it is our best ally to the extent that we have been missing opportunities to protect the public and the environment from hazards that have not been well understood or well enough controlled. It is our best chance to identify and to mitigate those, but it's also our best chance to avoid unnecessary burdens on the economy and unnecessary public fears that come from turning away from analysis and charging headlong into addressing the chemical or other crisis of the day.

And in that respect I think that the public interest community and the organized environmental movement need to shoulder some of the blame for allowing a new brand of risk assessment (one that "fixes" exaggeration by trivializing risks) to emerge. Risk assessment, to me at least, is what, in a less methodical way, Rachel Carson was doing in the 1950s and what some of the other heroes of the environmental movement were doing in the 1960s. The Environmental Defense Fund (EDF), one of the most influential groups, was founded by a group of scientists in the late 1960s around the DDT issue. And yet through much of the 1970s and the 1980s these groups were increasingly turning away from risk assessment because they saw it as a means for legitimizing pollution rather than eliminating it. Unfortunately their disdain—which I agree had some rational basis—for cost-benefit balancing of risks quickly expanded into an antipathy to risk assessment, and to some extent an aversion to quantitative scientific methods in general grew up as a result. For example, the Natural Resources Defense Council still has as its slogan "Law and Science for the Environment." The last time I checked, however, their payroll had 60 or 70 lawyers on it and two or three people who could be described as scientists, none of whom could fairly be described as a risk-assessment scientist. So by warning about the stakeholders who are embracing risk assessment and yet trying to pervert it, I am certainly not espousing a "mainstream" view that the environmental advocates would instantly endorse.

I think that a lot of the problem is that a vacuum has been created by the abdication of the public interest groups in the debate over how risks should be assessed, which has left in the minds of the media and the public the impression that these controversies involve science on the one side and values on the other. This has marginalized those of us who believe that the science of environmental protection and the values of people who want to err on the side of protecting the public are not in conflict at all. And yet the impression that has been given is that people advocating stronger protection don't have a leg to stand on, that all they have are facile emotional appeals to make. This is because what appear to be scientific facts are being countered in the political debate by what appear to be purely emotional responses. And that's been very unfortunate. As I will discuss below, I believe strongly that much of what is currently proffered as "value-free science" is both value-laden and unscientific; while the advocates of more stringent regulation have both facts and values on their side and should be willing to embrace the former and admit the latter.

Second, I think it's important to say at the outset that while I don't believe there exists widespread and systematic exaggeration of risk, I do think that overregulation does exist, both as a concept and in practice. It's quite possible that, even if we have been assessing risks fairly, we have been overreacting to certain kinds of risks as opposed to others. So I'm certainly not trying to make the case that, because I think risk assessment does a better job than the critics believe, there is no such thing as overregulation.

Certainly over the last 10 years OSHA has been accused not only of overregulating but also of overenforcing its regulations. There have been many horror stories told about OSHA, most of them untrue. However, they do point to a growing dissatisfaction with the way we, and to a large extent the EPA, go about our day-to-day business. As a result, in the last couple of years OSHA has made a renewed commitment to crack down on that kind of overzealous enforcement, because we want to focus more on the real hazards. But we will occasionally overstep, or react to serious hazards with remedies that could be much more cost-effective, just as we will occasionally impose limp remedies that do not do justice to the size of the hazard. This paper is a defense of risk assessment (as currently practiced), not of risk management in general, and certainly not of every regulation in specific.

And third, it would be foolish for me to say that the critics of risk assessment are completely off base; that there are no grains of truth in the warnings about exaggeration of risk. I even acknowledge that in the mix of cases where hindsight shows some risks have been exaggerated while others underestimated, some of the former cases were products of intentional steps designed to produce a desired effect. But I will argue these lapses should be corrected via specific remedies, not by ''fixing'' an entire system that isn't broken, at least not in the way the fixers think it is.

Before providing a brief recounting of how the ''conventional wisdom'' about risk exaggeration has spread, it may be helpful to see where that conclusion is having (or is about to have) profound and tangible influence. To a large extent, the academics' initial concern over ''junk science'' has encouraged three very influential strictures on regulatory risk assessment: regulatory ''reform'' legislation, Congressional appropriations riders, and Executive Branch oversight.

- In March 1995 the House passed a bill that essentially says that federal agencies are on the wrong track, that they have been wasting billions of dollars, and that they need to abandon this overconservative mode of risk assessment. The Senate was getting close to passing a similar version of the bill during 1995, but proponents fell two votes short of the 60 votes needed to force an up-or-down vote on the proposal. Both the Senate and House versions would, among many other provisions, have required agencies to document that the benefits of each regulation, as measured by putting a monetary value on the ''best estimate'' of risk (i.e., an estimate with all possible traces of conservatism removed), exceeded the costs thereof.[c] Interestingly, Congress was declaring that ''The [Judiciary] Committee also intends to stop the long-standing practice of presenting conservative (inflated) risk estimates'' (report on S.343, the Dole-Johnston bill) just one year after the first major National Academy of Sciences committee to study risk assessment methods in more than a decade (*Science and Judgment in Risk Assessment*) had concluded that ''risk assessment methods are fundamentally sound, despite often-heard criticisms.'' This committee, on which I had the pleasure of serving, was composed of a broad spectrum of experts, including one member from an environmental advocacy group and one from an industry research association. It agreed on over 70 specific recommendations to make risk assessments more transparent and scientifically rigorous—yet among these recommendations suggested a number of changes to current practice designed to *increase* the extent of conservatism (or to remove elements of ''anticonservative'' underestimation, depending on how you look at it). If any of the Congressional ''reformers'' were aware of the recent NAS study, this certainly was not reflected in the legislative findings or prescriptions; perhaps it was not accidental that none of the 24 experts who served on the committee was invited to testify at any of the hearings Congressional panels convened during 1995 to solicit views on the risk assessment legislation.
- The failure (to date) to pass omnibus risk assessment legislation has not, however, deterred Congress from ''fixing'' specific examples of what it considers overregulation via risk exaggeration. In each of the last several years, numerous appropriations riders have been attached to spending bills to prohibit agencies, particularly

[c] NOTE ADDED IN PROOF: In July 1997, the Senate considered a new regulatory reform bill (S.981, introduced by Senators Carl Levin and Fred Thompson), which contained fewer prescriptive procedures for ''fixing'' risk assessment, but which still emphasized reliance on ''most plausible'' (again, as opposed to exaggerated) risk estimates.

EPA and OSHA, from promulgating specific regulations, often with explanatory language added linking the prohibition to a perceived failure to estimate fairly the risks being regulated. In the case of OSHA's desire to explore ways to reduce work-related musculoskeletal disorders due to repetitive stress and other "ergonomic" factors, Congress has twice enjoined the agency from publishing a draft regulatory proposal, even though this is the very mechanism for *beginning* a scientific and economic review process that could identify and correct any flaws in the assessment of risks and costs. This preemptive behavior appears to reflect a view that risk exaggeration is so endemic that no amount of expert and public scrutiny can resist its siren song.

- And, even though the Clinton Administration has to date opposed the regulatory reform proposals and the specific regulatory prohibitions, the White House Office of Management and Budget is preparing to issue a comprehensive "best practices" guide to agency risk assessment that in part accepts and reinforces the view that smaller risk estimates are more "real."[d] For example, this guide instructs agency risk assessors that risk assessment procedures "should not reflect unstated or unsupported preferences for protecting public health or the environment, or unstated safety factors . . . such procedures may introduce levels of conservatism that cumulate across assumptions." In other words, exaggeration of risk has a gravitational pull of its own that must be vigilantly rooted out, and that doing so may require a change in "preferences" as well as in procedures.

THE MAKING OF A SNOWBALL

A brief chronology reveals how in just over a decade a plausible idea–that risks could be systematically overestimated if assessors were determined to do so despite evidence to the contrary–has "snowballed" into a wholesale indictment of risk-based regulation.

The first peer-reviewed article I remember on conservatism in risk assessment was written by two professors at the John F. Kennedy School of Government while I was a student there in the early 1980s. It was written by Richard Zeckhauser and Nick Nichols, two economists who had no training in science or experience conducting risk assessment, and was entitled "The Perils of Prudence: How Conservative Risk Estimates Distort Regulation." It made a number of very valid points about how risk management decisions *could be* distorted if risks *were* routinely exaggerated. It presented no evidence to suggest this was the case, but did point out isolated aspects of risk assessment practice that could well introduce elements of conservatism. The article was soon followed by a couple of books: one by Edith Efron, who wrote a book called the *Apocalyptics: Cancer and the Big Lie* in 1984. It was about 1000 pages of vitriol about overregulation. Others were by Elizabeth Whelan, who runs a group called the American Council on Science and Health in New York. They were part of a series with titles something like *Terror in the Kitchen* and *Panic in the*

[d] NOTE ADDED IN PROOF: This guidance document was released, with the quoted passage intact, in January 1996.

Pantry. The literary device used throughout was the construction and dismembering of a straw man: risk assessment procedures applied to common, healthy foodstuffs would make them deadly, so the procedure must be faulty.

In the late 1980s and early 1990s, Dan Koshland, who was until recently the editor of *Science*, and Phil Abelson, the former editor who still works there, started writing frequent editorials about the systematic and routine exaggeration of risk. Koshland invented a character called Dr. Know-it-All, who was his alter ego. He then wrote dialogues wherein he would answer all his own questions about how ridiculous regulation was, or about people who are afraid of all molecules and want to eliminate oxygen from the world.

Biochemist Bruce Ames, another famous participant in this debate, has been writing frequently in a similar vein, and he's been featured in *Science* on many occasions, generally arguing that carcinogens naturally occurring in foods are as risky as or riskier than synthetic compounds that enter the food supply, but that neither class of risk is large enough to worry much about.

This was at a point where every year the Office of Management and Budget put together a list of all the regulations, which included a series of essays describing thematic trends in regulation. In 1990, a piece by economist Richard Belzer about the out-of-control nature of risk assessment appeared as part of this compendium, and raised the volume to new levels of excess by claiming that "true risks" are often millions of times smaller than the exaggerators would have us believe.

Just a couple of other more recent examples. In 1993, Stephen Breyer wrote the book *Breaking the Vicious Circle: Toward Effective Risk Regulation.* Justice Breyer was a federal judge at that time, and he decided in the early 1990s to review the literature on risk assessment and write a book about the reinforcing cycle of public concern and exaggeration of risk. I had occasion to discuss these issues with him during the early stages of the writing, and it was clear to me at the time that his source material was largely drawn from secondary sources such as the editorials in *Science*.

And, of course, there have been any number of similar books written since Breyer's book was published. Probably the most recent one is by environmental journalist Gregg Easterbrook. Titled *A Moment on the Earth,* its thesis is that the earth is more resilient than we think. He also feels that the environmental laws and regulations have helped us out more than many people believe, and that the environmentalists should therefore not be on the defensive about the successes they have achieved. But the book's real message is that we should look back with success and stop driving forward to go after the smaller risks that remain. This is why I put it in the same general category with the other works that say that risk assessment and regulations are exaggerated.

In the national news media, the *New York Times* ran a five-part series on how regulation is out of control due to bad risk assessment. The *Los Angeles Times* published a similar series in September 1994, and *Smithsonian* magazine also just had a two-part series.

John Stossel, who is a reporter on ABC's weekly news magazine show *20/20,* did a one-hour documentary in 1993 called "Are We Scaring Ourselves to Death?" followed by a kind of town meeting that he hosted, with handpicked people sitting in an auditorium expressing their outrage at overregulation. Stossel has since been invited to congressional hearings, not as a journalist, but as an expert on risk assessment. This is apparently Congress's idea of an approach to making good public policy: "I'm not a scientist, but I played one once on TV."

More recently, I have been working on a review (1996, *American Scientist* **84:** 491–493) of a book by the late Aaron Wildavsky, who was a political scientist at Berkeley, called *But Is It True?* It's a compendium of several case studies that he and his graduate students all agreed were overblown hazards: arsenic, DDT, climate change, ozone depletion, toxic waste sites. In other words, the standard litany of things that, according to some, we have gone overboard on and shouldn't be worried about.

So perhaps a better analogy than a snowball picking up debris as it careens down a mountainside is that of a dog chasing its own tail. The leading edge of this debate is now being conducted by reporters who are writing stories based on editorials that they've read (often citing them as if they were found in the peer-reviewed portion of the journals they appeared in), editorials quoting books that the editorial writers have read, books that in some cases, but not in others, are quoting from primary research. But where is the scientific content? The actual primary articles in the specialty literature are now four or five generations behind where the debate is, and yet, for a lay reader, it looks like an unbroken chain of actual evidence and research content.

TWO UNIFYING CONCEPTS

Before discussing ten flaws I have identified in the standard denunciation of risk-assessment conservatism, there are two overarching ideas I want to flag. The first is the interplay of theoretical arguments and observational evidence. The two are complementary, and yet both critics of conservatism and defenders of current risk assessment practice tend to rely too heavily on one or the other, depending on which better suits their purpose in any particular case. Without continually looking to whatever evidence is available, it is easy to mislead oneself and one's audience by asserting that a given risk assessment result or a given procedure or assumption used by an agency is (or is not) overly conservative simply because a "better" theory yields a lower (or higher) risk estimate. Hence, for example, the dueling abstractions that occupied much of the specialists' time in the 1980s about whether exposures (and thus risks) should be scaled from laboratory animals to humans via the ratio of their respective body surface areas (a relatively more conservative procedure) or via their body weights (relatively less conservative). Until various data sets were eventually compiled and analyzed that allowed researchers to test the validity of each model, proponents of each procedure could only dismiss the alternative on the grounds that it was "unscientific" and motivated by a desire to influence the outcome one way or the other. Conversely, it is easy to assert conservatism or the lack thereof merely by comparing isolated outcomes to theoretical predictions—but the comparisons may not be representative or may not have enough statistical power to refute the practice they seem to cast doubt upon. A powerful set of comparisons between predictions and results, informed by a sound theoretical argument explaining the concordance or discordance, is our most useful ally for making risk estimates more scientifically sound, but such marriages of theory and evidence have been too sporadic during the heated debates (see below).

The second universal concept that will reappear throughout the remainder of this talk is the inevitability of uncertainty. Few laypeople appreciate, I contend, that even when risk assessment is sufficiently well developed to make reasonably accurate predictions, it is really only able to accurately quantify the range of uncertainty and identify specified quantities that exist within that range (e.g., the mean, median, 95th percentile upper bound). To know that on average, the magnitude of a risk is X, and/or to know that we can be 90 percent confident that the risk lies between Y and Z, is a very valuable input to risk management, but this should not be confused with knowing precisely how large the ''true'' risk is.

Here is a brief numerical example from a paper I published in *Environmental Health Perspectives* in April 1994. The basic idea was that in the late 1980s Bruce Ames and his colleagues were doing a lot of comparative risk assessment. They were publishing tables of values for the carcinogenic potencies of different substances and comparing them to each other. One of the most repeated comparisons that Ames made became very important during the debate over Alar in the late 1980s. He asserted that the natural carcinogen aflatoxin, which is, among other things, present in peanut butter, was 18 times more hazardous than the Alar in a glass of apple juice. The clear message was that the U.S. public should not be so worried about this pesticide in their apple juice supply when they were already tolerant of a naturally occurring risk that was by his estimation 18 times more dire than the synthetic risk was.

By tracing the effect of the uncertainties in the potency of the two substances, in the amount of apple juice and peanut butter different persons consume, and in the amount of each contaminant found in each foodstuff, I demonstated that the uncertainty in the relative risk extends over about six orders of magnitude. Ames's estimate of 18:1 is clearly one of the plausible points within that broad distribution (although I estimated that the midpoint of the range was much closer to 1:1), but any ''signal'' that either substance is riskier than the other is drowned out in the ''noise'' inherent in the comparison. It's possible that as a lower bound aflatoxin is about 400 times more hazardous than Alar was, but it's also equally likely that Alar was about 40 times riskier than aflatoxin. When you look at it this way, it suggests that there was something other than science going on in Ames's comparison.

So the relationship between uncertainty and conservatism is a multifaceted one: (1) since the very concept of conservatism is formally an expression of how large is the ratio of the estimated value of risk divided by its ''true'' value, precise pronouncements about the magnitude of this ratio are likely to be wrong given the underlying uncertainty in the risk being addressed–such pronouncements may be off the mark quantitatively, or may even be qualitatively incorrect (an estimate criticized for being much larger than the true value may in fact be smaller); (2) since every point within the distribution of uncertainty corresponds to a plausible value of risk, no single estimate can be ''correct''–instead, every estimate strikes a unique and value-driven balance between the consequences of overestimating versus underestimating the unknown true value (see item #2 below); and (3) two theories or assumptions that yield markedly different risk estimates may not be separable into one that is ''true'' and one that is ''untrue''–each may simultaneously be plausible given the uncertainty in the data used to discriminate among them (which arguably is the case in the example above regarding surface-area versus body-weight scaling).

TEN PROBLEMS WITH "CONVENTIONAL WISDOM"

I have written about the many oversimplifications and misimpressions the leaders of the conservatism bandwagon have fallen prey to at much greater length in a recent law review article critiquing Justice Breyer's book (1995, *New York University Environmental Law Journal* **3:** 295-381 [esp. 333-352]). I will summarize these arguments here; the first three relate to policy and management questions, the next five examine evidence regarding the actual conservatism of current risk assessment procedures, and the final two extend the discussion to conservatism in cost-benefit analysis.

1. Confusion between Two Kinds of Conservatism

Critics of conservatism are quite fond of setting up the entire debate as one pitting "unbiased" measures of risk (variously, the "true" values or average values or "most plausible" values) against "biased," inflated estimates. However, they almost invaribly ignore the two very different motivations behind deliberately using an estimate that exceeds the average, depending on whether uncertainty or interindividual variability in risk–or, as usual, both–are at work. When uncertainty is involved, the issue becomes whether it's better to be safe than sorry. This is fundamentally a question of, assuming you don't know what the true value of something is, how are you going to act under various assumptions about the range of values that are possible? Will you act as if the risk is higher than its average or lower than its average or at its average, according to what you are trying to do? And as we have seen, the allegation is that whenever there is uncertainty, risk assessment tries to take the conservative course and produce a risk estimate that's unbelievably high. I will examine the factual case for whether the estimates generated are in fact closer to the 95th, 99th, or higher (perhaps beyond the extreme uppermost bound of plausibility) percentiles of the distribution of uncertainty in risk than they are to central-tendency measures under uncertainty. The practical point, however, is that a 95th-percentile estimate of risk is not an "inflated" estimate of the average; it is an estimate that five percent of the time will still fail to be as large as the true risk and thence lead to decisions that are less protective of health and the environment than we would have chosen with perfect information.

The other phenomenon is that risks, in addition to being uncertain, are also variable across the exposed population, whether it's human beings who are exposed to different amounts of the particular substance, whether it's ecosystems that are at different levels of exposure, or whether it's people who by virtue of genetic makeup, environmental history, and other factors have different sensitivities to the exposures they face. It seems to me that the choice of an individual or a society to do something in the face of the reality that these risks vary across the population is not a matter of being safe rather than sorry, but is really a matter of having to decide who gets to be safe and who gets to be sorry, and those are hard choices. That is, it's a matter of confronting that in any of these cases, some people or some pieces of acreage or some ecosystems are going to be affected more than others and a line may need to be drawn; but when that line is drawn some people are one side and some on the other.

So when these new saviors of risk assessment come along and say they are going to replace bias with unbias, replace exaggeration with truth, and subjectivity with objectivity, hold on to your proverbial wallets. For one thing, are they saying we shouldn't be so worried about the possibility of everyone being at unacceptably high risk when in fact any conservatism that might exist is there to guard against the *certainty* that some will be sorry while others are safe? Or in the name of not overregulating on behalf of an unfortunate minority, would removing the conservatism in a risk estimate in fact subject all of us to a higher probability of being unsafe than we would willingly allow? To understand whether an assessment is too conservative, you have to be clear what consequences—for populations and/or for individuals—are being weighed.

2. No Estimates Are Biased; No Decisions Are Unbiased

The notion that conservatism is "policy" and its absence yields "good science" betrays an ignorance of the policy content of *any* estimate chosen from out of the umbra of uncertainty. From the point of view of a decision theorist (someone who is trained to look at problems and suggest the costs and benefits of different courses of action and the uncertainties therein), an estimate is "biased" only if it fails (on average) to correspond to the value it is designed to estimate, whether that value is itself a mean, a lower bound, an upper bound, whatever. On the other hand, any decision that flows from an estimate *is* biased in the colloquial sense of that word, because at best it can be a sound choice only contingent on an underlying policy choice the decision maker must impose upon the situation.

The example I would use, which I am borrowing from a group that was trying to make exactly the opposite point, is the everyday notion of traveling to the airport. A consortium of industry group researchers calling themselves the "Hazardous Waste Cleanup Project" wrote a report about the Superfund program a couple of years ago. Their main analogy was that the way EPA treats risks from hazardous waste is similar to somebody who would leave at midnight to drive to the airport for a flight that was leaving at noon the next day. The idea was that if this person started to ask about what things might go wrong on the way to making the plane, he might be told there could be traffic, his car could break down, his battery might be dead, he might get lost, there might be a long line at the ticket counter, and so forth. Thus, taking a worst-case estimate of each of those things and multiplying them all out, he ended up leaving at midnight for the noon flight.

Now, you wouldn't want to be so scared of missing the plane that you would lose touch with reality and allow so much time that it didn't make sense. But if you react to that in the extreme, which I guarantee you is where Congress wants to take it right now, the way out of this problem is to use what Congress calls "the best estimate." This has never been very well defined, but it can be either the mode of the probability distribution or the median or the expected value or some other measure of central tendency.

Therefore, if you gave each of those factors lower bounds, average values, and upper bounds, and combined them all, you might end up determining that on average it will take you about 20 minutes to get to the airport, that it could take you 5 minutes on a good day, and that occasionally it could take 2 hours on a bad day.

But the unbiased estimate of 20 minutes leads to a biased decision because it is the number that you would use only if your internal cost/benefit function was, "I want to arrive as close as possible to when the plane leaves. Every minute of being there early has a cost, and every minute of being there late has a cost, but I'm indifferent as to which direction the error is." Obviously that's the right idea if you are somebody who would rather be 4 minutes late than 5 minutes early to catch a plane. You have to choose some factor to balance the cost to you of each minute waiting for the plane to leave versus each minute of having the plane leave before you get there—to pretend not to choose is to stick yourself with a factor exactly equal to one, which is every bit as much a "preference" as a factor of 10 (you'd rather be 10 minutes early than one minute late), 100, or 0.01. An unbiased estimate of the 95th percentile of the distribution (allowing 2 hours in our hypothetical case) is the correct number to use if you regard each minute of lateness as roughly 20 times more costly than a minute spent cooling your heels.

With respect to environmental hazards, regulators have been trying to avoid saying that we are absolutely indifferent between underestimating risks, which could result in more human carnage than we would otherwise wish to have, and overestimating, which would cause more economic dislocation than we would otherwise knowingly tolerate. Thus any of those choices in that range has its own bias, but none of them is more biased than the other. They all reflect a different striking of that balance between being early or being late, or being careful with peoples' lives and being careful with money. A large number of factors I won't discuss here, including issues of irreversibility, social equity, and public perception, enter into such a calculus. Where one strikes that balance is a matter of personal or societal decision making. It's not a matter that the truth lies in the middle and everything else is untrue, which is, unfortunately, the way the debate has been twisted.

3. *"Common Sense" When People Are Different*

Common sense is a big item in the United States right now. On the best-seller list is a book called *The Death of Common Sense*, by Phil Howard, who is a lawyer in New York. It's made up of slightly (and not so slightly) misconstrued regulatory horror stories, such as the OSHA inspector who allegedly issued a citation for not labeling blackboard chalk as hazardous.

With common sense the ideal, what passes for it is the problem. When a risk cannot be reduced to a single number or a narrow range because it affects different people differently, again the "best estimate" is being held up as the right number to focus on. However, when people vary, the average is not the best estimate but is probably among the worst estimates because it obscures the reality of the situation under this veneer of objectivity.

For example, consider the need to build wooden ladders according to a regulation that says how strong the ladders have to be. It would be pretty bizarre if the code said that the ladder only had to hold 130 pounds because that's the weight of an average person. That would be fine for 50% of the people, which includes newborns and toddlers, all of whom are under that weight, but the other 50% of us could not use the ladders without breaking through them at our peril. Similarly, it does not seem commonsensical to build ladders that would support a 1500-lb person just because 1 out of every 100 million people might weigh that much. I think at some point you want to say this is more protection than we need. But to be drawn to the average because that's the "best," and to be told that you're extremist if you want to go up to (say) 200 lb because you would like to protect 95% of the population, I think that's twisting reality. Again, regulating to this level is not "exaggeration of risk," but recognition that a number higher than the universal average is exactly correct for some real people.

A more subtle example comes up both in the Clean Air Act and Superfund debates and also to some extent in OSHA. Here, it is tempting to draw a distinction between the behavior of an average person and an "upper-bound person" that leads to a nonsensical result. The EPA needs to make assumptions about how many years a person will live in proximity to a source of ambient air pollution or to a toxic waste site. Usually, EPA assumes that person will spend his or her entire life expectancy (70 years) in the location being modeled (be it the fenceline or some location with "reasonably high-end" exposure).

At OSHA we say the working lifetime is 45 years, so we model what would happen to someone if he or she were exposed for 45 years, because our statute explicitly requires this and because there are clearly many people who do work in the same job from age 20 to age 65. But suppose that objectively one could determine that nobody lives for 70 years in the same place. Let's say for the sake of argument that studies have been done showing that in the United States, on average people move from house to house about every 10 years.

The EPA is under a lot of pressure right now to divide all of their risk numbers by seven because they have allegedly overestimated the amount of time that somebody is in proximity to a pollutant source. At the same time we at OSHA are being told that people don't stay in the same job for 45 years, but move about every 15 years, so we should drop our risk estimate by a factor of three. Now even those critics who never met a risk estimate they didn't want to shrink presumably understand that such an adjustment would ruin perfectly good estimates of population risk, since as long as risk is proportional to total dose, the number of expected fatalities per year is invariant (as long as *someone* occupies the house or the job whenever it is vacated). But it does seem as if it's too conservative to assess *individual* risk via upper-bound estimates of working life span, until you stop to think about what would happen in a country where every smokestack was allowed to emit seven times more material on the grounds that nobody was exposed to any one smokestack for more than ten years. There would be seven times more pollution in the country, and unless you were moving either abroad or from Gary, Indiana, to Palm Springs, or someplace where there were no smokestacks around, your exposure is going to accumulate up to seven times what it would have been if you had stayed put and the regulation hadn't been weakened. And, of course, people who live near industrial parks or toxic waste sites in the first place will tend to be the least likely (or able) to move to pristine suburban neighborhoods or rural ranches; those who use chemical solvents in their jobs are unlikely to switch to office work.

Finally, the preceding discussions have implicitly made the charitable assumption that the uncertainty or interindividual variability is distributed continuously rather than in a discrete or "either-or" fashion. The lattter case is quite commonplace, however, and there replacing conservative estimates with average ones can lead to particularly bizarre results. "Either-or uncertainty" is common when there exist two or more fundamentally incompatible scientific theories to explain a key step in the risk assessment process; for example, the excess lifetime cancer risk from exposure to a substance might be as high as (say) 10^{-3} if tumors observed in laboratory animals are relevant to humans, and zero if they are not. And, variability is often "either-or" when males and females (or children and adults, etc.) have markedly different susceptibilities, or when exposure is strongly correlated with location (e.g., the risk of a plane crashing into your house is probably negligible unless you happen to live near an airport flight path, since most crashes occur during takeoffs and landings). If the alternative to being conservative in such cases is to choose the average, then not only is a policy of indifference to the type of error being imposed, but decision makers and the public may be unaware that the estimate chosen is guaranteed to be implausible. The risk of a substance that has "half a threshold," or the risk to a hypothetical person with the population average of one ovary and one testicle, would be clearly seen as nonsensical if those advocating such contrivances were honest about their ramifications.

4. "Fixing" the Part Can Ruin the Whole

Risk assessment can be thought of as the proverbial "black box," and a fairly intricate box at that. Inside that box there are at least several dozen assumptions that have to be made. And what's happening is that the critics are coming in and saying "I don't like the fact that you are assuming people live for 70 years; I don't like the fact that you are assuming people spend 24 hours a day out of doors when you really should say they spend only 8 hours a day out of doors."

What they are looking for are parts of the mechanism where there may be a tendency towards exaggeration, and they congratulate themselves when they find it. But what is not being looked at are the parts of the mechanism where the opposite effect is happening. If we assume for the moment that there are also aspects of risk assessment that lead to underestimation of risk, then it is perverse to go into the mechanism and "fix" the parts that are erring in one direction and not think about the parts that are erring in the other direction. In the extreme case, suppose that a specific risk assessment (or current procedures in general) happened to generate a highly accurate estimate of the true risk because the sum total of errors tending to introduce overestimation exactly equaled the magnitude of the errors of the opposite sign. Then by definition each selective "fix" of an error of the former type, even as it made that *portion* of the process more realistic, would make the *result* less realistic. Even if the estimates generated by a mix of imprecise assumptions do on balance tend to overestimate, it is still far from clear that rolling back only a hand-picked subset of assumptions deemed worthy of repair because they are too conservative will improve the result. This is not to suggest that risk assessors should not strive to improve the realism of each assumption they use, only that they should try insofar as possible to examine the "before and after" estimates to see if any external evidence sheds light on whether the procedural change would make the resulting risk estimate more or less plausible. A golfer's swing, after all, is made up of many separate components, and no teaching pro would insist on a series of adjustments based on watching the pupil take a practice swing; he would wait until he could see how well the pupil actually hit the ball.

In both cases it's the results that matter. The fact that there may be flaws in the process matters too, because the flaws may lead to flaws in the results, but only if you look at the whole picture and not just selected parts of it. I will return to this theme at the conclusion of this talk, when I will briefly set out the case that if we would bother to look at the performance of the whole process before tinkering with components thereof, we would be less driven to believe that any tinkering is necessary.

5. Fundamentally Sound Theories

The cornerstone of many of the attacks on risk assessment involves allegations that the basic theories used to estimate risks are implausibly conservative compared to more ''biologically based'' theories. Although many of the parameters that go into the risk assessment models chosen are sufficiently uncertain that it is possible to overestimate their mean values by a factor of 10 or perhaps even 100, the predictions arising from competing models can indeed differ by many orders of magnitude. An overly conservative approach to ''model uncertainty,'' therefore, could conceivably result in the millionfold overestimation of true risk that some have argued permeates the process. But are the models used really so outlandish? Just to take one example, consider the much-maligned assumption that the excess cancer risk from a relatively low dose of a carcinogen is roughly linearly proportional to the greater risk more easily observable at higher doses. Low-dose linearity, more than any other aspect of risk assessment, has taken a beating as the embodiment of ''junk science.'' In Aaron Wildavsky's recent book *But Is It True?* he constructs a clever analogy to ridicule this assumption, which he calls the ''milk room.'' The idea of the milk room is that if hundreds of people were standing in a sealed room that had 10 feet worth of milk in it, they would all surely drown. His point is that, following this logic, how many people would drown in one foot of milk? Would it be one-tenth that number? Then he takes it to its extreme. How many people would drown in one millionth of a foot of milk? Would it be one ten-millionth of the room's inhabitants, or exactly zero people (only a ''suicidal genius'' could manage to drown himself in this thin layer of milk, Wildavsky wrote). This analogy is unfair for any number of theoretical reasons, including: (1) the typical amount of downward extrapolation used to set regulatory exposure levels is far less heroic than the factor of 10^7 in the ''milk room''–often, especially in workplace settings, regulations allow humans to be exposed to levels only a factor of 100 or even a factor of 10 lower than the doses observed to cause a high incidence of serious adverse health effects in laboratory animals or among workers in highly contaminated locations; (2) even when exposed to identical concentrations of a toxic substance, humans exhibit widely varying degrees of risk due to biological and environmental factors influencing individual susceptibility, as I will discuss later; (3) ''low'' doses rarely constitute the first increment of biological stress, but cumulate against a background of exposure and risk that may compromise the exposed person's capacity to cope with the additional burden; and (4) the extra risk posed by the proverbial ''micron of milk,'' however small, may be unacceptable if it confers no benefit upon those exposed, but merely exists to benefit those who bear no risk. Thus, I believe a more reasonable parable would ask whether it is acceptable to add several inches of milk to a room already half-full, when some people are chest deep in the stuff while others are up to their necks in it.

The discussion of low-dose linearity does not have to stop with dueling parables, however, because we clearly have some empirical evidence to shed light on the reasonableness of this default assumption. Neither Wildavsky, Breyer, nor the many others who have made linearity a whipping boy made reference to one of the largest, longest, and most powerful human epidemiologic studies of a cancer-causing agent ever conducted—namely, the follow-up of the atomic bomb survivors in Japan. Five evaluations of these data over several decades by National Academy of Sciences committees have concluded that there exists no persuasive evidence of a threshold below which excess radiation confers zero increased risk, and that a linear extrapolation might well underestimate risk at lower doses. Similar evidence for linearity can be gleaned from the many studies on cigarette smoking and lung cancer. Nor have the critics acknowledged the fact that in the last 25 years there have been only two studies, one in the United States and one in the United Kingdom, with sufficient size and power to test the curvature of the dose-response function at reasonably low doses. These are the so-called megamouse studies, because instead of the 50 or 60 mice that are usually tested, thousands or tens of thousands of rodents were exposed to very low doses. In the more recent study, exposing 16 different dose groups yielded essentially a straight-line dose-response relationship for many of the tumor types going down to the lowest dose. This is just one example suggesting that even some of the things that are most widely criticized as being the most egregious examples of conservatism, if you go back to the science, may not be so.

6. The Kinship of Average and Conservative

If at least some of the models decried for exaggerating risk are unfairly branded as such, what about the parameters selected to implement these models? Here again, oversimplification and selective use of evidence can lead to a false verdict about the degree of conservatism. In some cases, regulators do deliberately choose a value from a parameter's distribution that is rather unlikely to be an underestimate. This does not mean, however, that the choice is necessarily conservative in absolute terms. Most of the uncertain parameters in risk assessment follow distributions that are symmetric (a "bell-shaped curve") on a multiplicative scale but that are skewed on a normal arithmetic scale. Suppose, for example, that the typical person in the United States earns $10,000 per year, and that everyone else earns some multiple (greater or less than one) of that amount, in equal multiplicative proportions—as many people earn $100,000 (10 times the midpoint) as earn $1,000 (one-tenth), and so on. If each standard deviation was a factor of 10 away from the midpoint, then about 68 percent of the population would earn between those two amounts. However, in absolute terms the richer group earns $90,000 more than the typical person, whereas the poorer group only earns $9,000 less. This means that, for example, 95 percent of the population earns less than $442,000, an amount 44 times that of the typical person, a conservative estimate, and one unlikely to be exceeded. However, if you take all of the earnings in the population and divide the sum by the number of people involved (i.e., compute the arithmetic average), the result is $142,000 per capita, because the five percent who earn more than $442,000–some who earn millions more–contribute much more to the average than the majority who earn less [if the units were risks instead of dollars, the expected number of fatalities (the "best estimate" of the aggregate risk) would be a function of the average value, not of the typical value]. The point of this example is to show that this "conservative" estimate of $442,000 is only three times larger than the actual average–and the more uncertainty that exists, the more likely it is that any upper bound will not significantly exceed the average.

Thus, when EPA uses the 95th percentile upper confidence limit on the number of tumors observed in an animal bioassay (10 rodents out of 50 tested may contract cancer, but simple statistics says that number has roughly a 5 percent chance of being as high as or higher than 14 out of 50 if we had the ability to repeat the experiment over and over again like flipping a coin), it is frequently accused of being overly conservative. Depending on the uncertainty, however, that upper bound may be only slightly higher than (or even lower than) the average. Hattis and Goble (*Risk Analysis,* 1991) have shown that for a typical bioassay design, it can never be more than about a factor of four greater than the average, a touch of conservatism but hardly a cause for panic.

The relationship between upper bound, average, and typical values is complicated and hard to explain concisely, but it is the kind of detail necessary to truly evaluate conservatism–which may explain why the critics gloss over it.

7. Other Parameters Underestimate Risk

In addition to steps in the process where what seem to be conservative choices may not in fact overestimate the average, current risk assessment practice involves other choices that are likely to understate the true or average values of the parameters they estimate. In exposure assessment, among other examples, scientists frequently tally up exposures from a complex mixture (e.g., effluent from a toxic waste site) by considering only a few "indicator chemicals" even though many others are known to be present.

"Anticonservative" aspects also crop up in dose-response analysis. One of the many examples is the fact that we test rats or mice for a large fraction of, but not for the entire span of, their lives. We start exposing them at about eight weeks of age after weaning. In the compressed mouse or rat life span this corresponds to about the first five years of a human life, and we know there is particular vulnerability to newborns and children in certain respects. And we also typically will end the experiment after 24 months, sacrifice the animals, and count the tumors.

Richard Peto, an eminent scientist in the United Kingdom, has shown that if, instead of testing what may be the equivalent of 70-year-old people, we let the rodents live several months longer, to the equivalent of 80 or 90 years old, we would be seeing, by a factor of up to seven, higher cancer risks per unit of dose in the animals. So there is a built-in nonconservatism in that part of the process. That one factor could cancel out most of the tendency towards overestimation contributed by the "24 instead of 8 hours outdoors" and the "95th percentile bioassay slope" assumptions.

8. Doing Nothing Can Underestimate Risk

The final example on the scientific side stems from what could be termed sins of omission, and what the 1994 National Academy of Sciences committee termed "missing defaults" in the process. There are at least two important examples wherein by not assuming anything, we are introducing an effect that, if anything, goes in the opposite direction from conservatism. In these cases, assessors have fallen into a logical trap by forgetting that not to choose is to choose; at every step in the process of assessing risk, to ignore a factor because its magnitude or influence can't be (precisely) quantified is to make the highly constraining assumption that it has a value of exactly zero. Many others have written about the problem that untested chemicals are assumed to have zero carcinogenic or toxicologic potency, a situation that may be causing more and more underestimation of cumulative risk to individuals as the number of newly introduced substances continues to outpace our ability to conduct even basic screening batteries of short-term tests, let alone full two-year bioassays. Risk assessors could remedy this situation by assigning probability distributions of uncertainty in potency to untested substances, drawing on whatever analogies can be reasonably inferred from the study of structurally similar compounds.

Where exposures to adequately tested substances predominate, this omission may not cause a significant tendency to underestimate risk. However, across the board a different "missing default" may seriously compromise our ability to avoid underestimation of individual risk, and perhaps even of aggregate population risk—the tacit assumption, which flies in the face of all we know of mammalian physiology, that all humans are identically sensitive to the carcinogenic effects of environmental toxicants. Even though we are all genetically, biochemically, and environmentally different from each other, risk assessors derive a single value for the cancer potency of each substance, in part because the test subjects (either small groups of inbred laboratory animals or small groups of exposed workers followed in epidemiologic studies) exhibit little or none of whatever interindividual variation is present in the diverse human population. That single value may adequately estimate the potency for the typical human, but if so it is bound to underestimate risk for the large fraction of the population more sensitive than the norm. How large an error might result?

Several rather preliminary studies on the basic biology of cancer suggest that in the "normal" human population—that is, factoring out the rare conditions where we know there is true hypersensitivity to cancer—there are subtle variations in sensitivity to carcinogenesis that may extend over 25-, 50-, 100-fold to either side of the norm just by virtue of different enzyme activities, different nutritional statuses, different ages, different immune responses, different DNA repair capabilities, etc. So right away we have built in a factor of 10 or 20 or 50 of underestimation for those people in the population who don't know that they are more sensitive but who may very well be. The 1994 National Academy report directed EPA risk assessors to do one of two things: either incorporate a reasonable estimate of the extent of interindividual variability into the cancer risk assessment process and generate estimates both for persons of average and above-average susceptibility, or else explicitly inform decision makers and the public that cancer risk estimates should not be interpreted as applying to any individual whose susceptibility differs substantially from the norm. As usual, even this consensus identification of a potentially dispositive source of underestimation of risk has not dissuaded the authors of academic critiques and federal legislation from their view that there is only one direction in which risk estimates can possibly err.

9. Uncertain Parameters Exaggerate Regulatry Cost

Now let's move from the benefits of regulation, namely the risks that we can reduce, to the costs of regulation, namely the economic side. There are profound problems with the field of regulatory economics, which is designed to come up with estimates of how much it will cost the economy to impose a particular regulation. You wouldn't know it to read the newspaper or listen to Congress, because the "conventional wisdom" has led to legislative proposals that direct scientists to get their act together, that call for peer review, that call for—unbelievable as it sounds—peer review of scientists by economists; but there is not a word suggesting that the economists developing the cost estimates also be subject to quality control, peer review, transparency, "best estimate" requirements, or public participation. Why is that? It's possible that economists are doing such a good job they don't need quality control, peer review, and so on, but I think the evidence says otherwise.

In particular, regulatory cost analysis suffers from a tendency to exaggerate cost. Just as in risk assessment, imprecision in cost analysis stems from parameter uncertainty as well as model uncertainty. Taking as given for the moment the basic theoretical models used, it is clear that some of the key parameters used in those models are vulnerable to exaggeration. For example, if you ask somebody how much it will cost to get the SO_2 out of a coal-fired power plant using a scrubber, the answer is going to depend on a variety of factors: whether the environmental engineers at the company have an incentive to not underestimate costs; whether the control technology is fully developed; whether competition for the controls and innovation in their design will cause their price to go down; whether the new hardware was going to be installed at the next major replacement of the boilers anyway—and all of these factors bias the answer in the direction of overestimation.

Looking at what regulations actually cost the regulated parties compared with the predictions that were made either by the industry itself or by a government agency, one commonly sees overestimation of cost, sometimes to a really staggering extent. One of the favorite examples at OSHA is the regulation of cotton dust. In 1978, exposure to cotton dust was causing something like 40,000 cases of brown lung disease or byssinosis in the United States every year. By today we've seen about a 95% drop to several hundred cases per year. In 1978, predictions were that it would cost hundreds of millions of dollars for the industry to comply with the regulation. However, at the time profitability in the United States textile industry was dropping by about 9% a year; but in the years following the OSHA regulation, profitability increased by about 4% a year into the 1980s. A lot of things were going on other than having to comply with OSHA controls, but the economists who look back largely believe that it was the investment in more modern equipment and the lower costs of workers' compensation, among other factors, that enabled that industry to drag itself out of an economic downturn.

Vinyl chloride is another example where both OSHA and the EPA regulated with great difficulty. Predictions at the time were that the vinyl chloride industry would suffer hundreds of millions of dollars in costs, but 18 months after the regulation took effect, the trade magazine, *Chemical Week,* ran the headline "Vinyl Chloride Rolls out of Jeopardy into Jubilation." It turns out that the equipment did not cost that much to install, and the savings in recovering more vinyl chloride, which was no longer going into the atmosphere or into the lungs of workers, paid for the controls in short order and caused net savings.

Of course, this is analysis by anecdote, and it's not satisfactory to say that that's what always happens. I will note, however, that a recent report issued by the Congressional Office of Technology Assessment examined eight major OSHA regulations issued in the 1970s and 1980s, and found that preregulatory estimates of compliance costs exceeded the actual expenditures in seven of the cases. For risk assessors to be told that their craft is bankrupt because sometimes they exaggerate assumptions and use 24 hours a day rather than 8, I think the answer is that maybe they are wont to introduce a factor of 2 or 5 or 10 that may confound the final result, but that economists often introduce much larger factors than that, and in a more predictable direction. The relevance to risk exaggeration is clear and direct: the main reason to be incensed about conservatism in risk assessment is its potential for impelling overregulation. But if *both* risks and costs are exaggerated by anywhere near the same factor, the regulatory solution that emerges will differ little from the one we would choose given perfect estimates of both.

10. Simplistic Economic Models Further Exaggerate Cost

The metaphor I would use to discuss the additional problem of model uncertainty in regulatory economics is that of throwing a stone into a pool of water. It's the waves that come from the impact of the stone hitting the water that really need to be measured, but economists have redefined the problem as "We want to know how big the stone was." In other words, they have decided that the cost of a regulation to society is defined as "you tell us the cost of the hardware needed to comply with the regulation, and we'll multiply that by how many pieces of hardware have to be purchased, and that's the cost." But that isn't always going to give the right answer. The money spent on the control technology, from the point of view of the firm facing the expense, is the proverbial stone; but from the vantage point of society in general, especially those who benefit economically from the demand for their products and services, the "stone" is not dead weight but opportunity.

There are economic models and assumptions that play a role here. For instance, the reason economists believe that the price charged for the scrubber is its true cost to the economy is that they use underlying assumptions such as full employment (there won't be any unemployed or underemployed people diverted to more productive uses by creating demand for scrubbers), perfect competition, and perfect information.

While these may be necessary assumptions, they are every bit as tenuous as low-dose linearity; yet you don't hear criticism of these ingrained economic assumptions because they have been around for so long. So long, in fact, that students are probably no longer being taught that they are assumptions, but that they are economic principles.

In this final example I hope to bring it all together. Returning to the Alar example, I think two lessons have been ignored in the follow-up to that controversy: what have we learned about the true risk of Alar and what have we learned about the true cost of doing without Alar? On the risk side, there was a study that was being conducted by the manufacturer at the time of the controversy, which wasn't finished until two years after the chemical was off the market. But when it came out, it showed that more mice contracted tumors at lower doses of Alar than were evident in the much-criticized study from 1973 that caused the EPA to look at the material in the first place. The potency calculations from the new study were actually fairly close to what the EPA had done at the time of the controversy. EPA had suggested that a child who drank two or three glasses of apple juice a day, which I understand is by no means a worst-case example, ran a risk that was on the order of 1 in 2000 or 1 in 3000. We could get into a discussion of whether that is a large risk or a small risk, but I wouldn't want to be in a room with 2000 or 3000 people and be told that one more of us was going to get cancer.

On the cost side, because the varieties of apple in the United States that were most dependent on this growth regulator to be economically profitable—the Red Delicious and the Macintosh, which between them controlled about 90% of the shelf space in the supermarkets—were temporarily harder to produce for the first year or so, supermarkets had to make room for less well-known varieties, which consumers discovered had many appealing qualities. As a result, the apple industry as a whole is now twice the size that it was six years ago. Both the prices commanded and the quantities demanded have gone up; we've gone from a one billion-dollar apple crop to a two billion-dollar apple crop in constant dollars. This is not to say that a lot of people in New York State and in Washington State did not suffer greatly economically from the dislocation of their varieties and the substitution. But there is something wrong when something that causes greater consumer satisfaction, greater producer satisfaction, and lower risk is reported as a debacle and a victory for the forces of chemophobia.

CONCLUSIONS

I referred earlier to the interplay between theory and evidence. The truth is we need a lot more evidence before we can reach a verdict on whether, when, and how much conservatism actually exists in risk assessment or risk-based regulation. The evidence for conservatism in regulatory cost accounting is, I believe, fairly compelling, although the "model uncertainty" has really yet to be explored and could cut the other way in important cases (if, for example, capital and labor markets really are working nearly optimally absent regulatory intervention, and mandating the purchase of risk-reducing technology has more of a negative effect on international competition and long-term investment than it has a positive effect on innovation and job creation). I have not discussed in any detail the evidence allowing "reality checks" to be made on dose-response and exposure assessment (there are detailed discussions of the relevant studies in my 1995 *New York University Environmental Law Journal* article), but if the critics looked more at these data and less at theoretical musings, their overconfidence in what's broken might wane. In particular, the few studies that have been done comparing human epidemiology results to prior predictions made from animal bioassay studies reveal that the numbers of humans who actually contracted cancer at given doses are roughly equal to what the allegedly "hyperconservative" way agencies interpret the animal data would have predicted. For some chemicals, fewer cases occurred in humans than would have been predicted, but on average the predictions turned out not to have been exaggerated. Similar sorts of studies exist comparing the predictions of exposure models to actual measurements, with the general result that although the models often overestimate average exposure, they tend *not* to overestimate true exposures to persons reasonably far, but not implausibly far, into the "tail" of the distribution of exposure variability.

Perhaps what we need in the short term is a truce in the dispute between those determined to stamp out risk assessment exaggeration (whether it exists or not) and those determined to frustrate this agenda by emphasizing the theoretical and observational evidence for underestimation of risk. If accompanied by a moratorium on decisions to weaken the amount of protection, if any, risk assessment procedures now afford to individuals and populations under the inevitable conditions of uncertainty and variability, such a cooling-off period might enable thoughtful advocates of improved risk-assessment science to work together to plan and conduct the research necessary to shed more light on the unresolved issues raised in this talk.

While we wait for this breakthrough, let me suggest—with full awareness that this might be an unfair oversimplification—that some of the pent-up energy devoted to trivializing risks might go into acknowledging and implementing "few regrets" strategies to actually control presumptively dangerous exposures. As I was editing the transcript of this talk for publication, OSHA promulgated a new occupational exposure limit for methylene chloride, replacing an older limit that state-of-the-art risk analyses suggested was posing lifetime excess cancer risks to nearly 250,000 workers ranging upwards of 1 chance in 100. The industry association that had opposed tightening the limit for more than a decade had also conducted very interesting research suggesting that existing risk analyses might have used overly conservative assumptions. OSHA ultimately determined that their conclusions were not sufficiently well developed or coherent to adopt in full. As part of the trade association's efforts to lobby Congress to overturn the rule, it highlighted the amount of money spent on the research, some $1.5 million, apparently to imply that OSHA had some responsibility to agree with the research findings proportional to the expense incurred. As a scientist, I acknowledge that assiduous research has an unmatched potential to improve regulation. However, I also reflected on the economic feasibility analysis accompanying the methylene chloride regulation, which documented that many of the workers exposed could receive substantial risk reduction via measures as inexpensive as installing window fans in work areas and providing long-handled brushes so that workers would not have to lean into solvent tanks to strip paint from furniture. It is hard for a regulator not to take time away from the fascinating intellectual debate over conservatism to wonder whether society couldn't afford to conduct this debate without letting it divert human and financial resources that could be better spent on progress toward public health.

A Memoir on Risk Assessment and Environmental Policy[a]

SHELDON WILFRED SAMUELS

Director Emeritus
Health, Safety and Environment
Industrial Union Department, AFL-CIO
and
Vice President
Ramazzini Institute for Occupational and Environmental Health Research
P.O. Box 1570
Solomons Island, Maryland 20688

THE COST OF REGULATION

The Supreme Court's benzene (or risk assessment) decision of 1980 in the case of the Industrial Union Department, AFL-CIO[5] versus the American Petroleum Institute unleashed creative forces within the international environmental sciences community. A new risk analysis discipline developed, replete with its own professional society, journals and–perhaps most telling–its own lines in the budget of the United States and other countries for personnel, research, professional training, and lay education.

Administratively and in proposals for sweeping laws, we are transforming past modes of regulating what we eat and breath, and how we work and play.

The court's decision initially was feared as a loss for the industrial unions who had petitioned the Occupational Safety and Health Administration (OSHA) for emergency action on a workplace standard that would yield more protection from the risk of cancer. The lawsuit was brought in defense of a standard that had already been highly compromised after more than a year of OSHA hearings and closeted labor-management negotiations.

Yet the standard has intense meaning for labor, since it is based in great part on research paid for by a fund created by the financial sacrifices of victims, rubber workers whose hard negotiations overcame the resistance of the major rubber manufacturers. The need for the fund was based on decades of courageous work during pre-OSHA days, when it could be done only at personal and professional risk, by Dr. Thomas Mancuso while he was Occupational Health Officer for the State of Ohio and, later, a research professor at the University of Pittsburgh. When the companies finally agreed to the fund, it was with the condition that Dr. Mancuso be excluded from doing any of the research. The primary contract went to the University of North Carolina. The companies even insisted that outside advisors could be excluded by their veto, as I was, from meetings of the joint university-labor-management committee that had oversight of the project.

[a] This paper is the fourth in a series of five.[1-4]

The Industrial Union Department petition was actually written by United Rubber Workers President Peter Bommarito, who had negotiated the fund, and his industrial hygienist, Louis Beliczky.

On its face, the decision was far from the disaster that many believed had taken place. The plurality on the court required OSHA to make a significant risk determination, not for titrating the level of control but for setting a priority in standards development, before proceeding with enforcement. However, the requirement was not to be "a mathematical straitjacket," but could be "based on policy considerations" that need not be supported "with anything approaching scientific certainty," "risking error on the side of overprotection rather than underprotection."

The fears of the labor and environmental movements arose–in hindsight with clear justification–from predicted distortions of the decision that until only recently have been a regulatory disaster: delays in standards development and promulgation that have resulted in thousands of lives shortened and hundreds of millions of dollars wasted each year. Farsighted efforts by a handful of scientists turned the disaster into a new paradigm of international regulation.

The passage of the 1967 (Muskie) amendments to the Clean Air Act and the 1970 Occupational Safety and Health Act brought an end to arbitrary, industry-dominated standard setting in the work and community environments. Within this legislated framework, retrogressive segments of industry failed in their efforts to continue imposition of crude, one-sided cost/benefit analysis methods of the past onto the regulatory process. The intellectual absurdities and moral abomination of their methods led to strong, effective opposition by a number of *ad hoc* coalitions of labor, public health, and environmental organizations. The OSHA/Environmental Network headed by Michael McCloskey of the Sierra Club and Howard Samuel of the Industrial Union Department was the largest of these coalitions.

The arguments of a lawyer's brief do not necessarily reflect his clients beliefs or actions. Having "won" the Supreme Court case, initial support for the paradigm by industry now wavers as their attempt to use it as a new angel's clothing for an aging cannibal fails. A heuristic paradigm is clearly evolving, and the first substantive management schemes are being proposed or applied. The retrogressive are reverting to their basic tool in risk assessment and management, brute political intimidation, because they correctly understand the basic nature of the paradigm, within which they are failing, once again, to win the regulatory battle. The battle is not over something called "objective science," but rather over the application of reason and logic.

Risk assessment models use, but are not themselves, abstract mathematical instruments of science. They are analytic structures dependent upon subjective assumptions laden with the cultural and moral values of the assessor and the manager, fed by selected and arbitrarily available "data." Any agency of government that uses a specific assessment model is pragmatically required to inject social constraints on the management of risk that externally shape and internally drive the connected risk assessment model. The social and ethical issues of regulation are not resolved, merely reconfigured, by the risk assessment-management concept.

REGULATORY MYTHOLOGY IN SOUTH CAROLINA

Evidence of unsettled social and ethical issues is found in the now-international mythology surrounding the purported risk assessment panacea. This was apparent at an international conference conducted (subsequent to the presentation of this paper) by the Medical University of South Carolina and sponsored by the Department of Energy.[b,6]

The keynote speaker, John Rimington, a former British regulator, gave as an example of the consequences of *not* using risk assessment methods the long drawn out debate in the United States on the ''Delaney'' clause of our food and drug protection laws, under which saccharin can be banned as a food additive.

He claims that saccharin, a widely recognized carcinogen, was not banned because of ''protests by diabetics.'' He believes that an amendment to the law substituting the United Kingdom Atomic Energy Authority (AEA) goal-oriented, risk-based model would have prevented the long controversy.

The National Academy of Science (NAS) Committee on Saccharin and Food Policy, on which I served, examined alternative approaches to the Delaney clause. We commissioned a risk assessment. The chemical had been developed as a varnish remover. Based on the public health practices of that day, unnecessarily eating untested chemicals was associated with unnecessary risk of disease; such chemicals were deemed unfit for human consumption until proved safe by the first Commission on Food Safety. This was during the administration of Theodore Roosevelt (prior to the passage of Delaney). The commissioner was fired by our rotund, saccharine-imbiding president. None of his successors have had the power to emulate the commissioner's action and remain in office.

An NAS assessment was done by University of California Professor David Goldsmith while on staff at the Academy. (Interestingly, he benefited from the United Rubber Workers' benzene project while a student at the University of North Carolina.) Largely unpublished but available in the NAS archive, this assessment established that the chemical is a weak carcinogen when the risk is diluted in the total population, but with magnified risks among school-age children, especially young blacks. This effect resulted from a combination of factors: long latency, the dietary habits of the impoverished, and targeted marketing by the grocery manufacturers and distributors. No dietary benefit was found. Most users in the industry-targeted group do not need the substitute. In fact, they may need the more-expensive (to the grocery manufacturer) sugar in their diet.

This assessment supports targeted regulation (not a ban) and is consistent with ''goal-oriented'' rules, leaving to the industry selection of specific methods of controlling their marketing behavior short of a total ban, with the goal of protecting the populations at magnified risk rather than the total population. Then why oppose a management scheme based upon the assessment?

[b] The author attended the meeting as a member of its steering committee. The edited proceedings excluded many of the quotations and paraphrases used here from the Rimington presentation because ''they were not true,'' according to a spokesman for the university. Important observations of Mr. Ward and the German presenters, Diethard Mager and Wolfgang Goldammer, documented here were also excluded.

Experience with laws that permit this approach to risk management–e.g., through OSHA's seldom-used variance procedure–demonstrates the requirement for specialized expertise in industry, which generally does not exist. A regulatory infrastructure that is immune from political pressures to monitor the variations and adequate inspectorate, funds, and staff are also required. These resources have never been available to any regulatory agency in the United States (or in Europe!). In the absence of these requirements, the coalition of consumer, environmental, and labor groups opposing any change of law is justified in its continuing opposition to change, since change in the current deregulatory climate would result in a reduction of the existing level of food protection.

Mr. Rimington and other speakers in the Medical University of South Carolina conference repeatedly denigrated the "litigious" nature of American society, seeing this as a bad effect of an alleged failure to use so-called goal-oriented risk assessment methods, purported to be based on supposedly objective "science" and pure reason. Ironically, our long-standing need for court action was identified by Edmund Burke in the British parliament nearly 250 years ago. It was he who first described our society as litigious, but he justified our need for a third avenue of appeal when the legislative and executive branches of government fail to protect human rights.

These needs–in the United States and in every democracy–find continued justification in views such as those of Mr. Rimington. In mimicry of their American soul mates, they propose for emulation by the government of the United States the assumption of thresholds of incommensurate, historically persistent risks viewed to be "tolerable," regardless of their necessity or the feasibility of their mitigation. A risk of one death per thousand among those in the caste of workers is deemed to be "acceptable," to use the parlance of the American proponents of this view, compared to a risk of one death per hundreds of thousands or even millions among those outside the caste. These risk values are coupled in use with the ALARA (as low as reasonably achievable) concept, correctly described by a discussant, David Ward, as "very vague and difficult to use." An imposed risk that is "reasonable" to an employer or regulator may not be to the worker at risk (who may be deprived of effective choice or effective representation in the assignment of risk). Reason is a purely deductive process only in mathematics. Beyond the fictional world of "as if," reason always integrates pleasurable self-interest and aversion of personal pain in its intuitive calculus.

THE HOPEWELL INCIDENT

In an incident at Hopewell, Virginia a major chemical producer many of whose workers were organized by affiliates of the Industrial Union Department, whose interests I represented at the time, ignored existing environmental, toxicological, and clinical evidence and, to reduce their legal liability, shifted production of Kepone (chlordecone), a cockroach pesticide, to a connected but corporately separate facility whose workers were without representation. More than half the workforce were severely poisoned over a two-year period and came to the attention of Commonwealth of Virginia and federal health authorities only through a routine report of a physician new to the community and uninfluenced by the code of silence imposed by the milieu of a company town.

Within days of notification, a thorough assessment was initiated by a team drawn from the Commonwealth Department of Health, Virginia Marine Science Institute, Virginia Commonwealth University, and an assortment of federal agencies. Based on the assessment, the plant was closed, registration of chlordecone canceled, fishing on the James River halted, and medical assistance provided to the workers. An effective, albeit partial, purge of the body burden of pesticide was developed using cholestyramine.

In the ensuing court action, a heavy fine was placed in trust to support research and education. The company upgraded its environmental competence and policies. The workers and their families were at least partially compensated.

The assessment and management of risk were successful, if too late for preventive measures, with the aid of traditional public health practices many of which have been relabeled "risk assessment." Consistent with this tradition, federal legislation mandating public release of an assessment, the Toxic Substances Control Act, was introduced by then Senator William Spong of Virginia and eventually passed through support of a coalition led by the Sierra Club and the Industrial Union Department. The National Toxicological Program and research programs that enabled the development of current risk assessment arose from this legislation.

The bottom of one of the largest and most productive estuarine systems in the world, providing critical food supplies and employment to millions of people, was not dredged. Nevertheless, today Kepone is difficult to detect in the food chain of the river or the Chesapeake Bay and generally cannot be found without resort to sophisticated core sampling of the bottom.

In the face of this history, a discussant in the Medical University of South Carolina conference, Robert Bernero, demonstrated how myths are created. Although confessing lack of knowledge, Dr. Bernero appeared to have mistakenly identified the hazard in the Hopewell, Virginia incident as dioxin. Another event may also have occurred in the same community, but if he was referring to the documented case, he mischaracterized the government action at Hopewell as a failure. In fact, it was a success, in part through court action. He also erroneously stated that an assessment had not been done and as a consequence action had not been taken.

OTHER FRUITFUL PARALLELS

The fact that the negative ethical and cultural values inherent in the assumptions of some assessment-management models, and thus in the models themselves, have been strongly rejected by the mainstream of the consumer, labor, and environmental movements does not mean that *all* methods employing risk assessment are equally unacceptable to them.

The Department of Energy's (DOE) UMTRA program in Grand Junction, Colorado, for example, where the major mill for the uranium mines of the Colorado Plateau was located, successfully used risk assessments identifiably inherent in the Environmental Protection Agency (EPA) and OSHA standards used as prescriptive goals in a complex remediation effort.

There are important risk management differences between the Grand Junction model and a model used by the Germans in similar uranium mine and mill remediation efforts in Saxony and Thuringia. Unlike the situation in the United States, in Germany responsibility for seeking or providing medical care and compensation for occupational risks is not shifted to the worker, but is assumed by the *berufgenossenshaft* (industry-labor-government association). Health care systems for the entire life span of workers generally are community provided, but special occupational clinics have been established serving their former and active uranium miners. When miners leave the region, a national network of university-based clinics is available. In the United States, only as a result of a lawsuit by DOE facility workers against the government, settled in 1995, was a lifetime medical surveillance program initiated. A coherent national plan of medical risk management has yet to be devised. Special legislation had to be passed to force medical assistance and compensation for some American miners and millers. Health insurance in the United States normally excludes coverage for occupational risks, which are subsumed in a separate and generally inferior system consistent with the caste status of American workers.

An assessment and attribution of risk based on dose reconstruction for every German miner and miller is being done by the *berufgenossenshaften* for the purpose of assigning responsibility for the costs of care and compensation for occupational disease between the government and the industry, not (as in the United States) between the industry and the worker. Occupational disease compensation (medical care costs and wage and pension replacement) in the United States is infrequent and usually occurs only after litigation between the worker and the industry.

The social costs involved in any cost/benefit analysis to determine the feasibility of site-specific remedial measures, extent of remediation, and prioritization can be excluded in the German model, since they are distributed first to the industry and then throughout the society as whole outside of the remediation budget. Thus the analysis is less likely to result in increased caste-driven economic or risk burdens on the worker and his/her family.

In the AEA model social costs would be assumed by the worker and the community and included, to the extent the wishes of the worker and community prevail, in the remediation budget. "Acceptable" or "tolerable" risks are allocated by caste.

Aside from these differences, there are strong similarities between the German model and the Grand Junction case. In both, population density was high; land use was intensive and historically derived; overall budgetary caps were determined legislatively in consultation with freely elected officials of municipal and state governments; elected workers' representatives and other "stakeholders" were directly involved in the risk allocation (which is not assigned on a caste basis, but is inherent in the differential of the workplace and community feasibility-based standards used in the United States and Germany).

SELIKOFF AND RISK ASSESSMENT

When the benzene decision came down, I sent it to Irving J. Selikoff at Mt. Sinai School of Medicine. He shared it with Cuyler Hammond, chief biostatistician for the American Cancer Society, upon whom he often relied for sophisticated statistical analysis. In my note accompanying the document, I asked for advice on what OSHA would need, from a scientist's perspective, to comply with the decision. Cuyler and Selikoff discussed the decision. Selikoff telephoned their reaction.

"Cuyler," Selikoff laughed, "doesn't think labor should worry too much, because he thinks all OSHA needs to touch up the assessment Roy Albert has done for EPA, is the back of an envelope and the stub of a pencil."

Dr. Albert, formerly of New York University's Institute of Environmental Medicine, who replaced Norton Nelson as chair of EPA's Science Advisory Board, calculated the risk of leukemia from benzene exposure in the community to guide proposed regulation from automobile and industrial emissions in the community. His success in doing this was used by the American Petroleum Institute in their argument against promulgation of the OSHA standard. OSHA considered Albert's work an incomplete basis for a workplace cancer standard.

Hammond was right. OSHA moved quickly (for OSHA) to comply with the decision, and the standard became law. Most of the delay in issuing the standard had nothing to do with the risk assessment, but with the management side of the regulatory process.

Selikoff did not let the issue rest with the benzene case. He was at the same time helping Eula Bingham fight off an attack on the development of a generic occupational cancer risk assessment and management policy by OSHA.

This project was initiated by a protegé of William Ruckelshaus, Marshall Lee Miller, Acting Assistant Secretary for OSHA in the first months of the Ford administration. It was continued by Morton Corn, who succeeded Miller, and completed by Bingham when she took Corn's place in the Carter administration.

OSHA had strong support from the directors of the National Cancer Institute (NCI), the National Institute of Environmental Health Sciences (NIEHS), and the National Institute for Occupational Safety and Health (NIOSH)–Arthur Upton, David Rall, and Jack Finklea, respectively–in pressing for a policy that would end the agent-by-agent approach to regulation that dominates OSHA and EPA standards development. A staff assessment justified the OSHA proposal, but drew heavy fire from the petroleum and chemical industries.

The proposed generic policy, however, never fully came to terms with a significant finding in a 1971 staff report to the surgeon general, the primary author of which was the late Marvin Schneiderman of the National Cancer Institute.[7] This report made it clear that threshold effects of even low levels of environmental carcinogens in populations had not been found. In the absence of threshold effects, regulation could not be based upon health effects alone. "Socially acceptable" levels of risk had to be determined. But the authors, correctly in the context of their mission, did not define socially acceptable risks. This void was filled by a concept of "acceptable risk" that included historically persistent and unnecessary risks–a notion that itself could never be socially acceptable because it is a morally repugnant concept.[8] For some proponents, the concept was simply a penultimate naiveté.[9] For others, especially the promotors of atomic energy in the Department of Energy and its dependents, it was a survival technique. Unfortunately, the concept of acceptable risk dominates the practice of risk assessment and management. The stench of cannibalism still clings to this vestige of the closed society from which we are evolving.

Industry advocates in Congress moved the now-defunct Office of Technology Assessment to attack the policy with a "scientific" risk assessment of occupational cancer. Sir Richard Doll, Warden of Green College, an industry-endowed portion of

Oxford University's scientific establishment, was selected to do the study. No Americans were trusted to be "objective" or credible.

The industry knew what the outcome would be. Doll's study[10] ravaged the OSHA proposal.

Selikoff never published his response to Doll, whom he considered to be the world's preeminent epidemiologist. What he called "mistakes" in Doll's assessment model[1] were in his view mistakes not of science, but of social perspective. Doll selectively rejected what he considered to be uncertain data, preferring to use uncertain personal factor data that burdened the worker and to exclude uncertain occupational data that burdened the employer. Thus, genetics and diet were arbitrarily given greater weight than occupation, because (Selikoff believed) Doll considered it more likely that more could be done about personal factors and less about industrial hygiene. The mistake was in claiming that this judgment was "scientific" or "objective" rather than social or moral and subjective.

Rather than publicly criticizing Doll, who he felt merely represented a cultural perspective from which Doll could not escape, Selikoff set in motion two separate actions.

In the first, he set out to show that Doll was wrong scientifically: the level of uncertainty of occupational data taken from death certificates in the United States did not justify their exclusion. He asked two retired collegues, Janet Kaffenburgh and Herbert Seidman, to help him examine the records of his asbestos worker studies. The result was a series of four papers, summarized in the last, which was also his last paper.[11] These papers drowned Doll's objections with hard data.

In his second course of action, Selikoff worked with William Nicholson, his closest colleague, to help him organize a platform for the views of the progressive scientific community. They put together a New York Academy of Sciences workshop on the scientific, legal, and social issues. Selikoff assigned to me the role of listening and reacting "from the perspectives of your prior papers on the 'fallacies' " (papers on the theoretical and moral fallacies of risk/benefit analysis and the concept of acceptable risk).

The paper that emerged[12] was an attempt to deal with uncertainties in scientific observation, in cultural interpretation, and in moral integration. Selikoff's own paper at that conference[13] focused on the scientific uncertainties. He answered the question in regard to reproductive effects, but his observation is perhaps equally applicable to all areas of scientific uncertainty: "Let's act on our suspicions, with incomplete data, because it is so important where reproduction is concerned."

At the time, Selikoff and I were newly appointed members of the National Cancer Institute's Advisory Board. He was approached by the Chairman and Richard Adamson (then Director of NCI's Division of Cancer Etiology) to chair a subcommittee that would look at the emerging techniques of quantitative risk assessment and the role of NCI in their use. He thought that was too narrow a scope and persuaded them to have me chair the committee (on which he agreed to serve) in an effort to reach the philosophical (moral and theoretic) questions with which I was (and still am) struggling. The result[14] documents a partial success. We never reached agreement on the moral issues, although we denounced, albeit in a footnote, the use of the terms *safe* and *cause,* because the former had "no scientifically demonstrable basis" and the latter "is commonly associated with the single cause-single effect paradigm."

We were able to pinpoint the scientific uncertainties in cancer risk assessment, and what NCI could do in their resolution, more clearly than had been done previously in a published government policy document. More importantly, we voiced Selikoff's approach to their resolution: the need to think in terms of multifactoral causation. In these discussions, he often paraphrased Ernst Mayr, whose evolutionary biology was Selikoff's theoretical framework. We rejected the simplistic single cause-single effect thinking that dominated risk management at the time and still does in law and rules that govern everything from clean air standards to workers' compensation. A paper he wrote for David Bates on multifactoral causation was critical in writing our report.[15]

Selikoff remained uneasy on the issue of causation. He began work on a concept of ''total burden of risk''—by which he meant a Darwinian web of physical, biological, social, cultural, and ethical risk factors. He held a workshop of the Collegium Ramazzini in Carpi, Italy on the concept, after which he asked me to write a paper on how the concept might be applied in environmental planning and regulation. His critiques of my work forced seven drafts. It was presented in summary form at a meeting of the René Dubos Center and reviewed again by Arthur Upton, whose criticisms resulted in still another draft. It is published in a collection of papers Upton edited.[16] Nevertheless, the paper failed to meet Selikoff's chief criticism: the absence of a model of *prospective developmental* risk assessment.

NELSON AND RISK ASSESSMENT

The version of risk assessment-management stimulated by the 1980 benzene decision was a radical departure from policies previously recommended by the National Academy of Science in two reports of the Academy published in 1975.[17,18] This effort was spearheaded by Norton Nelson, then Director of New York University's Institute of Environmental Medicine, although the second study, a policy document, emerged from a panel chaired by political economist Clarence Davies. Nelson placed me on the policy panel specifically to deal with the risk communications problem.

The NAS studies suggested methods of using toxicologic and epidemiologic quantification basic to any risk assessment model. These and other data were to be displayed in a framework, but not placed in a calculus with risk management data. This makes more difficult the distortions of scientific data to fit methods of cost-benefit economic analysis then and now being pressed by industry and its allies in the Congress and the administration. In fact, the report on decision making, or risk management, warned against such inappropriate quantification.

''Highly formalized methods'' were rejected (p. 44).[16] ''Value judgements about noncommensurate factors in a decision such as life, health, aesthetics, and equity should be explicitly dealt with by the politically responsible decision makers and not hidden in purportedly objective data and analysis'' (p. 51).[16]

Working quietly through ''the establishment'' was typical of Nelson. You had to look carefully to see his footprints. But they were everywhere. He was the real father of both NIOSH and NIEHS, the legislative campaigns for which he led.

Nelson was the only person labor, management, government, and academia could trust to chair the OTA advisory panel convened to review the Doll and other studies commissioned to refute the cancer policy. Peg Seminario of the AFL-CIO and Mike Wright of the steelworkers served on the panel, as did Vaun Newill of Exxon. Newill, a former government scientist, was recruited by the late Norbert Roberts (Exxon's medical director) specifically to provide a credible voice in the councils of his company and to moderate industry claims. Newill succeeded. The panel report[19] essentially rejected the simplistic cost-benefit analysis sought by the lowest common denominators in the petrochemical industries. Unfortunately, the price was a recommendation for still more studies and panels. It did defuse the confrontation.

The NAS studies were Nelson's basic answer to the assessment needs of the Toxic Substances Control Act. They were also his answer to Richard Doll's social pessimism. While the NAS process was churning, he wrote a brilliant rebuttal. Acknowledging personal factors, Nelson pinpointed what he called "the added burden (and fair distribution) of *occupationally* attributable risk":

> The reduction of the frequency of human cancer from occupational exposures to an insignificant level is a practical and attainable objective . . . work assignments (should) be open to all persons mentally and physically capable of fulfilling the task regardless of special genetic or sex limitations . . . controls should be sufficiently strict so that even the most sensitive components of the population are protected.[20]

RUCKELSHAUS AND RISK ASSESSMENT

When the benzene decision came down, more than delay was experienced at the Environmental Protection Agency, the nation's environmental policy pacesetter since its shaping under William Ruckelshaus in 1970. Shortly after the court acted, Ruckelshaus had returned to reign again at the EPA. He was called back to restore public confidence in an agency that had been gutted in the early years of the Reagan Administration. This he accomplished. He restored integrity to the agency. He also wanted to end a gridlock in regulation and toxic waste remediation, stemming from continuous confrontation in the courts and in the Congress between industry and a coalition of environmental and labor organizations. This he did not accomplish.

To end the gridlock, he queried scientists in academia and industry. Many suggested a risk assessment-management process as a means of developing consensus or a less disputable basis for agency action. An EPA-chartered NAS committee (which included Frank Mirer of the United Autoworkers Union) recommended a separation between assessment and management. This was meant to protect from distortion the purported objectivity of science in the regulatory process, as if scientists could divorce knowing how a risk would be managed from the design of the assessment models they use.[21] The futility of a total separation is evident in the NAS report, which made clear the importance of revealing the policy ramifications of the assessments.

Ruckelshaus, however, in his public embrace of the NAS report as a means of ending the EPA's regulatory problems, chose to believe that the policy ramifications could be put aside in assessment. Prior to a major public meeting he called at the Academy to announce his new policy, he circulated a draft of his speech to many of us in the regulatory community. I hand-delivered a reply on the day of receipt, hotly taking issue with the assumptions of inappropriate quantification, fallacious objectivity, and cannibalistic "acceptable" risks latent in the model he was adopting *as it existed at that time.*

Sitting in the back of the hall on the day of the meeting, I wondered if my criticisms had had any effect, or even had been read. The industry representatives appeared to be too happy.

I had been among the original core staff of civil servants around which Ruckelshaus built the EPA. Working with him personally, I sensed a Republican in the same pragmatic tradition of environmental activism and social justice as Russell Train and Nelson Rockefeller.

When I told him in February 1971 that I was leaving the agency to work for the industrial unions, Ruckelshaus said: ''But those are the guys who want to redistribute all the wealth in our country!'' ''As they should,'' I said, ''but they also demand and gain *respect* for the needs of the common man.'' He smiled and seemingly nodded in agreement. His door was always open to representatives of the labor movement. He was responsible for the EPA decision to require trained workers on Superfund sites, setting in motion the largest government-union training program since World War II.

But I was deeply disappointed in what he said at the Academy that day.

''Nothing will erode public confidence faster than the suspicion that policy considerations have been allowed to influence the assessment of risk,'' he said. Ruckelshaus clearly believed that there is ''an objective way to assess risk.'' Of course, he added, ''there is no purely objective way to manage it.''[22]

Ruckelshaus failed to understand that inherent in any assessment model is a set of subjective assumptions stemming in part from the value judgments of the assessor and in part by the fact that, while assessment and management can—and perhaps should—be administered separately, the needs of the manager teleologically drive the design of the assessment.

EMOTION, SCIENCE AND COMMUNITY

''Risk assessment'' and ''risk management'' are styles that have replaced the labels of similar past attempts at planning and regulating the human niche. Probably, they will be replaced by newer styles and newer labels in the future. If we look at them all, from Hippocrates' simple treatises on the air and water to the complex reports of CRESP (the Consortium for Risk Evaluation with Stakeholder Participation, a massive state-of-the-art enterprise operated by Bernard Goldstein, Gilbert Omenn, and Charles Powers, and guided by Arthur C. Upton), a broad pattern of need emerges.

We find a need to broaden our thinking beyond the carcinogen of the day, the Superfund site of the week, the management style of the month, and focus on developing a comprehensive model that fits the characteristics of our niche beyond our generation.

In doing so, we find a recurring mistake, the reason why a malconnection, if not a disconnection, persists between assessment of risk its management. This is the false expectation that science can meet the needs of the environmental manager, indeed the manager of any issue in human affairs, without dealing with the fundamental characteristic of humans. A pure mathematic—as distinct from moral—calculus has been promised, but not found, that would represent a connected assessment-management system that could yield a computation that could determine environmental priorities, such as the priority of action function of risk assessment established by the Supreme Court's plurality decision.

Analytically, the questions are obvious: different levels of scope (management tends to be broader), quantification (minute titration is less relevant in control than in establishing dose-response relationships), certainty (prudence and *p*-values may have little in common), incommensurability of both methods and data (even if you can assign a value to present life, the same value would not apply to future life), and definition (are cultural and ethical values relative or absolute?)

The result: problems supposed to be solved are not solved. The pace of regulation has not been quickened: renewed trials and repeated errors place the actual schedules of toxic waste remediation and toxic substance regulation decades behind published schedules.

The analytic questions are understood, but never fully addressed because of our reluctance to deal with a much more profound challenge. The heart of the issue is the subjectivity that rules us, the aorta of which is emotion.

We expect our actions to be rational, by which many of us mean without emotion. But reason is rife with antimony. Cold inference is exercised within the heated capsule of pain and fear, pleasure and satisfaction.

The expectation that emotion can somehow be surgically removed from the human, or at least separated, cannot be met. At the base of the most persistent arguments for the employment of risk assessment-management are ancient appeals for the exclusion of emotion through the application of what is believed to be scientific—by which the believers mean mechanistic—reason, to the exclusion of "demogogic politics." There was, and is, a demand for the exercise of impossible rules of reason that would exclude the logic of behaviors that avoid pain and fear, the substrate of risk avoidance, as if the life-protective purpose of reason can be defeated.

The argument is for release from the human bondage, from passion, and access to a world of detached fact and absolute objectivity. The language of chance is used. "Accident" becomes the favored cause of environmental disease and injury, as if life is only a cherry blossom moved by vagrant winds that know no master.

The scientist is pressured to abstract his work from the common culture, an effort that fails because culture has evolved at the same time, and in the same way, and has become integrated with the machinery of the human creature. Bonded by norms the being of which is emotion itself, cultural values intertwine with the heuristic assumptions at the base of every construct that orders and explains the data the scientist is dedicated to generate.

The models of human and ecological risk, for assessment or management, are no exception. But if they are no exception, then the stated expectations in government and industry for an emotionless, detached discipline cannot be met.

What *can* be done is to exercise the art of mediating the emotions of the *polis,* within the nest of the socially structured and politically defined community. It is by understanding the concept of community that we connect assessment and management of human and ecological risk.

Assessing risk can be a way of looking at effects without determining cause. In the absence of omniscience, that may often mean that it is a useful tool. Combined with cause, it can be more useful, and more useful still if its structure is brought closer to the structure of causation in the real world.

The real world is not composed of atomistic creatures. It is composed of communities. Communities are hierarchically structured. Darwin's web of causation is not that of a spider weaving a single strand on a single dimension. It is multistranded, multidimensional. It is the whole, not just the machinery, but also the emotions.

SELIKOFF AND DARWIN

A revolution in how we see the work and community environments "really began with Darwin," Selikoff the optimist used to say.[23] When he began a new career in his retirement years, he focused on the molecular biology of cancer. This was primarily for practical, short-term reasons: early detection and early intervention. Selikoff never stopped being a family physician. The immediate needs of his patients came first. But it was also for devising a broader concept of assessing and managing risk from the perspectives of the life history of the individual and of the species in a biological, cultural, and physical dynamic. To understand how to do this, he began to reread not only Darwin, but the disciples of Darwin, especially Mayr. What he could not do himself, he expected the young people he mentored, such as his former student William Rom and physician-geneticist Antonio Giordano, to do for him.

And he never stopped reading and questioning, trying to understand. On one of my last visits, as he lay on his hospital bed in great pain, I found him trying to read a history of philosophy by the Durants.

"Why a history?" I asked.

"It's short," he said, "and I'm looking for some philosophic tradition that will help us!"

A "tradition that will help us!" The words of the son of a Talmudic scholar.

"That tradition," I said, "is not in the history books. It exists, but is not taught. It would have to be reinstated." And I described what I thought it was: Darwin's observations and beliefs interpreted, tempered, and expanded through the reconstructed minds of two predecessors, Baruch de Spinoza and Johann Wolfgang Goethe, and our modern evolutionists—especially the early social ecologists and population geneticists at the Universities of Michigan and Chicago and his own Columbia—as well as Bergson and Freud.

"Spinoza, Goethe, and *Darwin?*" he laughed. He laughed with greater force than I had heard from him in weeks. "Maybe. Maybe not. Maybe it's not so crazy. Will the scientists believe you? Who knows. Try it anyway."

But how do we reinstate a tradition, the resurgence of which will connect risk and its control, a tradition that seeks the whole of continuous nature in the vital association of the community, within which, Freud taught us, the hierarchical structure of mental life is an analog of physical life?

We can write a philosophic *ex cathedra* polemic that might or might not be read, and that almost surely will pose still more versions of old questions we never answer. Or we can do what we have always done to make progress in the face of uncertainty: we can play the game of "as if."

What is both the simplest and most profound characteristic of the ancient Euclidean science we choose to mimic in our models is not widely understood: the arbitrariness, the fiction of the assumption in any axiomatic method. This mistake also is understandable. Black boxes, blinking lights, and printouts of confidence computations easily confuse us. Yet, in the systems upon which they are built, only heuristic values that vet or select our constructs prevail in the face of intractable conceptual mystery and persistent factual uncertainty.

The origin of modern science was in a Cartesian universe of discourse in which mechanical bodies were bifurcated from atomistic minds preoccupied with themselves, wrenched from the systems of communities that are the whole human in the communities of humans in nature. This was—and remains—the dominant ideal of science.

Despite his careful documentation of the development in lower and higher species of instinctive simultudes of love and the desire to be loved, of anger and appeasement, of fear and its avoidance, even the great Darwin could change the contempt for emotion of only some of the social philosophers and fewer still of the biologists of his day. Still, generations later, the phylogeny of emotion described in Darwin's work and subsequently by some of his disciples—Bergson, Mead, Freud, Dewey, Lorenz, Simpson, Tinbergen, Herrick, Emerson, Dobzhansky, Wright, Gould, Dubos, Hawley and others—has been forgotten. Each of these would have approached human risk prospectively and developmentally, as sought by Selikoff in his concept of the total burden of risk. Yet each has had little impact on environmental policy.

After a century, Darwin's work stands like an unlit beacon on a lonely shore swept by swells from environmental storms far from reality. But then, as Selikoff pointed out, we are only at the beginning of the development of whole new disciplines of natural, social, and moral science.

REFERENCES

1. Samuels, S. W. 1994. An open systems approach to risk assessment. Presented at Mt. Sinai Hospital. New York, April 29, 1993. Am. J. Ind. Med. **25:** 447-453. Letter of correction. Am. J. Ind. Med. **26:** 427.
2. Samuels, S. W. 1997. Ethical and metaethical criteria for an emerging technology: Risk assessment. Invited paper presented at the Pacific Rim Conference on Occupational and Environmental Medicine. Sponsored by ACOEM/Australasian Faculty of Occupational Medicine. Sydney, October 4, 1995. J. Brit. Soc. Occ. Med. **47,** 4: 241-246.
3. Samuels, S. W. 1997. Community, communication and causation. Int. J. Health Serv. In press.
4. Samuels, S. W. 1997. Communicating risk to workers: Historical and ethical perspectives. Invited presentation at the ASTDR-DOE-EOHSI Conference on Risk Communication. Piscataway, NJ, December 6, 1996. *In* Risk Communication in a Changing World. T. Tinker, M. Pavlova, B. Arkin & A. Gotsch, Eds. Ramazzini Institute/OEM Press. Beverly Farms, MA. In press.
5. Industrial Union Department vs. American Petroleum Institute (1980); 448 0.5 607 U.S.S.C., Washington.
6. Nixon, B. & D. Hoel.1996. International Case Studies in Risk Assessment and Management. Sponsored by the Medical University of South Carolina, AEA Technology, and the United States Department of Energy. Charleston, SC, March 5-7, 1996. Transcript, June 1997.
7. Department of Health, Education, and Welfare/Public Health Service. 1971. Report to the Surgeon General of the Ad Hoc Committee on the Evaluation of Low Levels of Environmental Carcinogens. Government Printing Office, Washington, D.C.
8. Lowrance, W. 1976. Of Acceptable Risk. Kaufman. Los Altos, CA.

9. Samuels, S. 1978. The fallacies of acceptable risk in risk/benefit decisions and public health, HEW (FDA) 80-1069, February 1978. Government Printing Office. Washington, D.C.
10. Doll, R. & R. Peto. 1981. The causes of cancer: Quantitative estimates of avoidable risks of cancer in the United States today. J. Nat. Cancer Inst. **66:** 1193-1308.
11. Selikoff, I. J. 1992. Death certificates in epidemiological studies, including occupational hazards: Inaccuracies in occupational categories. Am. J. Ind. Med. **22:** 493-504.
12. Samuels, S. W. 1981. The uncertainty factor. *In* Management of Assessed Risk for Carcinogens. W. J. Nicholson, Ed.: 269-282. Vol. 363, Annals of the New York Academy of Sciences. New York.
13. Selikoff, I. J. 1981. Carcinogenic risk management. *In* Management of Assessed Risk for Carcinogens. W. J. Nicholson, Ed.: 283-293. Vol. 363, Annals of the New York Academy of Sciences. New York.
14. Samuels, S. W. & R. H. Adamson. 1985. Quantitative risk assessment: Report of the Subcommittee on Environmental Carcinogenesis, National Cancer Advisory Board. J. Nat. Cancer Inst. **74**(4): 945-951.
15. Selikoff, I. J. 1983. Multiple factor intervention in environmental disease. *In* Symposium on Assessment and Perception of Risk to Human Health in Canada, October 1982. J. T. Rogers & D. V. Bates, Eds.: 171-179. Royal Society of Canada. Toronto.
16. Samuels, S. W. 1995. Living on the crust of the earth. *In* The City as a Human Environment. D. G. LeVine & Arthur C. Upton, Eds.: 171-186. Greenwood. Westport, CT.
17. National Academy of Sciences-National Research Council. 1975. Principles for Evaluating Chemicals in the Environment. National Academy Press. Washington, DC.
18. National Academy of Sciences-National Research Council. 1975. Decisionmaking for Regulating Chemicals in the Environment. National Academy Press. Washington, DC.
19. Office of Technology Assessment. 1981. Assessment of Technologies for Determining Cancer Risks from the Environment. OTAS-H-137. Government Printing Office. Washington, DC.
20. Nelson, N. 1981. A personal view of occupational cancer and its prevention. N. Nat. Cancer Inst. **67:** 227.
21. National Academy of Sciences-National Research Council. 1983. Risk Assessment in the Federal Government: Managing the Process. National Academy Press. Washington, DC.
22. Ruckelshaus, W. 1983. Risk, science and public policy. Science **221:** 1026-1028.
23. Samuels, S. W., Ed. 1992. The Selikoff Agenda (film). Ramazzini Institute. Solomons Island, MD.

The Use of Economics in Environmental Decision Making[a]

HOLLY STALLWORTH[b]

Office of Policy, Planning and Evaluation
U.S. Environmental Protection Agency
Mail Code 2184
401 M Street, S.W.
Washington, D.C. 20460

THE CURRENT ECONOMICS PARADIGM AT EPA

The use of economics at the Environment Protection Agency is largely defined by administrative decree. Since 1981, EPA has been required to do a cost-benefit analysis for "major" regulations (defined as those with economic impacts exceeding $100 million) as part of a Regulatory Impact Analysis. President Reagan's Executive Order (EO) 12291 imposed by administrative decree a decision criterion of maximizing net benefits over costs, regardless of whatever health- or technology-based standards were specified in the statute. The Office of Management and Budget (OMB) was given the task of reviewing these regulatory impact analyses for conformity with the EO's requirements. Thus began a decade-long conflict between EPA, which was charged with carrying out health- or technology-based standards in statutory mandates, and OMB, charged with enforcing the EO and the primacy of cost-benefit calculations. Frequently, regulations would remain locked in this bureaucratic hornet's nest until lawsuits and resulting court-ordered deadlines forced them out. In the middle of this entanglement, environmental economics at EPA took form.

The EO introduced not only intractable conflict between EPA and OMB, it ushered in a new kind of political economy in regard to environmental issues—one where the environmental quality was treated less as a ***public good*** *subject to value-based decisions* but as a ***private good*** *where price-based calculations were deemed to best inform.* This departed significantly from other public policy issues such as police or fire protection or national defense—where decisions arose from society's values, beliefs, common needs, sense of social justice or risk aversion. Public goods theory, developed since the days of Adam Smith, long recognized the need for government intervention in a number of select areas plagued by the "free rider" problem—also called the "tragedy of the commons." A classic example is the fisherman who is unwilling to curtail his harvest from an overexploited fishery because his private gains from overfishing run counter to society's long-run interest in main-

[a] This paper was previously published in *New Solutions, A Journal of Environmental and Occupational Health Policy,* Fall 1996, pp. 8–13. It is reprinted with permission. The opinions expressed herein are strictly those of the author and do not represent any official policy or opinion of the U.S. Environmental Protection Agency.

[b] Phone: 202/260-5247; fax: 202/260-2704; e-mail: stallworth.holly@epamail.epa.gov

taining the fishery. Many environmental goods and services meet the test of a public good–indivisibility of ownership or consumption. Therefore, private parties, acting on the basis of self-interest, will not have sufficient incentive to pay their fair share or protect a common property resource.

The historical treatment of public goods in economic theory presumed a need for government intervention where common property resources would not be adequately protected by private interests. Ignoring this, the cost-benefit requirement imposed a traditional supply-and-demand analysis on environmental goods. To comply with this EO, EPA's economists and consultants to EPA began what is now a 15-year-old experiment in constructing demand curves (monetary values) for environmental goods.

It may be that the EO's have left EPA little choice, but, as I've argued in previous writings,[1] a powerful asymmetry was created by this requirement for cost-benefit analysis: the "burden of proof" was placed on EPA to demonstrate dollar-based "benefits" exceeding costs. The market-based paradigm discounted, even ignored, nonquantified beliefs and values. Regulatory impact analyses became a Sisyphean task of constructing a patchwork of environmental and human health information to construct dose-response functions, followed by an attempt to "value" the regulation by placing a monetary number on the avoided damages to human health and the environment. In so doing, policy makers were forced to state a dollar value for lives saved, diseases avoided, trees left standing, clean air, clean water, visibility, scenic beauty, intrinsic value, value to future generations, and so forth. The multiplicity of effects, the numbers of people involved, and the psychic nature of many of the issues all combined to make the measurement problem extremely difficult, highly uncertain, and sensitive to starting assumptions. Traditional cost-benefit analysis originating from the 1930's and 1940's for water resources investments became increasingly strained as EPA faced large-scale problems with complex and uncertain ecological consequences. All of these empirical problems became grist for OMB's critical review and intervention in the rule-making process.

While there are certainly effects of policy choices that can be measured in dollars terms (e.g. jobs, profits, sales, etc.), the great bulk of this work has gone to extraordinary lengths to convert nonmarketed goods and services into consumer-based preferences that can be priced. Douglas MacLean[2] has argued, quite persuasively I think, that the willingness-to-pay monetized approach is the "low road" to the task of comparing different values. Instead, MacLean prefers moral inquiry and moral reasoning for resolving what are essentially moral conflicts. Similarly Sagoff[3] has pointed out that the values that guide consumer preferences may be different from those that drive political choices and desires for what the government might do. Both MacLean and Sagoff protest the attempts to capture in dollar terms such things as the loss of ecological resources for future generations or the spiritual comfort we might derive from protecting old-growth forests. While most enthusiasts of cost-benefit analysis will acknowledge the presence of these nonmonetizable effects, their allegiance to the monetized version of cost-benefit analysis remains strong. In practice, most neoclassical economists continue to recommend options with positive net benefits and dismiss policies with negative net benefits despite their acknowledgments of the numerous caveated shortcomings and flaws in a monetized analysis.

Although the EO of the Reagan-Bush administrations was replaced in October 1993 with Clinton's version, Executive Order 12866, the new Clinton EO preserved the basic structure of the cost-benefit requirement. Originally, the Clinton Administration did allow some room for those benefits that could not be monetized and placed some procedural reforms into the regulatory review process such as a time limit on OMB's review of regulations. However, recent new guidelines emanating from Clinton's OMB have turned the tide back in favor of the monetized standard. This "guidance" issuing from the Clinton Administration OMB aims at standardizing the way agencies "value" (i.e., monetize) the impacts of their programs.

Whatever the politics that have elevated cost-benefit analysis, it poses nightmarish difficulties for policy analysis and debate at EPA. In addition to the troublesome aspects of valuing human life and impacts on human health, the dollar-based standard for environmental policy faces a daunting array of ecological effects for which we can never hope to have dollar values. Ecological functions like nutrient cycling, carbon sequestration, oxygen production, groundwater recharge, air purification, sediment control, erosion control, and climate regulation all comprise elements of the planet's life support systems for which the *precautionary principle* might be a more appropriate standard.

GOAL SETTING BASED ON THE PRECAUTIONARY PRINCIPLE

The precautionary principle asserts that action should be taken in advance of scientific proof when further delay may prove unacceptably costly to society and nature. This principle simply turns the burden of proof in the opposite direction and says that society must be willing to take preventive action in the context of risk and uncertainty. Full scientific certainty is *not* required to justify protective actions that safeguard ecological functions that support and maintain life on earth. To be " precautious" means recognizing and respecting the margins of tolerance in ecological systems; and certainly not broaching them.

Although it is unlikely that a single principle will ever provide adequate direction for hundreds and thousands of environmental policy questions, the precautionary principle at least offers a directionally correct sensibility for restoring the burden of proof to those forces that exert change on the ecosystem.

Applying the precautionary principle to the cost of environmental regulation would mean treating the cost of regulation as something more like an insurance premium than a payment for tangible, measurable, proven benefits. Properly used, *benefit* implies something that promotes our well-being, whereas protection of human health and the environment is more often the avoidance of harm. This distinction may appear semantic until one considers that since the early 20th century, neoclassical economic theory has recognized the fundamental asymmetry between losing something and gaining something. The marginal disability of having your bicycle stolen exceeds the marginal utility you might experience from receiving a new bicycle. The "willingness to pay" standard from the monetized approach typically undervalues this underlying psychological fact that so often accompanies environmental degradation. As a perspective, precaution is clearly needed for an issue like global warming, where a decade of foot-dragging in the United States has been justified by calls for full scientific proof and more research. Admittedly precaution as a standard lacks a definition from which to prescribe specific standards and actions, yet it seems directionally more prudent than our current dollar-based, cost-benefit standard—with its bias toward waiting for more data and calling for more research. The precautionary principle meshes better with the *timing* issues involved in environmental policy—where the cost of waiting can be high.

Precaution is more important when prediction is difficult. Ecological systems have been shown not to be smooth and continuous but rather to have discontinuities that defy our linear predictions. For issues like biodiversity conservation and the preservation of ecosystem functions, the thresholds of tolerance embraced in the precautionary principle are based primarily on ecological information. Rather than treating ecosystem protection solely as a consumer issue, economists must look to others who can best express the ecological basis of sustainability. We must look to foresters for indicators of sustainable forestry; agronomists for indicators of sustainable agriculture; aquatic biologists for indicators of sustainable fisheries; terrestrial ecologists for direction on sustainable rangeland management, etc. In a truly interdisciplinary economics that is rooted in our dependency on natural resources, these biophysical indicators of sustainability need to be elevated on a par with more traditional economic measures of success: growth rates of output, sales, labor productivity, etc.

Whatever its merits, the precautionary principle may not save us from the wrenching moral, ethical, and economic dilemmas that are part of modern environmental decision making. But at least with precaution, debate shifts to this more sober perspective that recognizes the risk of significant and irreversible harm. Rather than debating until all uncertainties are removed, our policy analysis would be better served with a focus on the technical requirements of maintaining options for future generations in terms of biological diversity, ecological integrity, and resource productivity. Full scientific certainty should not be required to justify government intervention to safeguard ecological functions that support and maintain life on earth.

What follows are some suggestions for research efforts in the economics of environmental policy that can better capitalize on the true usefulness of economics.

ALTERNATIVE DIRECTIONS

While much of EPA's economics is defined by the laws passed by Congress and imposed by presidential EO, it is important that the Agency not limit itself to the cost-benefit/monetization paradigm but rather develop other approaches that "push the envelope" toward an economics that is more solution oriented. Rather than pounding square pegs into round holes with the monetary hammer, environmental economics can contribute to the search for solutions, e.g., by searching for efficient, cost-minimizing solutions and tracing real economic impacts.

Over two decades ago, William Baumol and Wallace Oates[4] declared that we would never have enough information to estimate the dollar benefits of pollution control. Baumol and Oates felt that the search for the Pareto optimal point (which required full monetization of the externality) was a fool's errand that should be abandoned. They advocated instead what they called a "sub-optimizing" approach—

i.e. searching for the most efficient means of achieving a *predetermined* environmental goal, a goal set by whatever political, social, and scientific processes pertain to the problem at hand. Although Baumol and Oates called it "least cost theory," today it might be recognized as *cost-effectiveness analysis,* and this can take many forms.

Cost-effectiveness analysis was the centerpiece of the old Carter executive guidance on regulatory matters. Accepting that social values and other noneconomic criteria must play a starring role in setting environmental goals, a cost-effectiveness analysis falls within what Baumol and Oates called the *suboptimizing approach.* Rather than seeking the *optimal point* or environmental goal, economics is best used to find the least-cost solution for predetermined environmental goals. Accepting that people want to preserve old growth forests and the species who live there for reasons that cannot be monetized, cost-effectiveness analysis yields to the social forces, scientific information, stakeholder negotiations, and political debate. After a goal has been set, the economist's tools of the trade—optimizing, marginal analysis, etc.—are then applied.

Cost-effectiveness analysis (seeking the least-cost solution for a given environmental goal) and *incremental cost analysis* are now touted by the United States Army Corps of Engineers. In a recent set of publications from its Institute for Water Resources, the Corps has discarded the monetization framework in favor of nonmonetary goals, such as preserving ecosystem structure/function or socially valued services. Methods such as the habitat evaluation procedure and the wetlands evaluation technique are used to express environmental goals. Principles of constrained optimization from economics are then used to choose from among various water resource plans.

Another alternative framework is *economic impact analysis.* Rather than converting complicated human health, ecological and quality of life effects into a dollar-based metric, economic impact analysis addresses only the market activity that results from some regulation, development, or government action and is thus limited to what can be measured in dollar terms. As a subset of this, *fiscal impact analysis* addresses impacts on government revenues. But note that tracing dollar-based *impacts* of policy choices is a different game from translating complex effects on human health, quality of life, and ecological systems into dollar-based estimates. In much the same way toxicology is used to trace effects of a pollutant on human mortality or morbidity, or ecotoxicology is used to define effects on an animal population, economic impact analysis defines effects on those groups in society that may gain or lose in economic terms. Unlike cost-benefit analysis, it restricts attention to economic effects that can be measured in market terms (jobs, profits, prices) and does not attempt to construct surrogate markets to convert the entire realm of policy consequences—ecological, human health or quality of life—into dollar values. Economic impact analysis does not attempt to convert social values into dollar-based estimates.

Rather than total effects (total costs minus total benefits), we need to begin our analysis with a sense of the "winners and losers" in environmental policy—i.e., who benefits and who gains from particular options, programs, or prices. Economists know that the marginal utility of a dollar (or other gain) is not constant across groups; thus it is necessary to have disaggregated information so that we can see the conflict played out between real stakeholders with starkly different economic characteristics. Consider the vast socioeconomic differences between the indigenous fish-consuming populations of the Columbia River Basin and the Bonneville Power Company, which profits from subsuming most of the water rights for hydroelectric power. Consider also the differential impacts of restoring the oyster beds of the Chesapeake Bay. In this case, a proper economic impact analysis should aim to show the relative impacts on two main user groups: Virginia's oyster fishing industry and Maryland's. Currently, these two sides are at loggerheads over the introduction of an oyster species from Japan that is more resistant to the protozoan diseases that have plagued the current oyster. Since Virginia's oyster industry is failing and Maryland's is still viable, Maryland has not wanted to undertake the risk (potential environmental injury) associated with introducing this non-native mollusk into the Chesapeake Bay.

Tracing the effects of environmental policy to different consuming and producing sectors is the basis of a more sober use of economics. With an eye toward equity, a comprehensive economic impact analysis identifies the groups, firms, and communities most likely to realize gains, losses, or both.

While the cost-benefit framework addresses the policy choice only in a "yes-no" fashion (to protect or not to protect), a more useful analysis would be directed at the full set of trade-offs and consequences of various policy choices. We might call this *trade-offs analysis,* although the term has little currency beyond one Corps of Engineers report (1995), which constructs a framework for trade-offs analysis combining stakeholder participation, multiobjective planning, game theory, and group processes.[5] Under this rubric, the Corps offers a framework for their task of setting the operating schedule of a dam.

No doubt policy frameworks will need to be adapted in response to specific policy questions. It would not be surprising if what works for the Corps of Engineers' need to determine water levels for a dam does not work for the Environmental Protection Agency trying to establish water quality standards under the Safe Drinking Water Act. Policy menus and tools vary widely. The full set of trade-offs can be quite complex, extending into many dimensions and platforms. For an issue such as logging in the Pacific Northwest, some platforms on which trade offs should be defined include: local quality of life (hunting and trapping, fish consumption), esthetic values and spiritual beliefs, ecosystem health (such as possible loss of salmon habitat, effects on soil erosion and water quality), and jobs/income (fishing jobs vs. logging jobs; income/profits relative to financial strength) in both the long run and the short run. These platforms for assessing trade-offs will likely have to be tailored to each specific problem.

CONCLUSION

The fundamental policy question is a difficult one: whether one state of the world is better than another. Treating this issue merely as a consumer problem does not do justice to the extraordinary dimensions of environmental policy. We operate on a stage marked by intergenerational impacts and effects on nonhuman species. Even when combined with other disciplines in a holistic analysis, economics cannot save us from these difficult decisions. Economists can only hope to make the trade-offs of policy choices clear.

Sustainability, that word so much in vogue in environmental policy, is a construct that properly shifts our attention to a concern for future generations; but the sustainability movement needs more precise empirical terms. Theoretical discussions of sustainability must give way to facts about particular sectors or economic activities: energy, agriculture, transportation, forestry. These particular problems require particular solutions, not conceptual or theoretical frameworks that can ill accommodate the facts associated with a particular issue. Sustainability may ultimately be the product of a thousand little pieces of a puzzle strung together.

The enormous task facing my discipline is to come to grips with the ecological conditions for sustainability–namely, to live off our "income" from natural resources while protecting "natural capital." With each unique policy question, this will have to be approached from a thousand different directions. When applied to the search for solutions and consequences, economics can contribute to a more holistic policy analysis that points us to the "best" policy–in the sense of achieving the greatest good for the greatest number for the longest period of time.

REFERENCES

1. STALLWORTH, H. 1995. The cost-benefit paradigm for environmental protection: An economist's perspective on the methodological, theoretical and ethical problems. New Solutions. Fall 1995: 14-19.
2. MACLEAN, D. E. 1981. Comparing values in environmental policies: Moral issues and moral arguments. Regulation Magazine. Jan.-Feb. 1981: 83-106.
3. SAGOFF, M. 1981. Economic theory and environmental law. Michigan Law Review **79:** 1393-1401.
4. BAUMOL, W. J. & W. E. OATES. 1971. The use of standards and prices for protection of the environment. Swed. J. Econ. March: 42-54.
5. CORPS OF ENGINEERS, INSTITUTE FOR WATER RESOURCES. 1995. Evaluation of Environmental Investments Procedures Manual, Interim: Cost Effectiveness and Incremental Cost Analyses. IWR Report 95-R-1, May 1995.

ADDITIONAL REFERENCES

CORPS OF ENGINEERS, INSTITUTE FOR WATER RESOURCES. 1995. Trade-off analysis for environmental projects: An annotated bibliography. IWR Report 95-R-8. August 1995.

DALY, H. E. & J. B. COBB. 1989. For the Common Good: Redirecting the Economy toward Community, the Environment and a Sustainable Future. Beacon Press. Boston.

EBERLE, D. W. 1996. Valuation of nonmarket goods: A methodology for public policy making. Dissertation, Boise State University, Bosie, ID.

ECO NORTHWEST. 1994. A method for estimating the economic effects of habitat protection. Final report for U.S. Fish and Wildlife Service. Portland, OR. January 1994.

KING, D. M., C. C. BOHLEN & P. R. CROSSON. 1995. Natural resource accounting and sustainable watershed management: With Illustration for the Upper Mississippi River watershed. A report for the President's Council on Sustainable Development. UMD Ref. No. UMCEES CBL-95-037. February 1995.

LIPTON, D. W., K. F. WELLMAN, I. C. SHEIFER & R. F. WEIHER. 1995. Economic valuation of natural resources: A handbook for coastal resource policymakers. National Oceanic and Atmospheric Administration, Coastal Ocean Office. Decision Analysis Series No. 5. NOAA Coastal Ocean Office. Silver Spring, MD. June 1995.

SKRZYCKI, C. 1996. Agencies question OMB's cost-benefit balancing act. Washington Post, November 3, 1996, p. B1.

YOUNG, T. F. & C. H. CONGDON. Plowing new ground: Using economic incentives to control water pollution from agriculture. Undated Environmental Defense Fund report.

A National Estimate of the Cost of Occupationally Related Disease in 1992[a]

MARIANNE C. FAHS,[b–e] STEVEN B. MARKOWITZ,[f] J. PAUL LEIGH,[g] CHONG-GAK SHIN,[h] AND PHILIP J. LANDRIGAN[i]

[c]*Health Policy Research Center*
Robert J. Milano Graduate School of Management and Urban Policy
New School for Social Research
New York, New York 10011

[d]*International Longevity Center (U.S.)*

[e]*Department of Health Policy*
[f]*Division of Environmental and Occupational Medicine*
[i]*Department of Community Medicine*
Mount Sinai School of Medicine
City University of New York
New York, New York 10029

[g]*Department of Economics*
San Jose State University
San Jose, California

[h]*Korea Institute for Health & Social Affairs*
Seoul, Republic of Korea

INTRODUCTION

With the prominence of economic concerns in health policy discussions, increasing attention has been paid to the economic costs of illness. Expert assessments of policies to confront major health problems now routinely include consideration of illness costs. In occupational health policy, however, this is not the case. Illness costs have been routinely excluded from consideration in the debates over controversial proposals for workplace safety regulations.

The National Institute of Occupational Safety and Health (NIOSH) is mandated by Congress to study the economic impact of proposed industry regulations. However, NIOSH has limited the economic impact analysis to econometric forecasts of labor

[a]This research was supported in part by the National Institute of Occupational Health and Safety Contract #U6OCCU902886-07. Portions of this research have been published in summary form in "Occupational Injury and Illness in the United States: Estimates of Costs, Morbidity, and Mortality," *Archives of Internal Medicine* 157: 1557–1568, 1997.

[b]Address for correspondence: Marianne C. Fahs, Ph.D., M.P.H., Director, Health Policy Research Center, Robert J. Milano Graduate School of Management and Urban Polity, New School for Social Research, 66 Fifth Avenue, New York, New York 10011. Phone: 212/229-5678; fax: 212/229-5335.

market dynamics. Consideration of the dynamics of the health care market, including the economic benefits of healthier workers, has been omitted from the economic impact assessments.[1] Consequently, the econometric models currently developed for NIOSH tend to *underestimate* the net social benefits of occupational risk reduction in the labor force, by omitting the benefits to the economy of healthier, more productive workers. Conversely, the models tend to *overestimate* the social costs of industry regulation, since potential savings in averted health care costs are ignored for workers whose occupational disease is prevented. These incomplete models of the labor market generate economic impact assessments that produce biased information for policy makers. The bias systematically devalues occupational disease prevention strategies, tending to support the status quo of industry standards.

To guide government policy formation that is in the best interests of the public, predicted economic outcomes of disease prevention strategies, such as industry regulations, should include estimates of the direct and indirect costs of occupationally related disease averted.

However, the literature on the economic costs of occupationally related disease remains underdeveloped. Despite frequent calls from national advisory groups and health policy analysts for national-level studies,[2–4] studies are either limited to specific diseases, such as work-related hypertension care[5] and upper extremity cumulative trauma disorders,[6,7] or to specific geographic regions, such as the states of Pennsylvania, New York, or Michigan.[8–10] A national investigation into the economic consequences of occupational disease is called for. It is of some urgency that resources be applied to the development of the health economic and epidemiologic research necessary to improve science-based policy in occupational health.

To begin to address this concern, this paper investigates data sources and develops cost-of-illness accounting methods to present a preliminary and partial estimate of the economic costs of occupationally related illness in the United States. The results presented here are drawn from a comprehensive report prepared for NIOSH.[11] In preparing this estimate, we rely on epidemiologic estimates of occupational illnesses developed by Markowitz and Landrigan.[12] We focus our attention on the six leading causes of death from occupationally related disease—that is, cancer, nervous system disorders, pneumoconioses, chronic respiratory disease, cardiovascular and cerebrovascular disease, and renal disorders. We supplement the economic estimates of these six occupational illnesses with partial estimates of the cost of illness for chronic, nonfatal occupational illness. Thus, we begin to assemble a composite framework for understanding the magnitude of the economic costs of occupationally related disease.

METHODS AND DATA

Two approaches can be used in estimating the costs of illness by the human capital method. Prevalence-based costs provide an estimate of the direct and indirect economic burden in a period of time (the base period) as a result of the prevalence of disease, a period most often a year in length. Included are the costs of the base-year manifestations of sequelae of disease that may have had its onset in the base year or any time prior to the base year. Prevalence costs measure the value of resources used or lost during a specified period of time, regardless of the time of disease onset.

Incidence-based costs represent the lifetime costs resulting from the disease or illness. In the aggregate, incidence costs in a given base year refer to the likely course of a disease and its duration, including survival rates since onset, medical care that will be used and its cost during the duration of the disease, and the impact of the disease on employment, housekeeping, and earnings.

Relatively few incidence-based studies exist, but the state of the art is illustrated by three studies. Hartunian, Smart, and Thompson[13] estimated the lifetime costs of cancer, coronary heart disease, stroke, and motor vehicle injuries. Policy Analysis, Inc. conducted a study for the National Center for Health Statistics.[14] This report examines the incidence-based costs of breast cancer, diabetes mellitus, rheumatoid arthritis, stroke, and acute lymphocytic leukemia. Oster, Colditz, and Kelly (1984) estimated the costs of smoking and the benefits of quitting in their book, *The Economic Costs of Smoking and Benefits to Quitting.*[15]

These studies investigate direct and indirect costs by modeling the disease process from onset until cure or death, including the trends of important parameters such as incidence, survival, use and cost of medical care, and time lost from work and housekeeping. In each of these studies, a great deal of effort was expended in locating and making the most of available data, which often were originally gathered for other purposes, were incomplete, and had to be modified to meet the needs of incidence costs analysis. These studies are impressive in their demonstration that incidence-based costs are methodologically feasible, and in their use of extensive sensitivity analyses to reveal the impact of alternative assumptions and parameter values on estimated costs.

For the incidence-based lifetime costs of occupational disease, data are needed on the number of *new* cases of cancer, heart disease, respiratory disease, renal disorders, and so on that are caused by or associated with various unhealthy occupations. To obtain estimates of lifetime costs of these *new* cases, one must have information on the severity of disease from onset, the direct medical costs incurred from onset to death, the productive time lost during this period, and the lag time between diagnosis and death. Owing to idiosyncrasies in the manner by which most occupational diseases are managed and recorded, accurate data both on incidence and cost are difficult to secure. Without substantial primary data collection and analysis, which were outside the resource constraints of the NIOSH project, the current data limitations for age-specific and sex-specific incidence rates and severity of occupational disease preclude the development of an incidence-based cost of illness estimate. The purpose of this report is to develop a reasonable appreciation for the potential magnitude of the economic cost of occupational disease in the United States in the face of less than optimal data.

The prevalence-based methodology estimates the direct and indirect costs of occupational disease using a step-down accounting strategy and available national data. The prevalence method is the more commonly used accounting strategy due to the less extensive data requirements. This method is primarily concerned with costs during a fixed period of time, normally a calendar year. The economic costs associated with occupational disease are estimated in this analysis using a prevalence-based methodology, following the work of Rice and colleagues.[16–18] The cost of disease is measured by the cost of resources consumed as the result of the disease during one year, and by the value of the lost productivity resulting from morbidity and premature mortality caused by the disease during that year. In estimating the economic burden resulting from the prevalence of disease, the conventional prevalence methodology attributes the future costs of premature mortality to the year in question, using discounting techniques to estimate the present value of future losses.

Following the prevalence-based method, we apply cost of illness accounting techniques to calculate the present value of the direct and indirect costs associated with occupational disease. Using the National Hospital Discharge Survey,[19] we calculated the total number of days spent in the hospital by patients with a primary diagnosis for each of the attributable occupational illness groups defined by specific ICD-9 codes for the occupational diseases most responsible for worker mortality presented earlier.[12] Total days of hospitalization by disease group were transformed to obtain standardized proportions of national hospital utilization attributable to occupational disease. We applied these proportions to the national health expenditure accounts (minus nursing home costs), estimated by the Health Care Financing Administration,[20] to obtain an estimate of direct medical costs. The direct costs of nursing home care for occupationally related disease were estimated using the National Nursing Home Survey.[21] These cost estimates, using diagnosis-specific nursing home length-of-stay data, were added to medical expenditure estimates to obtain an estimate of total direct costs.

Indirect costs were estimated using age-specific, sex-specific, and disease-specific mortality data from the National Center for Health Statistics,[22] life table estimates,[23] and expected earnings and labor force participation data from the Bureau of Labor Statistics.[24] By applying the attributable risk proportions developed by Markowitz and Landrigan[12] to the total estimates of individual costs by disease, the present value of the indirect costs of premature mortality due to occupational disease is estimated for the base year 1992. Finally, we calculated national disease-specific trends over time in the ratios of morbidity costs to direct costs, and morbidity costs to mortality costs[17,25] to obtain an estimate of the morbidity costs for the occupational diseases that comprise the major causes of death from occupational disease. All economic estimates are presented in 1992 dollars. Assumptions regarding age-specific labor force participation rates, discount rates, and administrative costs can be found in the complete report.[11]

In addition to estimating the economic costs associated with the occupational diseases responsible for major causes of death in the United States, we investigated the costs of specific nonfatal occupational diseases, including skin diseases and carpal tunnel syndrome, as reported to the Bureau of Labor Statistics. Industry-specific wage rates were applied to lost work time to obtain a conservative estimate of indirect costs. Direct costs were based on estimates obtained from published data from the National Council on Compensation Insurance.[8]

RESULTS

The annual economic cost of occupational disease in the United States is greater than $25.5 billion in 1992 dollars. Fatalities due to occupational diseases comprise

TABLE 1. Summary of Costs of Selected Occupationally Related Diseases—1992 (Costs in 000s)

Economic Cost	Cost of Fatal Occupational Diseases	Cost of Nonfatal Occupational Diseases	Total Cost of Occupational Diseases
Direct	$10,699,670	$5,370,452	$16,070,122
Indirect	$8,992,864	$472,336	$9,465,200
Mortality	$7,003,204	—	
Morbidity	$1,989,661	$472,336	
Total	$19,692,534	$5,842,788	$25,535,322

SOURCES: U.S. Health Care Financing Administration, Health Care Financing Review, Fall 1994; National Hospital Discharge Survey, National Center for Health Statistics, 1992; National Nursing Home Survey, National Center for Health Statistics, 1985; Medical Care Component, Consumer Price Index, Bureau of Labor Statistics, Department of Labor, 1995; Money Income of Households, Families and Persons in the United States, 1992; U.S. Bureau of the Census, 1993; and, Tables 2-6, Chapter 6: National costs of occupationally-related disease, in Costs of Occupational Injuries and Illnesses. NIOSH Final Report. Contract #U60CCU902886-07. Internal Document, 1995.

77 percent of the total. Of the $19.7 billion losses due to deaths from occupational disease in 1992, 54 percent are direct costs, 36 percent are mortality costs, and 10 percent are morbidity costs. Direct costs comprise 92 percent of total losses for reported nonfatal occupational illness. These results are summarized in TABLE 1.

The distribution by diagnosis of total economic costs for fatal occupational disease shows that the greatest losses are caused by cancer, diseases of the circulatory system, and chronic respiratory disease, accounting for $9.4 billion, $5.8 billion, and $3.9 billion, respectively. Together these three diseases accounted for 97 percent of the economic costs of fatal occupational illness.

TABLE 2 presents the range of total costs of occupational illness by disease, for fatal occupational illness, estimated at $19.7 billion dollars, with a high estimate of $24.2 billion and a low estimate of $15.2 billion. Range estimates are determined by applying the attributable risk proportions of Markowitz and Landrigan[12] to the disease-specific economic cost calculations. Total estimated costs for cancer amount to $9.4 billion, with a high estimate of $11.7 billion to a low estimate of $7.0 billion. Total estimated costs for nervous system disorders amount to $286 million, with a high estimate of $429 million to a low estimate of $143 million.

Total estimated costs for pneumoconioses amount to $202 million. Total estimated costs for chronic respiratory disease amount to $3.9 billion. Total estimated costs for cardiovascular and cerebrovascular diseases amount to $5.8 billion, with a high estimate of $7.7 billion to a low estimate of $3.9 billion. Total estimated costs for renal disorders amount to $151 million, with a high estimate of $226 million to a low estimate of $15 million.

TABLE 3 presents the breakdown of direct and indirect costs for fatal occupational illness. Total direct costs amount to $10.7 billion, and indirect costs are $9.0 billion.

TABLE 2. Range of Total Costs of Occupational Fatalities, by Disease (Costs in 000s)

Disease[b]	Estimated Proportion Due to Occupation[c]	Total Cost Range[a]		
		Low Estimate	High Estimate	Midpoint Estimate
Cancer	6-10%	$7,030,400	$11,717,334	$9,373,867
Nervous System Disorders	1-3%	$143,060	$429,180	$286,120
Pneumoconioses	100%	$201,654	$201,654	$201,654
Chronic respiratory disease	10%	$3,904,621	$3,904,621	$3,904,621
Cardiovascular and cerebrovascular disease	5-10%	$3,850,293	$7,700,586	$5,775,439
Renal disorders	1-3%	$75,416	$226,249	$150,833
Total		$15,205,444	$24,179,623	$19,692,533

SOURCES: U.S. Health Care Financing Administration, Health Care Financing Review, Fall 1994; National Hospital Discharge Survey, National Center for Health Statistics, 1992; National Nursing Home Survey, National Center for Health Statistics, 1985; Medical Care Component, Consumer Price Index, Bureau of Labor Statistics, Department of Labor, 1995; Money Income of Households, Families and Persons in the United States, 1992; U.S. Bureau of the Census, 1993.

[a] All cost estimates are in 1992 dollars. Low and High Range Estimates are directly proportional to epidemiologic estimates of attributable risk.[12]

[b] Specific ICD-9 codes used to define diseases are listed in Appendix A.

[c] Estimated proportions are from Markowitz and Landrigan.[12]

The total mortality costs amount to $7.0 billion, and total morbidity costs amount to $2.0 billion.

The range of estimates for the total direct and indirect costs for fatal occupational illness is $25.6 billion, with a high estimate of $32.3 billion and a low estimate of $18.8 billion. The midpoint estimate for total direct costs is $10.7 billion, and that for total indirect costs is $9.0 billion. The midpoint estimate for mortality is $7.0 billion, and that for morbidity is $2.0 billion. These results are presented in TABLE 4.

TABLE 5 presents the number of new cases of occupational illnesses and morbidity costs by industry and category of illness in 1992. The total costs for morbidity are $472 million. TABLE 6 presents the number and estimated total medical costs of new cases of occupational illnesses by industry and category of illness. These costs amount to over $5 billion.

DISCUSSION

In many ways, the methodological challenges researchers must face in estimating the economic costs of occupationally related disease mirror the challenges of industrial regulation policy, where fragmented information systems diffuse and obscure the predictable health effects of occupational hazards. Occupational health policy analysis—that is, the ability to analyze the effect of disease prevention technologies and

TABLE 3. Range of Total Costs of Occupational Fatalities by Direct and Indirect Costs by Disease (Midpoint Estimates) (Costs in 000s)

	Cancer	Nervous System Disorders	Pneumoconioses	Chronic Respiratory Disease	Cerebrovascular and Cardiovascular Disease	Renal Disorders	Total
Direct Cost	$4,521,965	$241,740	$8,585	$2,634,150	$3,214,237	$78,993	$10,699,670
Indirect Cost	$4,851,902	$44,380	$193,069	$1,270,471	$2,561,202	$71,839	$8,992,863
Mortality	$4,160,602	$25,393	$77,470	$511,019	$2,196,282	$32,438	$7,003,204
Morbidity	$691,300	$18,987	$115,599	$759,452	$364,921	$39,402	$1,989,661
Total	$9,373,867	$286,120	$201,654	$3,904,621	$5,775,439	$150,833	$19,692,534

SOURCES: U.S. Health Care Financing Administration, Health Care Financing Review, Fall 1994; National Hospital Discharge Survey, National Center for Health Statistics, 1992; National Nursing Home Survey, National Center for Health Statistics, 1985; Medical Care Component, Consumer Price Index, Bureau of Labor Statistics, Department of Labor, 1995; Money Income of Households, Families and Persons in the United States, 1992; U.S. Bureau of the Census, 1993.

TABLE 4. Range of Direct and Indirect Costs of Occupational Disease Fatalities (Costs in 000s)

	Total Cost Range[a]		
Economic Cost	Low Estimate	High Estimate	Midpoint Estimate
Direct cost	$8,337,400	$13,061,940	$10,699,670
Indirect cost	$6,868,044	$11,117,682	$8,992,864
Mortality	$5,202,044	$8,804,364	7,003,204
Morbidity	$1,666,000	$2,313,319	$1,989,660
Total	$15,205,444	$24,179,623	$19,692,533

SOURCES: U.S. Health Care Financing Administration, Health Care Financing Review, Fall 1994; National Hospital Discharge Survey, National Center for Health Statistics, 1992; National Nursing Home Survey, National Center for Health Statistics, 1985; Medical Care Component, Consumer Price Index, Bureau of Labor Statistics, Department of Labor, 1995; Money Income of Households, Families and Persons in the United States, 1992; U.S. Bureau of the Census, 1993.

[a] All cost estimates are in 1992 dollars. Low and High Range Estimates are directly proportional to epidemiologic estimates of attributable risk.[12]

clinical detection and treatment systems on health outcomes, cost of resources, and ultimately on productivity—is severely hampered by the fragmented information systems that are associated with the over 1500 employer-based health insurance plans for working populations. In addition, the loss of continuous medical history and follow-up data due to the separation of Medicare, the insurer for the population 65 years and older, from private employer-based insurance information systems further limits the data accessibility that is necessary to understand the full spectrum of the costs of occupationally related disease over the life span.

In order to assess the reliability of our estimates, we performed a sensitivity analysis. We analyzed the effect on our results of the assumptions used to estimate morbidity costs. To perform the sensitivity analysis, we calculated morbidity costs two ways. In TABLES 2-4, we presented estimates based on the calculation of morbidity costs as a ratio to mortality costs. TABLES 7-9 present estimates based on the calculation of morbidity costs as a ratio to direct costs. We estimated the ratio as a *linear function* of 1980 and 1985 ratios, calculated by Rice and colleagues.[17,25]

We find the method used does not substantially affect the final estimate of the total costs of occupational disease. The total economic cost estimates vary by less than 10% at midpoint.

Estimates by disease will vary according to the relationship between direct costs and mortality costs within disease categories. For some diseases such as cancer, using a ratio for morbidity costs that is based on mortality costs, the total estimate of the costs of cancer is slightly lower. This is due to the high relative proportion of direct costs to mortality costs for cancer patients. This relationship is not true for pneumoconioses, which have much higher ratios of mortality costs to direct costs. Therefore, the estimate of total costs for pneumoconioses, using morbidity cost based

TABLE 5. Number of New Cases of Occupational Illnesses and Morbidity Costs by Industry and Category of Illness, 1992 (000s)

	Agriculture, Forestry, Fishing	Mining	Construction	Manufacturing	Transportation and Public Utilities	Wholesale and Retail Trade	Finance, Insurance, Real Estate	Services	Private Industry, All
Total illnesses	6.2	1.9	10.5	292.3	16.7	43.9	16.1	69.8	457.4
Skin diseases or disorders	2.7	0.2	2.4	31.2	2.9	5.6	1.1	16.9	63.0
Dust diseases of the lungs	0.0	0.6	0.1	1.0	0.0	0.2	0.5	0.5	2.4
Respiratory conditions due to toxic agents	0.4	0.1	1.0	10.0	1.1	3.3	0.9	6.8	23.6
Poisoning	0.1	0.0	0.5	3.5	0.4	1.0	0.9	1.4	7.0
Disorders due to physical agents	0.4	0.1	1.2	11.1	0.9	0.0	0.8	3.7	18.2
Disorders associated with repeated trauma	1.5	0.7	2.2	219.9	8.7	20.2	11.4	17.3	281.9
All other occupational diseases	1.1	0.2	3.2	15.7	2.5	9.6	1.9	23.3	57.5
Lost workday cases[a]									
Total (including restricted works)	1.8	0.5	3.6	119.9	6.6	16.2	6.7	22.1	177.4
Average lost workdays per lost workday case	19	27	28	34	30	39	39	27	33
Average hourly earnings[b]	10.6	11.5	14.5	14.1	13.5	9.3	10.8	10.5	10.6
Total morbidity costs[c]	$2,787,321	$1,215,330	$12,473,121	$314,954,299	$21,061,235	$46,698,107	$20,459,615	$52,687,368	$472,336,400

SOURCES: U.S. Bureau of Labor Statistics, Bulletin 2370, supplement to Employment and Earnings, July 1991; and Employment and Earnings, monthly.
ASSUMPTION: Average lost workdays come from Bureau of Labor Statistics 1991 data.
[a] We assume that restricted workdays are 20 percent of a workday.
[b] Includes 17% administrative cost.
[c] Agricultural industries' wages come from average hourly earnings.

TABLE 6. Number and Estimated Total Medical Costs of New Cases of Occupational Illnesses by Industry and Category of Illness (Costs in 000s)

Industry Division	Total Illnesses	Skin Diseases or Disorders	Dust Diseases of the Lungs	Respiratory Conditions due to Toxic Agents	Poisoning	Disorders due to Physical Agents	Disorders Associated with Repeated Trauma	All Other Occupational Illnesses
Private industry, all cases	457.40	63.00	2.40	23.60	7.00	18.20	281.90	57.50
Mean medical cost using Ohio Worker 's Compensation	—	$0.40	$5.70	$5.70	$5.70	$5.70	$5.15	$5.70
Mean medical cost using NCCI	—	$8.75	$8.75	$8.75	$8.75	$8.75	$8.75	$8.75
Total medical cost using Worker's Compensation	$2,838,576	$34,187	$18,516	$182,072	$54,004	$140,411	$1,965,779	$443,607
Total medical cost using NCCI	$5,370,452	$745,896	$28,415	$279,415	$82,877	$215,481	$3,337,589	$680,778

SOURCES: U.S. Bureau of Labor Statistics, Occupational Injuries and Illnesses in the U.S. by Industry, Bulletin 2424, Govt. Printing Office, Washington DC, 1993; The Industrial Commission of Ohio and Division of Safety and Hygiene, Average Costs of Occupational Injuries and Illnesses 1980–1983, State of Ohio, March 1986; Webster & Snook; Neumark *et al.*[8]

NOTE: Medical costs are updated from the base years using medical portion of the consumer price index.

TABLE 7. Range of Total Costs of Occupational Fatalities, by Disease Sensitivity Analysis: Assumptions for Morbidity Costs Based on Estimated Direct Costs (Costs in 000s)

Disease[b]	Estimated Proportion Due to Occupation[c]	Total Cost Range[a]		
		Low Estimate	High Estimate	Midpoint Estimate
Cancer	6-10%	$7,464,566	$12,440,943	$9,952,754
Nervous system disorders	1-3%	$145,141	$435,423	$290,282
Pneumoconioses	100%	$89,794	$89,794	$89,794
Chronic respiratory disease	10%	$4,170,959	$4,170,959	$4,170,959
Cardiovascular and cerebro-vascular disease	5-10%	$4,085,800	$8,171,600	$6,128,700
Renal disorders	1-3%	$59,246	$177,737	$118,491
Total		$16,015,505	$25,486,455	$20,750,980

SOURCES: U.S. Health Care Financing Administration, Health Care Financing Review, Fall 1994; National Discharge Survey, National Center for Health Statistics, 1992; National Nursing Home Survey, National Center for Health Statistics, 1985; Medical Care Component, Consumer Price Index, Bureau of Labor Statistics, Department of Labor, 1995; Money Income of Households, Families and Persons in the United States, 1992; U.S. Bureau of the Census, 1993.

[a] All cost estimates are in 1992 dollars. Low and High Range Estimates are directly proportional to epidemiologic estimates of attributable risk.[12]

[b] Specific ICD-9 codes used to define diseases are listed in Appendix A.

[c] Estimated proportions are from Markowitz and Landrigan.[12]

on mortality cost, is substantially higher than the estimate for pneumoconioses using morbidity costs based on direct costs. Overall, in the estimates presented, there appears to be a balancing out of these effects, so that the total estimate appears stable.

There are other assumptions that should be tested in future research. Specifically, the assumptions regarding homogeneity of occupational disease death rates with national average age-specific death rates should be examined. If, for instance, workers with occupationally acquired cancer die at an earlier age than patients whose cancers are caused by nonoccupational factors, our economic costs estimates are likely to be biased downwards. A faster transition time between stages of severity would be consistent with higher concentrations of exposure to hazards at the work place, if less concentrated exposures to similar hazards in the environment are characterized by a ''dilutional effect'' in triggering pathologic disease responses.

National surveys and data sets for describing medical care utilization patterns for the general population should be explored further for measures and data regarding costs and outcomes of occupationally related disease. These rich sources of clinical and socioeconomic data have not been examined, for the most part, for model building and testing of hypotheses regarding health status, medical expenditure, and occupational status. Research directed toward the sources of knowledge in data sets (such as the National Medical Expenditure Survey[20]) would be a productive use of health policy research dollars.

TABLE 8. Total Costs of Occupational Fatalities by Direct and Indirect Costs by Disease (Midpoint Estimates) Sensitivity Analysis: Assumptions for Morbidity Costs Based on Estimated Direct Costs (Costs in 000s)

	Cancer	Nervous System Disorders	Pneumoconioses	Chronic Respiratory Disease	Cerebrovascular and Cardiovascular Disease	Renal Disorders	Total
Direct cost	$4,521,965	$241,740	$8,585	$2,634,150	$3,214,237	$78,993	$10,699,670
Indirect cost	$5,430,790	$48,542	$81,209	$1,536,809	$2,914,463	$39,498	$10,051,311
Mortality	$4,160,602	$25,393	$77,470	$511,019	$2,196,282	$32,438	$7,003,204
Morbidity	$1,270,188	$23,149	$3,739	$1,025,790	$718,181	$7,060	$3,048,107
Total	$9,952,754	$290,282	$89,794	$4,170,959	$6,128,700	$118,491	$20,720,981

SOURCES: U.S. Health Care Financing Administration, Health Care Financing Review, Fall 1994; National Hospital Discharge Survey, National Center for Health Statistics, 1992; National Nursing Home Survey, National Center for Health Statistics, 1985; Medical Care Component, Consumer Price Index, Bureau of Labor Statistics, Department of Labor, 1995; Money Income of Households, Families and Persons in the United States, 1992; U.S. Bureau of the Census, 1993.

TABLE 9. Range of Total Direct and Indirect Costs of Occupational Disease Fatalities Sensitivity Analysis: Assumptions for Morbidity Costs Based on Estimated Direct Costs (Costs in 000s)

	Total Cost Range[a]		
Economic Cost	Low Estimate	High Estimate	Midpoint Estimate
Direct cost	$8,337,400	$13,061,940	$10,699,670
Indirect cost			$10,051,310
Mortality	$5,202,044	$8,804,364	$7,003,204
Morbidity	$2,476,061	$3,620,151	$3,048,106
Total	$16,015,505	$25,486,455	$20,750,980

SOURCES: U.S. Health Care Financing Administration, Health Care Financing Review, Fall 1994; National Hospital Discharge Survey, National Center for Health Statistics, 1992; National Nursing Home Survey, National Center for Health Statistics, 1985; Medical Care Component, Consumer Price Index, Bureau of Labor Statistics, Department of Labor, 1995; Money Income of Households, Families and Persons in the United States, 1992; U.S. Bureau of the Census, 1993.

[a] All cost estimates are in 1992 dollars. Low and High Range Estimates are directly proportional to epidemiologic estimates of attributable risk.[12]

In summary, the estimates presented in this report are conservative. The economic cost estimates associated with deaths due to occupational disease include morbidity costs, but do not include costs for persons diagnosed with potentially fatal occupationally related diseases who did not die during 1992. In addition, no economic costs were attributed to deaths due to occupationally related heart disease after age 65. Our supplement to the costs of fatal illness, the Bureau of Labor Statistics report of occupationally related chronic disease[24] is widely criticized as being underreported. Estimates from the literature indicate the underreporting may be as much as threefold.[10]

CONCLUSION

A full accounting of the social and economic costs of occupational disease should include an analysis of distributional equity. Economic theory predicts that society will underinvest in areas where the benefits of the investment reach beyond the immediate investors. Currently, financial responsibility for disease due to occupational hazards is shifted away from Workers' Compensation, where it properly belongs, toward future Medicare expenses. This shift results in a "hidden tax," in which costs of occupational disease are externalized and thus are funded by general and payroll taxes.

Correction of this situation would create private market incentives for prevention of occupational disease and thus would lead to an increase in efficiency of the Medicare health insurance system. Analyses demonstrating the comparative efficiencies of possible solutions to this distributional inequity would have significant health policy implications. However, cost of illness accounting methodologies, such as that presented in this paper, do not allow hypothesis-driven analysis of policy options addressing this hidden cost transfer from the private sector to the public sector.

The development of state-of-the-art health policy models is useful for economic forecasting and would contribute to our knowledge of the magnitude and scope of inefficiencies or inequities under current policy. Cost effectiveness analysis can simulate and compare the effects of alternate policy choices on workers' health outcomes and medical costs. However, such health policy analyses require the use of mathematical computer-based stochastic models of disease to simulate the dynamics of treatment protocols, patient outcomes, and costs. These policy models rely on clinical information of some detail, including characteristics of the episode of disease and treatment as well as the effect of the disease on the patient and the patient's family.

Occupational health policy models should include the hypotheses of the health services research literature concerning the effectiveness and costs of alternative primary and secondary prevention policies. Moreover, hypotheses of the biological sciences concerning occupational exposures, interactions of toxins with disease mechanisms, and duration of risk due to exposure also should be considered as parameters in health policy models. Data gathered to document both the social severity and the clinical severity of occupationally related disease would be extremely useful and would enhance the validity of economic projections. In particular, occupationally related cancer and heart disease require further specificity. Questions to address regarding occupationally related cancers include the following:

> Are there occupationally related cancers that differ systematically from similar cancers with no known occupational risk factors (1) in progression rates between stages? (2) in latency periods? or (3) in stage-specific duration?

The variables that define transition times and progression probabilities between stages of disease severity can substantially affect the economic estimates. For heart disease, a stochastic model that incorporated mathematical decay functions for the declining rate of mortality from heart disease after age 65 due to occupational hypertension acquired before age 65 would substantially improve the economic cost estimates.

In summary, the current economic burden of occupational disease appears to be significant. Further economic research should undertake the task of probabilistic computer-based modeling to advance the scientific basis of the estimates. Monte Carlo sampling methods can estimate the health and economic burdens with statistical precision. Research models developed with epidemiologic detail in a dynamic computer-based optimization environment will enrich the economic contribution to debates concerning occupational health policy.

REFERENCES

1. U.S. Department of Labor, Occupational Safety and Health Administration, Office of Regulatory Analysis. 1995. Unpublished economic and environmental analysis documents are available in: OSHA Docket Office Technical Data Center, Room S-6212, 200 Constitution Avenue NW, Washington, DC 20210.

2. Institute of Medicine. 1981. Costs of environment-related health effects: A plan for continuing study. National Academy Press. Washington, DC.
3. U.S. Department of Health and Human Services. 1993. Morb. Mortal. Wkly Rep. **42**(39): 757-772.
4. U.S. Department of Health and Human Services. 1993. Vital and Health Statistics: Health Conditions among the Currently Employed: United States, 1988. Series 10, No. 198, July 1993.
5. Ruchlin, H. S., L. A. Melcher & M. H. Alderman. 1984. A comparative economic analysis of work-related hypertension care programs. J. Occup. Med. **26**(1): 45-49.
6. Webster, B. S. & S. H. Snook. 1994. The cost of compensable upper extremity cumulative trauma disorders. J. Occup. Med. **36**(7): 713-715.
7. Tanaka, S., P. Seligman, W. Halperin *et al.* 1988. Use of workers' compensation claims data for surveillance of cumulative trauma disorders. J. Occup. Med. **30**(6): 488-492.
8. Neumark, D., R. W. Johnson, E. A. Bresnitz, H. Frumkin, M. Hodgson & C. Needleman. 1991. Cost of occupational injury and illness in Pennsylvania. J. Occup. Med. **33**(9): 971-976.
9. Fahs, M. C., S. B. Markowitz, E. Fischer, J. Shapiro & P. J. Landrigan. 1989. Health costs of occupational disease in New York State. Am. J. Ind. Med. **16:** 437-449.
10. Oleinick, A., K. E. Guire, V. M. Hawthorne *et al.* 1993. Current methods of estimating severity for occupational injuries and illnesses: Data from the 1986 Michigan Comprehensive Compensable Injury and Illness Database. Am. J. Ind. Med. **23:** 231-252.
11. Leigh, J. P., S. Markowitz, M. Fahs, C. Shin & P. Landrigan. 1996. Cost of occupational injuries and illnesses. *In* Costs of Occupational Injuries and Illnesses. NIOSH Final Report. Contract #U60CCU902886-07.
12. Markowitz, S. B. & P. J. Landrigan. 1996. Counting occupational illness. Chapter 3. *In* Costs of Occupational Injuries and Illnesses. NIOSH Final Report. Contract #U60CCU902886-07.
13. Hartunian, N. S., C. N. Smart & M. S. Thompson. 1981. The Incidence and Economic Cost of Major Health Impairments. D. C. Heath. Lexington, MA.
14. Policy Analysis, Inc. 1981. Evaluation of Cost of Illness Ascertainment Methodology. Final Report, DHHS Pub. No. 233-79-2048.
15. Oster, Colditz & Kelly. 1984. The Economic Costs of Smoking and Benefits to Quitting. Lexington Books, D. C. Heath. Lexington, MA.
16. Rice, D. P. 1966. Estimating the Cost of Illness. Health Economic Series. U.S. Department of Health Education and Welfare. PHS Pub. No. 974-6. Public Health Service, No. 6. Washington, DC.
17. Rice, D. P., T. A. Hodgson & A. N. Kopstein. 1985. The economic costs of illness: A replication and update. Health Care Financing Rev. **7**(1): 61-80.
18. Hodgson, T. A. & M. Meiners. 1982. Cost of illness methodology: A guide to current practices and procedures. Milbank Mem. Fund Q. **60**(3): 429-462.
19. U.S. Department of Health and Human Services. 1991. Vital and Health Statistics: Detailed Diagnoses and Procedures, National Hospital Discharge Survey.
20. U.S. Department of Health and Human Services, Agency for Health Care Policy and Research. 1994. 1987 National Medical Expenditure Survey. Washington, DC.
21. U.S. Department of Health and Human Services, National Center for Health Statistics. 1985. National Nursing Home Survey, 1985. Washington, DC.
22. U.S. Department of Health and Human Services, National Center for Health Statistics. 1993. Work Table I. Deaths from Each Cause by 5-year Age Groups, Race and Sex: United States, 1991. Vital Statistics of the U.S., annual and unpublished data. Washington, DC.
23. U.S. Department of Health and Human Services, National Center for Health Statistics. 1994. Life Tables. Vital Statistics of the U.S., 1990. Volume II, Sec. 6, Pub No. 94-1104. Washington, DC.

24. U.S. BUREAU OF LABOR STATISTICS. 1991. Bulletin 2370, supplement to Employment and Earnings, July 1991; and Employment and Earnings, monthly.
25. RICE, D. P., T. A. HODGSON & F. CAPELL. 1989. The economic burden of cancer, 1985: United States and California. Chapter 3. *In* Cancer Care and Cost. DRGs and Beyond. R. H. Scheffler & N. C. Andrews, Eds.: 39-59. Health Administration Press Perspectives. Ann Arbor, MI.

Can Protecting Human Health and the Environment Be Justified on Cost-Benefit Grounds?

RUTH RUTTENBERG

Ruth Ruttenberg & Associates, Inc.
5107 Benton Avenue
Bethesda, Maryland 20814

Cost-benefit analysis, to be accurate, should eliminate externalities and reach out to measure all costs and all benefits associated with a pending program. Clearly, any policy to protect human health and the environment should have more advantages than disadvantages. How these costs and benefits are counted and what is counted are key. The cost-benefit debate can not be ignored. The benefits to workers; to the community; to local, state, and federal government; and often to the business community as well nearly always exceed costs. The full impact of an individual's death or disabilities can be staggering. It is important to build models and data bases to make the full costs and benefits clear to decision makers and to present these full costs and benefits in academically sound and analytically rigorous ways.

Dictionary definitions of *cost* focus not on dollars, but on sacrifice, distress, pain, and suffering. Likewise, definitions of *benefits* focus on value and welfare.

Cost-benefit analysis should be changed in two majors ways: (1) how measurements are made and (2) the paradigms used to make measurements.

CHANGE HOW MEASUREMENTS ARE MADE

Proactive approaches for redefining cost-benefit analysis from neoclassical models to full and realistic accounting are needed. Costs and benefits for a number of stakeholders, not just the business community, should be measured. More than short-run, direct costs that can be measured in dollars must be part of the accounting. Any accounting should include:

- long-run costs and benefits–definitely beyond reports on quarterly profits or year-end balance sheets;
- indirect costs and benefits–including effects on families when a worker is injured or becomes chronically ill; the economic effect on a community when, because of badly polluted air, it becomes difficult to recruit new businesses;
- the positive as well as the negative impacts of a regulation–with a focus on the economic and social assets of healthy workers and healthy community residents;

- nonquantitative costs and benefits as well as those that are not best expressed in dollars–including life, good health, and a longer life.

Fuller use of already existing numbers is important and is a straightforward task. For example, according to the National Safety Council, workplace accidents cost United States businesses and society more than $115 billion per year.[1] This includes such costs as wage and productivity losses of $62.5 billion, administrative expenses of $14.5 billion, and lost work time to employers of $10.2 billion. Avoiding workplace accidents not only would save lives, it would save the businesses of this country billions of dollars every year. Few, if any, would argue that expenditure for compensation is preferable to expenditure for prevention of death, disease, and injury. Yet, the manager who pays for compliance technology may not be the same manager that pays for disability, and so no trade-off analysis is ever performed. In addition, once compliance technology is in place, one can rarely identify the injury or illness that has been diverted as a result of creating a safer and more healthful workplace. Well over half the costs of workplace accidents according to the National Safety Council were for lost productivity and administrative expenses. It is simply not economically responsible to talk about the benefits of a foregone incident without making the full value of such losses central to analysis.

CHANGE THE PARADIGMS USED TO MAKE MEASUREMENTS

There are many established models that can be used as a springboard for new measurement models.

Human Resource Damage Assessment

As natural resource damage assessments (NRDA) gain in usage, so too should we develop human resource damage assessments. Just as damage to natural resources may have long-term irreparable impact, so may damage to a person.

The death or permanent disability of an individual human being leaves society with just as much of an irreplaceable natural resource as the loss of a vista or a recreational site or the abundance of a particular plant cover. If the unique and irreplaceable assets of an individual worker, not lost work days, were the focus of analysis, worker protection might be stronger.

The "nonuse" value of human health deserves the same consideration as the nonuse value of natural resources. Just as professionals have come to acknowledge that more is lost from natural resources than just their commercial value and use, more that their "commercial value" is lost to individuals, their families, and communities when individuals are "damaged." Lost work days are but one measurement of use value or loss.

The intrinsic value of natural resources should be an inherent part of all Natural Resource Damage Assessments. Likewise, the intrinsic value of an individual's health should be an inherent part of any "human resource damage assessment" that is part of regulatory and policy analysis.

Regulation and Improvements in Technology and Productivity

Regulation can and should be technology forcing. There are many instances in which regulation has literally been the "mother of invention." Regulation can be productivity enhancing, and we must increasingly document those examples that show that with carefully designed regulation, productivity and technology improvements can be the rule rather than the exception.

Regulation of the Grain Handling Industry

Dust in grain elevators was killing dozens of grain mill and grain elevator workers and destroying tens of millions of dollars of business property every year until OSHA began to develop safety regulations for the industry. In one month alone in the late 1970s six grain explosions and fires killed 56 people and caused over $100 million of damage. Since promulgation of the OSHA standard, death and damage from grain elevator explosions have declined significantly. And there is no evidence that the OSHA grain handling rule has posed hardship on industry. Threats of facility closures have not materialized. Instead, investment in plant and equipment is up; wages are up; and, at least from the perspective of employees, company profits are up as well.

Despite the concerns of industry spokespersons and many small business men and women, grain elevators and grain mills have not gone out of business. In 1993 the OSHA docket on grain dust was reviewed, and 60 companies were identified that had written directly to the Secretary of Labor during rule making to argue that their business might be forced to close if the grain dust rule was promulgated. Each of these 60 companies[2] was called, and at least 59 of them were still in business. (One had a disconnected telephone, and so its business status could not be determined). For at least 59 of 60 businesses to be still operating when all 60 felt they were in jeopardy due to a threatening regulation is an important story. Most were small businesses. The facilities were in 16 states–including Illinois, Indiana, Michigan, Minnesota, Missouri, Nebraska, Ohio, Pennsylvania, Tennessee, and Texas.

Regulation of the Vinyl Chloride Industry

Exposure to vinyl chloride during its production greatly increases the chances of a worker's developing angiosarcoma, a cancer of the liver. When OSHA began rule making, vinyl chloride producers claimed that the entire multibillion dollar industry was going to collapse and the producing firms would be forced to close down their operations. What happened? Within 18 months of promulgating the OSHA standard, new and more productive facilities were on line,[3] with at least six technological changes to make operations more efficient.

Regulation of the Cotton Textile Industry

Cotton dust has been responsible for the choking death and total disability of thousands of textile workers in the United States. Industry spokespersons foretold economic disaster if the proposed OSHA cotton dust regulation were promulgated. What happened? Industry was virtually in compliance in a matter of months, more than a year faster than the regulation required—with the textile industry modernized and more competitive than ever.[4] The postregulatory view of controlling cotton dust is a very different one from the prepromulgation debate. Rather than the predicted use of retrofits, add-ons, and enclosures, compliance was achieved primarily through the use of designed-in engineering controls. Cotton textile manufacturing is now more technologically consolidated, fully eliminating some of the processes that had previously been responsible for a substantial amount of worker exposure. New machine systems operate faster and with fewer breakdowns and errors. Energy efficiency, space efficiency, and materials efficiency have been achieved, and product quality has improved as well. Was small business adversely affected? A 1983 study for OSHA found that "there are not believed to be major economies of scale associated with . . . capital costs per unit of textile output."[4]

Regulations to Include Public Employees under OSHA

Extending OSHA coverage to all public sector employees, according to a study in 1994,[5] would actually save state and local governments across the United States more than $600 million a year, perhaps as much as $2.1 billion per year. It would also save the lives of hundreds of public employees and spare thousands of workers and their families the pain and suffering that comes with death and disability. Public-sector employees suffer 3.5 times as many work-related deaths as private-sector workers and 25 percent more injuries, yet they have OSHA protection in only half the states of this country. The lesson: save lives and save money.

Regulations that Mandate Worker Training

Worker training mandated by OSHA regulation can easily be credited with saving lives, health, and company property. A recent study of outcomes associated with training those who work with hazardous materials reported lives and health saved as a result of basic training.[6] A few brief examples:

- A training program in New York state that taught those who work in confined space to monitor the air in that space before entering it is credited with saving at least two lives. Two workers, upon returning from training, insisted on monitoring the air of a space they were about to enter and found lethal levels of chemicals. Days before, they would not have hesitated before entering the space, to their almost certain death.
- Just a few hours of awareness training may well have avoided a disaster similar to one that resulted in dozens of deaths in Hamlet, North Carolina. Workers returning from training found gates chained closed. Inside the gates where they worked were two rail cars filled with chlorine. Worker petitions led to the gates' being opened.

- HAZMAT training for some Michigan workers meant that when they experienced a spill of sulfuric acid, there was a rapid evacuation of the affected plant, with nausea the only adverse health effect.
- Active health and safety training following a disastrous petrochemical fire in California in the 1980s meant that when a similar fire occurred at the same facility 10 years later, the damage to plant and equipment was millions of dollars less than would have otherwise been the case, and quick action was credited with saving at least 5-6 lives.
- A worker returning to her Minnesota job after hazardous materials training realized that the procedure being used to pour mustard oil was extremely unsafe. After finding a responsive manager, she was thanked by management, because a spill of even a very small amount of the mustard oil would have caused an evacuation of the entire plant.

Noise Regulations

Many businesses have extended the useful life of their equipment in the process of complying with OSHA noise regulations. Two professors from North Carolina State testified before OSHA administrative law hearings that for less than one dollar and no down time the substitution of a piece of plastic for a piece of metal not only reduced noise, but also reduced vibration, thus adding years to the useful life of the affected equipment. Much of their work was with small businesses in the metal stamping and textile industries.

Similarly, when the noise level is reduced in compressed air tools–those used both in construction and industrial settings–the result is a lower level of vibration and longer useful life for the equipment.

GROWTH OF POLLUTION CONTROL AND HAZARD ABATEMENT INDUSTRIES

The pollution control and hazard abatement industries have been growth areas throughout the United States economy, and much of the growth has been in small and emerging businesses. The contribution of regulation to this growth in sales, revenue, jobs, and economic base should not be excluded from any matrix.

The impact of regulation on business is not only on the regulated companies. Many United States businesses license and sell hazard abatement technology and equipment. Pollution control and hazard abatement are among the fastest growing markets for industry in the United States. From safety boots to air scrubbers, from improved monitoring equipment to built-in engineering controls, the genius of United States creativity and entrepreneurship is generating hundreds of millions of dollars in new sales, and hundreds of new businesses have been spawned.

The promulgation of regulations creates identifiable market niches for new and emerging small businesses. For example, a conference held by EPA shortly after issuing regulations on asbestos brought over 500 businesses together, many of them small, to explore potential markets and a variety of compliance technologies. Or, to cite just one other example, many small and minority businesses have been created to help in compliance with lead abatement regulations. Saving a child from lead poisoning may save the child's future; it may also avoid expensive health and educational interventions for the affected child.

SUMMARY

The way to win the cost-benefit debate is to have clearly defined outcome measures. Most critical is a full accounting–i.e., long and short run, indirect and direct, nonquantitative and quantitative costs and benefits to all the relevant stakeholders. In this way externalities are eliminated, and eliminating externalities is a goal of every economist, regardless of political persuasion.

REFERENCES

1. National Safety Council. 1993. Accident Facts. National Safety Council. Itasca, IL.
2. Ruttenberg, R. 1994. Compliance with the OSHA Grain Handling Rule: Safety Measures Save Lives and Dollars. Contract K3-0841.0. U.S. Office of Technology Assessment. Washington, DC.
3. Dirks-Mason, S. & R. Ruttenberg. 1979. The effects of the OSHA vinyl chloride standard on the vinyl chloride industry. Prepared for the OSHA Policy Office. Washington, DC.
4. Ruttenberg, R. 1983. Compliance with the OSHA Cotton Dust Rule: The Role of Productivity Improving Technology. No. 233-7050.0. U.S. Office of Technology Assessment. Washington, DC.
5. Ruttenberg, R. 1994. Saving Money, Saving Lives: OSHA Coverage for Public Employees. American Federation of State, County, and Municipal Employees, Washington, DC.
6. Ruttenberg, R. 1993. Outcomes of HAZMAT Training. Draft prepared for National Institute of Environmental Health Sciences. Research Triangle Park, NC.

Mechanistic Modeling of Multiple Tumorigenesis: An Application to Data on Lung Tumors in Mice Exposed to Urethane[a]

A. Y. YAKOVLEV[b,c] AND L. V. PAVLOVA[d]

[b]*Department of Oncological Sciences*
Huntsman Cancer Institute
University of Utah
546 Chipeta Way, Suite 1100
Salt Lake City, Utah 84108

[d]*Department of Applied Mathematics*
St. Petersburg Technical University
29 Polytechnicheskaya Street
St. Petersburg 195251, Russia

INTRODUCTION

The strain A mouse lung tumor bioassay, developed as early as 1940,[1] has been used for the testing of hundreds of environmental chemicals for carcinogenic activity.[2] In particular, numerous experimental studies have amassed a large body of data on the formation of tumors, commonly referred to as adenomas, in the lungs of mice receiving different schedules of urethane. It is generally believed that the development of these benign tumors is irreversible and that they may progress to malignant carcinomas. The usual experimental practice is to count recognizable tumor foci in the lungs of mice sacrificed at different time intervals from the start of exposure. Clearly, both the tumor counts and the time of tumor latency provide a useful source of information on carcinogenic potency. A long-standing question is how can this information be utilized to make quantitative inferences about unobservable processes underlying multiple tumorigenesis. This challenge motivated Neyman and Scott[3] to develop a stochastic model of carcinogenesis aimed at the study of lung tumors induced by urethane. However, the authors limited their analysis of real data to qualitative conclusions about the expected values of tumor counts and their variations with time. Grosser and Whittemore[4] invoked distributional assumptions to analyze the number and size of lung tumors in outbred Swiss mice receiving urethane in their drinking water. Two hypotheses were tested to gain insight into the effects of chronic exposure. The first hypothesis postulates that each two-week exposure to urethane (which is thought of as the acute experiment) induces tumors independently of all other such exposures. The second hypothesis postulates that tumor growth is

[a]The research of A. Y. Y. is supported in part by National Cancer Institute Grant PO1-CA76466.
[c]Phone: 801/585-9543; fax: 801/585-5357; e-mail: yak@genetics.utah.edu

independent of the exposure rate at which urethane is administered. Both hypotheses were rejected by the likelihood ratio test, indicating that more complex biological mechanisms must be introduced to provide a realistic description of urethane-induced lung carcinogenesis.

A stochastic model of carcinogenesis developed by Yakovlev and Polig[5] is a good candidate for that purpose. Having been designed primarily for the analysis of radiation-induced carcinogenesis, this model describes and explains a wide range of experimental findings documented in the radiobiological literature, including dose-rate effects. The key feature of the model by Yakovlev and Polig is that it allows for radiation-induced cell killing to compete with the process of tumor promotion. The effects of cell toxicity are known to be inherent in the processes of chemical carcinogenesis as well. The model also contains parameters that account for the processes of lesion repair. In this paper, we apply the model proposed in Reference 5 to experimental data on urethane-induced carcinogenesis. In doing so, we extend the model to allow for multiplicity of tumors and interindividual variations in the initiation rate.

THE MODEL

According to the stochastic model proposed by Yakovlev and Polig[5] the cumulative number of tumors produced within the time interval $(0, t)$ is a Poisson random variable with the expected value given by

$$\Lambda(t) = \theta_1 \int_0^t h(u)\left(\int_0^{t-u} f(x) e^{\theta_2 \int_0^{u+x} h(z)dz}\, dx\right) du, \qquad \textbf{(1)}$$

where $h(u)$ is the dose rate (the rate of administration of a carcinogen), $f(x)$ is the promotion time distribution density, θ_1 and θ_2 are parameters that describe the sensitivity of cells to carcinogenic and toxic (cell-killing) modes of action, respectively. More specifically, $\theta_1 h(t)$ is the mean number of initiated cells per unit time given the dose rate $h(t)$. Similarly, the quantity $\theta_2 h(t)$ refers to the mean rate of formation of the lesions responsible for cell death.

In experiments with protracted exposures, the dose rate is usually kept constant over the exposure period T. In this case we can write

$$h(t) = \frac{D}{T}, \qquad 0 \le t \le T,$$

$$h(t) = 0,\ t > T, \qquad \textbf{(2)}$$

where D is a total dose of carcinogen. With $h(t)$ given by formula 2, formula 1 assumes the form:

$$\Lambda(t;T) = \theta_1 \varphi(t;T) = \frac{\theta_1 D}{T}\left[\int_0^T e^{-\frac{\theta_2 D}{T}x}\left(\int_0^{T-x} f(z)\, e^{-\frac{\theta_2 D}{T}z}\, dz\right) dx \right.$$

$$\left. + e^{-\theta_2 D}\left(\int_0^T F(t-x)dx - \int_0^T F(x)dx\right)\right] \text{ for } t > T, \qquad \textbf{(3)}$$

where $F(x)$ is the promotion time cumulative distribution function.

Formula 3 refers to experimental situations where animals are sacrificed at times larger than the period of exposure to urethane. A modification of formula 3 can readily be derived for $t \leq T$.[5] The sensitivity parameters θ_1 and θ_2 implicitly account for repair processes. An explicit description of the functioning of the repair system can be developed in terms of queuing theory,[5,6] but in the analysis of dose-rate effects it makes sense to regard θ_1 and θ_2 as constants in order to infer the contribution of lesion repair by the indirect route.

From the above model it follows that the number of tumors at time t is a Poisson process with the integral intensity $\Lambda(t;T)$. Grosser and Whittemore[4] noted an overdispersion effect, which may be attributed to pronounced interindividual variations in the adenoma counts. We observed a like effect when analyzing experimental data on urethane-induced tumorigenesis published by Shimkin *et al.*[7] This analysis suggested that a negative binomial distribution rather than a Poisson distribution of the number of tumors is consistent with the data. To obtain negative binomially distributed tumor counts under the model, we assume that the sensitivity parameter θ_1 (the mean number of initiated cells per unit dose) is a random variable that follows a gamma distribution, with a and $1/b$ standing for the shape and scale parameters of this distribution. Let $N(t;T)$ be the number of tumors per animal at time $t > 0$ given the period of exposure T. The corresponding randomization procedure results in the following distribution of this variable:

$$P(k) = \Pr\{N(t;T) = k\} = \binom{a+k-1}{k}\left[\frac{1}{1+b\varphi(t;T)}\right]^a \left[\frac{b\varphi(t;T)}{1+b\varphi(t;T)}\right]^k, \qquad (4)$$

with the parameter $\theta_1^* = ab$ representing the mean number of initiated cells per unit dose.

ESTIMATION OF THE MODEL PARAMETERS

Let t_i, $i = 1, \ldots, n$, be the sacrifice times, m_i, $i = 1, \ldots, n$, the number of animals sacrificed at t_i, and k_{ij}, $i = 1, \ldots, n, j = 1, \ldots, m_i$ the number of tumors observed in the jth animal sacrificed at t_i. Based on distribution 4, the likelihood function for these data is given by

$$L = \prod_{i=1}^{n}\prod_{j=1}^{m_i}\binom{a+k_{ij}-1}{k_{ij}}\left[\frac{1}{1+b\varphi(t_i;T)}\right]^a \left[\frac{b\varphi(t_i;T)}{1+b\varphi(t_i;T)}\right]^{k_{ij}}, \qquad (5)$$

where $\varphi(t;T)$ is specified by formula 3. It remains to specify the promotion time distribution involved in formula 3 and consequently in formula 5. To this end, the function $f(u)$ in formula 3 was assumed to be a gamma distribution density with scale parameter α and shape parameter β because this distribution, quite simple as it is, provides a good fit to various experimental and clinical data when incorporated in stochastic models of tumor latency.[8–10] To find the maximum likelihood estimates $\hat{a}$, $\hat{b}$, $\hat{\theta}_2$, $\hat{\alpha}$, $\hat{\beta}$ of the model parameters, the likelihood $L = L(a, b, \theta_2, \alpha, \beta)$ was maximized numerically by computer, using the algorithm BIFLEX from Reference 11. The maximum likelihood estimate of θ_1^* is given by $\hat{\theta}_1^* = \hat{a}\hat{b}$. To ensure stability of the estimation procedure, the search for estimates of the parameters a and α was

TABLE 1. Maximum Likelihood Estimates of the Model Parameters

T (days)	$\hat{\alpha}$	$\hat{\beta}$	$\hat{\tau} = \hat{\alpha}/\hat{\beta}$	$\hat{a}$	$\hat{b}$	θ_2
1	2	0.024	83	28	13.3 (3.50, 22.10)	2.75 (2.05, 3.45)
8	3	0.039	76	35	12.8 (6.20, 19.40)	3.21 (2.01, 4.41)
16	3	0.400	75	21	11.9 (4.50, 19.30)	2.67 (0.57, 4.77)
32	8	0.106	75	12	13.0 (3.50, 22.50)	2.36 (0.86, 3.86)

NOTE: The 0.95 confidence limits for b_1^* and θ_2 are given in parentheses.

limited to the set of positive integers. The confidence intervals for b and θ_2 were constructed using the asymptotic distribution of the likelihood ratio statistic.

ANALYSIS OF EXPERIMENTAL DATA

We applied the model described above to experimental data on urethane-induced lung tumors reported by White, Grendon, and Jones.[12] In these experiments, female strain A/J mice received injections of urethane according to different time and dose schedules, furnishing an opportunity to study the effect of dose rate on the tumor yield. With a fixed total dose, urethane was administered either once or in equal fractions every other day over periods of 8, 16, or 32 days. The animals were sacrificed at 56, 84, 112, 140, and 168 days following the single or first dose of urethane, and the number of pulmonary tumors was counted. At the time of sacrifice each group consisted of 10 animals. Further details of experimental methods and design can be found in Reference 12.

Shown in TABLE 1 are the model parameters estimated by the maximum likelihood method from the experimental data for $D = 1$ mg/g body weight and different values of T. As is evident from the table, the dose rate has little effect on the parameters b and θ_2. The same is true for the mean promotion time $\tau = \alpha/\beta$ as well as for the corresponding variation coefficient $v = 1/\sqrt{\alpha}$. In view of this fact, the number of unknown parameters can be substantially reduced. In doing so, we keep a, b (or a and θ_1^*), α, and β constant for all administration regimens, so that we have only eight parameters to be jointly estimated from the four samples under study. The values of the common parameters thus estimated were: $\hat{b} = 14$, $\hat{a} = 18$, $\hat{\alpha} = 5$, and $\hat{\beta} = 0.071$. This gives $\hat{\theta}_1^* = 252$, which is equal to the estimated total number of initiated cells. The estimated values of θ_2 and the corresponding 0.95 confidence intervals were as follows: $\hat{\theta}_2 = 2.47$, (1.57, 3.37), for $T = 1$; $\hat{\theta}_2 = 2.69$, (1.39, 3.99), for $T = 8$; $\hat{\theta}_2 = 2.71$, (1.91, 3.51), for $T = 16$; $\hat{\theta}_2 = 2.92$, (2.12, 3.72), for $T = 32$. The expected number of tumors per animal was computed with these values of the model

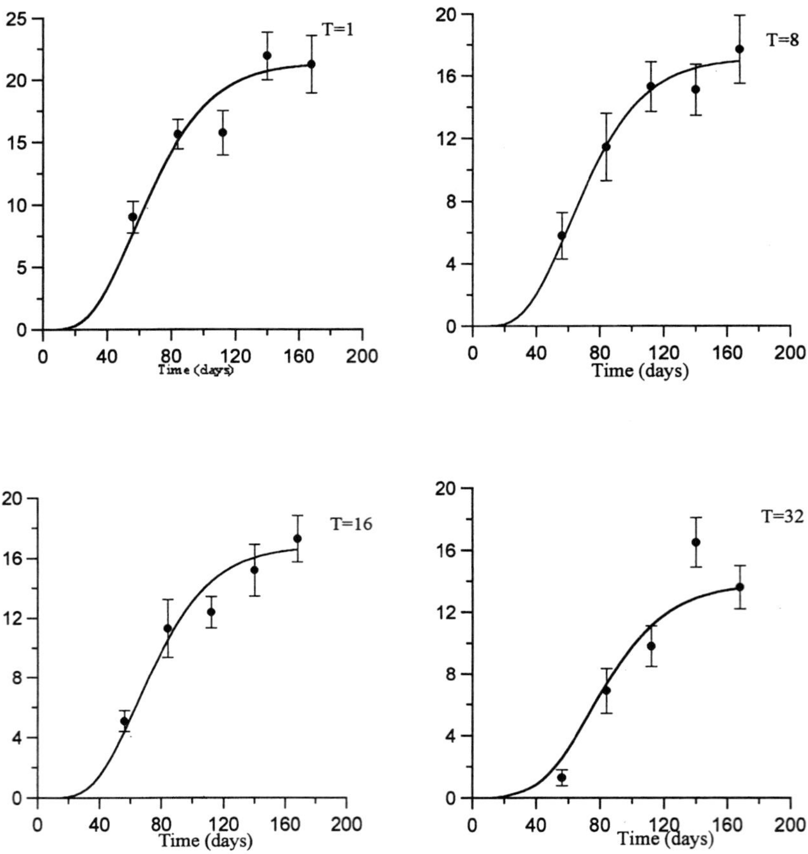

FIGURE 1. Expected number of tumors as a function of time for different exposure periods. Theoretical curves are shown with *solid lines,* experimental data are represented by the *sample mean values, bars* indicate one standard error for each experimental point.

parameters for each exposure period and compared with the sample mean tumor counts at various times after the first injection of urethane. Depicted in FIGURE 1, these theoretical curves simultaneously show good agreement with experimental data for all groups of animals. Very similar results were obtained for a total dose of 0.5 mg/g body weight.

It is interesting to note that even after some parameters had been pooled, the parameter θ_2 remained unaffected by the dose rate. This fact can be attributed to inefficient repair of lesions responsible for cell death. Since the parameter θ_1^* also appears to be independent of dose rate, the above analysis suggests that both precancerous lesions and the cell-killing component of urethane-induced damage are not subject to repair processes. While the conclusion regarding precancerous lesions is in full agreement with our earlier findings resulting from a similar analysis of experimental data on radiation-induced osteosarcoma and malignant lymphoma in mice,[9] the same cannot be said of the cell-killing damage. Specifically, it was found that at a dose as low as 0.2 Gy of protracted high LET (^{224}Ra) radiation *in vivo* almost all potentially lethal damage can be repaired. This interpretation, however, cannot be considered as a conclusive inference but rather as a hypothesis to be tested in direct experiments.

The analysis of time-to-tumor data and multiplicity of tumors induced by chemical carcinogens utilizes only a part of the information available in such studies. Another useful source of information can be provided by data on the time-dependent tumor size distribution. To extend the above approach to this type of data would require an explicit description of the expansion of initiated cell clones. Dewanji *et al.*,[13,14] Luebeck and Moolgavkar,[15] and Moolgavkar *et al.*[16,17] have developed methods based on birth-death stochastic processes for this purpose. It seems worthwhile to invoke similar methods for the incorporation of clonal expansion into the model discussed in the present paper, thereby taking advantages of both approaches.

SUMMARY

This paper discusses an application of the stochastic model of carcinogenesis proposed by Yakovlev and Polig[5] to the analysis of experimental data on multiple pulmonary tumors induced by urethane. The results of this analysis suggest that the rate of administration of urethane has no effect on the mean number of initiated cells per unit dose. Likewise, the formation of lesions responsible for cell death appears to be unaffected by the dose rate.

REFERENCES

1. Shimkin, M. B. 1940. Induced pulmonary tumors in mice. II. Reaction of lungs of strain A mice to carcinogenic hydrocarbons. Arch. Pathol. **28:** 239–255.
2. Stoner, G. D. 1991. Lung tumors in strain A mice as a bioassay for carcinogenicity of environmental chemicals. Exp. Lung Res. **17:** 405–423.
3. Neyman, J. & E. L. Scott. 1967. Statistical aspect of the problem of carcinogenesis. *In* Proceedings of the Fifth Berkeley Symposium on Mathematical Statistics and Probability, Vol. 4: 707–719. University of California Press. Berkeley, CA.
4. Grosser, S. & A. S. Whittemore. 1990. Transformation and growth of lung adenomas in mice exposed to urethane. *In* Scientific Issues in Quantitative Cancer Risk Assessment. S. H. Moolgavkar, Ed.: 176–195. Birkhäuser. Boston.
5. Yakovlev, A. Y. & E. Polig. 1996. A diversity of responses displayed by a stochastic model of radiation carcinogenesis allowing for cell death. Math. Biosci. **132:** 1–33.
6. Myasnikova, E. M., S. T. Rachev & A. Y. Yakovlev. 1996. Queueing models of potentially lethal damage repair in irradiated cells. Math. Biosci. **135:** 85–109.
7. Shimkin, M. B., R. Wieder, D. Marzi, N. Gubareff & V. Suntzeff. 1967. Lung tumors in mice receiving different schedules of urethane. *In* Proceedings of the Fifth Berkeley Symposium on Mathematical Statistics and Probability, Vol. 4: 707–719. University of California Press. Berkeley, CA.
8. Klebanov, L. B., S. T. Rachev & A. Y. Yakovlev. 1993. A stochastic model of radiation carcinogenesis: Latent time distributions and their properties. Math. Biosci. **113:** 51–75.
9. Yakovlev, A. Y., W. A. Müller, L. V. Pavlova & E. Polig. 1995. A Stochastic Model of Radiation Carcinogenesis Allowing for Cell Death and its Biological Implications.

Technical Report No. 567. Department of Statistics, Ohio State University. Columbus, OH.
10. Yakovlev, A. Y. & A. D. Tsodikov. 1996. Stochastic Models of Tumor Latency and their Biostatistical Applications. World Scientific Publ. Singapore.
11. Himmelblau, D. M. 1972. Applied Nonlinear Programming. McGraw-Hill. New York.
12. White, M., A. Grendon & H. B. Jones. 1967. Effects of urethane dose and time patterns on tumor formation. *In* Proceedings of the Fifth Berkeley Symposium on Mathematical Statistics and Probability, Vol. 4: 721–743. University of California Press. Berkeley, CA.
13. Dewanji, A., D. J. Venzon & S. H. Moolgavkar. 1989. A stochastic two-stage model for cancer risk assessment: II. The number and size of premalignant clones. Risk Anal. **9:** 179–187.
14. Dewanji, A., S. H. Moolgavkar & E. G. Luebeck. 1991. Two-mutation model for carcinogenesis: Joint analysis of premalignant and malignant lesions. Math. Biosci. **104:** 97–109.
15. Luebeck, E. G. & S. H. Moolgavkar. 1991. Stochastic analysis of intermediate lesions in carcinogenesis experiments. Risk Anal. **11:** 149–157.
16. Moolgavkar, S. H., E. G. Luebeck, M. De Gunst, R. E. Port & M. Schwartz. 1990. Quantitative analysis of enzyme-altered foci in rat hepatocarcinogenesis experiments. I: Single agent regimen. Carcinogenesis **11:** 1271–1278.
17. Moolgavkar, S. H., E. G. Luebeck, A. Buchmann & K. W. Bock. 1996. Quantitative analysis of enzyme-altered liver foci in rats initiated with diethylnitrozamine and promoted with 2,3,7,8-tetrachlorodibenzo-p-dioxin or 1,2,3,4,6,7,8-heptachlorodibenzo-p-dioxin. Toxicol. Appl. Pharmacol. **138:** 31–42.

Results of Three Life-Span Experimental Carcinogenicity and Anticarcinogenicity Studies on Tamoxifen in Rats

CESARE MALTONI,[a] FRANCO MINARDI,[b] CARMINE PINTO,[b] FIORELLA BELPOGGI,[b] AND LUCIANO BUA[b]

[a]*Cancer Research Center*
European Ramazzini Foundation
of Oncology and Environmental Sciences
Bentivoglio Castle
40010 Bentivoglio (BO), Italy

[b]*European B. Ramazzini Foundation of Oncology and Environmental Sciences*
Bologna, Italy

INTRODUCTION

Tamoxifen is a drug that is widely used in medical oncology as an antiestrogen. This effect is due to its competitive action on estrogen receptors, but other mechanisms can be implied. Most likely, tamoxifen may also act via the hypophysis by lowering the production of ovarian estrogens.

The use of tamoxifen in oncology started in 1971,[1] and it has been progressively and gradually expanding. Up to the present day it seems that over 5 million women have undergone treatment with this drug. Ordinarily, tamoxifen is administered at the daily dose of 20 mg, but sometimes 30 or 40 mg are prescribed.

Tamoxifen has been found efficacious, and is therefore used in primary hormonotherapy for female and male mammary carcinoma and for endometrial cancer. Its use has also been proposed in other tumors, mainly melanomas.[2] Its therapeutic effect on mammary cancer has been proved with experimental animal models.[3]

Nowadays, tamoxifen is widely used in postsurgical adjuvant therapy for mammary carcinoma in women. There are at present 14 clinical trials on this use,[4–19] and the updated results seem to show an advantageous effect of the drug on disease-free survival time and on overall survival.

Tamoxifen has been shown to have chemopreventive effects on mammary cancers experimentally induced in rats, or in a strain of mice that develop mammary tumors spontaneously at a high incidence,[3,20–26] and on the spontaneous mammary cancers of the colony of Sprague-Dawley rats used in the Cancer Research Center at the Castle of Bentivoglio (BT) of the European Ramazzini Foundation.[27–39]

The results obtained on spontaneous mammary carcinomas in female Sprague-Dawley rats show a sharp chemopreventive effect of tamoxifen, and they are particu-

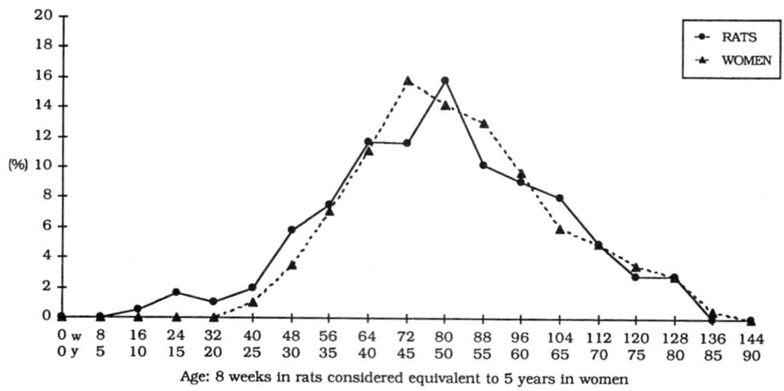

FIGURE 1. Comparative distribution by equivalent age of 232 mammary carcinomas observed among 2,000 untreated female Sprague-Dawley rats of the colony used at the CRC/ERF, and of 1,264 mammary carcinomas detected among 130,000 Bologna women under screening.

larly relevant for clinical extrapolation since this animal model must be considered human equivalent in its histological pattern, biological behavior, global incidence, and age-equivalent distribution of these tumors (FIG. 1).

The chemopreventive effect of tamoxifen on mammary carcinoma is also supported by the observation in mastectomized women of a protective effect of the drug on the contralateral mammary tumors, in the trials evaluating the effect of tamoxifen in adjuvant therapy. Of a total of 30,000 women included in those trials (180,000 woman-years), 379 cases of contralateral mammary carcinomas were observed in the control group, vs. 276 cases of these tumors in the tamoxifen-treated group, with an odds reduction of 35% (2P = 0.00001) (personal communication).

These experimental and clinical observations prompted three chemopreventive clinic trials, one in the United States on 16,000 women,[40–42] one in Italy on 20,000 women[43] and one in the United Kingdom on 15,000 women.[44,45] The daily dose employed in these trials is 20 mg/day.

Much is known about short- and middle-term wanted and unwanted effects of tamoxifen in treated women.[34,46–53] Much less is known of its long-term carcinogenic effects. Information on the carcinogenic potential of tamoxifen is, on the contrary, of primary relevance, because of the use of tamoxifen in adjuvant therapy, involving large groups of women who must be considered already cured by surgery alone, and because of the chemopreventive trials, which are now ongoing and whose results may eventually open the door to the adoption of tamoxifen treatment for chemoprevention of mammary cancer on large groups of women all over the world.

Careful pioneering observation in the Swedish adjuvant trial showed, even in 1989, an increase in endometrial carcinomas in women treated with tamoxifen at 40 mg daily.[54] The effect has now been confirmed also in women treated with the daily dose of 20 mg (the dose currently used).[55] In the total of 30,000 women of the ongoing adjuvant trials, at present 78 cases of endometrial carcinoma have been observed in treated women, vs. 21 in the control group (2P < 0.00001) (personal communication).

Five experimental studies in rats of different strains were performed to evaluate the carcinogenic effect of tamoxifen. The results, summarized in TABLE 1,[56–60] indicate that tamoxifen is indeed a hepatocarcinogen at very high doses. The still effective lower dose is 5 mg/kg b.w., which corresponds to 15 times the current clinical dose (considering 60 kg to be the weight of a woman, the current dose of 20 mg/day corresponds to 0.33 mg/day). It must be pointed out, on the other hand, that the maximum duration of these experimental hepatocarcinogenicity studies was 24 months.

To date there are no available results of long-term carcinogenicity bioassays of the types currently performed for industrial carcinogens and that follow the Good Laboratory Practices (GLP) (required for this type of testing). In 1988, 1989, and 1991, respectively, we started three life span experiments to evaluate the potential carcinogenic and anticarcinogenic effects of tamoxifen in all tissues and organs, following the rules of the GLP. The results of the three bioassays are herein presented. These three experiments are part of a wider project of 13 experimental studies, aimed at assessing the chemopreventive effects and carcinogenic risks of the drug, which was started in 1986.

MATERIALS AND METHODS

The tamoxifen tested is the one marketed by Zeneca, under the commercial name of Nolvadex®.

The tested animals were male and female Sprague-Dawley rats of the colony, which has been used for 25 years in the laboratories of the Cancer Research Center of the European Ramazzini Foundation of Oncology and Environmental Sciences, for which there is extensive information on expected nonneoplastic and neoplastic pathology available for about 10,000 controls.

In this strain, the incidence of mammary tumors is of the same order of that observed in women in industrial countries: mammary cancer arises in about 10% of the females (range 7–12%), and the number of mammary cancers per 100 animals usually ranges from 9 to 13 (since the same animal can bear more than one mammary malignancy). The distribution by equivalent ages in this animal model and in women overlaps (FIG. 1). The mammary cancers show all the various morphological and biological patterns that characterize the human types and subtypes.

For the purpose of the present studies, data are presented on selected tumors observed in 2 groups of untreated rats, respectively for 1,000 males and 1,000 females, born in 1988 (that is, at the same time as the animals of the herein-presented experiments), kept under control for their life span, and submitted to complete necropsy and systematic histopathological examination (TABLES 2 and 3).

The plans of the three experiments are presented in TABLE 4.

Tamoxifen was administered by stomach tube in water suspension; controls were gavaged with water alone.

The animals were submitted daily to observation, and weighed and clinically controlled periodically (weekly within the first 13 weeks of experiment, and then every 2 weeks).

At death, all animals were submitted to systematic necropsy. Specimens for histopathology include mammary glands, mammary tumors, brain, pituitary gland,

TABLE 1. Incidence of Hepatocarcinomas in Various Rat Strains Submitted to Long-term Treatment with Tamoxifen

Strain of Rats	Duration of Experiment (months)	Daily Dose (mg/kg b.w.)	No. of Animals		Hepatocarcinoma (Bearing Animals) (%)	Reference
			At Start	Corrected		
Sprague-Dawley	15	2.8	57	22	0	56
	15	11.3	57	11	45	
	12	45.2	55	4	75	
Wistar	24	5.0	52	51	16	57
	24	20.0	52	51	64	
	24	35.0	52	51	64	
Sprague-Dawley	12	11.3	84	36	44	58
	12	22.6	75	24	100	
Sprague-Dawley	15	11.3	5	5	60	59
	15	45.0	8	6	83	
Fischer F344	15	12.5	20	8	0	60

TABLE 2. Spontaneous Incidence of Selected Tumors in a Group of 1,000 Randomized Control Male Sprague-Dawley Rats

Type of Tumor	Animals Bearing Tumors		Incidence of Tumors	
	No.	%	No.	Per 100 Animals
Mammary				
Benign[a]	26	2.6	27	2.7
Malignant[b]	5	0.5	5	0.5
Hepatocarcinomas	11	1.1		
Testicular Leydig cell tumors	61	6.1		

[a] Fibromas and fibroadenomas.
[b] Carcinomas and sarcomas.

TABLE 3. Spontaneous Incidence of Selected Tumors in a Group of 1,000 Randomized Control Female Sprague-Dawley Rats

Type of Tumor	Animals Bearing Tumors		Incidence of Tumors	
	No.	%	No.	Per 100 Animals
Mammary				
Benign[a]	407	40.7	549	54.9
Malignant[b]	84	8.4	99	9.9
Hepatocarcinomas	0	—		
Uterine				
Carcinomas	16[c]	1.6		
Sarcomas	23	2.3		
Total malignant tumors	39	3.9		

[a] The great majority fibroadenomas and some fibromas.
[b] The great majority carcinomas and a few cases of sarcoma.
[c] Eleven adenocarcinomas and five squamous cell carcinomas.

TABLE 4. Plan of Three Experimental Studies

Experiment	1 (BT 5T)	2 (BT 8T)	3 (BT 12T)
Sex	Males and females	Females	Females
Age at start (weeks)	8	12	56
Route of administration	Oral[a]	Oral[a]	Oral[a]
Administered dose (mg/kg b.w.)	3.3	3.3	3.3
Schedule of treatment	6 days weekly, life span	8 days every 8 weeks, life span	6 days weekly, for 40 weeks
Duration of the experiment	Life span	Life span	Life span
Number of rats per group (treated and control)	100	150	139
Total number of animals	400	300	278
Duration of life span	167	166	143

[a] By stomach tube in water suspension.

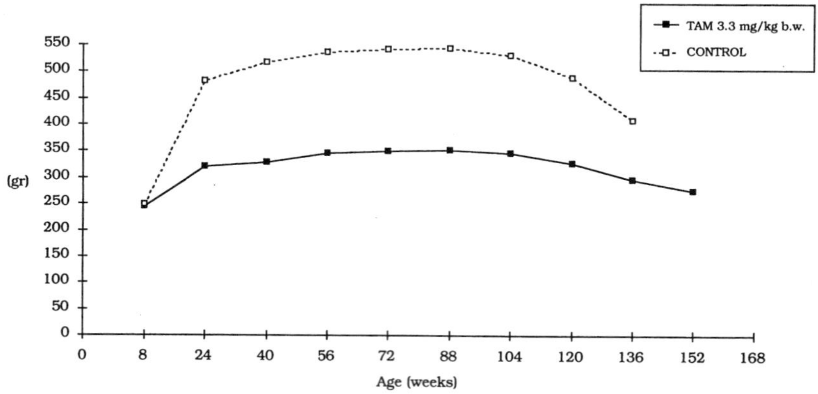

FIGURE 2. Mean body weight of males in experiment 1 (BT 5T).

Zymbal glands, salivary glands, Harderian glands, head (with oral and nasal cavities and external and internal ear ducts) (5 sections), tongue, thyroid and parathyroids, pharynx, larynx, thymus and mediastinal lymph nodes, trachea, lung and mainstem bronchi, heart, diaphragm, liver, spleen, pancreas, kidneys and adrenal glands, esophagus, stomach (fore and glandular), intestine (4 levels), bladder, prostate, uterus, vagina, gonads, interscapular fat pad, subcutaneous and mesenteric lymph nodes, femur, and any other organs and tissues with pathological lesions. All organs and tissues were preserved in 70% ethyl alcohol, except bones, which were fixed in 10% formalin and then decalcified with 10% formaldehyde and 20% formic acid in water solution. The normal specimens were trimmed, following the standard procedures of the BT laboratory: i.e., parenchymal organs were dissected through the hilus to expose the widest surface, and hollow organs were sectioned across the greatest diameter(s). The pathological tissue was trimmed through the largest surface, including normal adjacent tissues. The trimmed specimens were processed as paraffin blocks, and 3-5-micron sections of every specimen were obtained. Sections were routinely stained with hematoxylin-eosin. Specific stainings were performed when needed. The histological slides were examined independently by two pathologists, and then reviewed by a third pathologist.

RESULTS

Body Weight. In the animals treated with tamoxifen a reduction in body weight was observed: such reduction parallels the intensity of treatment (FIGS. 2-5). In the animals treated six times weekly since six weeks of age and for their life span (exp. 1/BT5T), a reduction of size among tamoxifen-treated animals of both sexes was observed.

Survival. In all three experiments, a moderate increase in the survival rate was observed in tamoxifen-treated groups with respect to control groups (FIG. 6-9).

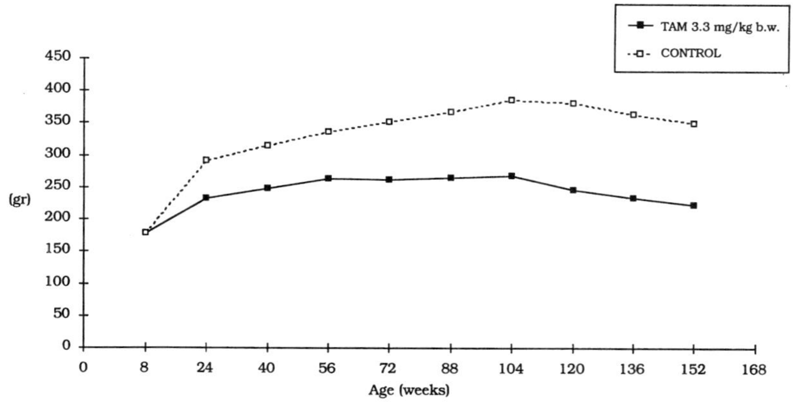

FIGURE 3. Mean body weight of females in experiment 1 (BT 5T).

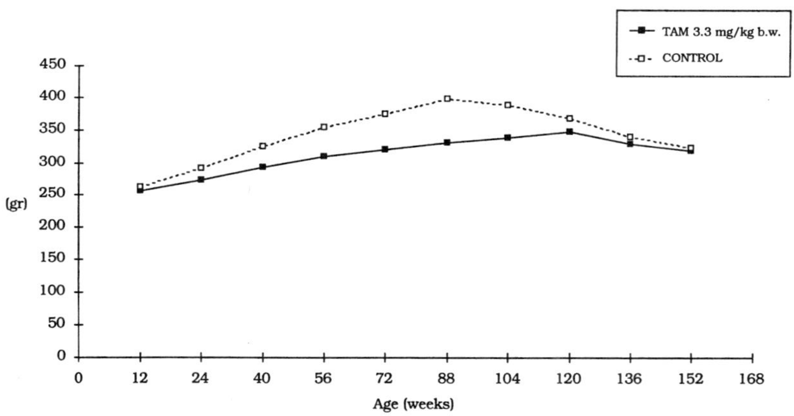

FIGURE 4. Mean body weight of females in experiment 2 (BT 8T).

Nononcological Changes. No evident behavioral changes were observed in tamoxifen-treated animals. In female rats, atrophic changes in cervical mucosa were observed at the histological examination, following continuous treatment with tamoxifen, started at a young age.

Carcinogenic and Anticarcinogenic Effects. Multiple tumors of the same site (monolateral and bilateral organs) and type were plotted only once, apart from the mammary and adrenal tumors of the same type, whose multiplicity has been taken into account.

Experiment 1 (BT5T)

The overall results are shown in TABLES 5 and 6. In the tamoxifen-treated groups there was a sharply decreased incidence of total benign tumors (TABLE 7), while no

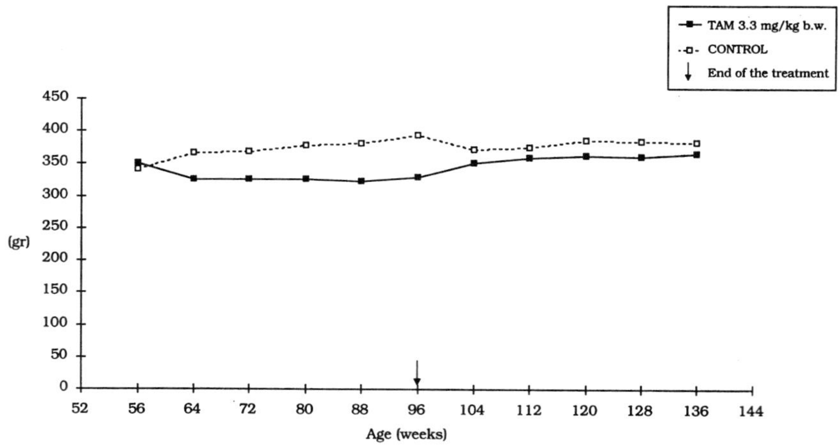

FIGURE 5. Mean body weight of females in experiment 3 (BT 12T).

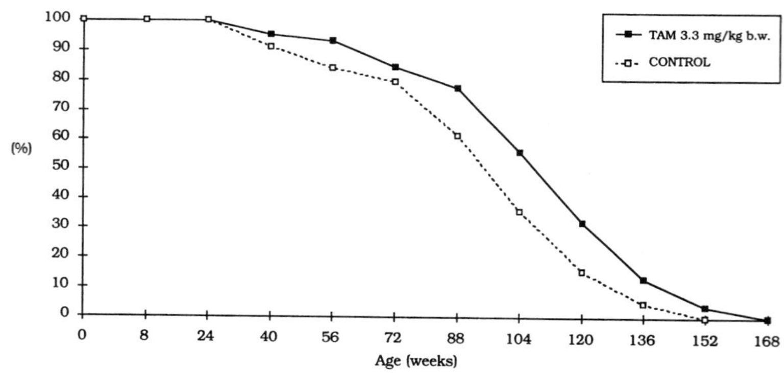

FIGURE 6. Survival of males of experiment 1 (BT 5T).

remarkable difference in the incidence of total malignant tumors was observed between treated and control males and females (TABLE 8). With respect to single tumors, tamoxifen was found: (1) to increase benign and malignant mammary tumors in males, and sharply decrease/inhibit benign and malignant tumors in females (TABLES 9, 10); (2) to decrease the pituitary gland tumors in males and females (TABLE 11), the medullary adrenal pheochromocytomas in males and females (TABLE 12), the islet cell pancreatic tumors in males (TABLE 13), the Leydig cell testicular tumors (TABLE 14) and the polyps of the uterus (TABLE 15); and (3) to slightly increase tumors and correlated oncological lesions of the liver among males and females (TABLE 16), and tumors of the uterus and vagina (TABLE 17). One pheochromoblastoma was found among treated males and treated females, while none were observed among

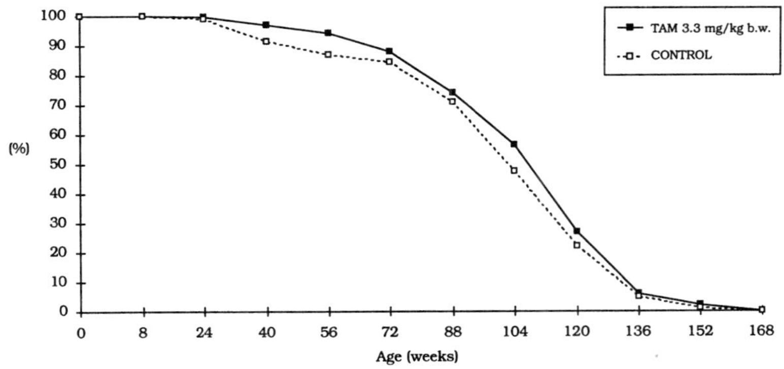

FIGURE 7. Survival of females of experiment 1 (BT 5T).

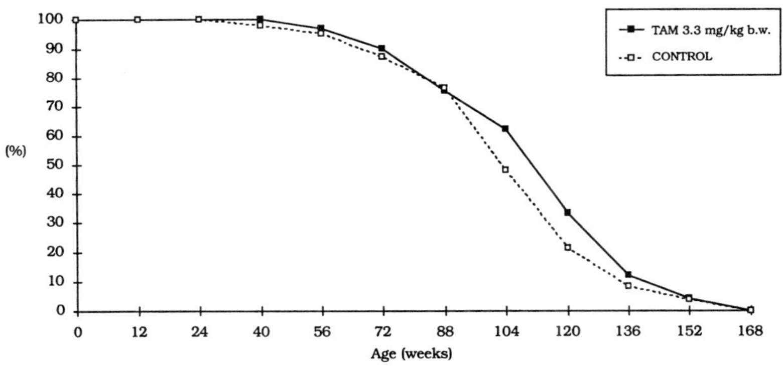

FIGURE 8. Survival of females of experiment 2 (BT 8T).

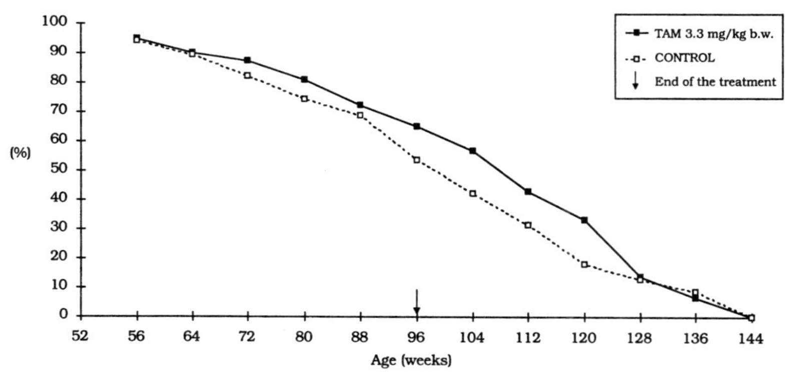

FIGURE 9. Survival of females of experiment 3 (BT 12T).

TABLE 5. Results of Experiment 1 (BT 5T): Number and Percentage of Male Sprague-Dawley Rats Bearing Various Types of Benign and Malignant Tumors[a]

Site	Histotype	Groups: I: 3.3 mg/kg b.w. No.	I: %	II: 0 (control) No.	II: %
Skin	Keratoacanthoma	0	—	1	1.0
Subcutaneous tissue	Fibroma	0	—	2	2.0
	Rhabdomyosarcoma	1	1.0	0	—
	Angiosarcoma	0	—	2	2.0
	Osteosarcoma	0	—	1	1.0
Mammary gland[b]	Fibroma and fibroadenoma	6	6.0	1	1.0
	Adenocarcinoma	2 (3)	2.0	0	—
Zymbal glands	Carcinoma	1	1.0	0	—
Ear ducts	Carcinoma	2	2.0	2	2.0
Nasal cavities	Olfactory neuroblastoma	1	1.0	0	—
Larynx	Squamous cell carcinoma	1	1.0	1	1.0
Trachea	Squamous cell carcinoma	0	—	1	1.0
Intestine	Leiomyoma	1	1.0	1	1.0
Liver[c]	Hepatoadenoma	1	1.0	0	—
	Hepatocarcinoma	2	2.0	0	—
Pancreas[d]	Islet cell adenoma	1	1.0	7	7.0
	Islet cell adenocarcinoma	0	—	1	1.0
Kidneys	Adenoma	2	2.0	0	—
Testes[e]	Leydig cell tumor	0	—	4	4.0
Peritoneum	Mesothelioma	1	1.0	0	—
Pituitary gland[f]	Adenoma	5	5.0	11	11.0
Thyroid gland	C-cell carcinoma	1	1.0	0	—
Adrenal glands[g]	Cortical adenoma	0	—	1	1.0
	Pheochromocytoma	16 (17)	16.0	19 (27)	19.0
	Pheochromoblastoma	1	1.0	0	—

Bones					
Cranium	Osteosarcoma	3	3.0	1	1.0
Soft tissues	Fibrosarcoma	0	–	1	1.0
Spleen	Fibroangioma	4	4.0	1	1.0
Hemolymphoreticular tissues[h]	Lymphomas and leukemias	11	11.0	14	14.0

[a] Numbers in parentheses indicate the number of tumors (one animal can bear more than one tumor).
[b] See TABLES 9, 10.
[c] See TABLE 16.
[d] See TABLE 13.
[e] See TABLE 14.
[f] See TABLE 11.
[g] See TABLE 12.
[h] Including spleen.

TABLE 6. Results of Experiment 1 (BT 5T): Number and Percentage of Female Sprague-Dawley Rats Bearing Various Types of Benign and Malignant Tumors[a]

		Groups			
		I: 3.3 mg/kg b.w.		II: 0 (Control)	
Site	Histotype	No.	%	No.	%
Skin	Dermatofibroma	1	1.0	0	–
	Sebaceous gland adenoma	1	1.0	0	–
	Fibrosarcoma	0	–	1	1.0
Subcutaneous tissue	Fibrosarcoma	1	1.0	0	–
	Liposarcoma	1	1.0	0	–
Mammary gland[b]	Fibroma and fibroadenoma	0	–	37 (55)	37.0
	Adenocarcinoma	0	–	8 (12)	8.0
	Fibrosarcoma	0	–	1	1.0
Zymbal glands	Carcinoma	1	1.0	1	1.0
Ear ducts	Carcinoma	2	2.0	3	3.0
Oral cavity, lips and tongue	Carcinoma	1	1.0	1	1.0
Larynx	Squamous cell carcinoma	0	–	1	1.0
Intestine	Adenocarcinoma	1	1.0	0	–
Liver[c]	Hepatoadenoma	1	1.0	0	–
	Cholangioma	0	—	2	2.0
	Hepatocarcinoma	3	3.0	0	–
Pancreas[d]	Islet cell adenocarcinoma	0	–	1	1.0
Bladder	Rhabdomyosarcoma	1	1.0	0	–
Ovaries	Fibroangioma	1	1.0	0	–
Uterus[e]	Polyp	0	–	13	13.0
	Fibroma	2	2.0	0	–
	Fibroangioma	1	1.0	0	–
	Angioma	0	–	1	1.0
	Adenocarcinoma	0	–	1	1.0

	Squamous cell carcinoma	1	1.0	0	–
	Sarcoma	3	3.0	2	2.0
Vagina[e]	Squamous cell carcinoma	1	1.0	0	–
Peritoneum	Mesothelioma	1	1.0	0	–
Pituitary gland[f]	Adenoma	2	2.0	16	16.0
Thyroid gland	Papillary adenocarcinoma	1	1.0	1	1.0
	C-cell carcinoma	0	–	1	1.0
Adrenal glands[g]	Cortical adenoma	5	5.0	6	6.0
	Pheochromocytoma	12 (19)	12.0	17 (25)	17.0
	Cortical adenocarcinoma	1	1.0	0	–
	Pheochromoblastoma	1	1.0	0	–
Major peripheral nerves	Malignant Schwannoma	1	1.0	0	–
Bones					
Cranium	Osteoma	1	1.0	0	–
	Osteosarcoma	1	1.0	1	1.0
Thymus	Squamous cell carcinoma	0	–	1	1.0
Spleen	Fibroangioma	1	1.0	0	–
	Angiosarcoma	1	1.0	0	–
Hemolymphoreticular tissues[h]	Lymphomas and leukemias	11	11.0	9	9.0

[a] Numbers in parentheses indicate the number of tumors (one animal can bear more than one tumor).
[b] See TABLES 9, 10.
[c] See TABLE 16.
[d] See TABLE 13.
[e] See TABLES 15, 17.
[f] See TABLE 11.
[g] See TABLE 12.
[h] Including thymus and spleen.

TABLE 7. Results of Experiment 1 (BT 5T): Incidence of Total Benign Tumors in Males and Females

				Benign Tumors			
		Animals		Animals Bearing Tumors		Tumors	
Group No.	Dose (mg/kg b.w.)	Sex	No.	No.	%	No.	Per 100 Animals
I	3.3	M	100	29	29.0	37	37.0
		F	100	26	26.0	35	35.0
II	0	M	100	33	33.0	56	56.0
		F	100	57	57.0	118	118.0

TABLE 8. Results of Experiment 1 (BT 5T): Incidence of Total Malignant Tumors in Males and Females

				Malignant Tumors			
		Animals		Animals Bearing Tumors		Tumors	
Group No.	Dose (mg/kg b.w.)	Sex	No.	No.	%	No.	Per 100 Animals
I	3.3	M	100	26	26.0	28	28.0
		F	100	31	31.0	34	34.0
II	0	M	100	24	24.0	24	24.0
		F	100	27	27.0	37	37.0

TABLE 9. Results of Experiment 1 (BT 5T): Incidence of Benign Mammary Tumors in Males and Females

Group No.	Dose (mg/kg b.w.)	Animals		Benign Mammary Tumors			
				Animals Bearing Tumors		Tumors	
		Sex	No.	No.	%	No.	Per 100 Animals
I	3.3	M	100	6	6.0	6	6.0
		F	100	0	—	0	—
II	0	M	100	1	1.0	1	1.0
		F	100	36	36.0	55	55.0

TABLE 10. Results of Experiment 1 (BT 5T): Incidence of Malignant Mammary Tumors in Males and Females

Group No.	Dose (mg/kg b.w.)	Animals		Malignant Mammary Tumors			
				Animals Bearing Tumors		Tumors	
		Sex	No.	No.	%	No.	Per 100 Animals
I	3.3	M	100	2	2.0	3	3.0
		F	100	0	—	0	—
II	0	M	100	0	—	0	—
		F	100	9	9.0	13	13.0

TABLE 11. Results of Experiment 1 (BT 5T): Incidence of Pituitary Gland Tumors in Males and Females

Group No.	Dose (mg/kg b.w.)	Animals		Animals Bearing Pituitary Gland Adenomas	
		Sex	No.	No.	%
I	3.3	M	100	5	5.0
		F	100	2	2.0
II	0	M	100	11	11.0
		F	100	16	16.0

TABLE 12. Results of Experiment 1 (BT 5T): Incidence of Adrenal Glands Pheochromocytomas and Pheochromoblastomas in Males and Females

Group No.	Dose (mg/kg b.w.)	Animals		Pheochromocytomas				Pheochromoblastomas			
				Animals Bearing Tumors		Tumors		Animals Bearing Tumors		Tumors	
		Sex	No.	No.	%	No.	Per 100 Animals[a]	No.	%	No.	Per 100 Animals
I	3.3	M	100	16	16.0	17	17.0	1	1.0	1	1.0
		F	100	12	12.0	19	19.0	1	1.0	1	1.0
II	0	M	100	19	19.0	27	27.0	0	—	0	—
		F	100	17	17.0	25	25.0	0	—	0	—

[a] In several animals pheochromocytomas were observed in both adrenal glands.

TABLE 13. Results of Experiment 1 (BT 5T): Incidence of Islet Cell Pancreatic Tumors in Males and Females

Group No.	Dose (mg/kg b.w.)	Animals		Animals Bearing Tumors: Islet Cell Adenomas		Animals Bearing Tumors: Islet Cell Adenocarcinoma	
		Sex	No.	No.	%	No.	%
I	3.3	M	100	1	1.0	0	–
		F	100	0	–	0	–
II	0	M	100	7	7.0	1	1.0
		F	100	0	–	1	1.0

TABLE 14. Results of Experiment 1 (BT 5T): Incidence of Leydig Cell Testicular Tumors

Group No.	Dose (mg/kg b.w.)	Animals		Animals Bearing Leydig Cell Tumors	
		Sex	No.	No.	%
I	3.3	M	100	0	–
II	0	M	100	4	4.0

TABLE 15. Results of Experiment 1 (BT 5T): Incidence of Polyps of the Uterus

Group No.	Dose (mg/kg b.w.)	Animals		Animals Bearing Tumors	
		Sex	No.	No.	%
I	3.3	F	100	0	–
II	0	F	100	13	13.0

TABLE 16. Results of Experiment 1 (BT 5T): Incidence of Tumors and Other Lesions of Oncological Interest of the Liver in Males and Females

				Animals Bearing Liver Changes							
		Animals		Nodular Hyperplasias		Nodular Dysplasias		Hepatoadenomas		Hepatocarcinomas[a]	
Group No.	Dose (mg/kg b.w.)	Sex	No.	No.	%	No.	%	No.	%	No.	%
I	3.3	M	100	9	9.0	2	2.0	1	1.0	2	2.0
		F	100	6	6.0	1	1.0	1	1.0	3	3.0
II	0	M	100	4	4.0	0	–	0	–	0	–
		F	100	6	6.0	0	–	0	–	0	–

[a] All with small deviation (low grade).

TABLE 17. Results of Experiment 1 (BT 5T): Incidence of Malignant Tumors of the Uterus and Vagina

				Animals Bearing Tumors											
		Animals		Uterus				Vagina				Total			
				Carcinomas		Sarcomas		Carcinomas		Sarcomas		Carcinomas		Sarcomas	
Group No.	Treatment (mg/kg b.w.)	Sex	No.	No.	%	No.	%	No.	%	No.	%	No.	%	No.	%
I	3.3	F	100	1	1.0	3	3.0	1	1.0	0	–	2	2.0	3	3.0
II	0	F	100	1	1.0	2	2.0	0	–	0	–	1	1.0	2	2.0

control animals (TABLE 12). No relevant changes were found in the incidence of the other detected tumors as a whole (TABLES 18, 19).

Experiment 2 (BT8T)

The overall results are shown in TABLE 20. In the tamoxifen-treated group there was again a clearly decreased incidence of total benign tumors (TABLE 21), while only a slight and not remarkable difference in the incidence of total malignant tumors was observed (TABLE 22). With respect to single tumors, tamoxifen was found: (1) to markedly decrease benign and malignant mammary tumors (TABLES 23, 24) (2) to decrease the pituitary gland tumors (TABLE 25), the medullary adrenal tumors (TABLE 26), the islet cell pancreatic tumors (TABLE 27), and the polyps of the uterus (TABLE 28) (3) not to affect the incidence of tumors and oncological lesions of the liver (TABLE 29); and (4) to increase the uterine-vagina sarcomas (TABLE 30). No relevant changes were found in the incidence of the other detected tumors as a whole (TABLES 31, 32).

Experiment 3 (BT12T)

The overall results are shown in the TABLE 33. In the tamoxifen-treated group there was again a clearly decreased incidence of total benign tumors (TABLE 34) and a slight and not remarkable decrease of total malignant tumors (TABLE 35). In the tamoxifen-treated group a reduction in benign mammary tumors was observed, both at the end of the treatment and thereafter (TABLE 36). After 40 weeks of treatment, complete protection against mammary cancer was observed; the protective effect also lasted after stopping the treatment (TABLE 37). A reduction in the incidence of pituitary gland tumors (TABLE 38), of the islet cell pancreatic tumors (TABLE 39), and of the polyps of the uterus (TABLE 40) was also observed. No decreased incidence of adrenal gland pheochromocytomas was detected (TABLE 41). No carcinogenic effect of tamoxifen was found on the liver (TABLE 42) and the uterus and vagina (TABLE 43). No relevant changes were found in the incidence of the other detected tumors as a whole among treated and control animals (TABLE 44, 45).

CONCLUSIONS

Under the tested experimental conditions, the results of our three experiments show that:

1. tamoxifen has a strong inhibiting (chemopreventive) effect on mammary cancer in females;
2. such chemopreventive effect also lasts when the treatment is stopped;
3. tamoxifen reduces the incidence of other tumors (including pituitary, medullary adrenal, islet cell pancreatic and Leydig cell testicular tumors, and polyps of the uterus);

TABLE 18. Results of Experiment 1 (BT 5T): Incidence of Benign Tumors Not Including the Ones Decreased[a] or Increased[b] by Tamoxifen Treatment

				Benign Tumors			
		Animals		Animals Bearing Tumors		Tumors	
Group No.	Dose (mg/kg b.w.)	Sex	No.	No.	%	No.	Per 100 Animals
I	3.3	M	100	7	7.0	7	7.0
		F	100	13	13.0	13	13.0
II	0	M	100	6	6.0	6	6.0
		F	100	8	8.0	9	9.0

[a] Decreased benign tumors: mammary tumors in females, pituitary gland adenomas, pheochromocytomas, islet cell pancreatic tumors, Leydig cell testicular tumors, polyps of the uterus (see TABLES 9–15).

[b] Increased benign tumors: mammary tumors in males, liver hepatoadenomas (see TABLES 9 and 16).

TABLE 19. Results of Experiment 1 (BT 5T): Incidence of Malignant Tumors Not Including the Ones Decreased[a] or Increased[b] by Tamoxifen Treatment

				Malignant Tumors			
		Animals		Animals Bearing Tumors		Tumors	
Group No.	Dose (mg/kg b.w.)	Sex	No.	No.	%	No.	Per 100 Animals
I	3.3	M	100	22	22.0	22	22.0
		F	100	24	24.0	25	25.0
II	0	M	100	23	23.0	23	23.0
		F	100	18	18.0	20	20.0

[a] Decreased malignant tumors: mammary tumors in females, islet cell pancreatic tumors (see TABLES 10 and 13).

[b] Increased malignant tumors: mammary tumors in males, pheochromoblastomas, hepatocarcinomas, tumors of the uterus and vagina (see TABLES 10, 12, 16, and 17).

TABLE 20. Results of Experiment 2 (BT 8T): Number and Percentage of Female Sprague-Dawley Rats Bearing Various Types of Benign and Malignant Tumors[a]

		Groups			
		I: 3.3 mg/kg b.w.		II: 0 (Control)	
Site	Histotype	No.	%	No.	%
Subcutaneous tissue	Lipoma	1	0.7	1	0.7
Mammary gland[b]	Fibroma and fibroadenoma	41 (55)	27.3	68 (93)	45.3
	Fibrolipoma	1	0.7	0	–
	Adenocarcinoma	5	3.3	12 (13)	8.0
	Fibrosarcoma	0	–	2	1.3
	Fibrohistiocytosarcoma	0	–	1 (2)	0.7
Zymbal glands	Carcinoma	1	0.7	1	0.7
Ear ducts	Carcinoma	7	4.7	3	2.0
Lung	Osteosarcoma	0	–	1	0.7
Stomach					
Glandular stomach	Adenoma	0	–	1	0.7
	Adenocarcinoma	0	–	1	0.7
Intestine	Adenocarcinoma	0	–	1	0.7
Liver[c]	Hepatocarcinoma	0	–	1	0.7
Pancreas[d]	Islet cell adenoma	1	0.7	6	4.0
Ovaries	Fibroma	0	–	1	0.7
	Fibroangioma	1	0.7	4	2.7
Uterus[e]	Polyp	3	2.0	13	8.7
	Fibroma	1	0.7	2	1.3
	Fibroangioma	0	–	1	0.7
	Squamous cell carcinoma	1	0.7	0	–
	Sarcoma	5	3.3	1	0.7
Vagina[e]	Squamous cell carcinoma	1	0.7	1	0.7
	Sarcoma	2	1.3	0	–
Peritoneum	Mesothelioma	1	0.7	1	0.7

Pituitary gland[f]	Adenoma	22	14.7	45	30.0
Thyroid gland	C-cell adenoma	3	2.0	2	1.3
	C-cell carcinoma	0	—	1	0.7
Adrenal glands[g]	Cortical adenoma	8	5.3	9	6.0
	Pheochromocytoma	8	5.3	18 (20)	12.0
	Cortical adenocarcinoma	4	2.7	1	0.7
	Pheochromoblastoma	1	0.7	1	0.7
Central nervous system					
Brain	Ependimoma	1	0.7	0	—
Meninges	Meningioma	2	1.3	0	—
Major peripheral nerves	Malignant Schwannoma	1	0.7	0	—
Bones					
Cranium	Osteosarcoma	2	1.3	1	0.7
Other	Osteosarcoma	0	—	2	1.3
Soft tissues	Fibrosarcoma	0	—	1	0.7
Spleen	Fibroangioma	0	—	3	2.0
Hemolymphoreticular tissues[h]	Lymphomas and leukemias	11	7.3	13	8.7

[a] Numbers in parentheses indicate the number of tumors (one animal can bear more than one tumor).
[b] See TABLES 23, 24.
[c] See TABLE 29.
[d] See TABLE 27.
[e] See TABLE 28, 30.
[f] See TABLE 25.
[g] See TABLE 26.
[h] Including spleen.

TABLE 21. Results of Experiment 2 (BT 8T): Incidence of Total Benign Tumors

				Benign Tumors			
		Animals		Animals Bearing Tumors		Tumors	
Group No.	Dose (mg/kg b.w.)	Sex	No.	No.	%	No.	Per 100 Animals
I	3.3	F	150	66	44.0	106	70.6
II	0	F	150	108	72.7	201	134.0

TABLE 22. Results of Experiment 2 (BT 8T): Incidence of Total Malignant Tumors

				Malignant Tumors			
		Animals		Animals Bearing Tumors		Tumors	
Group No.	Dose (mg/kg b.w.)	Sex	No.	No.	%	No.	Per 100 Animals
I	3.3	F	150	40	26.7	43	28.7
II	0	F	150	38	25.3	48	32.0

TABLE 23. Results of Experiment 2 (BT 8T): Incidence of Benign Mammary Tumors

Group No.	Dose (mg/kg b.w.)	Animals		Benign Mammary Tumors			
				Animals Bearing Tumors		Tumors	
		Sex	No.	No.	%	No.	Per 100 Animals
I	3.3	F	150	42	28.0	55	36.7
II	0	F	150	68	45.3	93	62.0

TABLE 24. Results of Experiment 2 (BT 8T): Incidence of Malignant Mammary Tumors

Group No.	Dose (mg/kg b.w.)	Animals		Malignant Mammary Tumors			
				Animals Bearing Tumors		Tumors	
		Sex	No.	No.	%	No.	Per 100 Animals
I	3.3	F	150	5	3.3	5	3.3
II	0	F	150	15	10.0	17	11.3

TABLE 25. Results of Experiment 2 (BT 8T): Incidence of Pituitary Gland Tumors

Group No.	Dose (mg/kg b.w.)	Animals		Animals Bearing Pituitary Gland Adenomas	
		Sex	No.	No.	%
I	3.3	F	150	22	14.7
II	0	F	150	45	30.0

TABLE 26. Results of Experiment 2 (BT 8T): Incidence of Adrenal Gland Pheochromocytomas and Pheochromoblastomas

Group No.	Dose (mg/kg b.w.)	Animals		Pheochromocytomas: Animals Bearing Tumors		Pheochromocytomas: Tumors		Pheochromoblastomas: Animals Bearing Tumors		Pheochromoblastomas: Tumors	
		Sex	No.	No.	%	No.	Per 100 Animals	No.	%	No.	Per 100 Animals
I	3.3	F	150	8	5.3	8	5.3	1	0.7	1	0.7
II	0	F	150	18	12.0	20	13.3	1	0.7	1	0.7

TABLE 27. Results of Experiment 2 (BT 8T): Incidence of Islet Cell Pancreatic Tumors

Group No.	Dose (mg/kg b.w.)	Animals		Animals Bearing Tumors			
				Islet Cell Adenomas		Islet Cell Adenocarcinoma	
		Sex	No.	No.	%	No.	%
I	3.3	F	150	1	0.7	0	—
II	0	F	150	6	4.0	0	—

TABLE 28. Results of Experiment 2 (BT 8T): Incidence of Polyps of the Uterus

Group No.	Dose (mg/kg b.w.)	Animals		Animals Bearing Tumors	
		Sex	No.	No.	%
I	3.3	F	150	3	2.0
II	0	F	150	13	8.7

TABLE 29. Results of Experiment 2 (BT 8T): Incidence of Tumors and Other Lesions of Oncological Interest of the Liver

Group No.	Dose (mg/kg b.w.)	Animals		Animals Bearing Liver Changes: Nodular Hyperplasias		Nodular Dysplasias		Hepatoadenomas		Hepatocarcinomas	
		Sex	No.	No.	%	No.	%	No.	%	No.	%
I	3.3	F	150	10	6.7	0	—	0	—	0	—
II	0	F	150	6	4.0	1	0.7	0	—	1	0.7

TABLE 30. Results of Experiment 2 (BT 8T): Incidence of Malignant Tumors of the Uterus and Vagina

Group No.	Treatment (mg/kg b.w.)	Animals		Animals Bearing Tumors: Uterus				Vagina				Total			
				Carcinomas		Sarcomas		Carcinomas		Sarcomas		Carcinomas		Sarcomas	
		Sex	No.	No.	%	No.	%	No.	%	No.	%	No.	%	No.	%
I	3.3	F	150	1	0.7	5	3.4	1	0.7	2	1.3	2	1.3	7	4.7
II	0	F	150	0	—	1	0.7	1	0.7	0	—	1	0.7	1	0.7

TABLE 31. Results of Experiment 2 (BT 8T): Incidence of Benign Tumors Not Including the Ones Decreased[a] by Tamoxifen Treatment

				Benign Tumors			
		Animals		Animals Bearing Tumors		Tumors	
Group No.	Dose (mg/kg b.w.)	Sex	No.	No.	%	No.	Per 100 Animals
I	3.3	F	150	16	10.7	16	10.7
II	0	F	150	23	15.3	24	16.0

[a] Decreased benign tumors: mammary tumors, pituitary gland adenomas, pheochromocytomas, islet cell pancreatic tumors, polyps of the uterus (see TABLES 23–28).

TABLE 32. Results of Experiment 2 (BT 8T): Incidence of Malignant Tumors Not Including the Ones Decreased[a] or Increased[b] by Tamoxifen Treatment

				Malignant Tumors			
		Animals		Animals Bearing Tumors		Tumors	
Group No.	Dose (mg/kg b.w.)	Sex	No.	No.	%	No.	Per 100 Animals
I	3.3	F	150	28	18.7	29	19.3
II	0	F	150	26	17.3	28	18.7

[a] Decreased malignant tumors: mammary tumors, hepatocarcinomas (see TABLES 23 and 29).
[b] Increased malignant tumors: tumors of the uterus and vagina (see TABLE 30).

TABLE 33. Results of Experiment 3 (BT 12T): Number and Percentage of Female Sprague-Dawley Rats Bearing Various Types of Benign And Malignant Tumors[a]

		Groups			
		I: 3.3 mg/kg b.w.		II: 0 (Control)	
Site	Histotype	No.	%	No.	%
Skin	Squamous cell carcinoma	0	–	1	0.7
Subcutaneous tissue	Fibrosarcoma	0	–	1	0.7
	Angiosarcoma	0	–	1	0.7
Mammary gland[b]	Fibroma and fibroadenoma	48 (65)	35.2	65 (100)	46.8
	Adenocarcinoma	2	1.4	10 (13)	7.2
	Fibrosarcoma	2	1.4	1	0.7
	Liposarcoma	0	–	1	0.7
Sebaceous gland	Adenocarcinoma	0	–	1	0.7
Zymbal glands	Squamous cell carcinoma	1	0.7	0	–
Ear ducts	Squamous cell carcinoma	3	2.1	7	5.0
Nasal cavities	Squamous cell carcinoma	1	0.7	0	–
Oral cavity	Squamous cell carcinoma	2	1.4	0	–
Larynx	Rhabdomyosarcoma	0	–	1	0.7
Lung	Adenocarcinoma	1	0.7	0	–
Liver[c]	Fibroangioma	1	0.7	0	–
	Cholangioma	0	–	1	0.7
Pancreas[d]	Islet cell adenoma	2	1.4	7	5.0
	Fibrosarcoma	1	0.7	0	–
Ovaries	Granulosa and theca cell tumors	3	2.1	1	0.7
	Adenocarcinoma	1	0.7	1	0.7
Uterus[e]	Polyp	7	5.0	14	10.1
	Fibroma	0	–	2	1.4
	Fibroangioma	1	0.7	2	1.4
	Adenocarcinoma	2	1.4	3	2.1
	Squamous cell carcinoma	3	2.1	0	–
	Sarcoma	5	3.6	6	4.3

Vagina[e]	Squamous cell carcinoma	0	—	1	0.7
Peritoneum	Fibrosarcoma	1	0.7	0	—
	Mesothelioma	0	—	1	0.7
Pituitary gland[f]	Adenoma	27	19.4	44	31.6
Thyroid gland	C-cell adenoma	0	—	1	0.7
	Follicular carcinoma	1	0.7	1	0.7
	C-cell carcinoma	2	1.4	1	0.7
Adrenal glands[g]	Cortical adenoma	7	5.0	8	5.7
	Pheochromocytoma	13 (15)	9.3	15 (16)	10.8
	Cortical adenocarcinoma	1	0.7	0	—
	Pheochromoblastoma	1	0.7	0	—
Central nervous system					
Brain	Oligodendroglioma	1	0.7	2	1.4
Meninges	Meningioma	2	1.4	0	—
Major peripheral nerves	Malignant Schwannoma	1	0.7	0	—
Bones					
Cranium	Osteosarcoma	3	2.1	2	1.4
Others	Osteosarcoma	0	—	1	0.7
Soft tissues	Fibrosarcoma	1	0.7	0	—
Spleen	Fibroangioma	0	—	3	2.1
	Angiosarcoma	0	—	1	0.7
Hemolymphoreticular tissues[h]	Lymphomas and leukemias	15	10.8	12	8.6

[a] Numbers in parentheses indicate the number of tumors (one animal can bear more than one tumor).
[b] See TABLES 36, 37.
[c] See TABLE 42.
[d] See TABLE 39.
[e] See TABLES 40, 43.
[f] See TABLE 38.
[g] See TABLE 41.
[h] Including spleen.

TABLE 34. Results of Experiment 3 (BT 12T): Incidence of Total Benign Tumors

				Benign Tumors			
		Animals		Animals Bearing Tumors		Tumors	
Group No.	Dose (mg/kg b.w.)	Sex	No.	No.	%	No.	Per 100 Animals
I	3.3	F	139	69	49.6	130	93.5
II	0	F	139	92	66.2	199	143.2

TABLE 35. Results of Experiment 3 (BT 12T): Incidence of Total Malignant Tumors

				Malignant Tumors			
		Animals		Animals Bearing Tumors		Tumors	
Group No.	Dose (mg/kg b.w.)	Sex	No.	No.	%	No.	Per 100 Animals
I	3.3	F	139	45	32.4	53	38.1
II	0	F	139	43	30.9	59	42.4

TABLE 36. Results of Experiment 3 (BT 12T): Incidence of Benign Mammary Tumors

		Animals			Benign Mammary Tumors			
					Animals Bearing Tumors		Tumors	
Group No.	Dose (mg/kg b.w.)	Sex	No.	Biophase (weeks)	No.	%	No.	Per 100 Animals
I	3.3	F	139	96[a]	21	15.1	28	20.1
				143[b]	48	35.2	65	46.8
II	0	F	139	96[a]	39	28.0	66	47.5
				143[b]	65	46.8	100	71.9

[a] End of tamoxifen treatment.
[b] Life span.

TABLE 37. Results of Experiment 3 (BT 12T): Incidence of Malignant Mammary Tumors

		Animals			Malignant Mammary Tumors			
					Animals Bearing Tumors		Tumors	
Group No.	Dose (mg/kg b.w.)	Sex	No.	Biophase (weeks)	No.	%	No.	Per 100 Animals
I	3.3	F	139	96[a]	0	—	0	—
				143[b]	4	2.8	4	2.8
II	0	F	139	96[a]	8	5.7	10	7.2
				143[b]	12	8.6	15	10.8

[a] End of tamoxifen treatment.
[b] Life span.

TABLE 38. Results of Experiment 3 (BT 12T): Incidence of Pituitary Gland Tumors

Group	Dose	Animals		Biophase	Animals Bearing Pituitary Gland Adenomas	
No.	(mg/kg b.w.)	Sex	No.	(weeks)	No.	%
I	3.3	F	139	143[a]	27	19.4
II	0	F	139	143[a]	44	31.6

[a] Life span.

TABLE 39. Results of Experiment 3 (BT 12T): Incidence of Islet Cell Pancreatic Tumors

Group	Dose	Animals		Biophase	Animals Bearing Tumors			
					Islet Cell Adenomas		Islet Cell Adenocarcinoma	
No.	(mg/kg b.w.)	Sex	No.	(weeks)	No.	%	No.	%
I	3.3	F	139	143[a]	2	1.4	0	–
II	0	F	139	143[a]	7	5.0	0	–

[a] Life span.

TABLE 40. Results of Experiment 3 (BT 12T): Incidence of Polyps of the Uterus

Group No.	Dose (mg/kg b.w.)	Animals		Biophase (weeks)	Animals Bearing Tumors	
		Sex	No.		No.	%
I	3.3	F	139	143[a]	7	5.0
II	0	F	139	143[a]	14	10.1

[a] Life span.

TABLE 41. Results of Experiment 3 (BT 12T): Incidence of Adrenal Gland Pheochromocytomas and Pheochromoblastomas

Group No.	Dose (mg/kg b.w.)	Animals		Biophase (weeks)	Pheochromocytomas				Pheochromoblastomas			
					Animals Bearing Tumors		Tumors		Animals Bearing Tumors		Tumors	
		Sex	No.		No.	%	No.	Per 100 Animals	No.	%	No.	Per 100 Animals
I	3.3	F	139	143[a]	13	9.3	15	10.8	1	0.7	1	0.7
II	0	F	139	143[a]	15	10.8	16	11.5	0	—	0	—

[a] Life span.

TABLE 42. Results of Experiment 3 (BT 12T): Incidence of Tumors and Other Lesions of Oncological Interest of the Liver

Group	Dose	Animals		Biophase	Animals Bearing Liver Changes							
					Nodular Hyperplasias		Nodular Dysplasias		Hepatoadenomas		Hepatocarcinomas	
No.	(mg/kg b.w.)	Sex	No.	(weeks)	No.	%	No.	%	No.	%	No.	%
I	3.3	F	139	143[a]	8	5.7	0	—	0	—	0	—
II	0	F	139	143[a]	8	5.7	0	—	0	—	0	—

[a] Life span.

TABLE 43. Results of Experiment 3 (BT 12T): Incidence of Malignant Tumors of the Uterus and Vagina

Group	Treatment	Animals		Biophase	Animals Bearing Tumors											
					Uterus				Vagina				Total			
					Carcinomas		Sarcomas		Carcinomas		Sarcomas		Carcinomas		Sarcomas	
No.	(mg/kg b.w.)	Sex	No.	(weeks)	No.	%	No.	%	No.	%	No.	%	No.	%	No.	%
I	3.3	F	139	143[a]	5	3.6	5	3.6	0	—	0	—	5	3.6	5	3.6
II	0	F	139	143[a]	3	1.2	6	4.3	1	0.7	0	—	4	2.9	6	4.3

[a] Life span.

TABLE 44. Results of Experiment 3 (BT 12T): Incidence of Benign Tumors Not Including the Ones Decreased[a] by Tamoxifen Treatment

				Benign Tumors			
		Animals		Animals Bearing Tumors		Tumors	
Group No.	Dose (mg/kg b.w.)	Sex	No.	No.	%	No.	Per 100 Animals
I	3.3	F	139	25	18.0	29	20.9
II	0	F	139	29	20.9	34	24.5

[a] Decreased benign tumors: mammary tumors, pituitary gland adenomas, islet cell pancreatic tumors, polyps of the uterus (see TABLES 36, 38, 39, and 40).

TABLE 45. Results of Experiment 3 (BT 12T): Incidence of Malignant Tumors Not Including the Ones Decreased[a] by Tamoxifen Treatment

				Malignant Tumors			
		Animals		Animals Bearing Tumors		Tumors	
Group No.	Dose (mg/kg b.w.)	Sex	No.	No.	%	No.	Per 100 Animals
I	3.3	F	139	40	28.8	47	33.8
II	0	F	139	36	25.9	44	31.6

[a] Decreased malignant tumors: mammary tumors (see TABLE 37).

4. when given at the dose of 3.3 mg/kg b.w., 10 times the ordinary dose in women, continuously for the life span, tamoxifen caused a slight increase in liver tumors. A borderline increase in malignancies of the uterus and vagina was also observed;
5. when the drug is given at the same dose, intermittently for the life span, an increase in uterine cancers (mainly sarcomas) was observed, but no carcinogenic effect on the liver was detected;
6. when the drug was given at the same dose, continuously but for a limited period of time, in adult female rats, no carcinogenic effect was detected; it must be pointed out that in this experiment, not only is the dose 10 times higher than the current clinical dose, but the length of treatment, with respect to the life span of the animal tested, is much longer than that considered in adjuvant therapy and in the chemoprevention of mammary cancer, with respect to the average age of women; and
7. tamoxifen increases the oncological pathology of the mammary gland in males.

On the basis of our data and of the experimental and clinical information from the scientific literature, the carcinogenic effects of tamoxifen on the liver and uterus appear to be related to the total dose. Such a dose relationship is clearly demonstrated for liver carcinogenesis in rats (TABLE 1) and, to some extent, also for uterine carcinogenesis in women: in fact, it is not by chance that the first evidence of endometrial uterine cancer was detected in the Swedish adjuvant therapy trial, in which tamoxifen was administered at the dose of 40 mg/day.

The chemopreventive effect of tamoxifen on mammary carcinoma is specifically effective in the control of breast cancer. However, even the carcinogenic side effects cannot be underestimated. As very often occurs in medical practice, the problem now is to assess whether there is a dose of the drug that is effective for chemoprevention, but that does not entail serious carcinogenic risks. There are two facts that support the expectation that such a dose may exist. Our data show that life-span treatment with tamoxifen at a dose 10 times higher than the one ordinarily employed in medical practice entails only marginal carcinogenic effects (Experiment 1), which, however, do not emerge in the experiment where the drug was given for a limited period, although still at a high dose and with continuous administration (Experiment 3). On the other hand, another series of experiments in our project (now ready for publication) have shown that 0.1 mg/kg b.w. of tamoxifen, corresponding to 6 mg daily in women, still completely inhibited the onset of spontaneous mammary cancer in our colony of rats, therefore demonstrating that doses much lower than 20 mg daily may still be effective in adjuvant therapy. The time has come to review the tamoxifen posology, in order to continue to benefit from its chemopreventive/therapeutic effect without creating risk situations.

SUMMARY

Tamoxifen was submitted to carcinogenicity bioassays on Sprague-Dawley rats (of the colony used at the Cancer Research Center in the Castle of Bentivoglio of the European Ramazzini Foundation of Oncology and Environmental Sciences) at the dose of 3.3 mg/kg b.w., by stomach tube, in three experiments.

In the first experiment the drug was administered once daily, 6 days a week to male and female rats, 8 weeks old at start for their life span. In the second experiment, the drug was administered to female rats, 12 weeks old at start, once daily for 8 consecutive days every 8 weeks for their life span. In the third experiment the drug was administered to female rats, 56 weeks old at start, 6 times weekly for 40 weeks; and then the animals were kept alive for their life span.

In the first experiment, a mild increase in hepatocarcinomas with low grading was detected. In the first and second experiments, a borderline increase in uterine malignancies was found. No carcinogenic effect was observed in the third experiment.

In the three experiments, tamoxifen showed a strong, long-lasting chemopreventive effect on mammary benign tumors and cancers. The presented data also indicate that tamoxifen treatment reduces the incidence of other tumors: pituitary adenomas, adrenal pheochromocytomas, islet cell pancreatic tumors, Leydig cell testicular tumors, and polyps of the uterus.

REFERENCES

1. Cole, M. P., C. T. A. Jones & I. D. H. Todd. 1971. A new anti-oestrogenic agent in late breast cancer. An early clinical appraisal of ICI 46474. Br. J. Cancer **25:** 270-275.
2. Furr, B. J. A. & V. C. Jordan. 1984. The pharmacology and clinical uses of tamoxifen. Pharmacol. & Ther. **25:** 127-205.
3. Jordan, V. C. 1976. Effect of tamoxifen (ICI 46,474) on initiation and growth of DMBA-induced rat mammary carcinomata. Eur. J. Cancer **12:** 419-424.
4. Ludwig Breast Cancer Study Group. 1984. Randomized trial of chemo-endocrine therapy and mastectomy alone in postmenopausal patients with operable breast cancer and axillary node metastases. Lancet **1:** 1256-1260.
5. Senanayake, F. 1984. Adjuvant hormonal chemotherapy in early breast cancer: Early results from a controlled trial. Lancet **2:** 1148-1149.
6. Cummings, F. J., R. Gray, T. E. Davis *et al.* 1985. Adjuvant tamoxifen treatment of elderly women with stage II breast cancer. A double blind comparison with placebo. Ann. Intern. Med. **103:** 324-329.
7. Palshof, T., B. Carstensen, H. T. Mouridsen *et al.* 1985. Adjuvant endocrine therapy in pre- and postmenopausal women with operable breast cancer. Rev. Endocrine Rel. Cancer **17** (Suppl.): 43-50.
8. Rose, C., S. M. Thorpe, K. W. Andersen *et al.* 1985. Beneficial effect of adjuvant tamoxifen therapy in primary breast cancer patients with high estrogen receptor values. Lancet **1:** 16-19.
9. Breast Cancer Trials Committee, Scottish cancer trials office. 1987. Adjuvant tamoxifen in the management of operable breast cancer: The Scottish trial. Lancet **2:** 171-175.
10. Delozier, T., J.-P. Julien, P. Juret *et al.* 1987. Adjuvant tamoxifen in postmenopausal breast cancer: Preliminary results of a randomized trial. Breast Cancer Res. Treat. **7:** 105-110.
11. Pritchard, K., J. W. Meakin, N. F. Boyd *et al.* 1987. Adjuvant tamoxifen in postmenopausal women with axillary node positive breast cancer: An update. *In* Adjuvant Therapy of Cancer. S. E. Salmon, Ed.: 391-400. Grune and Stratton. Orlando, FL.
12. Rutqvist, I. E., B. Cedermark, U. Glas *et al.* 1987. The Stockholm trial on adjuvant tamoxifen in early breast cancer. Breast Cancer Res. Treat. **10:** 255-266.
13. Bianco, A. R., C. Gallo, S. Marinelli *et al.* 1988. Adjuvant therapy with tamoxifen in operable breast cancer: 10 year results of the Naples (GUN) study. Lancet **2:** 1095-1099.

14. CRC Adjuvant Breast Trial Working Party. 1988. Cyclophosphamide and tamoxifen as adjuvant therapies in the management of breast cancer. Br. J. Cancer **57:** 604-607.
15. Nolvadex Adjuvant Trial Organization. 1988. Controlled trial of Tamoxifen as a single adjuvant agent in the management of early breast cancer. Br. J. Cancer **57:** 608-611.
16. Ribeiro, G. & R. Swindell. 1988. The Christie Hospital adjuvant tamoxifen trial. Status at 10 years. Br. J. Cancer **57:** 601-603.
17. Fisher, B., J. Costantino, C. Redmond *et al.* 1989. A randomized clinical trial evaluating tamoxifen in the treatment of patients with node-negative breast cancer who have estrogen-receptor-positive tumors. N. Engl. J. Med. **320:** 479-484.
18. Cummings, F. J., R. Gray, D. C. Tormey *et al.* 1993. Adjuvant tamoxifen versus placebo in elderly women with node-positive breast cancer: Long-term follow-up and causes of death. J. Clin. Oncol. **11:** 29-35.
19. Fisher, B., J. Costantino, L. Wickerham *et al.* 1993. Adjuvant therapy for node-negative breast cancer: An update of NSABP findings. Proc. Am. Soc. Clin. Oncol. **12:** 79.
20. Jordan, V. C., K. E. Allen & C. J. Dix. 1980. Pharmacology of tamoxifen in laboratory animals. Cancer Treat. Rep. **64:** 745-759.
21. Pento, J. T., R. A. Magarian & M. M. King. 1982. A comparison of the efficacy for antitumor activity of the non-steroidal antiestrogens analog II and tamoxifen in 7,12-dimethylbenz[a]nthracene-induced rat mammary tumors. Cancer Lett. **15:** 261-269.
22. McCormick, D. L. & R. C. Moon. 1986. Retinoid-tamoxifen interaction in mammary cancer chemoprevention. Carcinogenesis **7:** 193-196.
23. Gottardis, M. M. & V. C. Jordan. 1987. Antitumor actions of keokifene and tamoxifen in the N-nitrosomethylurea-induced rat mammary carcinoma model. Cancer Res. **47:** 4020-4024.
24. Teelmann, K. & W. Bollag. 1988. Therapeutic effects of the arotenoid Ro 15-0778 on chemically-induced rat mammary carcinoma. Eur. J. Cancer Clin. Oncol. **24:** 1205-1209.
25. Ratko, T. A., C. J. Detrisac, N. M. Dinger, *et al.* 1989. Chemopreventive efficacy of combined retinoid and tamoxifen treatment following surgical excision of a primary mammary cancer in female rats. Cancer Res. **49:** 4472-4476.
26. Jordan, V. C., M. K. Lababidi & D. M. Mirecki. 1990. Anti-oestrogenic and anti-tumour properties of prolonged tamoxifen therapy in C3H/OUJ mice. Eur. J. Cancer **26:** 718-721.
27. Maltoni, C., C. Pinto & G. Paladini. 1988. Project of experimental bioassays on chemoprevention agents performed at the Bologna Institute of Oncology: Report on tamoxifen control of spontaneous mammary tumors on Sprague-Dawley rats. Cancer Invest. **6:** 643-658.
28. Maltoni, C., M. Soffritti, C. Pinto, *et al.* 1988. Il contributo sperimentale alla chemioprevenzione. *In* Atti del XIV Congresso Nazionale di Oncologia: Il ruolo della terapia chirurgica in oncologia. Vol. II. F. Morino, L. Caldarola, A. Mussa, P. Calderini, D. Carretti & C. Maltoni, Eds.: 1073-1100. Monduzzi. Bologna.
29. Maltoni, C., C. Pinto, A. Mobiglia *et al.* 1989. La chemioprevenzione dei tumori: Bilanci, ricerche in corso e prospettive. *In* Aggiornamenti in Oncologia Medica. G. Rasà, C. Maltoni, S. Amato, G. Castiglione, G. Grasso, M. L. Palmeri & F. Cuva, Eds.: 3-89. Monduzzi. Bologna.
30. Maltoni, C., C. Pinto, M. Soffritti *et al.* 1989. La chemioprevenzione dei tumori della mammella: Acquisizioni disponibili, con particolare riguardo ai dati sperimentali. *In* I tumori della mammella. C. Maltoni, D. Marrano, S. Rubini, D. F. Rivelli & V. Patella, Eds.: 305-359. Monduzzi. Bologna.
31. Maltoni, C., F. Minardi, C. Pinto *et al.* 1990. Long-term bioassays on the toxic, carcinogenic and tumour chemopreventive effects (particularly on mammary carcinomas) of tamoxifen on Sprague-Dawley rats: Ongoing studies and early results. Acta Oncol. **11:** 289-305.

32. MALTONI, C., C. PINTO, A. MOBIGLIA *et al.* 1990. La chemioprevenzione dei tumori: Lo stato attuale delle conoscenze ed il progetto di ricerca dell'Istituto di Oncologia di Bologna. *In* Aggiornamenti in oncologia medica. T. Battelli, Ed.: 111-169. Monduzzi. Bologna.
33. MALTONI, C., C. PINTO, M. SOFFRITTI *et al.* 1990. Chemioprevenzione dei tumori della mammella. Argomenti di Oncologia **11:** 1-22.
34. MALTONI, C., F. MINARDI & C. PINTO. 1991. Il tamoxifen come potenziale agente chemiopreventivo nel carcinoma mammario nella donna: Scenario, presupposti scientifici, recenti acquisizioni sperimentali e studi clinici disponibili e in programmazione. *In* Progressi in oncologia clinica, Tamoxifene, Vol. I. G. Robustelli della Cuna & F. Pannuti, Eds.: 117-138. EDIMES. Pavia.
35. MALTONI, C., F. MINARDI, C. PINTO *et al.* 1991. Un nuovo approccio al controllo del carcinoma mammario nella donna: La chemioprevenzione. Adria Medica **2:** 11-50.
36. MALTONI, C., F. MINARDI, C. PINTO *et al.* 1991. La chemioprevenzione del carcinoma mammario: Bilancio delle conoscenze e prospettive. Atti delle Giornate Medico-Chirurgiche Internazionali in onore di Achille Mario Dogliotti, Vol. I: 91-172. Minerva Medica. Torino.
37. MALTONI, C., F. MINARDI, C. PINTO *et al.* 1992. La chemioprevenzione del carcinoma mammario: Basi scientifiche e orientamenti. *In* Atti del XVIII Congresso Nazionale di Oncologia, Il cancro della mammella alle soglie del Duemila, Vol. I. T. Battelli, P. Manocchi, R. Mattioli, A. Pilone, S. Delprete, S. Rossini, G. De Signoribus, R. R. Silva, D. Carretti & C. Maltoni, Eds.: 127-142. Monduzzi. Bologna.
38. MALTONI, C., F. MINARDI, M. SOFFRITTI *et al.* 1992. La prevenzione del carcinoma mammario: Presupposti scientifici e programmi. Acta Oncol. **13:** 523-530.
39. MALTONI, C., F. MINARDI, M. SOFFRITTI *et al.* 1994. The role of experimental research in cancer chemoprevention using human-equivalent animal models: A project on tamoxifen. *In* Sex Hormones and Antihormones in Endocrine Dependent Pathology: Basic and Clinical Aspects. M. Motta & M. Serio, Eds.: 319-329. Elsevier. Amsterdam.
40. FISHER, B. 1992. The evolution of paradigms for the management of breast cancer: A personal perspective. Cancer Res. **52:** 2371-2383.
41. LOVE, R. R. 1993. The National Surgical Adjuvant Breast Project (NSABP) Breast Cancer Prevention Trial revisited. Cancer Epidemiol. Biomarkers Prev. **2:** 403-407.
42. LIPPMAN, S. M., S. E. BENNER & W. K. HONG. 1994. Cancer chemoprevention. J. Clin. Oncol. **12:** 851-873.
43. VERONESI, U. & C. MALTONI. 1992. Protocollo di chemioprevenzione del carcinoma mammario con tamoxifen.
44. CUZICK, J. 1992. Protocol for the UKCCCR National Multicentre Tamoxifen Breast Cancer Prevention Trial.
45. POWLES, T. J., A. L. JONES, S. E. ASHLEY *et al.* 1994. The Royal Marsden Hospital pilot tamoxifen chemoprevention trial. Breast Cancer Res. Treat. **31:** 73-82.
46. BLACKBURN, A. M., S. A. AMIEL, R. R. MILLIS *et al.* 1984. Tamoxifen and liver damage. Br. Med. J. **289:** 288.
47. CLARYSSE, A. 1985. Hormone-induced tumor flare. Eur. J. Cancer Clin. Oncol. **21:** 545-547.
48. DIVER, J. M., I. M. JACKSON & J. D. FITZGERALD. 1986. Letter to the editor, Tamoxifen and non-malignant indication. Lancet **1:** 733.
49. SMITH, I. 1988. Adjuvant tamoxifen for early breast cancer. Br. J. Cancer **57:** 527-528.
50. LOVE, R. R. 1989. Prospects for antiestrogen chemoprevention of breast cancer. J. Natl. Cancer Inst. **82:** 18-21.
51. POWLES, T. J., J. R. HARDY, S. E. ASHLEY *et al.* 1989. Chemoprevention of breast cancer. Breast Cancer Res. Treat. **14:** 23-31.
52. POWLES, T. J., J. R. HARDY, S. E. ASHLEY *et al.* 1989. A pilot trial to evaluate the acute toxicity and feasibility of tamoxifen for prevention of breast cancer. Br. J. Cancer **60:** 126-131.

53. Powles, T. J., C. R. Tillyer, A. L. Jones *et al.* 1990. Prevention of breast cancer with tamoxifen—An update on the Royal Marsden Hospital Pilot Programme. Eur. J. Cancer **26:** 680–684.
54. Fornander, T., L. E. Rutqvist, B. Cedermark *et al.* 1989. Adjuvant tamoxifen in early breast cancer: Occurrence of new primary cancer. Lancet **1:** 117–120.
55. Fisher, B., J. P. Costantino, C. K. Redmond *et al.* 1994. Endometrial cancer in tamoxifen-treated breast cancer patients: Findings from the National Surgical Adjuvant Breast and Bowel Project (NSABP) B-14. J. Natl. Cancer Inst. **86:** 527–537.
56. Williams, G. M., M. J. Iatropoulos, M. V. Djordjevic *et al.* 1993. The triphenylethylene drug tamoxifen is a strong liver carcinogen in the rat. Carcinogenesis **14:** 315–317.
57. Greaves, P., R. Goonetilleke, G. Nunn *et al.* 1993. Two-year carcinogenicity study of tamoxifen in Alderley Park Wistar-derived rats. Cancer Res. **53:** 3919–3924.
58. Hard, G. C., M. J. Iatropoulos, K. Jordan *et al.* 1993. Major difference in the hepatocarcinogenicity and DNA adduct forming ability between toremifene and tamoxifen in female Crl: CD (BR) rats. Cancer Res. **53:** 4534–4541.
59. Hirsimäki, P., Y. Hirsimäki, L. Nieminen *et al.* 1993. Tamoxifen induces hepatocellular carcinoma in rat liver: A 1-year study with two antiestrogens. Arch. Toxicol. **67:** 49–54.
60. Dragan, Y. P., S. Fahey, K. Street *et al.* 1994. Studies of tamoxifen as a promoter of hepatocarcinogenesis in female Fischer F344 rats. Breast Cancer Res. Treat. **31:** 11–25.

Recent Developments on the Avoidable Causes of Breast Cancer

DEVRA LEE DAVIS,[a] MONTIRA J. PONGSIRI,[b] AND MARY WOLFF[c]

[a]*Strang Cornell Cancer Research Laboratory*
The Rockefeller University
1230 York Avenue
New York, New York 10021
and
World Resources Institute
1709 New York Avenue, N.W.
Washington, D.C. 20006

[b]*Department of Public Health*
Yale University School of Forestry and Environmental Studies
New Haven, Connecticut

[c]*Mount Sinai School of Medicine*
1 Gustave L. Levy Place
New York, New York 10029

INTRODUCTION

Breast cancer remains a puzzling disease of enormous public health importance. While incidence of many cancers has declined in the past two decades, the rates of breast cancer and related deaths have been rising steadily. In the United States, 44,000 women die of breast cancer every year, and each of them loses nearly two decades of life. This is translated into the equivalent loss of almost one million woman-years of life. Increased levels of screening alone cannot account for the worldwide jump in breast cancer rates. Routine mammography screening is available only in some developed countries and cannot account for increased deaths in developing regions.[1] This section highlights new developments in the effort to identify avoidable causes of breast cancer. It provides recent updates from several leading researchers working on experimental and epidemiologic analysis, drawing upon the 1997 *Environmental Health Perspectives* monograph "Hormones, Hormone Metabolism, Environment, and Breast Cancer."

There are important differences in the disease profiles between ethnic groups both across and within geographical borders. While there has been recent progress in reducing deaths in American women under 65, new cases are appearing in older white and African-American women. Four out of five white women versus three out of five African-American women survive disease. In addition, socioeconomic differences exist in the stage distribution of disease. Forty-six percent of low-income women are diagnosed at Stages 0 and 1 compared with 59% in the high-income group.[1]

Compared to Asian countries, rates of breast cancer are much higher among United States women, but they are increasing rapidly in those areas. In 1980, the incident rate of breast cancer in white women in the United States was upwards of four times higher than the rate in China, Japan, and the Philippines.[1] Other migration studies have confirmed that lifestyle and environment are important factors in breast cancer risk. Asian women who have migrated to the United States develop breast cancer rates comparable to those of their new country over time. Furthermore, Asian-American women who were born and raised in the United States had a 60% higher risk of disease than women who had immigrated.[2]

Most cases of breast cancer cannot be explained by established risk factors, including early menarche and genetic predisposition (see TABLE 1). In fact, fewer than 10% of cases are related to inherited genetic abnormalities. At most, only half of all reported cases occur in women with known risk factors.

XENOHORMONE THEORY

A common feature of most of the established risk factors of breast cancer is exposure to hormones. We have proposed that the remaining unknown causes may include exposure to environmental chemicals, which can produce breast cancer by two distinct paths: one path chiefly involves estrogen or other hormones, while the other works principally by affecting genetic events[3] (see FIGURE 1). Based on a series of recent experimental and epidemiological findings, it is believed that some incidence of breast cancer arises from the action of endogenous or exogenous hormones. The exogenous hormones, coined *xenohormones,* have the ability to disrupt normal cellular functions through both hormonal and genetic mechanisms. These xenohormones may mimic the action of natural estrogen and even androgen, which can influence the ultimate production and metabolism of estrogen.

Davis *et al.* have hypothesized that breast cancer may be linked to the metabolism of estrogen. Depending on the exclusive pathway by which estrogen is broken down by p450, signals for breast cell proliferation can be induced. Pathway I leads to the formation of 2-hydroxyestrone, which binds weakly to the estrogen receptor and is excreted relatively rapidly from the body. Alternatively, pathway II yields 16-alphahydroxyestrone, which tends to persist in the body and can tightly and irreversibly bind to the estrogen receptor, leading to some cancer-causing events[4] (FIGURE 2). *In vivo* evidence has shown that 16-alphahydroxyestrone levels are higher in breast cancer patients than in those with reduction mammoplasty. Interestingly, 16-alphahydroxyestrone levels are lower in Asian women, who traditionally have lower rates of breast cancer incidence.[5]

Once xenoestrogens reach the inside of a cell, they may affect the balance between the key metabolites by enhancing the production of the "bad" 16-alphahydroxyestrone estrogens or, through binding with the estrogen receptor, can turn on the genes that regulate cell growth. Xenoestrogens, including chlorinated organics and some polycyclic aromatic hydrocarbons (PAHs), and other agents that alter the ratio of 2-hydroxyestrone to 16-alpha-hydroxyestrone production and bioavailability could set the stage for tumor growth. As relatively more 16-alpha-hydroxyestrone is produced, there is a greater chance for it to physiologically affect many normal functions. In

TABLE 1. Established Risk Factors for Breast Cancer in Women[a]

Factor	High-risk Group	Low-risk Group
	Relative Risk Greater than 4.0	
Age	Old	Young
Country of birth	North America, Northern Europe	Asia, Africa
Mother *and* sister with history of breast cancer, especially if diagnosed at an early age	Yes	No
Atypical epithelial cells in nipple aspirate fluid	Yes	No fluid produced
Mutations in BRCA1 and BRCA2, breast cancer at early age	Yes	No
	Relative Risk of 2.1-4.0	
Nodular densities on mammogram	Densities occupying >75% of breast volume	Parenchyma composed entirely of fat
History of cancer in one breast	Yes	No
Mother *or* sister with history of breast cancer	Yes	No
Biopsy-confirmed benign proliferative breast disease	Yes	No
Hyperplastic epithelial cells without atypia in nipple aspirate fluid	Yes	No fluid produced
Radiation to chest in moderate to high doses	Yes	No
	Relative Risk of 1.1-2.0	
Socioeconomic status	High	Low
Marital status	Never married	Ever married
Place of residence	Urban	Rural
Place of residence (within United States)	Northern	Southern
Race/ethnicity, breast cancer ≥45 years of age	White	Hispanic, Asian
Race/ethnicity, breast cancer <40 years of age	Black	Hispanic, Asian
Religion	Jewish	Seventh Day Adventist, Mormon
Removal of ovaries before age 40	No	Yes
Parity, breast cancer ≥40 years of age	Nulliparous	≥4
Parity, breast cancer <40 years of age	Parous	Nulliparous
Age at first full-term pregnancy	≥30	<20
Age at menarche	≤11	≥15
Age at menopause	≥55	<45
History of primary cancer in endometrium, ovary	Yes	No
Weight, breast cancer ≥50 years of age	Obese	Thin

[a] From Kelsey *et al.*[19]

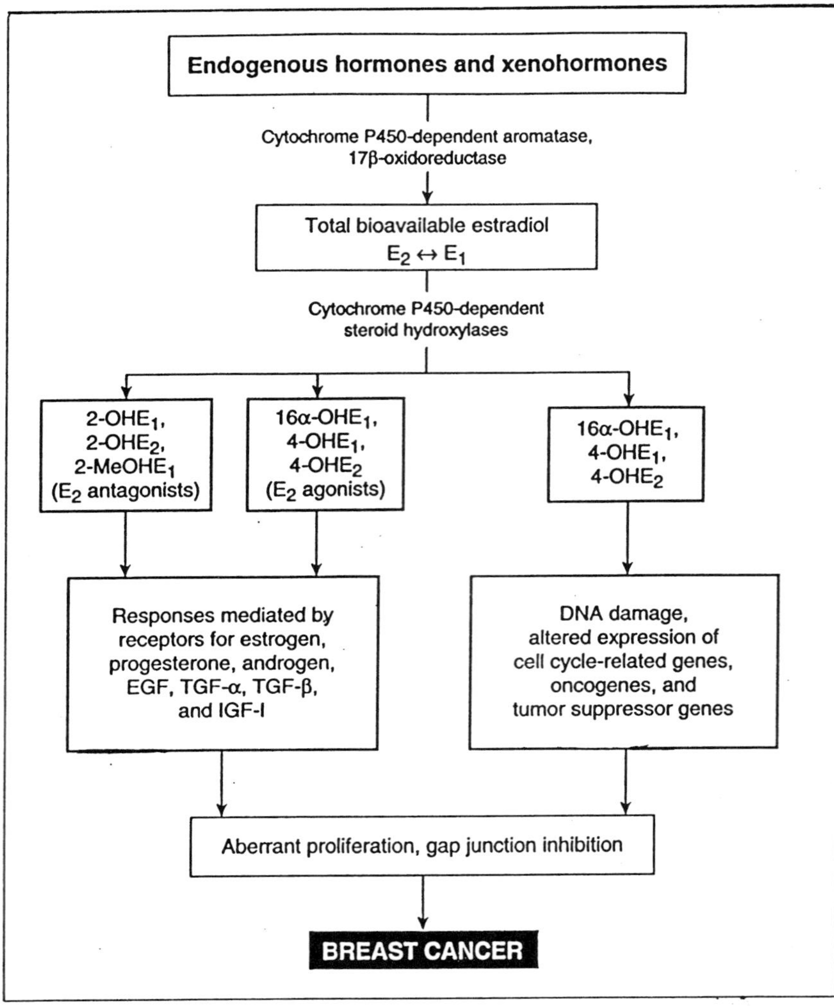

FIGURE 1. Reported differential effects of estrogen metabolites on receptor-mediated responses and directly on DNA suggest the possibility of developing biologic markers to identify women at risk of breast cancer. Examples of such markers might be radical-induced DNA damage and ratios of estrogen metabolites. (Reprinted with permission from Davis *et al.*[1])

addition to this hormonal path to breast cancer, 16-alphahydroxyestrone has the ability to affect genetic events relevant to breast cancer. It can alter the integrity of DNA by up-regulating oncogenes *jun* and *fos,* which lead to genetic instability. 16-Alphahydroxyestrone may even lead to structural or functional damage by disrupting the sequences of bases that comprise DNA or otherwise compromise the ability of DNA

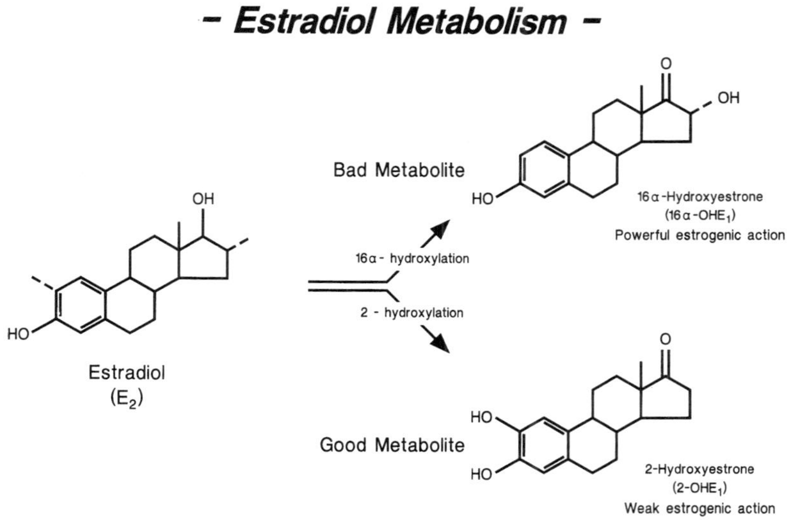

FIGURE 2. Metabolic pathways of estrogen. (Reproduced with permission from the World Resources Institute website.[5])

to direct repair.[5] In addition, reduction-oxidation at the 4-position of estrogen during its metabolism yields 4-hydroxyestrone, which may also covalently bind with the estrogen receptor (ER) and induce carcinogenesis through radical-induced DNA damage [2] (see FIGURE 1). Furthermore, some materials may not affect ER but instead directly alter p450, which is responsible for the formation of 16-alphahydroxyestrone. Both hormonal and genetic pathways result in the up-regulation of aberrant proliferation and development of breast cancer.[3]

Receptors for several major hormones, including estrogen, progesterone, and androgen, appear to be more commonly expressed in breast cancer cases. The complex interrelationships among these hormones remain to be elucidated. One study of human breast cancer found that the androgen receptor was the sex hormone receptor most frequently found both in primary and secondary breast cancer, and occurred much more frequently in metastatic cases.[6] Another recent study of cultured MCF-7 human breast cancer cells reported that androgens prevent the estrogen-dependent augmentation of the cytoplasmic progesterone receptor. Women with lower levels of androgens in their urine had a significantly greater rate of recurrence of disease.[7]

The development of the human breast involves a number of steroid hormones, including "male" hormones, such as androgen and testosterone, and "female" steroids, 17B estradiol (E2) and progesterone. Kelce *et al.* reported that p,p DDE acts as a potent anti-androgen in male rats.[8] It is possible that agents that function like male hormones in the female can increase the production of bioavailable estradiol by signaling the pituitary to produce estrogen and progesterone above normal levels. In that manner, anti-androgens might elevate circulating estradiol through the hypothalamic-gonadal-pituitary axis. Against a perceived deficit of androgen, the body could produce greater levels of estrogen.[8]

ANIMAL EVIDENCE

Although we may at best extrapolate from animal data, they are important in supporting epidemiological evidence and alerting us to potential carcinogens. Many chemicals, including pesticides and polycyclic aromatic hydrocarbons, have been shown to promote breast cancer in rodents, and these can guide us in evaluating their roles in human disease (see TABLE 2). Of course, there are important differences between animal and human systems to be noted when we generalize animal results. Not all compounds that are carcinogenic in animals cause cancer or even pose high risks in humans. In addition, none of the chemicals tested by the National Cancer Institute to promote mammary tumor growth in animals is specific to just the breast. Therefore, it is critical to consider the dose, exposure level, and site of tumor development in the model. The animal studies reported to date have implicated a number of environmental chemicals as causes of breast cancer.[9]

Organochlorines and chemically related pesticides are especially persistent in the environment and in the body, as their use patterns are widespread, leading to long-term exposures. Despite the carcinogenic labels given to many, only DDT has been linked to mammary gland tumors in animals.[9] Much attention has recently been drawn to the reproductive effects of DDT on wildlife.

PAHs, which originate from cigarette smoke, smoked food products, and air pollution, cause mammary gland tumors in animals, but have not yet convincingly been associated with breast cancer in humans. One reason is that PAHs have shorter lifetimes than DDT, and cannot directly be measured for cumulative exposures. PAHs may promote tumors long before detection is possible, so markers of exposure at critical time periods have to be determined.[9]

One instance of a short-lived, but potent breast carcinogen is diethylstilbestrol (DES). DES was prescribed to pregnant women before the 1970s in order to prevent spontaneous abortions and to maintain healthy fetuses. It has been shown to cause mammary gland tumors in rats and mice. 1,2-Dibromoethane (EDB) also induces breast tumors in both rats and mice, and at every exposure level applied to males and females. Interestingly, dermal, inhalation, and oral routes of exposure produced tumors at sites of application as well as at far removed sites for some compounds. Ted Colton *et al.* reported that mothers who used DES during pregnancy had a 50% increased risk of breast cancer, based on very short exposures during pregnancy.[10] 1,2-Dibromo-3-chloropropane (DBCP) is a widely used agricultural insecticide that promotes mammary tumor growth in female rats and is implicated in a number of reproductive disorders.[9]

EXPERIMENTAL STUDIES

There are two mechanisms by which xenoestrogens may directly influence breast tumor growth. They can affect cell proliferation via receptor-independent mechanisms involving structural/functional alterations in DNA. They can also directly bind to the estrogen receptor, which acts as a transcription factor regulating growth. The estrogen receptor can regulate genes such as c-*fos,* c-*jun,* and c-*myc,* which are involved in breast cell proliferation. 16-alpha-hydroxyestrone binds to the estrogen receptor

TABLE 2. NTP-Evaluated Chemicals Associated with Mammary Gland Cancer in Laboratory Animals (as of July 1997)[a]

TR No.	Chemical
049	Acronycine
289	Benzene
452	2,2-Bis(bromomethyl)-1,3-propanediol
288	1,3-Butadiene
434	1,3-Butadiene
379	2-Chloroaceto phenone (CN)
467	Chloroprene
405	C.I. Acid red 114
285	C.I. Basic red 9 monohydrochloride
091	Clonitralid
207	Cytembena
162	2,4-Diaminotoluene (2,4 toluene diamine)
028	1,2-Dibromo-3-chloropropane
210	1,2-Dibromoethane
400	2,3-Dibromo-1-propanol
066	1,1-Dichloroethane
055	1,2-Dichloroethane
263	1,2-Dichloropropane (propylene dichloride)
342	Dichlorvos
372	3,3′-Dimethoxybenzidin dihydrochloride
390	3,3′-Dimethylbenzidine dihydrochloride
054	2,4-Dinitrotoluene
326	Ethylene oxide
356	Furosemide
374	Glycidol
092	Hydrazobenzene
032	Isophosphamide
306	Methylene chloride
146	Nithiazide
118	5-Nitroacenaphthene
337	Nitrofurazone
461	Nitromethane
358	Ochratoxin A
060	Phenesterin
019	Procarbazine hydrochloride
193	Reserpine
115	Sulfallate
251	2,4- & 2,6-Toluene diisocyanate
153	O-Toluidine hydrochloride
384	1,2,3-Trichloropropane

Number of chemicals causing tumors in mammary gland: 40

[a] From electronic communication with James Huff, National Institute of Environmental Health Sciences, Research Triangle Park, NC 27709.

covalently and irreversibly and may affect these same genes. The estrogen receptor is also implicated in the down-regulation of tumor suppressors, such as p53 and Rb.[2] Other functional damage of the DNA that may result involves the activation of telomerase, which protects chromosome ends from degradation, ensuring proper replication and preventing the activation of DNA damage checkpoints. Telomerase activity is not detected in normal somatic cells, but is present in immortal, cancerous ones, so that replication is stable and continuous.[11] Others have studied the links between 16-alpha-hydroxyestrone and a decrease in gap junction communication, also involved in cellular growth. And, 16-alpha-hydroxyestrone induces DNA repair synthesis, which is a well-established marker of DNA damage. High levels of this metabolite may prove to be useful as a flag for the early stages of breast cancer.[2]

Not all xenoestrogens disrupt normal endocrine functioning. Xenoestrogens in some synthetic chemicals and foods can bind to the estrogen receptor and cause cell proliferation. However, they differ in their ability to produce certain estrogen metabolites and regulate the cell cycle. *Persistent* xenoestrogens, such as those found in pesticides, fuels, and plastics, tightly bind to the estrogen receptor and promote aberrant cell growth. These effects can be additive or synergistic.[2] Other xenoestrogens, which are *not persistent* and are rapidly excreted from the body, can downplay the effects of the estrogen receptor. These include plant products, such as soy, cauliflower, and broccoli. These "good" xenoestrogens may serve as antioxidants. In addition, they may inhibit angiogenesis, protease, or kinase, reducing the propensity of aberrant breast cells to proliferate, increasing DNA repair, or producing other changes in the genetic or hormonal microenvironments.[12] Despite the beneficial effects of these particular xenoestrogens, there is growing human evidence that the persistent xenoestrogens play an important role in the etiology of breast cancer.

HUMAN EVIDENCE

Xenoestrogens, such as DDT and organochlorines, may act through 16-alpha-hydroxyestrone and the estrogen receptor to cause cancer. There have been a number of case-control studies that have attempted to establish links between DDT levels and breast cancer. A study by Wolff *et al.* in 1992 found that DDT tissue levels were almost 50% greater in breast cancer patients compared with controls. They determined a relative risk of about 3 for the highest quartile of exposure compared to the lowest. These results were confirmed in a later study, where there were significant differences in DDT levels between women with breast cancer and matched controls. Here, women with the highest exposure levels had a fourfold increased risk of cancer compared to those in the lowest category of exposure. Krieger's large study of 150 cases and controls also found a strong association between DDT tissue levels and elevated breast cancer risk. They examined blood collected long before diagnosis and found marked differences in exposure related to ethnicity. Caucasians, African-Americans, and Asians were sampled in the study. Taken as an entire cohort, no remarkable findings were made. However, after separating out the Asian women, they were able to link DDE levels and breast cancer in the other two groups.[9]

A recent Dutch study reported that breast cancer patients actually had lower levels of DDE in their fat tissue than did controls. These results are surprising if we expect

DDT and its derivatives to play a role in disrupting regular hormonal functions. From aggregated data across five Western European countries, they determined that the DDE concentration was 1.35 μg/g among cases and 1.51 μg/g within the control group, finding an inverse association between DDE levels and breast cancer risk. However, the samples were measured after diagnosis, and the average patient was stage II or III. This means that the cancers were 10–20 years old at the time when fat tissue was analyzed for residues. Therefore, it is possible that cancer could have altered the body's metabolism of DDT by mobilizing stores into the bloodstream before clinical diagnosis. A secondary effect of cancer may be lower DDE concentrations in fat. The authors concede that although serum and adipose DDE levels are highly correlated in healthy women, the same may not be true in women with breast cancer.[13] Therefore, these findings could reflect the *consequences* of cancer, rather than the causes.

There are critical windows of time during which regulatory genes respond to exposures. Susceptibility to exposure is a function of the rate of cell division. When exposures occur may be just as important as the levels of exposure. High levels of estrogens *in utero* may predispose the embryo to some types of breast cancer. In adolescence, estrogens may influence developing breast cells in making them more vulnerable to cancer-causing agents. And postmenopausal women may be more susceptible because they have endured longer exposures to the active form of estradiol over the years.[5]

NEW EVIDENCE

The biggest increase in breast cancer rates has occurred among the number of estrogen-dependent tumors, those that are mediated by hormonal factors. Glass *et al.* reported that in the Kaiser Permanente HMO there had been an average 131% increase in the incidence of estrogen receptor-positive (ER+) tumors during the 25-year study.[14] Dewailly *et al.* recently found that over the last 20 years, the median number of estrogen receptors in breast tumors has increased greater than fourfold, from 14 to 58 fmol/mg of protein. During this same period, high exposures to organochlorine compounds were widespread. Testing for a possible link between these two events, their group compared DDE concentrations in breast fat tissue of 18 patients in an earlier case-control study with documented estrogen receptor levels over time. A Spearman rank correlation coefficient adjusted for tumor size and patient age showed a clear relationship between DDE in adipose and estrogen receptor levels in the breast. These results suggest that organochlorines acting through the estrogen receptor may be involved in greater estrogen receptor levels, and perhaps in the rising incidence of ER+ breast cancer.[15]

Denzo and his colleagues at Vanderbilt University have recently discovered that many of the pollutants thought to be estrogen mimickers may also act through the androgen receptor as well as through different binding proteins. Using a competitive binding assay, they measured the ability of a mix of pollutants, including DDT, nonylphenol, dieldrin, and atrazine, to attach to a variety of receptors and binding proteins in the presence of natural estrogens and androgens. A higher than expected number of environmental chemicals, namely DDT and its derivatives, atrazine and dieldrin, bound to the androgen receptor; and most of the test compounds bound to at least one of the binding proteins. These results have major implications for hormone-mediated responses. Chemicals that can mimic the action of hormones may have a variety of mechanisms at their disposal and work synergistically to cause harm.[16]

In addition, recent studies have shown that results may be sensitive to the testing model. Bisphenol-A was more potent when applied to human cells than to animal cells.[17] Bisphenol-A is a by-product of polycarbonate, commonly found in some plastics. It leaches from plastics when heated to certain temperatures. These results could have important ramifications for public health. The traditional paradigm of using animal cell models to support government regulations may underestimate the long-term effects of exposures to pesticides and other environmental hazards.

CONCLUSION

Breast cancer arises when cells undergo mutations that allow them to proliferate beyond control; each of the pathways to disease will ultimately affect a person's genetic makeup. It is very important to consider the epidemiological, environmental, and genetic evidence together in order to target risk factors and develop effective prevention strategies. Although the human evidence is inconsistent, public policy demands proactive measures to prevent harm, rather than waiting for definitive scientific proof of the causes of breast cancer. At the very least, the science to date is very compelling and calls for additional, and precautionary action to reduce suspect exposures. For every dollar spent on the treatment of breast cancer, only a penny is spent on prevention.[18] Fueled by heightened concern over this disease, an unprecedented coalition of environmental and feminist groups has emerged, demanding more efforts at prevention. These organizations include the National Breast Cancer Coalition, National Action Plan on Breast Cancer, Community Breast Health Project, Breast Cancer Action, Silent Spring Institute, Massachusetts Breast Cancer Coalition, Women's Community Cancer Project, and the Women's Environment and Development Organization.

Many of the interventions proposed to reduce breast cancer risk involve radical modifications in diet, lifestyle, and even reproductive behavior. These will not be easily changed by social policy. Increasing consumption of fruits and vegetables and reducing animal fat and exposure to pesticide residues remain fundamental objectives in protecting public health. However, the endocrine system may be far more vulnerable than we had thought, especially since other possible effects such as decreased sperm counts worldwide have recently captured much attention. In addition, some pesticides have been linked to a number of illnesses in workers, including breast cancer, as well as cancer and behavioral problems in their children. We need to encourage studies on the biological mechanisms by which environmental chemicals affect us. We can also design products that will result in less pollution and waste. And finally, we need to endorse policies that will do a better job at minimizing our exposures to suspect materials and to raise public awareness so people may be empowered to take steps to reduce their risks.

REFERENCES

1. DAVIS, D. L., D. AXELROD, M. OSBORNE & N. TELANG. 1997. Environmental influences on breast cancer risk. Sci. Med. **4**(3): 56-63.
2. DAVIS, D. L., D. AXELROD, M. OSBORNE, N. TELANG, L. BRADLOW & E. SITTNER. 1997. Avoidable causes of breast cancer: The known, unknown, and the suspected. Ann. N.Y. Acad. Sci. **833.** In press.
3. DAVIS, D. L. *et al.* 1997. Medical hypothesis: Bifunctional genetic-hormonal pathways to breast cancer. Environ. Health Perspect. **105**(Supplement 3): 571-577.
4. DAVIS, D. L., H. L. BRADLOW, M. WOLFF, T. WOODRUFF, D. G. HOEL & H. ANTON-CULVER. 1993. Medical hypothesis: Xenoestrogens as preventable causes of breast cancer. Environ. Health Perspect. **101**(5): 372-377.
5. WORLD RESOURCES INSTITUTE. 1997. Web Page. Environmental Links to Breast Cancer. Http://www.wri.org/health/
6. DORGAN, J. F. *et al.* 1997. Serum sex hormone levels are related to breast cancer risk in postmenopausal women. Environ. Health Perspect. **105**(Supplement 3): 583-585.
7. THOMAS, B. S., R. D. BULBROOK, J. L. HAYWARD & R. R. MILLIS. 1982. Urinary androgen metabolites and recurrence rates in early breast cancer. Eur. J. Cancer Clin. Oncol. **18:** 447-451.
8. KELCE, W. R., C. S. STONE, S. C. LAWS, L. E. GRAY, J. A. KEMPPAINEN & E. M. WILSON. 1995. Persistent DDT metabolite, p,p′-DDE is a potent androgen receptor antagonist. Nature **375:** 581-585.
9. WOLFF, M., G. COLLMAN, J. C. BARRETT & J. HUFF. 1996. Breast cancer and environmental risk factors: Epidemiological and experimental findings. Annu. Rev. Pharmacol. Toxicol. **36:** 573-596.
10. PIKE, M. C. *et al.* 1981. Oral contraceptive use and early abortion as risk factors for breast cancer in young women. Br. J. Cancer **43:** 72-76.
11. HIYAMA, E. *et al.* 1996. Telomerase activity in human breast tumors. J. Nat. Cancer Inst. **88**(2): 116-122.
12. ZAVA, D., M. BLEN & G. DUWE. 1997. Estrogenic activity of natural and synthetic estrogens in human breast cancer cells in culture. Environ. Health Perspect. **105**(Supplement 3): 637-645.
13. VAN'T VEER, P. *et al.* 1996. DDT and postmenopausal breast cancer in Europe. The Lancet. In press.
14. GLASS, A. G. & R. N. HOOVER. 1990. Rising incidence of breast cancer: Relationship to stage and receptor status. J. Nat. Cancer Inst. **82**(8): 693-696.
15. DEWAILLY, E., P. AYOTTE & S. DODIN. 1997. Could the rising levels of estrogen receptor in breast cancer be due to estrogenic pollutants? J. Nat. Cancer Inst. **89**(12): 888.
16. RALOFF, J. 1997. Hormone mimics get harder to pigeonhole. Sci. News **151:** 254.
17. STEINMETZ, R., R. BIGSBY, N. BROWN, D. ALLEN & N. BEN-JONATHAN. 1997. The environmental estrogen bisphenol-A stimulates prolactin release *in vitro* and *in vivo*. Endocrinology **138**(5): 1780-1786.
18. MONTAGUE, P. 1997. Cancer trends. Rachel's Environ. Health Weekly #500. June 12, 1997.
19. KELSEY, J. L. *et al.* Epidemiology and prevention of breast cancer. Annu. Rev. Public Health **17:** 58.

Dietary Fiber, Hispanics, and Breast Cancer Risk?

LOVELL A. JONES,[a] ROSIE GONZALEZ, PATRICIA C. PILLOW, SARAH A. GOMEZ-GARZA, CATHERINE J. FOREMAN, JANICE A. CHILTON, ADRIANA LINARES, JOHN YICK, MAYHAR BADREI, AND RICHARD A. HAJEK

Center for Research on Minority Health
Experimental Gynecology/Endocrinology
The University of Texas M. D. Anderson Cancer Center
Houston, Texas 77030

INTRODUCTION

The relationship between the nutritional habits of ethnic groups and their differences in breast cancer rates may provide us with important information on the role that diet might play in the etiology of breast cancer. In the United States, the breast is the single most common site of cancer among Hispanic and non-Hispanic women, across all geographic regions.[1] However, Hispanic women consistently have lower rates of breast cancer than do non-Hispanic women in most geographic areas.[1,2] For example, the incidence rate of breast cancer among Hispanic women in the United States ranges between 107.4 cases per 100,000 in Illinois and 33.5 per 100,000 in the Lubbock, Texas area. In certain regions of the United States, such as Illinois, the Hispanic population actually has a higher rate of breast cancer than do non-Hispanic women from other regions, such as the cities of Lubbock and El Paso, Texas; Dade County, Florida; and the state of New Mexico.[1]

Breast cancer mortality rates for immigrant Hispanic women are also lower than those for white and black women. Rosenwaike[3] published the mortality differentials of immigrant Hispanic populations collected during 1979 to 1981. The highest mortality rate resulting from breast cancer for these populations was among native Cubans (24.1 per 100,000). Other immigrant populations, such as native Puerto Ricans, had the lowest rate (16.1 per 100,000), followed by Mexicans (17.7 per 100,000). As

[a] To whom request for reprint should be addressed: Lovell A. Jones, Ph.D., Director, Experimental Gynecology/Endocrinology, University of Texas M.D. Anderson Cancer Center, Box 304, 1515 Holocombe Boulevard, Houston, Texas 77030. Phone: 713/792-3316; fax: 713/794-5553; e-mail: lovell_jones@gnnonc.mdacc.tmc.edu

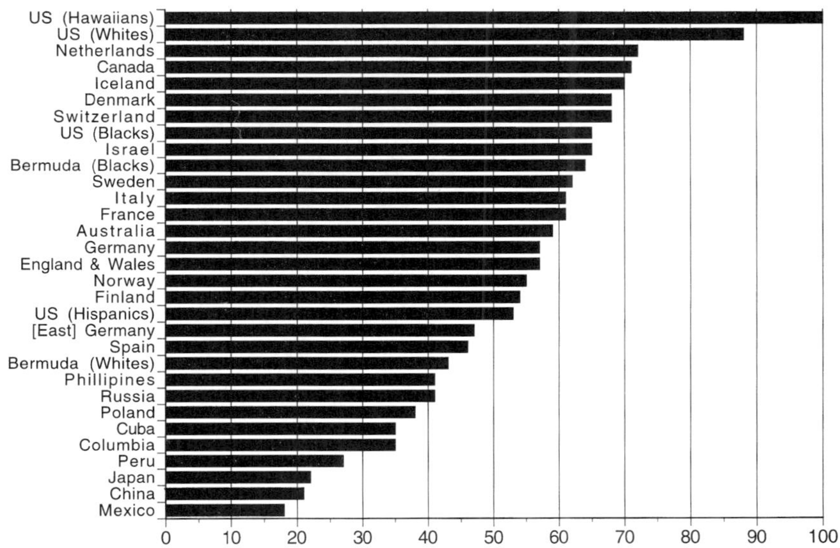

FIGURE 1. Mortality rate (number of deaths per 100,000 persons) from breast cancer by country of origin. (Based on information provided in References 4 and 5.)

FIGURE 1 shows, these rates are not significantly different from those of the country of origin.[4,5] When comparisons are made across the regions and among various heterogeneous Hispanic populations, there is tremendous variation and significant differences in breast cancer incidence rates.[1] Interestingly, Hispanic countries such as Mexico, Colombia, and Cuba, and Hispanic regions such as El Paso and Lubbock tend to have the lowest breast cancer incidence rates.[4,5] These national and regional variations in breast cancer incidence rates among all ethnic groups, as well as among Hispanic populations, may be explained by dietary factors.

Researchers generally agree that reproductive hormones, specifically estrogens, are involved in the etiology of breast cancer.[6] What is now well known is that over 65% or more of the women who develop breast cancer have no known risk factors and that family history accounts for only 5 to 10% of all cases. However, what all breast cancers have in common is estrogens. For instance, (a) breast cancer develops almost exclusively in females;[7] (b) administration of exogenous estrogens have been associated with breast cancer in men;[8] (c) early oophorectomy results in a reduction in the risk of breast cancer and also reduces the growth of human breast cancer tumors;[9,10] and (d) the plateau in the age-incidence curve for breast cancer occurs in the premenopausal period.[11] However, the specific role of estrogen as it relates to dietary factors, such as fat and fiber, continues to be a topic of great interest and controversy. Although estrogen is a central factor, researchers should take into account that the mechanism(s) by which fat, fiber, and estrogen are involved in the initiation/promotion of breast cancer may be multifocal. For instance, as shown in FIGURE 2, fat and fiber each have a different effect on both the total circulating estrogen level as well as on the bioavailable level.

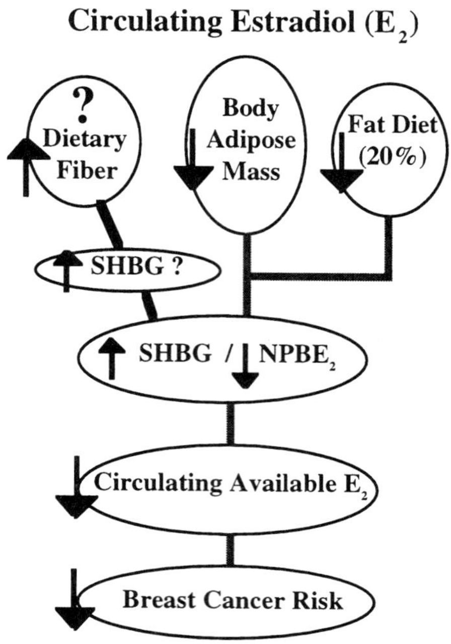

FIGURE 2. Diagram of model indicating effects of dietary fiber and fat on circulating estradiol (E_2), and thus on breast cancer risk. It is hypothesized that dietary fiber increases the percentage of E_2 bound to SHBG and thus decreases the circulating levels of bioavailable E_2. SHBG = sex hormone binding globulin; $NPBE_2$ = non-protein bound estradiol.

Several studies have demonstrated that a reduction of dietary fat is associated with a decrease in the level of circulating estrogen.[12,13] However, the distribution of estradiol bound to serum proteins (albumin, sex hormone binding globulin) and that which is freely circulating may be more critical to breast cancer risk than the total amount of circulating estrogen.[14] In a recent dietary intervention study, we found that a reduction of total dietary fat intake to approximately 20% results in a decrease in the level of non-protein-bound estradiol.[15]

A recent study by Cohen *et al.*[16] reported that a 1:1 combination of wheat bran and psyllium, when added to a high-fat diet, effectively reduced the development of mammary tumors in rats. Although most breast cancer and nutrition research has focused on the role of dietary fat, recent epidemiological evidence indicates that a protective effect from fiber occurs independently of the effects of a low-fat diet.[17–20] According to one hypothesis, a correlation between dietary fiber, steroids, and breast cancer exists because dietary fiber binds estrogens in the small intestine, causing a reduction in their enterohepatic circulation.[21,22] Therefore, bacterial activity is very important in the enterohepatic circulation of estrogens. In support of this mechanism, Adlercreutz and colleagues have reported that a disruption of the normal intestinal microflora results in a reduction of urinary estrogen excretion.[22,23]

In addition to the effects of intestinal bacteria on estrogen metabolism, another proposed mechanism involves direct binding of fiber to the unconjugated estrogens within the gut.[6,22] Schultz and Howie demonstrated that unconjugated estrogens readily bind to some types of fibers *in vitro*.[24] In addition, water-insoluble fibers, which are present in high concentrations in foods typically consumed by vegetarians, have a high affinity for binding estradiol and estrone.[25] There is also evidence that plant lignans may influence the formation and metabolism of estrogen.[20] Plant lignans, not to be confused with the dietary fiber lignin, can be synthesized by intestinal bacteria from specific insoluble components of grains and other fiber-rich foods. Interestingly, the concentration of urinary lignans increases as dietary fiber intake increases.[6,20,22]

Although data on the Hispanic diet are scarce in the United States, especially fiber data, there is evidence from national studies that Hispanics are consuming a diet that is higher in dietary fiber than that of most other ethnic groups.[26,27] A study conducted in Texas supports these findings and has shown that Hispanics living in certain regions of this state are adhering to a more traditional diet, consuming foods such as beans, rice, and corn tortillas.[28] These traditional, fiber-rich dietary habits may be the answer to the lower incidence of breast cancer among some Hispanic populations.

This report provides some much-needed information regarding the dietary fiber intake and consumption patterns in the female Hispanic population. While these data may only begin to help explain the lower incidence of breast cancer among this population, we hope that our current long-term breast cancer prevention trial with a larger study population will further clarify this controversial association between breast cancer and dietary factors, specifically fiber. The methodology developed with the vanguard study will go a long way in aiding us in this endeavor.

METHODS

Selection of Study Population

The study participants recruited were community senior citizens from a Houston area YWCA as well as employees from both the Houston YWCA and The University of Texas M. D. Anderson Cancer Center, and represented the following range of characteristics, as shown in TABLE 1. This diverse trial criteria was established in order to adequately test the dietary instruments across a variety of variables. Selected subjects also had to meet minimal criteria for literacy in order to adequately complete trial questionnaires and three-day food records. A total of 23 participants completed three-day food records and food frequency questionnaires.

Data Collection Procedures

Southwest Food Frequency Questionnaire (SWFFQ)

The participants completed two SWFFQ's, one month apart (SWFFQ1 and SWFFQ2), in order to test the instrument's reliability and to compare "intra" differences between the two food frequency questionnaires and "inter" differences between

TABLE 1. Sociodemographic Characteristics of Hispanic Women from the Vanguard Study

Characteristic	(*n*)	Mean	Std. Dev.	Median	Mode	Range
Age (years)	22	52.045	(±16.45)	58.5	30	(30–72)
Education (years)	22	10.841	(±4.56)	12.0	12	(1–18)
Income range	22	$10,000–$20,000		$10,000–$20,000	$10,000–20,000	(>$10,000–>$51,000)
Born in United States	13 (59.1%)					
Born in Mexico	6 (27.3%)					
Born in Central America (El Salvador)	2 (9.1%)					
Born in South America (Columbia)	1 (4.6%)					
Years lived in United States if born in another country	(8 of 9 reported years)	29.375	(±15.901)	25.0	10.0	(10–51)
Language						
Bilingual	18 (81.8%)					
Spanish only	4 (18.2%)					
English only	0 (0%)					

the food frequency questionnaires and the food record. The participants were asked to report dietary intake for the previous month. This would allow both instruments to comparably capture similar foods of the current season. Based on results obtained by Dr. Gladys Block with The Supplemental Foods Program for Woman, Infant, and Children dietary assessment validation study, the instrument was administered by interview.[29,30] All of the interviewers were trained by the research dietitian, and most were bilingual. Most of the Hispanic participants were also bilingual, with five preferring to speak Spanish (TABLE 1). One participant completed the SWFFQ by self-administration. This subject was provided with brief instructions for completing the questionnaire. However, due to errors in completing the questionnaire and overreporting of food intake, this participant's data was excluded from the final data analysis.

Food Records

The participants were assigned three randomly selected days (including two weekdays and one weekend day, all nonadjacent, over a three-week period) for which to keep a food record. The subjects had to participate in a one-hour group training session, taught by the bilingual research dietitian, in order to maintain accurate reporting of foods consumed, portion sizes, and preparation methods. Although the literature underlines the many challenges involved in obtaining accurate reports of food intake, particularly in a low-literacy, Hispanic population, there were only a few cases where a participant did not adequately complete her food record. The research dietitian reviewed each food record with the participant for completeness, and when necessary the research dietitian assisted the subject with recall of food intake. It is the opinion of the nutrition research team that the thorough food record training session made a significant difference in the accuracy and completeness of the food records.

Dietary Analysis: SWFFQ and Food Records

Data entry of the SWFFQ questionnaires was completed in Arizona by a trained nutrition staff using a system provided by the Nutrition Core Unit at the Arizona Cancer Center. Dietary analysis was conducted at the Arizona Cancer Center using their proprietary nutrient analysis software and database. Nutrient calculations were performed using the Minnesota Nutrition Data System (NDS) software, developed by the Nutrition Coordinating Center (NCC), University of Minnesota (Minneapolis, MN; Food Database version 10A; Nutrient Database version 2.8).[31,32] If an analytic value is not available for a nutrient in a food, NCC calculates the value based on the nutrient content of other nutrients in the same food or on a product ingredient list, or estimates the value based on the nutrient content of similar foods. A missing value is allowed only if (1) the value is believed to be negligible, (2) the food is usually eaten in very small amounts, (3) it is unknown if the nutrient exists in the food at all, or (4) there is no way to estimate the value because the food is unlike any other. Statistical analysis of both the three food records and the two SWFFQ's were conducted using SPSS for Windows Release 6.1.[33] Descriptive statistics were applied and Wilcoxon matched-pairs signed-ranks tests were conducted to test for

TABLE 2. Mean Intake of Total Dietary Fiber, Soluble Fiber, and Insoluble Fiber by Dietary Assessment Instrument

Energy and Nutrient	Three-Day Food Record	SWFFQ1[a]	SWFFQ2[b]	SWFFQ[c]
Energy (kcal)	1526	2031	1809	1920
Total dietary fiber (g)	16.16	23.04	19.05	21.05
Soluble dietary fiber (g)	4.87	DF	DF	DF
Insoluble dietary fiber (g)	10.87	DF	DF	DF

[a] First administration of Arizona Food Frequency Questionnaire.
[b] Second administration of Arizona Food Frequency Questionnaire.
[c] Mean of both food frequency questionnaires.
[d] DF = Data forthcoming.

significant differences in mean energy and fat intake as measured by the three-day food records and the two food frequencies (TABLE 2). Analysis of variance was used to compare the mean intakes of dietary fiber by food subgroup (TABLE 3).

RESULTS

The distribution of the 22 study participants across various characteristics are presented in TABLE 1. Of the 23 women who completed both food frequency questionnaires and the three-day food record, one was omitted from final analysis due to errors in completing the questionnaires and overreporting of food intake. The average age of this cohort of Houston area Hispanic women was 53 years. Regarding birth country, 13 were born in the United States, 6 in Mexico, 2 in Central America, and one participant was born in South America. For the 41% born outside of the United States, the average length of time in the United States was 29 years. Most of the participants were bilingual. The average level of education was a little over 10 years, and 64% of the participants fell into the lower income category of \$10,000-\$20,000 per year.

TABLE 2 provides the mean dietary fiber, soluble fiber, and insoluble fiber values (grams) by dietary assessment instrument. Mean total dietary fiber intake was 16 g/day according to the three-day food record and 21 g/day according to the food frequency questionnaire. The differences in total fiber values between the three-day food record and the SWFFQ1 were statistically significant. TABLES 3 and 4 show that the highest percentage of fiber was in the form of insoluble fiber (10.87 g/day) rather than soluble fiber (4.87 g/day).

In analyzing the different food subgroup contributions of dietary fiber according to the food frequency questionnaires (TABLE 3), a few important food categories stand out as the major contributors of dietary fiber. This Hispanic female population received most of its dietary fiber from the following subgroup categories: fruits; vegetables; breads/tortillas, cereals, and crackers; and beans, nuts, and seeds. Small amounts (~1

TABLE 3. Mean Food Subgroup Contributions of Dietary Fiber for SWFFQ1 and SWFFQ2

Food Subgroup	Mean (SD) SWFFQ1	Median SWFFQ1	Mean (SD) SWFFQ2	Median SWFFQ2
Beans, nuts, seeds	2.77 (2.73)	1.90	2.07 (3.01)	1.21
Beverages	0.002 (0.01)	0	0.002 (0.01)	0
Breads/tortillas, cereals, crackers	5.12 (4.70)	3.90	5.53 (4.34)	4.02
Cakes, cookies, pastries	0.12 (0.23)	0.04	0.07 (0.08)	0.04
Fruits	6.43 (6.54)	4.05	4.03 (3.08)	3.44
Juices	0.37 (0.29)	0.46	0.33 (0.35)	0.23
Meat	0.02 (0.07)	0	0.01 (0.01)	0
Mixed dishes	0.96 (0.85)	0.63	0.78 (0.64)	0.63
Salty snacks	0.96 (1.49)	0.31	0.76 (1.20)	0.22
Soups	0.92 (1.17)	0.47	0.73 (1.01)	0.35
Starchy side dishes	0.94 (0.52)	0.52	0.79 (1.03)	0.40
Sweets, candy, syrups	0.15 (0.41)	0.03	0.02 (0.04)	0.01
Vegetables	4.29 (3.50)	3.80	3.94 (2.32)	3.60

TABLE 4. Mean Intake of Dietary Fiber, Soluble Fiber, and Insoluble Fiber by Daily Food Records

Dietary Fiber	Day 1	Day 2	Day 3	X[a]
Total dietary fiber	17.48	14.88	16.11	16.16
Soluble fiber	11.65	10.58	10.39	10.87
Insoluble fiber	5.44	3.97	5.21	4.87

[a] Three-day mean dietary of fiber intake.

g/day) of fiber were provided by mixed dishes, soups, salty snacks, and starchy side dishes. Meat, condiments, sweets, juices, and beverages contributed minimal amounts (<1 g/day) of dietary fiber to the total intake.

As shown in TABLE 5, based on the SWFFQ, significant differences in dietary fiber intake were found from some of the different food subgroups depending on the birth country. The participants born outside the United States consumed significantly ($p = 0.05$) more fiber from the soups/gravies/sauces and beans/nuts/seeds categories than those born in the United States. Those born outside the United States also consumed slightly more fiber from vegetables and side dishes. Fiber consumption for those participants born in the United States was slightly higher within the fruits, salty snacks, cakes/cookies, and mixed dishes food categories.

DISCUSSION

The data on cancer among Hispanics in the United States is very limited, particularly regarding dietary practices. However, from studies currently available,[6,13,17,34]

TABLE 5. Mean Food Subgroup Contributions of Dietary Fiber for SWFFQ1 and SWFFQ2 by Participants Born in and Outside of the United States

Food Subgroup	Born in USA SWFFQ1 (g)	Born Outside of USA SWFFQ1 (g)	Born in USA SWFFQ2 (g)	Born Outside of USA SWFFQ2 (g)
Total dietary fiber	20.40	26.86	19.69	18.14
Beans, nuts, seeds	1.68	4.34[a]	1.50	2.90
Beverages	0.000	0.004	0.001	0.003
Breads	4.45	6.09	7.05	3.33[a]
Cakes, cookies, pastries	0.15	0.07	0.10	0.04
Fruits	7.05	5.54	4.08	3.95
Juices	0.35	0.40	0.30	0.37
Mixed dishes	1.05	0.83	0.84	0.70
Salty snacks	1.00	0.89	1.10	0.27
Side dishes	0.75	1.21	0.53	1.16
Soups, sauces, gravies	0.51	1.53[a]	0.59	0.94
Sweets	0.22	0.04	0.03	0.01
Vegetables	3.16	5.92	3.58	4.47

[a] $p = 0.05$.

there is evidence of a clear association between dietary intake patterns, specifically that of dietary fiber, and the lower rates of breast cancer. For instance, a recent study by Trapido *et al.*[1] indicates that the incidence of breast cancer correspondingly increases as the distance from the Mexico-United States border increases. The only exception to this seems to be large metropolitan areas such as New York City. These same areas have both readily available traditional ethnic foods and strong community ties to the country of origin. This may contribute to maintaining strong dietary practices. In addition, epidemiological evidence that confirms the effects of high-fiber diets on blood estrogen concentrations support this association.[17,34] The protective role of dietary fiber is further indicated by the fact that the risk for developing breast cancer is lower among populations, such as Asians, who consume a high-fiber diet—higher than in the Western world, where the diet is high in animal fat and low in fiber.[35]

Our current study is consistent with previous reports that Hispanic women consume more dietary fiber than the general population in the United States.[26] The dietary fiber (16 g/day via food record and 21 g/day via SWFFQ) consumed by this population of Hispanic women represents a fiber intake that is even higher than that reported for Hispanic women and men (10 g/day and 14 g/day, respectively) in an earlier national report.[26] The women participating in our study were generally older of lower socioeconomic status and literacy than the subjects of this earlier report.

Thompson *et al.*[27] reported that the major fiber sources for women are foods in the fruit, vegetable, and grain food groups as well as the items in those food groups eaten in mixtures, such as soups and rice-based dishes. These data suggest that the dietary fiber food sources consumed by this population are predominately water-insoluble fibers.[27,36] As indicated by the data presented in TABLE 3, the current study also found that the food subgroups of fruits; vegetables; breads/tortillas, cereals, and crackers; as well as beans, nuts, and seeds provide for most of the participants' dietary fiber intake. Consequently, the fiber the participants consumed had a ratio of insoluble vs. soluble fiber (10.87 vs. 4.87 g/day) that is consistent with that recommended by the Federation of American Societies for Experimental Research.[37] Several researchers who have hypothesized on the mechanisms of dietary fiber suggest that it is the insoluble fiber that provides protection against breast cancer.[6,36,38] This further supports the protective role of dietary fiber in the Hispanic population.

These food subgroups, as classified in the SWFFQ, with their protective insoluble fiber, represent some of the staples of the traditional Hispanic diet.[39,40] Thus, these data suggest that this small cohort of predominately United States-born Hispanic women are adhering to some of the traditional dietary habits and consumption patterns of their Mexican-born ancestors. This is significant because researchers who have analyzed the effects of acculturation on dietary intake indicate that the traditional Hispanic diet is healthier than the mainstream or "typical" American diet in regard to breast cancer.[39,40] This is further supported in the current study by the fact that overall our nine Mexico-born participants consumed slightly more dietary fiber than their United States-born counterparts. This is true for most major food categories contributing dietary fiber, and it is significant for the bean and soup food subgroups (TABLE 5). Even across different regions of the United States this pattern is evident. Areas that follow a more traditional Hispanic diet, such as El Paso and Lubbock, have the lowest breast cancer rates when compared with areas, such as Illinois, that are less likely to follow this dietary pattern.[1] These large variations in breast cancer incidence rates across different regions of the United States further support the protective role of the traditional Hispanic diet.

Although the dietary information available on the Hispanic diet is limited, the dietary fiber information in this report provides more support for the growing evidence that dietary factors contribute significantly to the reduced breast cancer incidence rate in the Hispanic population. In addition, our study supports the need for culturally specific dietary instruments. Although the data was not presented, we recommend the use of focus groups to detect the differences in recognition of particular food groups among Hispanics in different regions. For example, when measuring the consumption of tuna it is imperative to distinguish between a can of tunafish and the locally available cactus fruit that is commonly called tuna, especially when measuring dietary fiber. As our group continues to study the food consumption patterns in this population, we look forward to the dietary information that will be provided, and we hope to contribute to the knowledge base of the relationship between a traditional Hispanic diet and low incidence of breast cancer.

What implication does this have with regard to addressing the expectations, attitudes, and beliefs about dietary fiber and health and the perceptions of external influences on food choice, especially those for the indigenous and immigrant populations? As the opening paragraph stated, unless one takes into account the importance of diet and culture as it relates to cancer prevention, we will never be able to discern the true role of diet and the factors involved.

SUMMARY

The cancer rates of immigrant populations in the United States must be taken into account when looking at the importance of diet and culture as it relates to cancer prevention. Unfortunately, some nutrition studies targeted toward nontraditional white populations have not adequately confronted the issue of cultural meaning in efforts to gather dietary data accurate enough to support nutritional analyses, identify marginal diets, or relate risk to dietary patterns. The study presented here resolves many of the culturally specific issues utilizing awareness, attention, and judicious combination of culturally sensitive qualitative and quantitative research techniques. The importance of such a study in an Hispanic population is based on the fact that the age-adjusted rate of breast cancer in countries such as Mexico is among the lowest in the world. In addition, although one of the fastest-growing minority groups in the United States, Hispanic women living in this country have been shown to have the lowest incidence of and mortality rates from this disease across most geographic regions of the United States. Therefore, one might speculate that dietary factors, which have been shown to play a role in breast cancer prevention, may account for this difference. It is well recognized that the traditional Hispanic diet is rich in protective nutrients such as dietary fiber. It is known that through complex mechanisms, dietary fiber works to reduce the amount of estrogens in the body. Research also indicates that it is the level of endogenous estrogen in the body that may influence the onset of breast cancer. In order to better understand how dietary factors may be associated with breast cancer in Hispanic women, it is important that one develop the proper tools to discern any potential differences. Therefore, we developed an approach to obtaining dietary fiber information from a small cohort of 22 Houston-area Hispanic women as a vanguard study for a larger breast cancer prevention trial. Two separate dietary assessment instruments were utilized, a three-day food record and the Southwest Food Frequency Questionnaire. The mean intake of dietary fiber was 16 g/day according to the food record and 21 g/day according to the SWFFQ. Fruits, vegetables, breads, cereals, and beans provided for most of the participants' dietary fiber intake. These results support evidence that the Hispanic population's dietary fiber intake is higher than that for other groups, and this may help explain the lower incidence of breast cancer among some Hispanic populations.

REFERENCES

1. Trapido, E. J., B. Valdez, J. L. Obeso, N. Strickman-Stein, A. Rotger & E. J. Pérez-Stable. 1995. Epidemiology of cancer among Hispanics in the United States. J. Nat. Cancer Inst. Monogr. **18:** 17-28.
2. National Cancer Institute. 1988. Cancer among blacks and other minorities: Statistical profile. U.S. Department of Health and Human Services, National Institutes of Health. Bethesda, MD.
3. Rosenwaike, I. 1987. Mortality differentials among persons born in Cuba, Mexico, and Puerto Rico residing in the United States, 1979-81. Am. J. Public Health **77**(5): 603-606.
4. Secretaria de Salud. 1991. Compendio de Informacion Epidemiologica de Cancer 1982-1988. Dírección General de Epidemiologica. Mexico.
5. Parkin, D. M., C. S. Muir, S. L. Whelan *et al.* 1992. Cancer incidence in five continents, Vol. 6. International Agency for Research on Cancer (IARC Scientific Publication 120). Lyon.

6. ROSE, D. P. 1992. Dietary fiber, phytoestrogens, and breast cancer. Nutrition **8:** 47-51.
7. WATERHOUSE, J., C. MUIR, P. CORREA & J. POWELL. 1976. *In* Cancer Incidence in Five Continents, No. 15, Vol. 3: 584. International Agency for Research on Cancer. Lyon.
8. SYMMERS, W. S. 1968. Carcinoma of breast in trans-sexual individuals after surgical and hormonal interference with the primary and secondary sex characteristics. Br. Med. J. **2:** 83-85.
9. BEATSON, G. T. 1896. On the treatment of inoperable cases of carcinoma of the mamma: Suggestion for a new method of treatment with illustrative cases. Lancet **2:** 104.
10. FEINLEIB, M. 1968. Breast cancer and artificial menopauses. A Cohort study. J. Natl. Cancer Inst. **41:** 315.
11. PETRAKIS, N. L., V. L. ERNSTER & M. C. KING. 1982. *In* Cancer Epidemiology and Prevention. D. Schottenfeld & J. F. Fraumeni, Eds.: 855-870. Saunders. Philadelphia.
12. ROSE, D. P., A. P. BOYAR, C. COHEN & L. E. STRONG. 1987. Effect of a low-fat diet on hormone levels in women with cystic breast disease. 1. Serum steroids and gonadotropins. J. Natl. Cancer Inst. **78:** 623-626.
13. GOLDIN, B. R., M. N. WOODS, K. L. SPIEGELMAN, C. LONGCOPE, A. MORRILL-LABRODE, J. T. DWYER, W. GUALTIERI, E. HERTZMARK & S. L. GORBACH. 1994. The effect of dietary fat and fiber on serum estrogen concentrations in premenopausal women under controlled dietary conditions. Cancer **74:** 1125-1131.
14. JONES, L. A., D. M. OTA, A. J. GILCHRIST, G. A. JACKSON, P. M. JACKSON, K. KEMP, D. E. ANDERSON, S. K. MCCAMANT, & D. H. BAUMAN. 1987. Bioavailability of estradiol as a marker for breast cancer risk assessment. Cancer Res. **47:** 5224-5229.
15. DIPAOLO, D., W. INSULL, J. YICK, D. JOHNSTON, R. SHALLENBERGER, V. VOGEL, A. BERKOWITZ, W. KLISH & L. A. JONES. 1995. Effects of a low-fat diet on bioavailable E_2 (NPBE) levels in an ethnic diverse population. Proc. Am. Cancer Res. **36:** 277 (Abstr.).
16. COHEN, L. A., Z. ZHAO, E. A. ZANG, T. T. WYNNS, B. SIMI & A. RIVENSON. 1996. Wheat bran and psyllium diet: Effects of N-methyinitrosourea-induced mammary tumorigenesis in S344 rats. J. Nat. Cancer Inst. **88:** 899-907.
17. ADLERCREUTZ, H. 1984. Does fiber rich food containing animal lignan precursors protect against both colon and breast cancer? An extension of the "fiber hypothesis." Gastroenterology **86:** 761-766.
18. GOLDIN, B. R., H. ADLERCREUTZ, S. L. GORBACH *et al.* 1982. Estrogen excretion patterns and plasma levels in vegetarian and omnivorous women. N. Engl. J. Med. **307:** 1542-1547.
19. GOLDIN, B. R., L. SHERWOOD & S. L. GORGACH. 1988. Effect of diet on the plasma levels, metabolism, and excretion of estrogens. Am. J. Clin. Nutr. **48:** 787-790.
20. ANDERSON, J. W. & W. & W. CHEN. 1979. Plant fiber, carbohydrate, and lipid metabolism. Am. J. Clin. Nutr. **32:** 346-363.
21. KRITCHEVSKY, D. 1983. Fiber, steroids, and cancer. Cancer Res. (Suppl.) **43:** 2491s-2495s.
22. ADLERCREUTZ, H., T. FOTSIS, C. BANNWART, K. WAHA, T. MAKELA, G. BRUNOW & T. HASE. 1986. Determination of urinary lignans and phytoestrogen on various habitual diets. J. Steroid Biochem. **25:** 791-797.
23. ADLERCREUTZ, H., F. MARTIN, M. J. TIKKANEN & M. PULKKINEZ. 1975. Effect of ampicillin administration on the excretion of twelve oestrogens in pregnancy urine. Acta Endocrinol. **80:** 551-557.
24. SHULTZ, T. D. & B. J. HOWIE. 1986. In vitro binding of steroid hormones by natural and purified fibers. Nutr. Cancer **8:** 141.
25. WHITTEN, C. G. & T. D. SHULTZ. 1988. Binding of steroid hormones in vitro by water-insoluble dietary fiber. Nutr. Res. **8:** 1223-1235.
26. BLOCK, G. & A. F. SUBAR. 1992. Estimates of nutrient intake from a food frequency questionnaire: The 1987 National Health Interview Survey. J. Am. Diet. Assoc. **92:** 969-977.

27. Thompson, F. E., M. F. Sowers, E. A. Frongillo & B. J. Parpia. 1992. Sources of fiber and fat in diets of U.S. women aged 19 to 50: Implications for nutrition education and policy. Am. J. Public Health **82:** 695-702.
28. Borrud, L. G., P. C. Pillow, P. K. Allen, R. S. McPherson, M. Z. Nichaman & G. R. Newell. 1989. Food group contributions to nutrient intake in whites, blacks, and Mexican Americans in Texas. J. Am. Diet. Assoc. **89**(8): 1061-1069.
29. Block, G. 1995. Personal letter regarding an unpublished validation study among low-income Hispanic women, March, 1995.
30. U.S.D.A. Food and Nutrition Service. 1995. WIC Dietary Assessment Validation Study. U.S.D.A. Contract # 53-33198-2-032. Freeman Sullivan & Co. San Francisco.
31. Feskanich, D., B. H. Sielaff, K. Chong & I. M. Buzzard. 1989. Computerized collection and analysis of dietary intake information. Comput. Methods Programs Biomed. **30:** 47-57.
32. Schakel, S. F., Y. A. Sievert & I. M. Buzzard. 1989. Sources of data for developing and maintaining a nutrient database. J. Am. Diet. Assoc. **88:** 1268-1271.
33. SPSS Inc. Copyright 1989-1994. SPSS for Windows, Release 6.1. SPSS Inc. N. Michigan Ave., Chicago, IL 60611.
34. Reddy, B. S., L. A. Cohen, G. D. McCoy, P. Hill, J. H. Weisburger & E. L. Wynder. 1980. Nutrition and its relationship to cancer. Adv. Cancer Res. **32:** 237-245.
35. Adlercreutz, H., Y. Mousavi & K. Hockerstedt. 1992. Diet and breast cancer. Acta Oncologica **31:** 175-181.
36. Lanza, E., S. Shankar & B. Trock. 1992. Dietary fiber. *In* Macronutrients. Investigating Their Role in Cancer. M. S. Micozzi & T. E. Moon, Eds.: 293-319. Marcel Dekker. New York.
37. Pilch, S. M., Ed. 1987. Physiological Effects and Health Consequences of Dietary Fiber. Federation of American Societies for Experimental Biology. Bethesda, MD.
38. Bright-See, E. 1988. Dietary fiber and cancer. Nutr. Today **23**(4): 4-10.
39. Romero-Gwynn, E., D. Gwynn, L. Grivetti, R. McDonald, G. Stanford, B. Turner, E. West & E. Williamson. 1993. Dietary acculturation among Latinos of Mexican descent. Nutr. Today: 6-12.

Reproductive Determinants of Breast Cancer in Mexican Women[a]

LIZBETH LÓPEZ-CARRILLO,[b]
JAIME BRAVO-ALVARADO,
OFELIA POBLANO-VERASTEGUI, AND
DORIS ORTEGA ALTAMIRANO

National Institute of Public Health
Av. Universidad 655
Col. Santa María Ahuacatitlán, C.P. 62508
Cuernavaca, Mor. México

INTRODUCTION

In Mexico, breast cancer (BC) is the second cause of female mortality due to cancer. The mortality trend for this type of cancer shows a constant increase. It is estimated that the number of deaths due to BC that occurred in 1991 (2,379) represented an increase of 94% in relation to registered deaths due to this type of tumor in 1980 (1,226) in this country.[1]

Mexico BC incidence has also risen, as in developed countries, with late diagnosis in the majority of patients. According to information from the National Cancer Registry of the Mexican Ministry of Health, during 1989 1,521 new BC cases were reported, and only 2% of these (30 cases) were diagnosed in the *in situ* phase of the tumor.[2]

Exposure to endogenous estrogens is the risk factor with the strongest association to BC incidence. Various international studies have shown that early age at menarche,[3,4] late age at the birth of the first child and menopause,[3–7] childlessness,[3–6] and absence of breast feeding[3,4,8–10] increase the probability of developing this type of tumor.

Estrogen replacement therapy in postmenopausal women,[11–14] consumption of alcohol[15–17] and of saturated fats,[18–20] obesity,[21–23] and contraceptive use[14] are events with controversial links to an increased risk of BC. In spite of progress that has been made in knowledge of BC etiology, it is estimated that only 30% of breast tumors can be explained by the above-mentioned factors.[24]

In order to evaluate reproductive risk profiles of women with BC in Mexico, this article compares reproductive characteristics of women with BC and the profiles of women without breast disease. In addition, information is included about the contrast in the reproductive patterns of women with BC and women with benign breast disease (BBD).

[a] This work was supported by the MacArthur Foundation and the Ministry of Health of Mexico.
[b] Phone: 5273/11-01-11, ext. 2432; fax: 5273/11-23-38; e-mail: lizbeth@insp3.insp.mx

METHODS

During the period between March 1994 and August 1995 an epidemiological study of breast cancer incident cases and clinical controls was carried out in Mexico City to analyze the relevance of a set of known reproductive risk factors for breast cancer among Mexican women.

The study population was made up of 277 women with histologically confirmed BC diagnosis (cases), and 201 women without breast disease (controls). A general description of the reproductive characteristics of a third group of 326 women with benign breast disease was also included; this group is not used as a control since the benign disease patients are much younger than the breast cancer patients. Participating women were identified in three hospital units of the Ministry of Health (General Hospital, GEA Gonzalez Institute, and Cancerology Institute) and a Social Security hospital (PEMEX Picacho). Eligible women were asked for written informed consent to apply a questionnaire about sociodemographic, reproductive, obstetric, and dietary characteristics. In addition, each participant's weight and height were measured.

Based on the information obtained with the questionnaires, a socioeconomic index, a Quetelet index, and various breast feeding indexes were constructed.

The socioeconomic index was constructed based on two components: physical characteristics of the woman's home (type of floor covering, presence of running water and sewage system) and education of the head of the household. Due to the homogeneity of the women's housing conditions, greater weight was assigned to education (75% vs. 50%), a modification of the methodology originally proposed by Bronfman *et al.*[24] In addition, only three categories were considered: low, middle-low, and middle.

The Quetelet index was calculated by dividing weight (kg) by height squared (m^2) for each of the women. Finally, duration of breast feeding was determined by adding up the months of reported breast feeding for the first child and for all children (nonweighted breast-feeding indexes). The number of months of breast feeding was corrected by frequency (times per day) and duration of each feeding session (minutes per session) to create a weighted breast feeding index for the first and for all children.

The principal sociodemographic and reproductive characteristics for women with BC (cases), with BBD, and without breast disease (controls) are described using simple analyses. Likewise, results of crude and adjusted odds ratios for women with BC (cases) compared to women without breast disease (controls) are presented, which were obtained using logistic regression models. The dose-response behavior of the reproductive variables was evaluated by including them continuously in the corresponding logistic regression model. This analysis was performed with STATA statistical software.

RESULTS

TABLE 1 shows reproductive characteristics and socioeconomic level of women with BC or with BBD compared with the group of women without breast disease (controls).

As can be seen, on average BC occurred at later ages than BBD: the average age of BC patients was 50 years old, while for women with BBD it was 34. It should

TABLE 1. Reproductive Characteristics and Socioeconomic Level in the Study Population

Characteristic	Women with Breast Cancer	Women with Benign Disease	Women without Breast Disease
Age (years)			
X̄	50.1	34.2[a]	49.7[b]
D.E.	13.5	12.0	13.7
(*n*)	(277)	(326)	(201)
Menarche (years)			
X̄	13.2	13.1	13.1
D.E.	1.5	1.6	1.6
(*n*)	(274)	(325)	(200)
Natural menopause (years)			
X̄	46.86	46.34	46.50
D.E.	4.86	5.53	5.27
(*n*)	(104)	(26)	(69)
Surgical menopause (years)			
X̄	40.64	38.83	41.89
D.E.	9.55	7.91	7.56
(*n*)	(37)	(18)	(28)
Age at first birth (years)			
X̄	22.2[a]	20.8	20.6
D.E.	5	4.1	4.2
(*n*)	(226)	(222)	(177)
Number of live children			
X̄	4.0	2.9[a]	4.7
D.E.	2.8	1.9	2.9
(*n*)	(221)	(214)	(163)
Breast-feeding index for first child (months)			
X̄	6.5[a]	6.7	8.1
D.E.	7.1	7.0	7.9
(*n*)	(221)	(220)	(173)
Total breast-feeding index (months)			
X̄	31.0[a]	24.2[a]	42.9
D.E.	38.5	30.4	46.5
(*n*)	(221)	(220)	(177)
Weighted breast-feeding index for first child (minutes/feeding/day)			
X̄	206.4[a]	287.63	297.4
D.E.	248.1	275.3	307.0
(*n*)	(172)	(180)	(113)
Total weighted breast-feeding index (minutes/feeding/day)			
X̄	79,351.75[a]	84,273.3[a]	120,526.9
D.E.	128,382.8	127,360.7	158,876.8
(*n*)	(158)	(179)	(111)

TABLE 1. Reproductive Characteristics and Socioeconomic Level in the Study Population (*Continued*)

Characteristic	Women with Breast Cancer	Women with Benign Disease	Women without Breast Disease
Family history of breast cancer			
Yes (%)	11.9[c]	5.5	4.0
(*n*)	(277)	(326)	(201)
Quetelet index (kg/m^2)			
$\bar{X}$	27.25	25.7	26.56
D.E.	4.64	9.28	4.78
(*n*)	(266)	(323)	(193)
Socioeconomic index			
$\bar{X}$	1.45[d]	1.64[a]	1.25
D.E.	1.09	1.01	1.00
(*n*)	(237)	(285)	(1.71)

[a] $p < 0.05$, statistic t test for mean comparison.
[b] Within the design, controls were paired by age with breast cancer cases.
[c] $p < 0.05$, chi^2.
[d] $p = 0.0621$, chi^2.

be noted that due to matching by age used in the study design, the age of women with BC was the same as that for the control group.

Both age at menarche (approximately 13 years old) and at natural menopause (approximately 46 years old) were the same in the three groups studied. Only 5.5% of the women with BBD had surgical menopause, compared with around 13% of women with BC and controls. As expected, average age for this intervention was lower than the age observed for natural menopause.

On average, women with BC had their first child at 22 years old, while the average age at the birth of their first child of controls and women with BBD was 20 years old. This two-year difference was statistically significant. Parity was similar among women with BC (4.0) and controls (4.7), although among the former the percentage of nulliparous women was greater than for the latter (19.93% vs. 12.43%). Women with BBD had significantly fewer children (mean = 2.9) and included a larger percentage of nulliparous women (33.85).

In relation to the number of months of breast-feeding for the first child, the controls had a mean of 8.1 ± 7.9 months, which was significantly greater than the average length of breast-feeding for women with BC (6.5 ± 7.1 months). Similarly, when the number of months of breast-feeding for all breast-fed children was accumulated, women with BC and BBD breast-fed for less time. These differences were statistically significant.

The difference between breast-feeding practices by women with BC and controls intensified when, in addition to months breast-feeding, frequency by day and duration per feeding (weighted breast-feeding indexes) were considered, both for the first child index and for all children who were breast-fed.

A family history of breast cancer was more prevalent among women with BC (11.9%) as compared to controls (4%) ($p < 0.05$).

The body-mass index (Quetelet), was similar in the three groups of women, with a variation between them from 25.71 ± 9.28 to 27.25 ± 4.6 kg/m^2.

Women with BBD had on average a higher socioeconomic level than controls (1.64 vs. 1.25, $p < 0.05$), followed by women with BC, for whom the average score did not reach statistical significance (1.45 vs. 1.25).

The adjusted odds ratios for the reproductive variables between BC cases and women with no breast disease as controls are shown in TABLE 2. Age at menarche was not found to have an effect, using as a reference the 15-years-and-over age group, even when the menopause status was considered (TABLE 3). Among postmenopausal women, late age at menopause did not show an effect on breast cancer frequency either.

In contrast, it was estimated that women who had their first live birth after 20 years of age have a greater probability of developing BC than women who had their first child before this age (OR 1.84, 95% CI 1.23-2.75). This risk increased even more for nulliparous women (OR 2.63, 95% CI 1.45-4.77), with a statistically significant trend. The effect of childlessness and late age at first live birth remained when it was stratified by menopause status (TABLE 3).

Likewise, having a greater number of children had a protective effect in relation to BC, independent of age at first birth (data not shown here). Therefore, for those women who had fewer than five children, the probability of developing BC was 1.79 times greater than among women who had more than four children. As in the previous case, nulliparous women had the greatest risk (OR 2.59, 95% CI 1.43-4.91). This effect continued with a significant trend only among postmenopausal women, increasing for nulliparous women (OR 3.82, 95% CI 1.73-8.42).

In terms of breast-feeding of the first child, a strong protective effect was found in relation to BC, after three months of breast-feeding, compared with women who had children and did not breast-feed them (OR 0.42, 95% CI 0.22-0.79), with a significant test for trend. This result did not change after adjusting by parity (data not shown here). This effect continued to exist when considering the total number of months breast-feeding for all children, with odds ratios of 0.49 for 1 year of accumulated breast-feeding, and up to 0.32 for over 5 years and 4 months.

Breast-feeding was a protective factor in premenopausal women, because among postmenopausal women tests for trend were not significant.

After considering the number of times per day (frequency) and the duration of each breast-feeding (weighted breast-feeding indexes), the results showed a similar effect for the first child and for all children in premenopausal women.

A family history of cancer was a strong predictor of BC (OR 3.29, 95% CI 1.39-7.79). This effect was much greater among premenopausal women than among postmenopausal women (OR 6.04 vs. 2.21).

Finally, the body mass index did not show an important association with BC incidence, as was also true for the socioeconomic level index.

TABLE 2. Adjusted Odds Ratios for Reproductive Characteristics between Breast Cancer Cases and Age-Matched Controls

Variable	No. Cases	No. Controls	OR	95% CI	Test for Trend (*p*)
Menarche (years)					
≤15	36	42	1.0[a]	–	0.990
8–12	59	81	1.29	0.72–2.29	
13–14	82	102	1.20	0.69–2.08	
Age at first birth (years)					
≤20	102	96	1.0[b]	–	0.001
>20	75	130	1.84	1.23–2.75	
Nulliparous	20	49	2.63	1.45–4.77	
No. of children					
>4	70	66	1.0[b]	–	0.005
≤4	92	155	1.79	1.16–2.74	
Nulliparous	23	55	2.59	1.43–4.71	
Total breast-feeding duration for first child (months)					
0	72	35	1.0[b]	–	0.049
1–3	31	35	0.42	0.22–0.79	
4–8	42	34	0.61	0.33–1.12	
9–12	43	39	0.55	0.33–1.12	
13–48	33	30	0.54	0.28–1.03	
Total breast-feeding duration (months)					
0	36	12	1.0[b]	–	0.009
1–11	57	42	0.49	0.23–1.06	
12–30	52	42	0.42	0.19–0.93	
31–64	39	40	0.32	0.14–0.71	
65–240	37	41	0.32	0.14–0.72	

TABLE 2. Adjusted Odds Ratios for Reproductive Characteristics between Breast Cancer Cases and Age-Matched Controls (*Continued*)

Variable	No. Cases	No. Controls	OR	95% CI	Test for Trend (p)
Weighted breast-feeding duration for first child (minutes/feeding/day)					
0-192	106	55	1.0[b]	—	0.004
193-324	20	20	0.51	0.25-1.04	
325-750	36	19	0.97	0.50-1.87	
≥751	10	19	0.22	0.09-0.53	
Total weighted breast-feeding duration (minutes/feeding/day)					
0-24,000	75	39	1.0[b]	—	0.033
24,001-75,600	36	23	0.83	0.43-1.61	
75,601-194,400	26	25	0.55	0.23-0.95	
≥194,400	21	24	0.47	0.23-0.95	
Family history of cancer					
No	198	170	1.0[c]	—	—
Yes	28	7	3.29	1.39-7.79	
Quetelet index (kg/m2)					
≤24.34	75	64	1.0[b]	—	0.187
24.35-27.92	91	64	1.11	0.69-1.77	
≥27.93	100	65	1.25	0.79-1.98	
Socioeconomic index					
Low	64	52	1.0[a]	—	0.377
Middle-low	34	33	0.78	0.42-1.45	
Middle	97	67	1.02	0.62	

[a] Adjusted for age at first birth and family history of breast cancer.
[b] Adjusted for family history of breast cancer.
[c] Adjusted for age at first birth.

TABLE 3. Adjusted Odds Ratios for Reproductive Characteristics between Breast Cancer Cases and Age Matched Controls by Menopausal Status

	Premenopausal					Postmenopausal				
Variable	No. Cases	No. Controls	OR	95% CI	*p* Value Trend	No. Cases	No. Controls	OR	95% CI	*p* Value Trend
Menarche (years)										
≥15	11	15	1.0[a]	–	0.596	42	36	1.0[a]	–	0.572
8–12	43	28	2.21	0.85–5.76		81	59	0.91	0.43–1.92	
13–14	49	39	1.92	0.75–4.88		102	82	0.89	0.44–1.78	
Natural menopause (years)										
<45	–	–	–	–	–	24	18	1.0[b]	–	0.646
45–50	–	–	–	–	–	64	40	1.2	0.58–2.48	
50+	–	–	–	–	–	16	11	1.1	0.41–2.91	
Age at first birth (years)										
≤20	46	48	1.0[a]	–	0.007	50	54	1.0[c]	–	0.023
>20	58	34	1.71	0.94–3.10		71	41	1.92	1.11–3.32	
Nulliparous	16	10	1.59	0.64–3.92		33	10	3.71	1.65–8.34	
Number of children										
>4	20	21	1.0[c]	–	0.179	45	49	1.0[c]	–	0.015
≤4	82	53	1.54	0.75–3.14		73	39	2.07	1.18–3.65	
Nulliparous	18	12	1.48	0.56–3.91		37	11	3.82	1.73–8.42	
Breast-feeding duration for first child (months)										
0	37	14	1.0[c]	–	0.029	34	21	1.0[c]	–	0.446
1–3	22	22	0.37	0.15–0.88		9	13	0.41	0.15–1.14	
4–8	18	17	0.41	0.16–1.03		24	17	0.88	0.38–2.02	
9–12	11	15	0.27	0.10–0.75		32	24	0.85	0.39–1.32	
13–48	14	11	0.45	0.16–1.26		19	19	0.64	0.28–1.49	

TABLE 3. Adjusted Odds Ratios for Reproductive Characteristics between Breast Cancer Cases and Age Matched Controls by Menopausal Status (*Continued*)

	Premenopausal					Postmenopausal				
Variable	No. Cases	No. Controls	OR	95% CI	p Value Trend	No. Cases	No. Controls	OR	95% CI	p Value Trend
Total breast-feeding duration (months)										
0-11	53	32	1.0[c]	–	0.048	40	22	1.0[c]	–	0.05
12-30	25	22	0.65	0.31-1.36		27	20	0.74	0.34-1.01	
31-64	17	18	0.55	0.25-1.25		21	22	0.48	0.21-1.08	
65-240	7	10	0.42	0.14-1.25		30	31	0.54	0.26-1.12	
Weighted breast-feeding duration for first child (minutes/feeding/day)										
0-192	43	22	1.0[b]	–	0.029	32	17	1.0[c]	–	0.229
193-324	18	12	0.87	0.35-2.15		18	11	0.84	0.32-2.20	
235-750	8	12	0.41	0.14-1.15		18	13	0.71	0.28-1.81	
>751	6	9	0.34	0.10-1.14		15	15	0.54	0.21-1.38	
Total weighted breast-feeding duration (minutes/feeding/day)										
0-24,000	43	22	1.0[b]	–	0.029	32	17	1.0[c]	–	0.229
24,001-75,600	18	12	0.86	0.35-2.15		18	11	0.84	0.32-2.20	
75,601-194,400	8	12	0.41	0.14-1.15		18	13	0.71	0.28-1.81	
>194,400	6	9	0.34	0.10-1.14		15	15	0.54	0.21-1.38	
Family history of cancer										
No	90	80	1.0[d]	–	–	107	90	1.0[d]	–	–
Yes	14	2	6.04	1.32-27.65		14	5	2.21	0.76-6.48	
Quetelet index (kg/cm2)										
≤24.34	38	34	1.0[c]	–	0.629	36	30	1.0[c]	–	0.159
24.25-27.92	37	24	1.24	0.61-2.51		54	40	1.05	0.55-1.99	
≥27.93	40	35	0.94	0.48-1.81		60	30	1.62	0.84-3.11	

TABLE 3. Adjusted Odds Ratios for Reproductive Characteristics between Breast Cancer Cases and Age Matched Controls by Menopausal Status (*Continued*)

	Premenopausal					Postmenopausal				
Variable	No. Cases	No. Controls	OR	95% CI	*p* Value Trend	No. Cases	No. Controls	OR	95% CI	*p* Value Trend
Socioeconomic index										
Low	23	16	1.0[a]	–	0.690	41	36	1.0[a]	–	0.138
Middle-low	17	19	0.53	0.21–1.38		17	14	1.01	0.43–2.36	
Middle	48	38	0.68	0.30–1.52		49	29	1.34	0.70–2.58	

[a] Adjusted for age at first birth and family history of breast cancer.
[b] Nonadjusted.
[c] Adjusted for family history of breast cancer.
[d] Adjusted for age at first birth.

DISCUSSION

According to the results of this study, the principal risk factors for breast cancer among Mexican women are: childlessness and low parity, late age at birth of the first child, and a history of breast cancer in the patient's family. These results agree with those reported in the international literature. [3–10] Likewise, a protective effect of breast-feeding was found among premenopausal women, which is also consistent with international research suggesting the existence of this protective factor.[9,25]

Other studies have found that the early presentation of menarche (<12 years) increases the risk of having breast cancer, and it has been estimated that for every two years later that menstruation occurs, the probability of having breast cancer is reduced by 10%.[9] This finding was not replicated in Mexico. Two possible explanations for this could be the international difference that exists in terms of mean age for this event. For example, among Chinese women the average age at menarche is 17 years, while among Mexican women it is 13 years.[3] Other possible explanations are that the effect of age at menarche is very weak and random errors inherent in its measurement do not allow its detection.

Late age at menopause is another risk factor that has been identified in international studies, in which it has been estimated that for every five years difference in the occurrence of this event, the risk of having BC varies by 17%.[25] As with menarche, late age at menopause was not found to be an associated factor in studies carried out in Mexico.

Some authors have reported that an existing breast tumor could begin the accelerated growth stage in women who give birth to their first child after 30 years of age. Likewise, it has been suggested that conceiving a child protects breast tissue against agents that initiate carcinogenesis. However, the mechanisms that increase the risk of having BC in women who are older when they give birth to their first child have not been clearly defined.

The results of this study agree both with international and national findings.[26,27] Therefore, it can be established that the risk of having breast cancer among Mexican women is approximately two times greater for those women who had their first child after 30 years of age.

Childlessness is a risk factor for BC that has been consistently reported in the scientific literature. This effect has been observed principally in breast cancer diagnosed during postmenopause,[25] as was observed in this study, given that our results show an approximately 2.5 times greater risk when comparing childless women with those who had four or more children.

In relation to the effect of the number of children, independent of the age of the mother when the first child was born, international results are controversial.[25] In Mexico, our results suggest that multiparity is a reproductive characteristic that decreases the risk of BC, independent of age at first birth. Based on the decrease in fertility rates that has occurred,[28] this result implies that the percentage of women at risk of having breast cancer will increase in the future.

The most recent epidemiological studies on the subject suggest that breast-feeding is a protective factor in relation to breast cancer in premenopausal women;[25] these findings, confirmed in our study, show that an average of 60% protection exists with the first breast-fed child, and this is maintained when considering the number of months for all breast-fed children. These results were independent of parity and were not observed in postmenopausal women.

The mechanisms that have been proposed to explain the protective effect of breast-feeding on BC incidence include: an increase in anovulatory cycles, a decrease in estrogen production, a direct physical effect on mammary epithelial cells, or the elimination of carcinogens through this biological fluid.[25]

The association between family history of breast cancer and increased risk of having this disease is a consistent result in a number of studies, including this one, in which it is estimated that those women with a relative with this type of neoplasm had a 3.29 times greater risk. As expected, the observed effect was greater in premenopausal women, although a smaller but statistically significant effect was also found in postmenopausal women, which suggests that diagnosis in this subgroup might have been late.

Despite the importance of family history of breast cancer in the etiology of this disease, it is estimated that in the general population the fraction of breast cancer attributable to genetic origin is only approximately 6%;[25] this reflects the low prevalence-of the *BRCA1* gene, which has been identified as a predisposing factor for breast cancer.

Obesity, measured with the Quetelet index, was not associated with BC incidence in the population studied. In relation to this, first it should be noted that in general international results have not found a considerable increased risk of BC in postmenopausal women, and an inverse relation (that is, protective) has even been suggested in premenopausal women.[25] Second, in the study population there was insufficient variability to evaluate the effect of the body mass index mentioned, because the range was only about 3 units (24.34 to 27.3 kg/cm^2).

The socioeconomic level was not observed to have an effect, probably because the majority of the women who participated in this study were from two public hospitals, and had similar socioeconomic characteristics.

Finally, the importance of reproductive factors for breast cancer in Mexico has been confirmed in this article, and agrees with results reported in studies from many countries. In addition, the findings lend additional support to the promotion of maternal breast feeding.

ACKNOWLEDGMENTS

The authors are grateful for the valuable participation of Dr. Luisa Torres and Dr. Laura Torres in the supervision of the field work for this research project; to Dr. Ramón Alberto Rascón for his technical assistance; and to Ms. Reina Collado and Ms. Betania Allen for editing and translating this document, respectively.

REFERENCES

1. Secretaria de Salud. 1993. Perfiles estadísticos No 7: Tumores. Series Monográficas. México, D.F.
2. Secretaria de Salud. 1993. Morbilidad por neoplasias malignas 1982–1989. México, D.F.

3. HARRIS, J. R., M. E. LIPPMAN, U. VERONESI & W. WILLET. 1992. Breast cancer. N. Engl. J. Med. **327:** 319-328.
4. YUAN, J. M., M. C. YU, R. K. ROSS, Y. T. GAO & B. E. HENDERSON. 1988. Risk factors for breast cancer in Chinese women in Shanghai. Cancer Res. **48:** 1949-1953.
5. MACMAHON, B., M. PURDE, D. CRAMER & E. HINT. 1982. Association of breast cancer risk with age at first and subsequent births: A study in the population of the Estonian Republic. J. Nat. Cancer Inst. **69:** 1035-1038.
6. RAO, D. N., B. GANESH & P. B. DESAI. 1994. Role of reproductive factors in breast cancer in a low-risk area: A case-control study. Br. J. Cancer **70:** 129-132.
7. ROSNER, B., G. A. COLDDITZ & W. WILLET. 1994. Reproductive risk factors in a prospective study of breast cancer: The nurses' health study. Am. J. Epidemiol. **139:** 819-835.
8. ROMIEU, I., M. HERNANDEZ-AVILA, E. LAZCANO, L. LOPEZ & R. ROMERO-JAIME. 1996. Breast cancer and lactation history in Mexican women. Am. J. Epidemiol. **143:** 543-552.
9. MCTIERNAN, A. & D. B. THOMAS. 1986. Evidence for a protective effect of lactation on risk of breast cancer in young women. Am. J. Epidemiol. **124:** 353-358.
10. SISKIND, V., F. SHOFIELD, D. RICE & C. BAIN. 1989. Breast cancer and breast-feeding: Results from an Australian case-control study. Am. J. Epidemiol. **130:** 229-236.
11. COLDITZ, G. A., M. J. STAMPFER, W. WILLET, C. H. HENNEKENS, B. ROSNER & F. F. SPEIZER. 1990. Prospective study of estrogen replacement therapy and risk of breast cancer in postmenopausal women. JAMA **264:** 2648-2653.
12. ARMSTRONG, B. K. 1988. Estrogen therapy after the menopause: Boon or bane? Med. J. Aust. **148:** 213-214.
13. NEWCOMB, P., M. P. LONGNECKER & B. E. STORER. 1995. Long-term hormone replacement therapy and risk of breast cancer in postmenopausal women. Am. J. Epidemiol. **130:** 788-795.
14. HENDERSON, I. C. 1993. Risk factors for breast cancer development. Cancer **71:** 2127-2140.
15. NASCA, P. P., M. BAPTISTE, N. A. FIELD, B. B. METZGER, M. BLACK, C. S. KWON *et al.* 1990. An epidemiological case-control study of breast cancer and alcohol consumption. Int. J. Epidemiol. **19:** 532-538.
16. WILLET, W. C., M. J. STAMPFER, G. A. COLDITZ, B. A. ROSNER, C. H. HENNEKENS & F. E. SPEIZER. 1987. Moderate alcohol consumption and the risk of breast cancer. N. Engl. J. Med. **316:** 1174-1180.
17. DEN BRANDT, P. A., R. A. GOLDBOHM & P. VAN 'T VEER. 1995. Alcohol and breast cancer: Results from the Netherlands cohort study. Am. J. Epidemiol. **141:** 907-915.
18. KATSOUYANI, K., A. TRICHOPOULOU, S. STUVER, Y. GARAS, A. KRITSELIS, G. KYRIAKOU *et al.* 1994. The association of fat and other macronutrients with breast cancer: A case-control study from Greece. Br. J. Cancer **70:** 537-541.
19. SASAKI, S., M. HORACSEK & H. KESTELLOT. 1993. An ecological study of the relationship between dietary fat intake and breast cancer mortality. Prev. Med. **22:** 187-202.
20. WILLET, W. C., M. J. STAMPFER, G. A. COLDITZ, B. A. ROSNER, C. H. HENNEKENS & F. E. SPEIZER. 1987. Dietary fat and the risk of breast cancer. N. Engl. J. Med. **316:** 22-28.
21. KATOH, A., V. J. M. WATZLAF & F. D. AMICO. 1994. An examination of obesity and breast cancer survival in post-menopausal women. Br. J. Cancer **69:** 928-933.
22. TONKELAAR, I., J. C. SEIDEL, H. J. A. COLLETTE & F. WAARD. 1994. A prospective study on obesity and subcutaneous fat patterning in relation to breast cancer in post-menopausal women participating in the DOM project. Br. J. Cancer **69:** 352-357.
23. TORNBERG, S. A. & J. M. CARSTENSEN. 1994. Relationship between Quetelet's index and cancer of breast and female genital tract in 47,000 women followed for 25 years. Br. J. Cancer **69:** 358-361.
24. BRONFMAN, M., H. GUISCAFRÉ, V. CASTRO, R. CASTRO & G. GUTIÉRREZ. 1988. Estrategias para mejorar los patrones terapéuticos utilizados en diarrea aguda en unidades de atención médica primaria. II. La medición de la desigualdad: Una estrategia metodológica, análisis de las característica socioeconómicas de la muestra. Arch. Invest. Med. (Méx.) **19:** 351-360.

25. KELSEY, J. 1993. Breast cancer. Epidemiologic reviews. The Johns Hopkins University School of Hygiene and Public Health. Baltimore, MD.
26. TOVAR-GUZMAN, V. 1995. Factores de riesgo reproductivos de cáncer de mama en mujeres mexicanas. Un estudio de casos y controles hospitalarios. Thesis, Universidad Nacional Autónoma de México. México.
27. GARCÍA-SÁINZ, M. & R. BORREGO-ROMÁN. 1981. Factores de riesgo para el cáncer mamario. Un estudio epidemiológico retrospectivo. Gac. Med. Mex. **117:** 323–331.
28. OLAIZ, G., M. HERNÁNDEZ, E. LAZCANO, L. LÓPEZ-CARRILLO, J. OLVERA, P. PARES *et al.* 1994. Cáncer. Un encuentro con el futuro epidemiológico. Cuadernos de Salud No. 1. Secretaría de Salud. México.

Building Community Networks for Environmental Health

JANET A. PHOENIX[a]

Manager, Public Health Programs
National Safety Council
1025 Connecticut Avenue, N.W., Suite 1200
Washington, D.C. 20036

BRIDGING THE GAP BETWEEN RESEARCHERS AND AFFECTED POPULATIONS

All too often researchers in environment, health, and related disciplines engage upon research in the absence of meaningful input from communities, populations, and individuals who are directly affected by that research. By meaningful input, I mean involving those who are affected by the problem during the research planning phase. Research and the ultimate health of the communities we study depend upon the creation of a collaboration between academic institutions and communities. Communities know their needs and know what is acceptable to them. There are norms of behavior that every group uses to define acceptable and unacceptable behavior. When someone from the outside comes in, an acknowledgment of the existence of these norms is incumbent upon the outsider. A listening and observing process must take place in order for understanding and mutual agreement upon goals to occur.

ENVIRONMENTAL JUSTICE AND PUBLIC PARTICIPATION

When we work on environmental health issues in communities of color and in low-income communities, we are working on issues of environmental justice. One definition of environmental justice refers to the effort to preserve the planet by combating disproportionate impacts of pollution on people of color and low income communities. Another term commonly used to describe what currently exists in many communities is environmental racism. Environmental racism is defined as racial discrimination in environmental policy-making and the enforcement of regulations and laws, the deliberate targeting of communities of people of color for toxic waste facilities, the official sanctioning of the life-threatening presence of poisons and pollutants in our communities, and the history of excluding people of color from leadership in the environmental movement. Whatever definition of choice one uses, it is important to acknowledge that without inclusion of affected populations any efforts to do work to improve environmental conditions in communities of color can be viewed as illegitimate. This is the essence of a commitment to public participation.

[a]Phone: 202/974-2474; e-mail: leadctr@nsc.org

EXISTING ENVIRONMENTAL HEALTH NETWORKS

Geographic and ethnic environmental justice networks have been organized around the country to coordinate the efforts of small grassroots organizations and to provide networking opportunities and manage campaigns focused on specific environmental justice issues. These include but are not limited to the Southwest Network for Economic and Environmental Justice, The Asian and Pacific Islander Environmental Network, the Southern Organizing Committee for Environmental and Economic Justice, the Indigenous Environmental Justice Network, and the Northeast Environmental Justice Network. Some of these organizations have collaborated with academic institutions to conduct training and research activities.

MODELS OF ENVIRONMENTAL JUSTICE RESEARCH

I hope these remarks have served to provide a model of collaboration that can be used to build a credible and valuable program of environmental research at any institution. First and foremost is the notion of involvement of affected community members from the outset as the research project or program is planned. Second is the notion of community-driven priorities and benefits that should be derived from the research undertaking. Third is the notion of ongoing work with organizations that have a track record of working in the affected communities on issues that they have identified as priorities. While this may sound simple, accomplishing it may be more difficult than imagined. This model was put into effect in the Aquesasne nation in upstate New York. Native American midwives who were concerned about a nearby dioxin-producing facility contacted researchers at the State University of New York. The midwives wanted to know whether dioxin contamination in breast milk was linked to an increasing number of birth defects they were observing in newborns. Thus a collaboration was born that led to an ATSDR-funded research project in which the principal investigator is a Native American woman.

A less favorable example is the legacy left by a research project undertaken by the State of California's Department of Health. They studied lead contamination in soil, paint, and drinking water and obtained blood samples in three California counties. One of these counties was Alameda, which contained the East Oakland community just outside San Francisco. When residents learned of the study, they asked for the results to be released. Initially the State was reluctant to share the information with community residents. Only when the community organized around the issue and began to demonstrate at local hospitals, demanding routine lead screening for their children, did the situation improve and official test results were made available. It soon became clear that despite myths to the contrary, lead poisoning was very much alive in Oakland, California and in other areas of the state as well. The response of the community to what was perceived as an effort to withhold information from them concerning their welfare and the welfare of their children led to a lawsuit forcing the inclusion of routine lead screening in the Early Periodic Screening Detection and Treatment Program (EPSDT) under federal Medicaid law. While gains were made for the nation's poor children, trust that could have developed between researchers and community members was permanently damaged.

BIBLIOGRAPHY

1. 1992. Beyond the Green, Redefining and Diversifying the Environmental Movement. Environmental Careers Organization. Boston, MA.
2. Brown, P., Ed. 1996. Perspectives in Medical Sociology. Waveland Press. Illinois.
3. Bryant, B. & P. Mohai, Eds. 1992. Race and the Incidence of Environmental Hazards, A Time for Discourse. Westview Press. Boulder, CO.

Ethical Issues in Genetic Screening and Genetic Monitoring of Employees[a]

KAREL VAN DAMME,[b,c,d] PAOLO VINEIS,[e]
MARJA SORSA,[f] AND LUDWINE CASTELEYN [b,c]

[b]*Center for Human Genetics*
University of Leuven
Herestraat, 49
B-3000 Leuven, Belgium

[c]*Epidemiology and Community Medicine*
University of Antwerp
Antwerp, Belgium

[e]*Unit of Cancer Epidemiology*
Department of Biomedical Science and Human Oncology
University of Turin
Turin, Italy

[f]*Finnish Institute of Occupational Health, and*
Ministry of Education
PB 293
11717 Helsinki, Finland

MEDICAL TESTING OF WORKERS AND PREVENTION

Genetic screening and genetic monitoring are new tools in occupational health. Genetic testing is still used mainly for research purposes, but its use on a routine basis might represent a challenge for current prevention policies. This concern was the basis for a European Concerted Action, a research project funded by the European Commission, entitled "The Ethical, Social, and Scientific Problems Related to the Application of Genetic Screening and Genetic Monitoring for Employees in the Context of a European Approach to Health and Safety at Work" (Biomedical and Health Research Contract CT92-1213). One of the aims of the concerted action was to identify the rules of good practice and the legal requirements necessary to guarantee that use of the new techniques would reflect current European values and would be in the interests of workers. We also aimed to establish a European network of professionals and scientists to follow up future use of the techniques.

[a] This study was performed under a grant from the European Commission (Biomedical and Health Research Contract CT92-1213), and was coordinated at the Center for Human Genetics (Professor Herman Van den Berghe, Director) at the University of Leuven.

[d] Corresponding author. Phone/fax: 32 16 40 72 74; e-mail: Ludwine.Casteleyn pophost.eunet.bc

The following general approach was adopted to identify the ethical and social problems that might be raised by the introduction of genetic screening and genetic monitoring for workers. Certain medical selection and health surveillance practices used currently in occupational settings and possible future techniques were analyzed for their accuracy, relevance, necessity, and consequences. For this purpose, a model relating exposure, susceptibility, and health impairment was developed. "Necessity" was studied with regard to the relationship between primary prevention, medical selection, and surveillance. The "consequences" were considered at the level of both the individual and society. The values and principles commonly upheld in Western European countries, such as respect for human dignity, democratic participation, solidarity, and social justice, were identified on the basis of general political beliefs, and current and future practices in the selection of workers and health surveillance were checked for compliance with those principles. Current legislation for the protection of workers' health was evaluated for the accuracy with which it preserves these ethical values. Guidelines were established with respect to the socioethical aspects of selection and surveillance techniques that are destined for all parties involved in relevant regulatory activities.

A prevention policy has several objectives, some of which may be conflicting. The main objective may be to increase productivity in a company, for instance by reducing absenteeism or selecting a healthy work force; or to lower the costs of insurance or other compensation for victims of occupational and other diseases. Alternatively, prevention may consist of adapting workplaces to workers, such that virtually every worker can be considered fit for a job. Clear objectives and basic options that reflect socioethical values are preconditions for the relevance and acceptability of a practice that is part of a prevention policy.

An occupational prevention policy can involve three general tools:

- *Adaptation of workplaces to workers* (for instance, through industrial hygiene). Even if the extent of reduction of risk in a particular case cannot be quantified, it is clear that lowering exposures and substituting less dangerous substances for dangerous ones will usually reduce risk.
- *Medical surveillance of workers* (for instance, through periodical medical examination of workers at risk). The history of occupational medicine shows that medical surveillance has been a major impetus for better industrial hygiene. It is often forgotten that testing itself raises greater awareness of possible work-related risks and the need for industrial hygiene. Medical surveillance can, however, also be used wrongly to select out only the victims of occupational diseases at an early stage, without improving the working conditions.
- *Preemployment or preplacement examinations* (for instance, testing physical fitness or susceptibility to disease). A major problem with medical selection practices is that they are often of questionable relevance, in contrast to widespread opinion. New testing practices, including genetic susceptibility tests, can be developed that partially overcome this drawback.

The way in which these three tools are used and their complementarity reflect the basic options and the objectives to be attained. If the main objective is to reduce insurance costs, ruling out job applicants with increased susceptibility to disease will be emphasized at a preemployment examination, while medical surveillance may aim to rule out workers showing the first symptoms of a disease. In this case, industrial hygiene will be improved only in order to further reduce insurance costs. In a worker-orientated approach, preemployment medical examinations will be used to protect the worker, giving him or her a job that corresponds to his or her fitness and if necessary adapting the working conditions to the abilities of the applicant, perhaps through industrial hygiene and medical surveillance; the latter will also be used to check that working conditions are consistent with the abilities of the worker.

Differences in basic objectives may lead to the use of different medical tests, but these same tests may be used to attain different objectives. A practice must thus be evaluated for its contribution to the objectives. Differences in basic objectives may involve different approaches to similar risk factors, and the choice of priorities may be affected. The question at the root of socioethical debates is whether a particular practice makes sense. In the debate on the socioethical acceptability of medical selection practices, little attention is given to the accuracy and relevance of the practice for attaining the objective. Instead, the debate often starts directly from such considerations as the need for risk reduction measures or the social consequences of a testing practice, assuming that the practice is relevant. In the International Code of Ethics for Occupational Health Professionals of the International Committee for Occupational Health,[1] respect for human dignity is the *primum mobile,* emphasizing the importance of ensuring the health and well-being of individual workers and of the workforce as a whole. The improvement of working conditions is considered to be the central tool of occupational health professionals, in accordance with their central mission: protecting health. As Dr. Coppée said at the International Committee for Occupational Health conference in Nice in 1993, "The future of occupational health is perhaps to know how to resolve the conflict between values such as the right to health and the right to work at the level both of the individual and all workers, with the aim of protecting health and allowing employment." This thought corresponds broadly to the legislative frameworks of many Western European countries, although practice may not always correspond.

We first comment on the new genetic tools, genetic monitoring, and genetic screening, and then try to identify similarities and differences in current medical testing practices. We will then focus our attention on two issues that are often encountered in debates on the ethical aspects of medical testing in occupational settings: the relevance of the models used in clinical medicine for ethical analysis in occupational settings, and the relevance of the principle of informed consent for genetic and other testing.

GENETIC MONITORING: EXPERIENCES, POSSIBILITIES, AND APPLICATIONS IN OCCUPATIONAL HEALTH

Our understanding of toxicological processes at the molecular level has increased rapidly. Conventional biological monitoring has been bolstered by the new tools of genetic monitoring and molecular toxicology, for evaluation of biologically relevant doses and identification of risks in population groups and individuals. Genetic monitoring involves the use of genetic toxicology for measuring biomarkers of genetic effects and for assessing exposure to genotoxic substances in individuals with defined exposure at work, in the environment, or from their life style. When genetic biomonitoring shows that the genetic material has been damaged, the results can be used to estimate risk only at the level of the population. The results of cytogenetic tests do not allow prediction of individual risk for cancer. Genetic monitoring can potentially result in early identification of genotoxic exposures and thus enable identification of high-risk populations and priorities for intervention. Use of predictive biomarkers can save time and prevent unnecessary end effects, such as cancer.

Human peripheral blood lymphocytes are suitable for use in surveillance because they are readily accessible and because they integrate exposure over a relatively long period. Exposure to chemical mutagens may result in increased frequencies of chromosomal aberrations and/or sister chromatid exchanges in blood lymphocytes of exposed individuals. Genetic monitoring of the occupational environment usually involves cytogenetic techniques, which entail scoring of microscopically visible chromosomal damage, such as structural chromosomal aberrations, sister chromatid exchange, and micronucleated cells. Chromosome painting and use of chromosome-specific probes by fluorescent *in situ* hybridization techniques have considerably improved the sensitivity of cytogenetic monitoring.

Relevance of Genetic Monitoring to Cancer Risk

When cytogenetic tests on peripheral blood lymphocytes show that the genetic material has been damaged, the result can be used to estimate risk at the level of the population, and an increased frequency of chromosomal aberrations in a population should be considered an indication of an increased risk for diseases related to genetic damage, including cancer, in the exposed population.[2] Somatic genetic damage in peripheral blood lymphocytes has little or no effect on the health of the individual, however, since most lymphocytes carrying genetic damage die and are replaced.

In general, a concordance has been shown between human exposure to carcinogens and increased cytogenetic damage,[2] supporting the predictivity of cytogenetic biomonitoring for cancer risk. The number of agents that have repeatedly been shown to induce cytogenetic changes in humans is still relatively limited. For vinyl choride, benzene, ethylene oxide, and alkylating chemotherapeutic agents, the extent of damage has been shown to be a function of exposure level. Thus, even though cytogenetic end points are not very sensitive or specific for detecting exposures in present-day occupational settings, positive results in such tests have often prompted implementation of hygienic improvements, even in the absence of direct evidence of a relationship between somatic chromosomal damage and adverse health outcomes.

Data from human genetic monitoring are considered to be relevant for evaluating human cancer risk by The International Agency for Research on Cancer in the process of classifying the strength of evidence for human cancer risk. In several cases, this has led to a change in the classification of a compound. Strong evidence of a dose-related response in chromosomal aberrations and sister chromatid exchange in workers exposed to ethylene oxide raised the classification of the compound to the highest category, group 1, even though there was limited evidence from human cancer epidemiology.[3] Other well-documented genotoxins have similarly been reclassified–for example, cisplatin (group 2B to 2A[4]), spraying and application of insecticides (group 2B to 2A[5]), and styrene (group 3 to 2B).

From both the public health and scientific viewpoints, there should be increased integration of experimental techniques with epidemiological research strategies, so as to better focus cancer risk assessment. This will require collaborative, multidisciplinary work among experts in different disciplines.

Genetic Screening of Workers

The human body meets chemical challenges by a series of defence mechanisms that call upon enzymatic detoxification systems and on DNA repair enzymes. The capacity of these defence systems may differ considerably from one individual to another, and a poor capacity can lead to increased risk after exposure to a harmful substance, in comparison with other individuals exposed at the same level. Many studies have shown the modulating role of genetic metabolic polymorphism, for instance, in activating and deactivating carcinogens. Rapid progress in characterizing the human genome and advances in molecular genetics should allow identification of "susceptibility genes" for many diseases in healthy, asymptomatic individuals. Examples have been discussed elsewhere.[6] These well-known examples may explain the tendency to use genetic tests (genotype and phenotype testing) in order to distinguish between workers who have a greater and a lesser susceptibility to certain diseases after a particular exposure.

Unlike genetic biomonitoring, genetic screening addresses the hereditary genetic structure or the phenotype, which is the expression of genes (making an individual a slow or a fast acetylator, for example). These tests could, in principle, become part of preemployment testing. Susceptibility is also the result of acquired factors, however, and inherited susceptibility can be the result of a series of genetic factors other than that measured in the test. Acquired factors are environmental (other past or current occupational and nonoccupational exposure), biological (age, sex, previous or current diseases), or associated with life style (e.g., nutrition, tobacco, or alcohol consumption, and even stress).

A susceptibility model has been developed that makes it possible to correlate susceptibility, exposure, and disease and to locate the level of intervention of selection practices and medical surveillance.[1] This model should clarify the wide variation among individuals in their responses to toxic substances, which are determined only in part by genetic factors. Each step that occurs within the organism after exposure–from exposure to internal dose, internal dose to effective biological dose to early biological effect, to a structural or functional change possibly resulting in (clinical) disease)–is mediated by acquired and inherited susceptibility factors, and many genes could be involved at each step. For example, a weak capacity for DNA repair might affect the step from effective biological dose (e.g., DNA adducts) to early biological effect (mutation or chromosomal aberration) by resulting in a higher frequency of chromosomal aberrations after exposure to carcinogens. But other factors may be as important: After similar exposure, an individual in better physical condition will have a lower internal dose (due to reduced breathing for the same effort), which could lead to a much lower effective biological dose, and therefore to a lower risk, despite a poor capacity for DNA repair.

In evaluating the scientific credibility of a hypothesis of a particular genetic susceptibility to disease, a number of questions must be raised, in particular with respect to metabolic polymorphism. The authors of a recent review[1] concluded that with respect to the debrisoquine phenotype/genotype and *N*-acetyltransferase polymorphism, testing may be largely irrelevant, for several reasons. Van Damme *et al.*[6] proposed a framework for judging the acceptability of screening for susceptibility, identifying 10 points that reflect scientific, social, and ethical questions and that relate to the relevance, the accuracy, the need for and the consequences of a testing practice.

Despite the lack of evidence that genotypic and phenotypic screening tests are relevant for workers, the potential ethical implications of such screening is being discussed intensely. There is confusion, however, between genetic testing for scientific research purposes and testing on a routine basis as part of occupational health surveillance. The issues at stake may be different in the two cases. The debate is further confused by extrapolation of the ethical models widely used in clinical medicine to occupational settings. We address the latter problem.

SIMILARITIES AND DIFFERENCES BETWEEN THE NEW GENETIC TESTS AND CURRENT TESTING PRACTICES

There are some differences with regard to preemployment or preplacement testing between tests for genotypic and phenotypic susceptibility and what might be considered more traditional testing practices in occupational health, such as lung radiography for workers exposed to silicon dioxide or haematological examinations for workers exposed to benzene.

Biological markers are assumed to provide information on the risk for health impairment after exposure. In genotypic testing, the relationship between the marker and the risk for an effect—if based on more than a statistical correlation—is often indirect or putative. In more traditional tests, the association between the marker and the risk for health impairment is more evident, and the association with the effect determinants tends to be stronger, especially when there is clinical plausibility in the relationship between the marker and the effect. In genotypic tests, only one of the many intervening factors is isolated, while various intervening factors are already integrated in the results of more traditional tests. The latter are indicators of a later step in the continuum of biological events that can occur after exposure and therefore tend to identify a smaller number of persons as being at risk. Since genotypic tests seek inherited markers specific to the individual and unrelated to the environment, they do not stimulate better industrial hygiene; more traditional medical surveillance tests may do so, since they are more closely related to the exposure history of the person. For the same reason, genotypic testing will not result in financial compensation (for "having the wrong genes"), whereas traditional testing may sometimes do so, as it can indicate previous exposure to harmful working conditions.

Genetic biomonitoring, on the other hand, is more similar to traditional surveillance practices and may even fill the gap in occupational surveillance for early detection of malignancy or reproductive toxicity.

RELEVANCE FOR OCCUPATIONAL SETTINGS OF ETHICAL MODELS USED IN CLINICAL MEDICINE

Evaluation of Genetic Screening according to the "Georgetown Paradigm"

The Georgetown paradigm[7] is the most widely used ethical model in clinical medicine, which is applied, case by case, to ethically uncertain situations that arise in clinical practice. It is based on four general principles: beneficence, nonmaleficence, decisional autonomy of the patient, and equity. Conflicts readily arise among these principles, as discussed in textbooks of bioethics, such as that of Beauchamp and Childress.[7] For example, patients may not be able to express their will because of the pathological conditions by which they are affected (in this case, medical paternalism may be accepted in order to restore the patient's decisional autonomy). The Georgetown paradigm owes it popularity to the fact that it allows the physician to deal with most clinical situations without violating the main values of western tradition. By weighting the four values on a case-by-case basis, the physician uses the principal Western philosophical traditions: for example, Kantianism is reflected in equity, libertarianism in decisional autonomy, and utilitarianism in beneficence. Although the Georgetown paradigm is undoubtedly useful in the medical context, it has limitations in its public health applications, such as in (hypothetical) genetic screening.

A simplistic approach to genetic screening would be to weight the benefits and costs of genetic screening against those of primary prevention. The superficial conclusion might be that genetic testing is less expensive and generally more convenient than limiting exposure. Although it represents economic convenience, this approach is unacceptable, as beneficence itself involves an internal hierarchy of elements. According to Frankena,[8] beneficence (including nonmaleficence) has four elements:

1. not to inflict harm;
2. to prevent harm;
3. to repair harm;
4. to do good.

This hierarchy is both logical and ethical. Without it, many everyday actions would make no sense, and denial of this hierarchy makes ethics difficult to define. Acceptance of the hierarchy implies that primary prevention is an ethical obligation of the employer and should always be implemented. Lack of reference to these four elements and hierarchical organization would hamper proper use of the Georgetown paradigm.

Genetically based metabolic polymorphisms may be unevenly distributed among different ethnic groups: for example, the proportion of slow acetylators is 10% among Asians and 90% among Africans. Racial discrimination would thus be an immediate consequence of the inappropriate use of genetic screening, which might be aimed at excluding workers at preemployment examination.

A Critique of the Georgetown Paradigm

The Georgetown paradigm is used wrongly if its four principles are weighted equally, so that equity, for example, is given the same *a priori* weight as decisional autonomy. In this situation, the physician is left to decide how to weight the principles in different situations, according to personal preferences. Physicians more sensitive to decisional autonomy issues would be more careful in obtaining informed consent or would be more critical of medical practices that hamper the patient's will. Others would weight beneficence more heavily. Assigning equal *a priori* weight to the ethical principles is wrong because the four principles are not independent. In medical tradition, beneficence (doing good) is secondary to nonmaleficence (*primum non nocere*). Beneficence without decisional autonomy has only limited meaning, since subjects affected by the decision would not be able to appreciate the risks and benefits if they were deprived of their decisional autonomy. The conditioning of beneficence on decisional autonomy has been acknowledged in the ethical literature by statements that the only justification of the paternalistic attitude, that is, doing good without asking for the patient's agreement, is to restore the patient's ability to decide. This occurs, for example, with patients in coma. Similarly, decisional autonomy itself has no meaning in the absence of equity or fairness. If two patients are treated unfairly, that is, they do not receive the same treatment for the same disease (for example, as a consequence of "rationing" of health care), their decisional autonomy is not respected.

The principle of *primum non nocere* clearly indicates that primary prevention is the main obligation of society in the face of known causes of disease. The *prima facie* priority of decisional autonomy over beneficence means that the introduction of genetic screening should be preceded by an open debate about its scientific basis, its implications, and its advantages and disadvantages. The priority of equity over decisional autonomy means that the latter should not be conditioned on, for example, the labor market. In conditions of unemployment, such as exist in large areas of Europe today, job applicants may not be completely free to choose between being employed in a hazardous job and being unemployed.

Weighting beneficence, equity, and decisional autonomy is thus not really a question of individual preference or choice. The four general principles have at least a logical, if not an ethical, natural hierarchy. The Georgetown model has emerged as the main bioethical paradigm in medicine (particularly in the Anglo-Saxon context), not only because it allows the physician to refer to the principal western systems of thought, condensed in the four principles, but also because it represents a strongly individualistic approach.

More General Tendencies in Western Societies

The Georgetown paradigm has been used dogmatically and simplistically. Biomedical ethics emerged principally in response to various moral crises created by technology rather than as an expression of some universal, atemporal principle. The introduction of genetic screening requires adequate reactions, not a case-by-case evaluation based on the application of general principles. For example, the Georgetown paradigm is insufficient to meet certain tendencies in western societies.

- The Swiss theologian Bondolfi[9] described the transition of western societies in this century to "biological capitalism," consisting of large-scale exploitation of the biological world, while the last century was characterized by exploitation mainly of the mineral world.

- Preventive medicine is increasingly being challenged and substituted by predictive medicine–that is, there is an increasing tendency to classify individuals on the basis of their susceptibility to disease. Clearly, insurance companies play a crucial role in this process. As Nelkin and Tancredi have pointed out,[10] tests of susceptibility are becoming so numerous that completely "normal" subjects scarcely exist.

- Although the recent tradition of occupational medicine and psychology stresses the need for adapting jobs to humans and not *vice versa,* the introduction of genetic screening and emphasis on private insurance might reintroduce the opposite view, that work organization is the given element and human subjects are the dependent variable.

It would be erroneous for medicine, and particularly public health, to consider that "cost-benefit" calculations exhaust the ethical issues. The utilitarian point of view is the main philosophy of public health, which is based on a computation of the benefits of a certain action in relation to its social costs. More precisely, the utilitarian view is based on a linear combination of individual advantages and disadvantages, so that the benefits, risks, and costs for different individuals are computed on the same scale. The scale is usually an economic one, based on a money value of human life. Thus, for example, the causation of three cases of cancer in the American population as a consequence of exposure to a carcinogen is considered an "acceptable" event, in that the overall social benefits appear to outweigh the burden of disease (on a linear scale). As Rawlsians have pointed out, however, we cannot put all individuals in the same basket. The ethical perspective implies action in favor of the most disadvantaged sectors of society, in order to restore "primary social goods." Similar reasoning is currently acknowledged in clinical medicine, where paternalism is accepted in order to restore the will of the patient. Similarly, actions in favor of the disadvantaged have the goal of restoring decisional autonomy.

According to Rawlsians, there are symbolic aspects of human interactions, such as equity, that must be weighted more than others, that is, their violation counts more than the potential material advantages that can be achieved. This point of view, which belongs to the Kantian tradition, is consistent with the proposal of the philosopher John Searle to distinguish between "regulative" and "constitutive" rules in moral decision: regulative rules concern the most efficient ways of achieving a certain goal (they are instrumental to the goal), while constitutive rules concern the definitions of ethics itself in that they identify which values are at stake. This distinction further reinforces the idea that the four principles of the Georgetown paradigm cannot be placed at the same level.

RELEVANCE OF APPLYING THE PRINCIPLE OF INFORMED CONSENT TO GENETIC AND OTHER TESTING IN OCCUPATIONAL HEALTH

Application of the principle of individual informed consent for medical testing in an occupational context is problematic, for several reasons:

- The accuracy of the information provided may be limited.
- The authenticity of the consent may be questionable.
- The decision of an individual may conflict with the interests of others.

A prerequisite for reliable individual consent is obviously the provision of accurate, up-to-date information about the test. However, the accuracy of the information depends on knowledge about the relevance of the test and the accuracy of its results. The relevance of a test is defined by the strength of the association between its results and the risk for developing disease or other adverse health effect. The results should be interpretable as the relative risk or the probability that an individual will have an adverse health effect when exposed to an external risk factor. The limited relevance of tests is not always well understood: for instance, the level of exposure to a factor can have a considerable effect on its relevance as a predictor of relative risk. Thus, it is not only difficult to explain the concept of probability of risk to an individual who is being asked to give his or her consent, but it is even more difficult to explain the uncertainties engendered by factors that affect the strength of the association between a test result and the relative risk, particularly as so little is known about this subject. Uncertainty also arises from limitations to the reliability and validity of a test, that is, the accuracy of its results.

Even if the information given is as correct as possible, the authenticity of the consent may still be questionable, for several reasons:

- The authority of the person giving the information may affect the decision of the individual.
- Informed consent can be given only if the individual can understand the explanation correctly; but even a clear explanation cannot guarantee correct understanding.
- Individual decisional autonomy is not synonymous with the ability to decide.
- Individual decisional autonomy may be affected by lack of (degrees of) freedom to decide, owing to social constraints.
- The context in which a test is to be conducted, particularly objective and perceived inequalities of power between the provider and the receiver of information, may affect both the communication process and the decision.

Finally, the principle of informed consent makes an abstraction of possible conflicts between the individual's right to decide and the interests of third parties such as other employees, other job applicants, the work force in general, including the unemployed, and even society as a whole. The context of testing may be such that an individual's consent may directly or indirectly limit the possibility of others not to consent, and therefore their decisional autonomy. Whether this is so depends on the consequences for individuals who refuse the test. Because society has the duty to protect the freedom and rights of each individual, the freedom of some cannot be allowed to limit the freedom of others. This implies that decisions about work, health, and privacy should to some extent be taken by society and not left to the individual. The informed consent model leaves it up to the informed individual to balance his or her chances of getting a job, protecting his or her health, and protecting his or her privacy, and thus to decide whether to accept a test or not. To what extent can the work force as a whole, or job applicants in general, come to the same conclusion as the individual giving (or not giving) consent about the balance between work, health, and privacy? If the individual's decision to accept a particular practice is in conflict with what is considered to be the common interest, it would be wrong to allow introduction of the testing practice, even if informed consent is obtained. In addition, individual consent may not accord with the interests of society as a whole. The balance of values behind the testing practice may conflict with the principles upheld by a democratic society. Acceptance of underlying values of industrial practices that are in conflict with democratic values presents a challenge to the latter.

For all these reasons, individual consent cannot be considered a substitute for balancing values and interests and for making decisions about the acceptability of testing practices at the level of society. Social law and regulations should be the anchor of ethical principles and may thus help to increase the freedom of many people.

ACKNOWLEDGMENTS

The authors thank E. Heseltine for critical comments and help.

REFERENCES

1. International Commission on Occupational Health. 1995. International Code of Ethics for Occupational Health Professionals. ICOH. Singapore.
2. Sorsa, M., J. Wilbourn & H. Vainio. 1992. *In* Mechanisms of Carcinogenesis in Risk Identification. H. Vainio, P. N. Magee, D. B. McGregor & A. J. McMichael, Eds.: 543-544. International Agency for Research on Cancer. Lyon.
3. International Agency for Research on Cancer. 1991. IARC Monographs on the Evaluation of Carcinogenic Risks to Humans, Vol. 53, Occupational Exposures in Insecticide Application, and Some Pesticides. IARC. Lyon.
4. International Agency for Research on Cancer. 1994. IARC Monographs on the Evaluation of Carcinogenic Risks to Humans, Vol. 60, Some Industrial Chemicals. Lyon.
5. International Agency for Research on Cancer. 1987. IARC Monographs on the Evaluation of Carcinogenic Risks to Humans, Suppl. 7, Overall Evaluations of Carcinogenicity: An Updating of *IARC Monographs* Volumes 1 to 42. Lyon.

6. Van Damme, K., L. Casteleyn, E. Heseltine, A. Huici, M. Sorsa, N. van Larebeke & P. Vineis. 1995. Individual susceptibility and prevention of occupational diseases: Scientific and ethical issues. J. Occup. Environ. Med. **37:** 91-99.
7. Beauchamp, T. L. & J. F. Childress. 1989. Principles of Biomedical Ethics, 3d edit. Oxford Univ. Press. Oxford.
8. Frankena, W. 1973. Ethics. 2d edit. Prentice Hall. Englewood Cliffs, N.J.
9. Bondolfi, A. 1992. Primum non Nocere. Editions Alice. Geneva.
10. Nelkin, D. & L. Tancredi. 1989. Dangerous Diagnostics. Basic Books. New York.

Genetic Testing: A Technology Assessment Perspective

PAOLO VINEIS [a]

Unit of Cancer Epidemiology
Department of Biomedical Science and Human Oncology
Turin University and San Giovanni Battista Hospital
Via Santena, 7
10126 Turin, Italy

SCIENTIFIC AND PRACTICAL ISSUES IN GENETIC TESTING

From a scientific point of view, the idea that genes exert an important role in explaining human pathology has gained much popularity in recent decades. In the 1930s Lancelot Hogben, Professor of Social Biology at the University of London, gave a series of lectures on the relationship between genes and environment. His lectures in clinical genetics were published in 1933 with the title *Nature and Nurture,* a terminology that rapidly became popular.[1] He made an important statement, which is still valid today: ''In so far as a balance sheet of nature and nurture has an intelligible significance, it does not entitle us to set limits to changes that might be brought about by regulating the environment'' (quoted in Reference 2).

However, Hogben's message has not been taken seriously by other eminent scientists. Ronald Fisher, the most important statistician of this century, and a prominent figure in genetics himself, made several attempts to criticize the evidence related to the causal link between smoking and lung cancer. He claimed that such a link could not be considered causal because (1) there was no experimental proof, only observational evidence; and (2) scientists could not rule out that a genetic trait both induced people to smoke and caused lung cancer.[3] Both arguments have been proved faulty on the basis of a large amount of evidence: animal experiments; studies on biomarkers (including oncogenes) in humans; studies on twins; and other types of genetic investigations.[4] Unfortunately, evidence on the links between Fisher and the tobacco industry has also been provided. In fact, he was the paid consultant of the Tobacco Manufacturers' Standing Committee since 1956, and a smoker himself.[5] According to Stephen J. Gould, the ''genetic fallacy'' has been repeatedly used for exactly the reason that was feared by Hogben, to avoid environmental action: ''Are workplaces toxic? Screen workers and fire those with genetic predispositions to react badly . . . The genetic fallacy is generic—and applicable almost anywhere for the common and lamentable social aim of preserving an unfair status quo.''[5]

The availability of a test does not mean that it should be used. According to a scientific bias, all ''hypotheses'' should be tested. Many philosophers of this century have maintained that the sole basis for empirical justification are prediction and testing. However, medicine is not strictly (or not only) a science; the goal of medicine

[a] Phone: +39-11/670-6525; fax: +39-11/670-6692; e-mail: vineis@inrete.it

is the benefit of the individual. "Predictive" (including genetic) testing is even more dangerous than diagnostic testing, since the latter answers an immediate health question, whereas the former is used to predict potential disease in the future. Testing in medicine should be used cautiously. Resnik[6] has proposed five simple rules to consider before testing:

1. The specificity and sensitivity of the test(s).
2. The subjective probability of a diagnosis based on the evidence at hand, that is, the clinician's confidence in his or her diagnosis.
3. The consequence of making an incorrect diagnosis.
4. The patient's interests in not taking the test, that is, the avoidance of pain, harm, or risks of harm, inconvenience, or costs.
5. Society's interests in not conducting the test, that is, costs to society.

From this point of view, genetic testing is no different from other forms of medical testing.[7] Screening poses additional ethical and practical problems in comparison with testing. The use of genetic tests in screening and in diagnosis should not be confused. Cystic fibrosis is probably the only example of a population screening program based on DNA testing that can be justified.[7] However, it is unusual in that only a few mutations account for most cases of the disease.[7]

THE PERSPECTIVE OF TECHNOLOGY ASSESSMENT

The previous section has posed the problem of practical misuse of scientific discoveries, and of the need for guidelines on when and how genetic testing should be used. The transfer of research into practice is becoming a key issue in modern medicine. Renaldo Battista has proposed the metaphor of the bridge to describe the goals of "technology assessment" in health care; the bridge has the function of assuring communication between science and practice: "the scientific work may proceed unimpeded but not uninformed by the policy process and the policy process may proceed informed but not hijacked by the reductionist tendencies of scientific inquiries."[8] Technology assessment offers an avenue for organizing and communicating information from many domains that are potentially relevant to making choices in health care.

In the case of genetic screening, namely for mutations in BRCA1-BRCA2, the recently discovered genes that predispose to breast cancer, technology assessment implies answering at least five types of problems:

1. Issues related to tests:

   - Sensitivity and specificity.
   - Predictive value (depending on the prevalence of mutations in the groups tested).

2. Issues related to the population groups to test:

   - Criteria for selection (e.g., number of first-degree relatives with breast/ovarian cancer).

3. Issues related to the predictivity of mutations:
   - Cumulative risk of cancer in women testing positive (penetrance of the gene).
   - Genetic heterogeneity (hereditary tumors not due to BRCA1-BRCA2 mutations).
   - Added value of the search for mutations (in addition to the pedigree).
4. Issues related to actions to undertake among women testing positive:
   - Bilateral radical mastectomy?
   - Mammography under age 50?
   - Greater frequency of mammography?
     (need for further evidence concerning effectiveness in avoiding invasive cancers).
5. Ethical issues:
   - Groups involved: high-risk women; other women; daughters and future generations.
   - Values at stake: decisional autonomy (right not to know; right to know); beneficence; equity (cost/benefit for high-risk women, daughters, and future generations vs. alternative choices for the benefit of the general population).

False positive results may be obtained if irrelevant polymorphisms cannot be clearly distinguished from functionally relevant mutations. False negatives in genetic testing are caused by unidentified mutations in the same gene, while the term "genetic heterogeneity" is used for susceptibility attributable to other relevant genes. Penetrance is important since some genes strongly express the phenotype, thus clearly increasing the risk of cancer, while for others the linkage with phenotypic expression is much weaker.[9] As far as predictivity is concerned, according to family studies the cumulative risk of breast cancer in women with a mutation of the BRCA1 gene is 85% at age 80, while in BRCA1-negative women the risk is 8%.[10] However, it should be clear that the cumulative risk among women with the mutation is overstated, since it has been measured within families, that is, among women whose risk was already known to be increased.

Concerning the question of who should be tested, there is fair agreement on the criteria that should be used: women to test for mutations are those with (1) two first-degree relatives with breast cancer under age of 50; (2) two first-degree relatives with breast cancer, including one bilateral; (3) more than two first-degree relatives with breast cancer; (4) one first-degree relative with breast cancer under 50 and one with ovarian cancer; (5) two first-degree relatives with ovarian cancer.

However, once the mutation has been identified, more problems arise. According to a Dutch guideline, the following actions should be taken: (1) when the lifetime risk of breast cancer is greater than 15-20% (based on the family history), women should practice breast self-examination, should undergo a medical inspection every six months, and should undergo mammography once a year from the age of 25, while measurement of markers like CA125 and CA15.3 is optional; (2) when the lifetime risk is greater than 25-30%, mutations should be sought; (3) when the lifetime risk is greater than 50% (i.e., all women with germline mutations in BRCA1, BRCA2, or p53), the indication is radical mastectomy.[11] Other agencies, such as the American

National Cancer Institute, recommend prudence, partly as a consequence of scientific uncertainties.[12]

Ethical issues were sketched earlier, and relate to conflicts between the "right not to know" of the woman who is tested and the "right to know" of her daughters or future generations. Additional conflicts are related to the balance between the effectiveness of actions undertaken to avoid early death in those testing positive, the costs of screening, and the rights of other users of the health services. For example, genetic screening might prove incredibly expensive and might hamper extension of effective breast cancer screening in the general population (over age 50).

An application of the principles of technology assessment to genetic screening of workers, with an in-depth discussion of ethical issues, is presented in the contribution by Van Damme *et al.*[13]

To conclude, technology assessment of health care is a powerful tool, which, according to the metaphor of the bridge, may allow adequate interaction between science, policy, and clinical practice. A widespread prejudice is that science offers universal and objective knowledge that needs to be applied to a social context that in turn is value laden. At least in the case of medicine, a different perspective would consist of identifying the needs of the population and providing a well-designed strategy (based on scientific evidence) to answer such needs, thus overcoming the dichotomy between evidence provided by objective and universal scientific laws and the world of values. A model to consider is this century's architectural avant-garde (e.g. Gropius and Van Doesburg), which proposed a unity of technical design, materials to be used, and esthetic and functional goals of the objects or buildings designed, on the basis of social needs.

REFERENCES

1. HOGBEN, L. 1933. Nature and Nurture. Williams. Norgate, London.
2. DOLL, R. 1996. Nature and nurture: Possibilities for cancer control. Carcinogenesis **17:** 177-184.
3. FISHER R. A. 1958. Lung cancer and cigarettes? Nature **182:** 108.
4. VINEIS, P. & N. CAPORASO. 1995. Tobacco and cancer: Epidemiology and the laboratory. Environ. Health Perspect. **103:** 156-160.
5. GOULD, S. J. 1991. The smoking guns of eugenics. Natural History **12:** 8-17.
6. RESNIK, D. B. 1995. To test or not to test: A clinical dilemma. Theor. Med. **16:** 141-152.
7. WALD, N. J. 1996. What is genetic screening anyway? J. Med. Screening **3:** 57.
8. BATTISTA, R. 1996. Towards a paradigm for technology assessment. *In* Scientific Basis of Health Services. M. Peckham & R. Smith, Eds. BMJ Publishing Group. London.
9. PONDER, B. A. J. 1995. Genetic testing of the common cancers: Potential and problems. Eur. J. Cancer **31A:** 807-808.
10. FORD, D., D. F., EASTON, D. T. BISHOP, S. A. NAROD, D. E. GOLDGAR & THE BREAST CANCER LINKAGE CONSORTIUM 1994. Risks of cancer in BRCA1 mutation carriers. Lancet **343:** 692-695.
11. OOSTERWIJK, J. C. & J. G. M. KLIJN. 1995. Present guidelines for referral and management when familial/hereditary breast (-ovarian) cancer is suspected. South West Cancer News **1:** 10-12.
12. NELSON, N. J. 1996. Caution guides genetic testing for hereditary cancer genes. J. Nat. Cancer Inst. **88:** 70-72.
13. VAN DAMME, K., P. VINEIS & M. SORSA. 1997. Ethical issues in genetic screening and genetic monitoring in employees. Ann. N.Y. Acad. Sci. **837:** 554-565 (this volume).

The Long-lasting Legacy of Industrial Carcinogens: The Lesson of Asbestos

Irving J. Selikoff Memorial Lecture, 1995

CESARE MALTONI

Cancer Research Center
European Ramazzini Foundation
of Oncology and Environmental Sciences
Bentivoglio Castle
40010 Bentivoglio (BO), Italy

In memory of Dr. Irving J. Selikoff
the great defence advocate of asbestos victims

PREAMBLE

I wish to express my thanks to the President and to all Members of the Executive Council of the Collegium Ramazzini for having appointed me to deliver the first Selikoff Memorial Lecture. I am honored and moved at this recognition for a number of related reasons. For 30 years, from the '60s to the early '90s, Dr. Selikoff was the leading light in occupational medicine, a point of reference for the scientific community in his own country and throughout the world. His contributions to asbestos pathology are milestones in the history of medicine. Dr. Selikoff was an exceptional man: a rare blend of intelligence, culture, science, superb medical practice, commitment, intellectual integrity, and warmth. I expect most people will know that to me he was a great friend whose loss I constantly feel. His place can be taken by no one.

CANCER: A UNIQUE DISEASE

Cancer is certainly the main public health hazard of our time. It is a unique disease in its biological import, epidemiological scale, historical connection with the current development paradigm, and the peculiar nature of its pathogenesis (carcinogenesis). To ignore this is to misunderstand cancer.

Biological Import of the Disease

Cells have three possible destinies: (1) they can maintain their physiological integrity; (2) they can deteriorate and die as a consequence of their programmed life and/or of a series of aggressions of differing type and origin; or (3) they may adapt and survive by transforming themselves under exposure to agents that directly or

TABLE 1. Total Mortality and Mortality due to Malignant Tumors among Males (M) and Females (F) in the Province of Bologna in 1990[a]

	Sex		
	M	F	M + F
Inhabitants	437,297	474,418	911,715
Total mortality	5,351	5,206	10,557
Mortality due to malignant tumors			
No.	1,842	1,463	3,305
%	34.42	28.10	31.31
CR[b]	421.22	308.38	362.50
ASR(I)[b]	283.77	206.77	244.58
ASR(E)[b]	300.25	172.45	225.09
ASR(W)[b]	197.53	115.40	149.85
SMR	109.63	120.34	114.38

[a] From the Nominative Mortality Registry of Bologna and Province.

[b] The crude rates (CR) and the adjusted rates (ASR) [with reference to the Italian (I) European (E), and world (W) populations] refer to 100,000 people.

indirectly affect the cell genome. Cancer must be considered a/the prototype outcome of cell transformation. Tumors should be thought of not just as a particular disease, but as a cell destiny.

Present Epidemiological Scale

Cancer must be seen as the primary cause of death by a specific ascertained disease in the industrialized world. In 1990 in the Province of Bologna, an industrial area, the crude rate of mortality for all cancers, all ages, and both sexes, stood at 362.5/100,000 inhabitants (TABLE 1), and cancer was the cause of death in over 32% of all mortality of any kind, with a tendency to increase (FIG. 1). The cancer mortality rate rises with age, but at the same time cancer represents the leading cause of death among people under 70, with a growing incidence at younger ages.[1]

Cancer and the Historical Scenario

The scale of cancer and its tendency to increase and to strike earlier age groups depend on two factors: (1) the aging of the population; and (2) mainly the growing proliferation of cancer-causing agents in the human environment, which characterizes the industrial era. Cancer must therefore be viewed as a largely environmental disease, as many epidemiological surveys have demonstrated.[2]

The Projected Scale of Cancer

The Province of Bologna may be considered as a representative sample of the industrialized world, both for its general carcinogenic potential and for the age

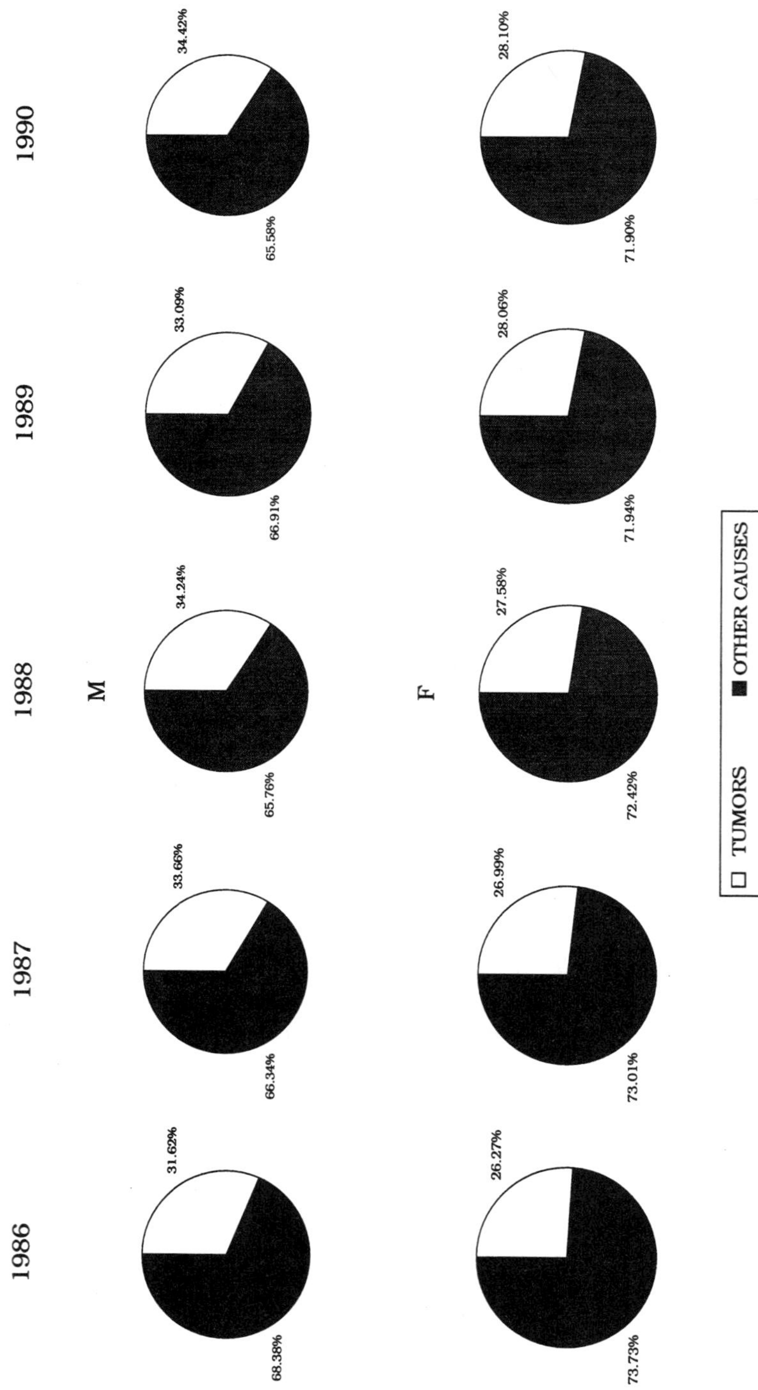

FIGURE 1. Mortality due to malignant tumors and all other causes in the years 1986, 1987, 1988, 1989, 1990 at various ages among males and females in the Province of Bologna. (From the Nominative Mortality Registry of Bologna and Province.)

distribution of its population. If we assume: (1) that the level of industrialization and the consumer economy in the emerging countries between 2020 and 2060 could be the same as that of the industrialized countries in the years from 1950 to 1990; (2) that the population distribution by age in the emerging countries in the year 2060 will be similar to the province of Bologna and the industrialized countries in general at the end of the 1980s; (3) that the world population in the '60s of the next century will have reached 10 billion inhabitants, mainly because of population growth in the emerging countries; and (4) that the efficacy of present cancer control strategy (with particular reference to prevention) do not sharply improve; then, applying cancer mortality rates in the Province of Bologna (crude rate) to the future population, world cancer mortality around 2060 will account for over 35 million deaths per year. However, this projected world cancer mortality may well be an underestimate, considering the continuous progress of industrialization in our society and the progressive aging of the already industrialized countries. These two factors are indeed expected to increase the incidence of cancer still further, and moreover to anticipate it by shortening the latency time, with a consequent increase in mortality and relative loss of years of life.

The Peculiar Nature of Carcinogenesis

Carcinogenesis, the mechanism by which cancer sets in, has features all its own. The changes produced by cancer-causing agents (carcinogens) are largely irreversible.

Nonetheless, from the time of exposure until the appearance of a tumor or its detectable pathologic precursors, there elapses a long time interval, the so-called latency period, characterized by its "silence."

The likelihood of cancer increases with the degree of exposure to one and the same carcinogen (dose), and also with exposure to several carcinogens through a syncarcinogenic effect.

Lastly, carcinogenesis is a stochastic process: no dose, however small, can be considered safe in principle.

THE PROBLEM OF INDUSTRIAL CARCINOGENS

From the last decades of the 19th century until today, directly or indirectly industry has set loose in our environment a countless series of agents not met with before or only at low concentrations. Only a tiny part of these agents have been properly screened for carcinogenicity.[3] Of what has been studied, the percentage found to be carcinogenic is dramatically high,[4] and even more alarming if one thinks of the host of agents whose carcinogenic potential remains unknown. Many such agents are being poured into the environment in vast quantities, measurable in millions, or tens of millions, or hundreds of millions of tonnes every year.

THE LONG-LASTING LEGACY OF INDUSTRIAL CARCINOGENS

It is only in recent years that a rule has been enacted subjecting new-generation industrial agents to carcinogenicity trials before production, employment, and dissemination in the environment. It follows that in the past a predictably high number of potential carcinogens must have been released into the environment for years on end, sometimes at high concentrations. Only in a few cases has production of these been suspended, after dramatic evidence of a cancer risk had forced itself on public awareness, and only after long, specious ponderings by bureaucrats and politicians, whose only role too often has been to put off taking control measures.

The result is that all societies on the planet Earth today have a weighty legacy of cancer risk.

The fact is hardly surprising. Consider:

(1) the enormous carcinogenic potential accumulating in the environment;
(2) the continuing production of many proven carcinogens, albeit under restrictive regulations (a classic example is vinyl chloride, which was produced at the rate of 10 million tonnes per year in the early '70s and whose annual production had reached 26 million tonnes in 1995);
(3) the failure as yet to identify potential carcinogens, which hence continue to be manufactured and circulated without control;
(4) the fact that carcinogenic effects, which are largely irreversible, manifest themselves after a long latency period, such that exposure today may give rise to cancer in 10, 20, 30, 40, or even 50 years' time;
(5) the fact that carcinogens may linger in the tissues and cells of the human organism, even when they are soluble chemical agents, owing to the formation of stable bonds between them and the biological substrate;
(6) the fact that many carcinogens hang about in the surrounding environment, where they can be traced even several decades after being introduced, thus continuing to attack the human organism; and
(7) the conjecture, not properly shown but not to be discounted, that genetic modifications may be transmitted to future generations, who may so have a greater propensity to contract specific types of cancer, or cancer in general. This kind of legacy may be the most frightening side to industrial carcinogens.

THE LESSON OF ASBESTOS

General Background

For a century asbestos has been widely and intensely used by industry. Tens and tens of millions of tonnes of various asbestos ores have been extracted, put to use, and scattered across the biosphere. Asbestos is reckoned to have been used in some 3,000 ways.[5]

Today it is found more or less everywhere: (1) wherever it is mined and milled; (2) wherever it is used by manufacturing; (3) wherever it and its products are installed (buildings, ships, rolling stock, cars, etc.); and (4) in the environment as a whole, which is permeated with manufactured goods in which it has been employed (public buildings, houses, car brakes, etc.), and then discarded as waste.

Since asbestos is virtually indestructible, it lingers endlessly in man's habitat.

The harm of asbestos to humans has been known since the dawn of the century. We recently came across a sentence of the civil and penal court of Turin (Italy) of 1906, in which the judge, in litigation between the British Asbestos Company and a local newspaper (which had reported on the health risk of asbestos), recognized the evidence for an increase in broncopneumonia among exposed workers.

For about 80 years we have known that asbestos produces a peculiar pulmonary fibrosis (asbestosis). The first report of its potential carcinogenic effect dates from 60 years ago, when Lynch and Smith[6] first associated asbestosis with lung carcinoma.

It has long been known that asbestos causes tumors of various kinds, especially mesothelioma of the pleura and peritoneum, carcinoma of the lung, larynx and oropharynx, carcinoma of the kidney, and carcinoma of the digestive tract.[7]

Despite this, asbestos and goods containing it go on being produced and used in many countries, above all in the Third World.

Once asbestos enters our organism, chiefly by the airways, traces of it remain in the structure of human and animal tissue practically for the rest of its life. This circumstance means that even short-and/or low-concentration environmental exposure actually carries a far higher exposure of the target cells, the dose being expressed by concentration multiplied by time of exposure. No wonder, then, that even low-concentration and/or short-duration exposure, whether occupational or environmental, can cause asbestos-related cancers.

As with all carcinogens, modifications induced by asbestos are on the whole irreversible.

A Paradigm Case

Asbestos thus represents the paradigm of a long-latency legacy from industrial carcinogens. The reasons are:

(1) the number of people potentially exposed to it one way or another is immense;
(2) those exposed yet apparently healthy are anyway at risk of cancer since they bear irreversible carcinogenic alterations, while asbestos continues to reside and work within their organisms;
(3) goods containing it go on being used;
(4) from where it is sited, asbestos migrates in powder form throughout the environment, by man's doing or through natural circumstance (wind, rain, acid rain, etc.), creating a situation of widespread exposure;
(5) now scattered across the biosphere, it lingers indefinitely in our habitat, a real risk for future generations;
(6) although the scientific community, the industries concerned, governments, and international agencies are aware of the grave risks posed by asbestos exposure, in many parts of the world the material continues to be employed, breeding new forms of pollution;
(7) if not expertly performed, the growing number of asbestos-stripping operations may be a further dramatic source of secondary pollution.

Identifying asbestos risks is made easier by the fact that among other tumors it produces mesothelioma; which was a complete rarity until the end of the Second World War.[8] The current epidemic of this tumor is almost entirely due to asbestos. Mesothelioma hence provides a pointer to the exposure risk of this material.

Our Experience

Our experience is based on cases of mesothelioma collected by the epidemiological unit of the European Ramazzini Foundation of Oncology and Environmental Sciences. This experience shows:

- the epidemiological magnitude of asbestos-related cancer in working categories already known to be at risk;
- the emergence of new risk categories following environmental exposure;
- risk following nonoccupational exposure in workplaces polluted with asbestos;
- the nonanecdotal frequency of mesothelioma following family exposure;
- risk following home or indoor exposure;
- risk following environmental exposure at large.

The Epidemiological Magnitude of Carcinogenic Risk in Working Categories Already Known to Be at Risk. The classic example is our study of the incidence of mesothelioma among railroad workers.

At present 181 cases have been reported from a number of countries besides Italy: South Africa, Rhodesia, the United States, Sweden, Canada, Switzerland, France.[9]

By simply collecting cases (without any systematic inquiry), we have identified 123 instances of mesothelioma among Italian workers occupationally exposed to asbestos used in railroads (TABLES 2-4). The occurrence of mesothelioma among these workers has increased year by year (FIGS. 2,3).

The Emergence of New-Risk Working Categories. Asbestos is used extensively for the insulation of thermo-hydraulic systems (boilers, pipes, etc.) and for furnaces in sugar refinery plants. In 1985, seven cases of mesothelioma were reported among sugar refinery workers in Sweden.

Since 1986 we have identified 11 cases of mesothelioma among sugar refinery workers in our region, which includes the province of Bologna and two others adjacent to it (TABLE 5).

Risk following Nonoccupational Exposure in Workplaces Polluted with Asbestos. Seven cases of ours concern mesotheliomas among clerical workers whose jobs did not entail contact with asbestos, but who were working in a workplace polluted with the mineral (TABLE 6).

The Nonanecdotal Frequency of Mesothelioma following Family Exposure. In seven cases from our series a mesothelioma set in after family exposure to asbestos (TABLE 7). In our opinion the onset of mesothelioma from exposure within the family

TABLE 2. Italian Cases (123) of Mesotheliomas following Job Assignment Exposure to Asbestos Used in Railroads

	No. of Cases of Mesotheliomas				
Category	Pleural	Pericardial	Peritoneal	Pleuroperitoneal	Total
Workers of the FS,[a] especially machinists	75	1	1	1	78
Rolling-stock machinists and workers engaged in the repair and demolition of the rails, at workshops not belonging to the FS	40	0	5	0	45
Total	115	1	6	1	123

[a] FS = Ferrovie dello Stato (Italian State Railroads).

TABLE 3. Distribution by Region of 123 Italian Cases of Mesotheliomas following Occupational Exposure to Asbestos Used in Rairoads

Region	Cases		
	FS[a]	Not FS	Total
Abruzzo	1	0	1
Campania	2	9	11
Emilia Romagna[b]	36	16	52
Friuli-Venezia Giulia	2	2	4
Lazio	0	3	3
Liguria	2	4	6
Lombardia	3	1	4
Marche	1	0	1
Piemonte	9	2	11
Puglia	4	0	4
Sicilia	2	0	2
Toscana	7	8	15
Trentino	1	0	1
Umbria	1	0	1
Veneto	7	0	7
All regions	78	45	123

[a] FS = Ferrovie dello Stato (Italian State Railorads).

[b] Where the European Ramazzini Foundation of Oncology and Environmental Sciences is located.

is underestimated. All seven of our cases were identified through painstaking follow-up of patient stories. Epidemiological investigation of deaths based on charts and certificates is unlikely to bring to light mesotheliomas caused by family contact.

Risk following Home or Indoor Exposure. In six cases of the series (all women) mesothelioma set in following prolonged exposure to asbestos contained in manufactured objects in the home (TABLE 8). This finding is worrying, as it proves asbestos may be a widespread risk indeed.

Risk following Environmental Exposure. Four cases of mesothelioma were observed in individuals living in an area polluted with asbestos (TABLE 9).

Data in the literature on the risk of asbestos following general environmental exposure are scanty and indirect. In such cases the connection of mesothelioma with asbestos exposure is difficult to establish without a careful inquiry, which can usually be conducted only within medical institutions (mainly in hospitals).

The series of mesothelioma cases is steadily growing at our Foundation, giving us important new insights into the magnitude of asbestos carcinogenesis.

CONCLUSION

From what we know and from the lesson of asbestos, industrial carcinogens may represent an unendingly bleak legacy of mankind. To be producing and circulating

TABLE 4. Latency Period and Age at Death, Respectively, of 47 and 40 Emilia Romagna Cases[a] of Mesotheliomas following Occupational Exposure to Asbestos Used in Railroads

	No.			Period of Latency (years)		Age at Death (years)	
Category	Total	Dead	Still Alive	Average	Range	Average	Range
FS[b] workers	35	30	5	33.6	16-51	60.7	39.77
Not FS workers	12	10	2	28.6	12-39	61.5	45-77
Total	47	40	7	32.3	12-51	61.0	39-77

[a] Out of 52.

[b] FS = Ferrovie dello Stato (Italian State Railroads).

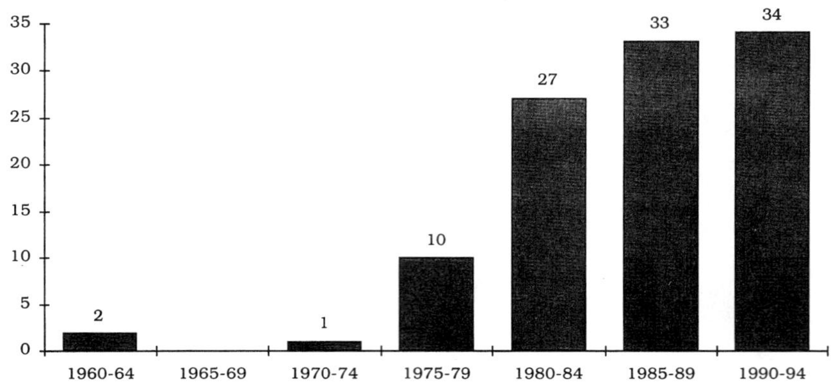

FIGURE 2. Italian cases of mesothelioma (107 out of 123 cases observed) following occupational exposure to asbestos used in railroads: distribution by death quinquennium.

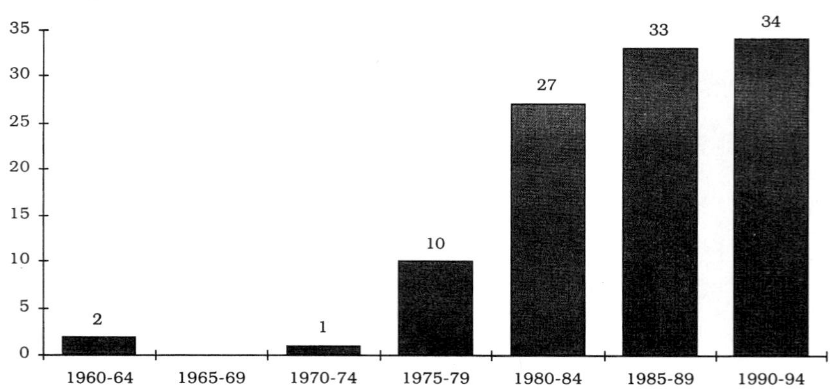

FIGURE 3. Emilia Romagna cases of mesothelioma (45 out of 52 cases observed) following occupational exposure to asbestos used in railroads: distribution by death quinquennium.

such carcinogens becomes not just a crime against the present generation of adults, but against their children and unborn generations as well.

TABLE 5. Italian Cases (11) of Mesothelioma following Occupational Exposure to Asbestos Used in Sugar Refinery Plants

Case No. (a)	Initials	Site of Sugar Refinery Plant	Sex	Job	Mesothelioma: Site	Latency Time (years)	Age at Onset (years)	Year of Diagnosis	Age at Death	Year of Death
1	LS	Crevalcore (Bologna)	M	Worker engaged in running centrifuges and in maintenance of refinery plants	Pleura	29	61	1986	62	1987
2	TL	Codigoro (Ferrara)	M	Various jobs (seasonal)	Pleura	31	49	1986	49	1986
3	FG	Bondeno (Ferrara)	M	Various jobs (his main place of work was under a boiler) (seasonal)	Pleura	28	44	1989	49	1994
4	BD	Molinella (Bologna)	M	Pipefitter	Pleura	41	65	1991	66	1992
5	GB	Bondeno (Ferrara)	M	Pipefitter	Pleura	34	54	1991	56	1993
6	DU	Classe (Ravenna)	M	Maintenance worker Pipefitter Responsible for thermal system	Pleura	41	62	1992	63	1993
7	CG	Molinella (Bologna)	M	Painter Engaged in the heating of sugar-beet sauce	Pleura	43	78	1993	78	1993
8	BA	Crevalcore (Bologna)	M	Mason engaged in the maintenance and repair of furnaces	Pleura	37	77	1993	78	1994
9	RF	Molinella (Bologna)	M	Porter	Peritoneum	41	80	1994	80	1994
10	MA	Bologna	M	Responsible for thermal system	Pleura	48	82	1994	82	1994
11	GA	Motencosaro Scalo (Macerata)	M	Boiler operator seasonal	Pleura	23	45	1995		Living
Mean						36.0	63.4		66.3[b]	

[a] According to year of diagnosis.
[b] Referred to the 10 cases already deceased.

TABLE 6. Italian Cases (7) of Mesothelioma following Asbestos Exposure in Workplace, Not due to Job Assignment

				Mesothelioma			
Case No.	Sex	Job	Source of Exposure	Site	Latency Time (years)	Age at Onset (years)	Year of Diagnosis
1	M	Military radar operator traveling on railroad rolling stock	Rolling stock polluted with asbestos	Pleura			1989
2	M	Post office clerk traveling on railroad rolling stock	Rolling stock polluted with asbestos	Pleura	44	64	1989
3	M	Sleeping car attendant traveling on railroad rolling stock	Rolling stock polluted with asbestos	Pleura			1989
4	M	Barber	Clients: asbestos-cement workers, polluted with asbestos	Pleura	34	57	1990
5	M	Farmer and breeder	Cowshed and outbuildings with asbestos-cement corrugated panel roof	Pleura	''Many years''	60	1992
6	M	Bank employee	Roof of the office heavely insulated with asbestos	Pleura	35	64	1993
7	M	Farmer and breeder	Cowshed and outbuildings with asbestos-cement corrugated panel roof	Peritoneum	34	61	1995

TABLE 7. Italian Cases (7) of Mesothelioma following Familial Asbestos Exposure due to Contact with Occupationally Polluted Members of the Family

			Mesothelioma			
Case No.	Kinship	Job Assignment of Exposed Member of Family	Site	Latency Time (years)	Age at Onset (years)	Year of Diagnosis
1	Daughter	Worker of a sugar refinery	Pleura	37	37	1988
2	Daughter	Switchman in railroad	Pleura	34	44	1988
3	Wife	Machinist	Pleura			1989
4	Wife	Machinist	Pleura			1993
5	Wife	Machinist on ship	Pleura	46	66	1993
6	Wife	Engine driver in railroad	Pleura	29	57	1994
7	Sister	Machinist	Pleura	30	30	1995

TABLE 8. Italian Cases (6) of Mesothelioma following Asbestos Exposure from Structures Present in Dwellings

Case No.	Sex	Working Activity	Source of Exposure	Mesothelioma Site	Latency Time (years)	Age at Onset (years)	Year of Diagnosis
1	F	Housewife	Presence in kitchen of asbestos-cement insulating panels	Pleura	"Many years"	66	1987
2	F	Farmer	House roofed with asbestos-cement corrugated panels	Peritoneum	30	63	1994
3	F	Worker at a wood packaging factory	House roofed with asbestos-cement corrugated panels	Pleura	33	64	1994
4	F	Teacher	House roofed with asbestos-cement corrugated panels	Pleura	45	71	1994
5	F	Teacher	House roofed with asbestos-cement corrugated panels	Pleura	62	62	1995
6	F	Hosier	House roofed with asbestos-cement corrugated panels	Pleura	20	64	1995

TABLE 9. Cases (4) of Mesothelioma following Asbestos Exposure from the Residential Area

Case No.	Sex	Working Activity	Source of Exposure	Mesothelioma Site	Mesothelioma Latency Time (years)	Mesothelioma Age at Onset (years)	Year of Diagnosis
1	F	Dressmaker	Dwelling located near a shipyard	Pleura	32	64	1990
2	F	Housewife	Dwelling located near a harbor	Pleura	68	68	1990
3	F	Teacher	Dwelling located near a busy railroad track	Pleura	64	64	1993
4	F	Porter[a]	Dwelling located near a rolling stock factory	Pleura	37	71	1995
Mean					50.3	66.8	

[a] Nonoccupationally exposed to asbestos.

REFERENCES

1. Maltoni, C., P. Carmentano & A. Palazzini. 1990. Cancer mortality trends analysis for Bologna and Province. Programs, methodology, objectives and early results. *In* Trends in Cancer Mortality in Industrial Countries. D. L. Davis & D. Hoel, Eds.: 110–130. Vol. 609, Annals of the New York Academy of Sciences. New York.
2. Doll, R. 1977. Introduction. *In* Origins of Human Cancer. Incidence of Cancer in Humans, Vol. 4, Book A. H. H. Hiatt, J. D. Watson & J. A. Winsten, Eds.: 1–12. Cold Spring Harbor Laboratory. Cold Spring Harbor, NY.
3. National Academy of Science. 1984. Toxicity Testing. Strategies to Determine Needs and Priorities. National Academy Press. Washington, DC.
4. Maltoni, C. 1995. The contribution of experimental (animal) studies to the control of industrial carcinogenesis. Appl. Occup. Environ. Hyg. **10**(9): 749–760.
5. International Agency for Research on Cancer. 1977. Monographs on the evaluation of carcinogenic risk of chemicals to man. Asbestos, Vol. 14.
6. Lynch, K. M. & W. A. Smith. 1935. Pulmonary asbestosis. III. Carcinoma of the lung in asbestos-silicosis. Am. J. Cancer **14:** 56–64.
7. Selikoff, I. J. & H. Seidman. 1991. Asbestos-associated deaths among insulation workers in the United States and Canada. *In* The Third Wave of Asbestos Disease: Exposure to Asbestos in Place. Public Health Control. P. J. Landrigan & H. Kazemi, Eds.: 1–14. Vol. 643, Annals of the New York Academy of Sciences. New York.
8. Mark, E. J. & T. Yokoi. 1991. Absence of evidence for a significant background incidence of diffuse malignant mesothelioma apart from asbestos exposure. *In* The Third Wave of Asbestos Disease: Exposure to Asbestos in Place. Public Health Control. P. J. Landrigan & H. Kazemi, Eds.: 196–204. Vol. 643, Annals of the New York Academy of Sciences. New York.
9. Maltoni, C., C. Pinto, R. Carnuccio *et al.* 1994. Mesotheliomas following exposure to asbestos used in railroads: 122 Italian cases. *In* Advances in Modern Environmental Toxicology. The Identification and Control of Environmental and Occupational Diseases: Hazards and Risks of Chemicals in the Oil Refining Industry, Vol. 23, M. A. Mehlman & A. Upton, Eds.: 635–659. Princeton Scientific Publishing Co. Princeton, NJ.

Index of Contributors

Alkaslassy, D., 307-318
Arteaga, M., 126-137

Badrei, M., 524-536
Belpoggi, F., 15-52, 77-95, 189-208, 469-512
Bingham, E., xiii
Blair, A., 246-256
Boland, B., xv
Brautbar, N., 96-104
Bravo-Alvarado, J., 537-550
Bua, L., 469-512
Burgaz, S., 122-125
Burger, J., 360-371, 372-386

Casteleyn, L., 554-565
Chilton, J. A., 524-536
Chow, W.-H., 114-121
Ciliberti, A., 15-52, 209-238
Cocco, P., 246-256
Congia, P., 246-256
Correa-Villasenor, A., 157-169
Crouch, E. A. C., 387-396

Davies, J. E., 257-268
Davis, D. L., 513-523
Dement, J. M., 53-76
Dickey, C., 353-359
Dosemeci, M., 114-121

Ecca, A. R., 246-256
Eden-Wynter, R. A., 176-188
El Haj, S., 269-290
Elliott, E., 157-169

Fahs, M. C., 440-455
Ferreira, A. J., 291-299
Filippini, F., 77-95
Finkel, A., 397-417
Francis, M., 157-169

Gasteyer, S., 269-290
Gitelman, A., 53-76
Goldsmith, J. R., 300-306
Gomez-Garza, S. A., 524-536
Gonzalez, R., 524-536
Grandjean, P., 239-245
Green, L. C., 387-396

Hajek, R. A., 524-536
Hay, A., 138-156
Hayes, R. B., 114-121
Hensley, L., 53-76

Jaqhabir, M., 269-290
Jones, L. A., 524-536

Karakaya, A., 122-125
Karakaya, A. E., 122-125
Klebanov, M., 307-318

Landrigan, P. J., 440-455
Lefemine, G., 209-238
Legator, M. S., 170-175
Leigh, J. P., 440-455
Lemesch, C., 307-318
Lenzi, A., 189-208
Lerman, Y., 307-318
Li, G.-L., 114-121
Linares, A., 524-536
Linet, M., 114-121
López-Carrillo, L., 537-550

Maltoni, C., xi, 1-14, 15-52, 77-95, 189-208, 209-238, 469-512, 570-586
Markowitz, S. B., 440-455
Marques, E. P., 291-299
Matanoski, G. M., 157-169, 176-188
Menarini, L., 15-52
Minardi, F., 469-512
Murthy, L. I., 319-352

Namatalla, G., 96-104

Ortega Altamirano, D., 537-550

Palmas, C., 246-256
Pavlova, L. V., 462-468
Pedro, I. S., 291-299
Perera, F. P., 353-359
Peterson, J. C., 257-268
Phoenix, J. A., 551-553
Pillow, P. C., 524-536
Pines, A., 307-318
Pinto, C., 15-52, 469-512
Poblano-Verastegui, O., 537-550
Pongsiri, M. J., 513-523

Rangan, U., 105-113
Ribak, J., 307-318
Richter, E. D., 269-290
Riojas-Rodríguez, H., 176-188
Rothman, N., 114-121
Ruttenberg, R., 456-461

Saavedra, D., 126-137
Saba, G., 246-256

Safi, J., 269-290
Samuels, S. W., 418-432
Santos-Burgoa, C., 157-169, 176-188
Shin, C.-G., 440-455
Snyder, R., 105-113
Soffritti, M., 15-52, 77-95, 189-208, 209-238
Sorsa, M., 554-565
Stallworth, H., 433-439

Tarrel, J., 138-156
Tao, X., 157-169
Tena, M., 126-137

Van Damme, K., 554-565
Vieira, D. N., 291-299
Vineis, P., 554-565, 566-569
Vojdani, A., 96-104

Wacholder, S., 114-121
Wolff, M., 513-523

Yakovlev, A. Y., 462-468
Yick, J., 524-536
Yin, S.-N., 114-121
Yücesoy, B., 122-125